*Atlas of*
# Allergies and Clinical Immunology

*Third Edition*

# Atlas of
# Allergies and
# Clinical Immunology

**EDITED BY**

## Philip Fireman, MD

Professor of Pediatrics and Medicine
University of Pittsburgh Medical Center and
Children's Hospital of Pittsburgh
Pittsburgh, Pennsylvania

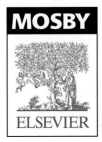

**MOSBY**

**ELSEVIER**

**MOSBY**
ELSEVIER

1600 John F. Kennedy Blvd.
Ste. 1800
Philadelphia, Pennsylvania 19103-2899

ATLAS OF ALLERGIES AND CLINICAL IMMUNOLOGY

ISBN-13: 978-0-3230-2495-2
ISBN-10: 0-323-02495-5

**Copyright © 2006, 1996 by Mosby, Inc.**

---

### NOTICE

Knowledge and best practice in this field are constantly changing. As new research and experience broaden our knowledge, changes in practice, treatment and drug therapy may become necessary or appropriate. Readers are advised to check the most current information provided (i) on procedures featured or (ii) by the manufacturer of each product to be administered, to verify the recommended dose or formula, the method and duration of administration, and contraindications. It is the responsibility of the practitioner, relying on their own experience and knowledge of the patient, to make diagnoses, to determine dosages and the best treatment for each individual patient, and to take all appropriate safety precautions. To the fullest extent of the law, neither the Publisher nor the Editor assumes only liability for any injury and/or damage to persons or property arising out or related to any use of the material contained in this book.

The Publisher

---

**Library of Congress Cataloging-in-Publication Data**
Altas of allergy and clinical immunology/[edited by] Philip Fireman.—3rd ed.
      p. ; cm.
   Rev. ed. of: Atlas of allergies. c1991.
   Includes bibliographical references and index.
   ISBN 0-323-02495-5
   1. Allergy—Atlases. I. Fireman, Philip, IL Atlas of allergies.
   [DNLM: 1. Hypersensitivity—Atlases. QW 517 A8811 2006]
   RC584.A845 2006
   616.97—dc22

Acquisitions Editor: *Rolla Couchman/Karen Bowler*
Developmental Editor: *Carla Holloway*
Project Manager: *Joan Sinclair*

Printed in China

Last digit is the print number:   9   8   7   6   5   4   3   2   1

*I dedicate this third edition of Atlas of Allergies and Clinical Immunology to someone who is very special to me because she has had the most profound influence on my life, my family, and my career. Without her support this book would not have been initiated nor achieved. She is the love of my life, my wife and best friend—Marcia Levick Fireman.*

# Acknowledgments

This third edition of *Atlas of Allergies and Clinical Immunology* would not have been possible without the contributions and collaboration of my professional colleagues who wrote or co-authored their respective chapters. I am most fortunate to have recruited an outstanding group of allergists and clinical immunologists who found time in their already busy careers and lives to help me complete this Atlas. These experienced clinicians, investigators, and educators provided the knowledge in aggregate to encompass the many varied aspects of these diseases that plague our mutual patients. I thank them all for their exceptional efforts.

To my administrative assistant, Mariann A. Stefanik, I must convey my heartfelt appreciation for all of her hard work. Without her excellent organizational, secretarial, and computer skills this venture could not have been completed. With her cheerful demeanor she kept me, as well as all of the contributors, focused on achieving our goals.

In addition, there are others without whose skills and persistence this third edition would never have been accomplished. I acknowledge with sincere gratitude the excellent editorial assistance from the publishing professionals at Mosby and now Elsevier, for the past 15 years. Specifically, I want to thank Cathy Carroll, Managing Editor, Todd Hummel who helped me to initiate and pursue this third edition, and editorial associates Dana Lamparello, Rolla Couchman, Joan Sinclair, and, especially, Carla Holloway, without whose expertise and guidance we could not have gotten through this project.

# Foreword

As co-editors of the first two editions of *Atlas of Allergies*, Dr. Fireman and I conceived of a visually appealing book that would not be relegated to the coffee table. We strove to provide accurate and practical information and the accompanying text of the Atlas, together with photographs, tables, and figures, proved to be well received by both specialists and primary care physicians. It was particularly satisfying that many readers told us they made use of the Atlas in their own teaching endeavors.

A number of academic responsibilities precluded my participation in this third edition of *Atlas of Allergies*, but I was delighted to see that Dr. Fireman has carried the torch so well. He has assembled a stellar group of nationally known authors and has greatly expanded the Table of Contents to better reflect the changing times in the field of Allergy and Immunology. For example, latex allergy was not even mentioned in our 1996 edition and now,

as an increasingly recognized cause of both occupational and non-occupational sensitivity, it occupies a separate chapter. Immunotherapy, the familiar practice of "allergy shots," occupied six paragraphs under allergic rhinitis in the last edition. With the extraordinary changes taking place in this area and the promise of exciting new developments in the near future, this subject certainly deserves its own space. Finally, recognizing that allergy and immunology extends beyond the convention allergic diseases, new chapters on rheumatologic diseases, HIV/AIDS, and immunization are now offered.

I predict that this third edition of *Atlas of Allergies* will meet with even more success than the previous editions and I extend my congratulations to Dr. Fireman and the other authors for a job well done.

*Raymond G. Slavin*

# Preface

This third edition of the *Atlas of Allergies and Clinical Immunology* was undertaken with the support, but without the active participation of my friend and professional colleague Dr. Raymond Slavin. Dr. Slavin and I co-edited the first two editions of *Atlas of Allergies* and it was most gratifying to both of us that the initial two editions were so well received. This positive response from so many who read the Atlas encouraged me to continue to pursue this endeavor. I appreciate and thank Dr. Slavin for his many contributions to the content of the earlier two editions. In his absence, I have recruited additional new contributors that include such eminent clinicians and investigators as Drs. Vincent Beltrani, Emil Bardana, Wesley Burks, Ira Finegold, Paul Greenberger, Kevin Kelly, Tom Medsger, William Shearer, and Ellen Wald.

The original editorial vision of this Atlas has not changed; however, the scope of this new *Atlas of Allergies and Clinical Immunology* has been enlarged to include other aspects of clinical immunology in addition to allergic diseases. Our intent continues to be to provide a concise and accurate description of the clinical aspects of allergic and clinical immunologic diseases by utilizing pictorial and graphic materials including charts, tables, illustrations, and photographs. The narrative text bridges the visual material with essential clinical information appropriate for understanding the basis, as well as the recognition, diagnosis, and management of these diseases.

This Atlas is directed to all clinicians whether the generalist, specialist, or student with the intent to provide a broad-based perspective on allergy and clinical immunology. The past 10 years have seen an almost unprecedented surge in progress in bio-medical science and technology with many new developments in understanding the many facets of the immunologic basis of these diseases and their management. In collaboration with the contributors we have incorporated this information in all of the updated and revised chapters. In addition, the content of the Atlas has been significantly expanded with new chapters on Latex Allergy and Immunotherapy of Allergic Diseases. The immunologic basis of allergic diseases has enlarged the scope of the specialty of allergy to include Clinical Immunology. Therefore, we have added chapters on Rheumatologic Diseases and Immunization, as well as a separate chapter on Acquired Immunodeficiency Disease, besides the chapter on Primary Immunodeficiency Disease.

I appreciate the efforts of our contributors to achieve the relevance and conciseness that this Atlas displays. Many colleagues in Allergy and Clinical Immunology have told me that they have utilized portions of the Atlas for their own teaching and lectures. I anticipate that this third edition will continue to be a significant resource to all of those interested in allergic and clinical immunologic diseases.

*Philip Fireman, MD*

# Contributors

ROBERT C. ARFFA, MD
Clinical Assistant Professor, Department of Ophthalmology, University of Pittsburgh, Pittsburgh, Pennsylvania; University of Pittsburgh Medical Center, Pittsburgh, Pennsylvania
Chapter 12: Allergic Immunologic Ocular Diseases

CHRISTOPHER S. BALIGA, MD
Clinical AIDS Research Fellow, Department of Pediatrics and Molecular Virology and Microbiology, Baylor College of Medicine, Houston, Texas; Clinical AIDS Research Fellow, Department of Allergy and Immunology, Texas Children's Hospital, Houston, Texas
Chapter 21: HIV/AIDS

EMIL J. BARDANA, JR., MD
Professor of Medicine, Division of Allergy and Clinical Immunology, Oregon Health and Science University, Portland, Oregon
Chapter 6: Occupational Allergies

SERGEI N. BELENKY, MD, PhD
Director, Division of Allergy, Asthma, and Immunology, Pediatric Alliance of Pittsburgh, Pittsburgh, Pennsylvania
Chapter 7: Hypersensitivity Pneumonitis

VINCENT S. BELTRANI, MD, FAAAAI
Associate Clincial Professor, Department of Dermatology, Columbia University, New York, New York; Visiting Professor, Department of Allergy and Rheumatology, University of Medicine and Dentistry of New Jersey, Newark, New Jersey
Chapters 14: Contact Dermatitis and 15: Atopic Dermatitis

A. WESLEY BURKS, MD
Professor and Chief, Pediatric Allergy and Immunology, Duke University Medical Center, Durham, North Carolina
Chapter 13: Food Hypersensitivity

MARGARETHA CASSELBRANT, MD, PhD
Interim Chief of Service, Division of Pediatric Otolaryngology, Children's Hospital of Pittsburgh, Pittsburgh, Pennsylvania
Chapter 11: Otitis Media

IRA FINEGOLD, MD, MS
Assistant Clinical Professor of Medicine, Columbia University, New York, New York; Chief of Allergy, Department of Medicine, St. Luke's-Roosevelt Hospital Center, New York, New York; Director, R.A. Cooke Institute of Allergy, Roosevelt Hospital, New York, New York
Chapter 22: Immunotherapy: Vaccines for Allergic Diseases

GILBERT A. FRIDAY, JR, MD
Clinical Professor of Pediatrics, University of Pittsburgh School of Medicine, Children's Hospital of Pittsburgh, Pittsburgh, Pennsylvania
Chapter 4: Anaphylaxis and Insect Allergy

CARL R. FUHRMAN, MD
Professor of Radiology, Chief, Division of Thoracic Radiology, Department of Radiology, University of Pittsburgh Medical Center, Pittsburgh, Pennsylvania
Chapter 7: Hypersensitivity Pneumonitis

DEBORAH A. GENTILE, MD
Assistant Professor of Pediatrics, Department of Pediatrics, Drexel University School of Medicine, Philadelphia, Pennsylvania; Member, Division of Allergy, Asthma, and Immunology, Department of Pediatrics, Allegheny General Hospital, Pittsburgh, Pennsylvania
Chapter 3: Diagnostic Tests in Allergy

LESLIE C. GRAMMER, MD
Professor of Medicine, Division of Allergy and Immunology, Northwestern University Feinberg School of Medicine, Chicago, Illinois
Chapter 17: Drug Allergy

DAVID P. GREENBERG, MD
Adjunct Associate Professor, Department of Pediatrics, University of Pittsburgh, Pittsburgh, Pennsylvania; Children's Hospital of Pittsburgh, Pittsburgh, Pennsylvania; Director, Scientific and Medical Affairs, Aventis Pasteur, Swiftwater, Pennsylvania
Chapter 23: Immunization

PAUL A. GREENBERGER, MD
Professor of Medicine, Department of Medicine, Division of Allergy-Immunology, Northwestern University Feinberg School of Medicine, Chicago, Illinois
Chapter 8: Allergic Bronchopulmonary Aspergillosis

KEVIN J. KELLY, MD
Professor of Pediatrics and Medicine, Associate Dean of Clinical Affairs, Department of Allergy and Immunology, Medical College of Wisconsin, Milwaukee, Wisconsin; Chief, Allergy and Immunology, Department of Medicine, Children's Hospital of Wisconsin, Milwaukee, Wisconsin
Chapter 16: Latex Allergy

MACY I. LEVINE, MD
Clinical Professor of Medicine, Department of Medicine, University of Pittsburgh School of Medicine, Pittsburgh, Pennsylvania; Attending Physican, Department of Medicine, University of Pittsburgh Medical Center, Pittsburgh, Pennsylvania
Chapter 18: Urticaria and Angioedema

ELLEN M. MANDEL, MD
Associate Professor, Department of Otolaryngology and Pediatrics, University of Pittsburgh, Pittsburgh, Pennsylvania; Research Pediatrician, Department of Pediatric Otolaryngology, Children's Hospital, Pittsburgh, Pennsylvania
Chapter 11: Otitis Media

THOMAS A. MEDSGER, JR, MD
Professor of Medicine, Division of Rheumatology and Clinical Immunology, University of Pittsburgh School of Medicine, Pittsburgh, Pennsylvania
Chapter 19: Rheumatologic Diseases

ANDREJ PETROV, MD
Instructor of Medicine, University of Pittsburgh School of Medicine, Division of Pulmonary, Allergy and Critical Care Medicine, Pittsburgh, Pennsylvania
Chapter 1: Immunology of Allergic and Clinical Immunologic Disorders

KLARA M. POSFAY-BARBE, MD, MS
Instructor, Department of Pediatrics, University of Pittsburgh School of Medicine, Pittsburgh, Pennsylvania; Division of Allergy, Immunology, and Infectious Diseases, Children's Hospital of Pittsburgh, Pittsburgh, Pennsylvania
Chapter 23: Immunization

THARAKNATH RAO, MD, MS
Associate Director, Department of Clinical R&D, Inflamation, Pfizer Global Research and Development, Pfizer Inc., Ann Arbor, Michigan; Clinical Adjunct Assistant Professor, Department of Internal Medicine/Rheumatology, University of Michigan, Ann Arbor, Michigan
Chapter 19: Rheumatologic Diseases

AMY M. SCURLOCK, MD
Clinical Instructor, Department of Pediatrics, University of Arkansas for Medical Sciences/Arkansas Children's Hospital, Little Rock, Arkansas
Chapter 13: Food Hypersensitivity

WILLIAM T. SHEARER, MD, PhD
Professor of Pediatrics and Immunology, Baylor College of Medicine, Houston, Texas; Chief, Allergy and Immunology Service, Texas Children's Hospital, Houston, Texas
Chapter 21: HIV/AIDS

DAVID P. SKONER, MD
Director, Allergy, Asthma, and Immunology, Vice Chair, Clinical Research, Department of Pediatrics, Allegheny General Hospital, Pittsburgh, Pennsylvania
Chapter 5: Asthma

RACHEL E. STORY, MD, MPH
Fellow, Department of Medicine, Division of Allergy and Immunology, Northwest University School of Medicine, Chicago, Illinois
Chapter 17: Drug Allergy

MICHAEL D. THARP, MD
Professor and Chairman, Department of Dermatology, Rush University Medical Center, Chicago, Illinois
Chapter 18: Urticaria and Angioedema

ELLEN R. WALD, MD
Professor of Pediatrics and Otolaryngology, University of Pittsburgh School of Medicine, Children's Hospital of Pittsburgh, Pittsburgh, Pennsylvania; Chief, Division of Allergy, Immunology, and Infectious Diseases, Children's Hospital of Pittsburgh, Pittsburgh, Pennsylvania
Chapter Ch 10: Sinusitis

LEE A. WILEY, MD
Associate Professor, Ophthalmology, West Virginia University Eye Institute, Morgantown, West Virginia
Chapter 12: Allergic Immunologic Ocular Diseases

# Contents

Foreword   ix

Preface   xi

1. Immunology of Allergic and Clinical Immunologic Disorders   1
Andre Petrov and Philip Fireman

2. Allergens   35
Philip Fireman

3. Diagnostic Tests in Allergy   55
Deborah Gentile

4. Anaphylaxis and Insect Allergy   65
Gilbert Friday and Philip Fireman

5. Asthma   81
David Skoner

6. Occupational Asthma and Allergies   115
Emil Bardana

7. Hypersensitivity Pneumonitis   125
Sergei Belenky and Carl Fuhrman

8. Allergic Bronchopulmonary Aspergillosis   137
Paul Greenberger

9. Allergic Rhinitis   147
Philip Fireman

10. Sinusitis   167
Ellen Wald

11. Otitis Media   179
Ellen Mandel, Margaretha Casselbrant, and Philip Fireman

12. Allergic Immunologic Ocular Diseases   195
Lee A. Wiley, Robert C. Arffa, and Philip Fireman

13. Food Hypersensitivity   213
Amy M. Scurlock and A. Wesley Burks

14. Contact Dermatitis   225
Vincent Beltrani

15. Atopic Dermatitis   243
Vincent Beltrani

16. Latex Allergy   259
Kevin Kelly

17. Drug Allergy   271
Leslie Grammer and Rachel Story

18. Urticaria and Angioedema   279
Michael D. Tharp, Macy I. Levine, and Philip Fireman

19. Rheumatologic Diseases   293
Tom Medsger and Tharaknath Rao

20. Primary Immunodeficiency Diseases   329
Philip Fireman

21. HIV/AIDS   351
Christopher Baliga and William Shearer

22. Immunotherapy: Vaccines for Allergic Diseases   369
Ira Finegold

23. Immunization   379
Klara M. Posfay-Barbe and David Greenberg

*Andrej Petrov and Philip Fireman*

# *1* Immunology of Allergic and Clinical Immunologic Disorders

Syndromes that are now identified as allergic or clinical immunologic diseases have been described for centuries, but the concept of an immunologic basis for these diseases was not introduced until the 20th century. During the past 50 years, advances in immunology have changed the practice of allergy and clinical immunology. We now understand the mechanisms for many of the diagnostic and therapeutic procedures that had developed empirically but without well-controlled documentation of efficacy over the previous 100 years. In addition, these important advances in immunology have influenced the professional organizations in allergy and immunology and the residency and fellowship training programs to such an extent that this branch of medicine is now frequently referred to as the specialty of "allergy and immunology" or "clinical immunology."

## TERMINOLOGY (DEFINITIONS)

It is important to define the terms common in clinical practice. The manner in which the words *immunology, immunity, autoimmunity, allergy, hypersensitivity,* and *atopy* are used has at times revealed confusion regarding their meaning. *Immunology* was initially described as the study of antigen–antibody interactions in which the host became resistant to disease, and the term implied a beneficial host defense induced by the antigen. This type of immunity is referred to as *adaptive* or *acquired immunity* to a specific antigen (Box 1-1). However, there are host defense mechanisms that are not specific to given antigens or microbes; this type of immunity is referred to as *innate* or *natural immunity.*

Whereas the limited definition of immunology given previously is appropriate for the study of infectious diseases, it does not describe the body's response to noninfectious environmental factors, such as pollens, drugs, and other potential antigens, including neoplasms. The basic property of the immune system is to distinguish nonself from self. This exists in a delicate balance between tolerance to self and the response to or rejection of nonself. *Autoimmunity* defines the condition in which tolerance to self is lost, and if these immune responses to the host occur with heightened reaction, autoimmune diseases can develop.

*Hypersensitivity* indicates a heightened or exaggerated immune response that develops after more than one exposure to a given antigen. *Hypersensitivity* is usually considered synonymous with *allergy.* An antigen responsible for an allergic reaction is an *allergen.* The term *allergy* was introduced by Clemens Von Pirquet in 1906 to designate an altered reactivity to a foreign substance after prior experience with the same material, whether this response was helpful or harmful to the host.[1] This concept of allergy, popularized by Gell and Coombs, may have merit in that it permits an organized and systematic approach to the pathogenesis of immunologic diseases.[2] Nevertheless, the term *allergy,* as commonly used in clinical practice, indicates an adverse reaction and describes the pathophysiologic responses that result from the interaction of an allergen with antibodies and/or lymphocytes in a patient previously exposed and sensitized to that allergen (Fig. 1-1). This immunologic definition of allergy is accepted by most but not all allergists, as nonimmune processes can influence the pathogenesis of allergic diseases with recognized immune etiologies.

The terms *atopy* and *atopic* are frequently used in reference to allergic diseases. Derived from the Greek word meaning "strange," they were introduced by Coca and Cooke in 1923 to describe allergic diseases, such as asthma, allergic rhinitis (hay fever), and atopic dermatitis (infantile eczema), that showed a familial predilection and an implied genetic predisposition.[3] Other allergic diseases, such as contact dermatitis and serum sickness, showed no familial tendency and were referred to as nonatopic. It was also recognized that serum from these allergic individuals contained a factor subsequently described as a skin-sensitizing antibody. This heat-labile serum factor could passively sensitize the skin of a nonsensitive individual and, after intradermal challenge with a specific allergen, the passively sensitized skin showed a positive wheal-and-flare reaction within 20 minutes (Fig. 1-2). This passive transfer test, also known as the Prausnitz-Kustner, or PK, test, provided documentation of the presence of a specific serum antibody important in the pathogenesis of allergic diseases. More than 90% of these antibodies are now identified as immunoglobulin (Ig) E.[4] Many allergists use the term *atopic* instead of *allergic* to identify those families and patients with hereditary predisposition toward asthma, hay fever, and/or infantile eczema.

---

**BOX 1-1**
**Human Immunologic System**

Innate immunity (natural immunity)
Adaptive immunity (specific immunity)

---

# HOST IMMUNE SYSTEM

A significant, but not the only, function of the immune system is defense against microbes that cause infection. Early host responses are initiated by innate immunity, and later responses involve the adaptive immune systems (see Box 1-1). Innate immunity (natural or native immunity) consists of mechanisms that are native to the host in that they exist even before infection and therefore respond rapidly when the host is exposed to microbes. In contrast to innate immunity, the adaptive (specific) immune responses are more highly evolved and once stimulated, increase in magnitude over days with subsequent exposure to the specific agent. However, these two immune responses are not mutually exclusive and function as an integrated system to protect the host. Whereas the adaptive immune response may take days to provide protection for the host, innate immunity is typically activated promptly and

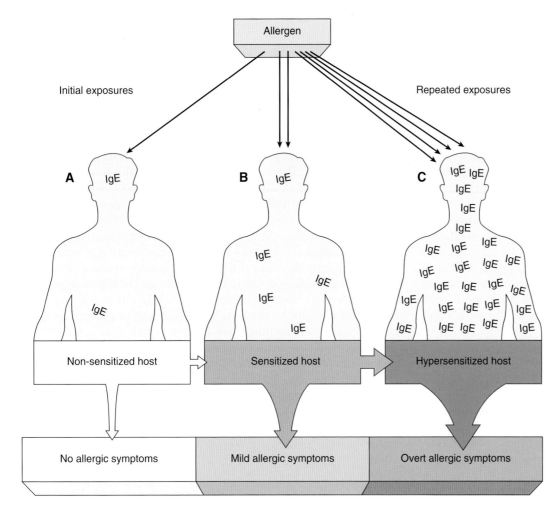

**Figure 1-1.** Hypersensitivity and allergy. *A,* On initial exposure to an allergen, there are no overt manifestations of allergic disease because the patient is nonsensitized. However, the allergen will initiate an immune response, which results in the synthesis of immunoglobulin E (IgE) and sensitization of the susceptible (atopic) host. *B,* On subsequent, repeated exposures, this sensitized individual synthesizes increased amounts of IgE, thus becoming hypersensitive. *C,* From this point onward, reexposure to this specific allergen provokes the overt manifestations of allergic disease.

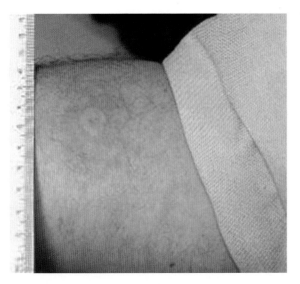

**Figure 1-2.** Immunoglobulin E (IgE)-mediated wheal-and-flare reaction of passively sensitized skin. This photo was taken 20 minutes after allergen injection into a skin site containing IgE antibodies to the allergen. This Prausnitz-Kustner test is no longer used in clinical practice, given the risk of passive transfer of viral diseases. The skin reaction is usually accompanied by pruritus. It begins within minutes after allergen is injected and peaks in 20 minutes. The reaction usually subsides within an hour, unless a late-phase IgE reaction ensues. The late phase IgE-reaction may have its onset at 2 to 6 hours after allergen exposure and persist for up to 24 hours.

contains the infection until the adaptive immune response resolves the infection.

The innate immune system recognizes and responds to a few highly conserved structures present on microbial organisms.[5] These structures are referred to as pathogen-associated molecular patterns (PAMPs). These PAMPs are produced only by the pathogens and not the host. They include bacterial lipopolysaccharides, mannons, bacterial RNA and DNA, and other microbial constituents. Receptors on the cellular components of the innate system, which include the neutrophils, macrophages, and natural killer (NK) cells, recognize these PAMPs. Once these pattern recognition receptors interact with a PAMP on a microbial organism, the effector cells (neutrophils or macrophages) respond immediately without the need for further proliferation or differentiation. This prompt response distinguishes it from the adaptive immune responses. There are three groups of pattern-recognition receptors: secreted, endocytic, and signaling.[6] The secreted pattern-recognition molecules function as opsonins and may activate complement. The signaling pattern-recognition receptors (also known as toll receptors) lead to expression of proinflammatory and immune-modulating cytokines. The endocytic group of pattern-recognition receptors mediates the uptake of microbes into the macrophages, which digest and present the microbial peptides as antigen. This serves as the link between the innate and adaptive immune system. The several components of the innate system are listed in Box 1-2.

The principal components of the adaptive immune response are lymphocytes and their secreted soluble products.[7] These secreted products include immunoglobulins and various cytokines. There are several specific characteristics of the adaptive immune response that distinguish it from innate immunity. These include specificity, diversity, memory, and feedback regulation that leads to discrimination between self and nonself antigen determinates. In the adaptive immune system, specific T-lymphocyte (T-cell) and B-lymphocyte (B-cell) receptors are generated during development and differentiation to endow each lymphocyte with a structurally unique receptor to recognize a microbial pathogen. Because these specific unique receptors are not encoded in the germ line, the diversity of the repertoire of receptors is generated randomly and expanded by clonal expansion on exposure to an antigen. This mechanism potentially gives rise to a very large number of antigen specificities; for example, $1 \times 10^{15}$ for B-cell receptors and $1 \times 10^{18}$ for T-cell receptors. The several components of the adaptive immune system are listed in Box 1-3.

# CLASSIFICATION OF IMMUNOLOGIC REACTIONS IN ALLERGIC DISEASES

The manifestations and expressions of allergic disease are dependent on many variables, which include the genetic constitution of the sensitized individual, the nature of the allergen involved, the route of allergen administration to the sensitized subject, the biologic properties of the antibodies or sensitized cells, and the local tissue response to the allergen–antibody interaction. If a suspected allergen is applied to or injected into the skin of a previously sensitized allergic subject, several different responses occur. The allergic or hypersensitivity cutaneous reactions can be classified as immediate hypersensitivity (IgE early- and late-phase) reactions and T-cell (48 hours) hypersensitivity reactions.

## IMMEDIATE HYPERSENSITIVITY RESPONSES

The immediate cutaneous hypersensitivity reaction usually develops within 20 minutes of challenge with the antigen and is manifested as a wheal-and-flare skin response (see Fig. 1-2). Studies have demonstrated that an antibody (typically IgE immunoglobulin) present in either serum or tissues binds to the specific antigen and initiates secretion of mediators of inflammation and cytokines that are responsible for the immediate hypersensitivity response.

Biopsy and microscopic examination of an immediate cutaneous hypersensitivity reaction at 15 to 30 minutes reveals little cellular infiltrate—perhaps a few neutrophils and occasional eosinophils and some local edema. It is the immediate hypersensitivity reaction that is the basis for much of the allergy skin testing performed by clinical allergists and immunologists.

## LATE PHASE AND DELAYED RESPONSES

Depending on IgE antibody and allergen concentrations, a subset of allergy patients shows a late (2 to 6 hours) cutaneous allergic IgE response in addition to the immediate (15 to 30 minute) reaction. Biopsy of the late-phase IgE reaction reveals moderate cellular inflammation and an increased number of neutrophils and lymphocytes, with many basophils and eosinophils.

---

**BOX 1-2**
**Human Innate Immunologic System**

Neutrophils
Macrophages
Dendritic cells
Natural killer cells
Mast cells
Complement cytokines

---

**BOX 1-3**
**Human Adaptive Immunologic System**

T cells
B cells
Immunoglobulins (antibodies)
Eosinophils
Mast cells, basophils
Complement cytokines

The T-cell–mediated cutaneous delayed hypersensitivity reaction typically peaks 48 to 72 hours after antigen challenge and is characterized by local erythema and induration (Fig. 1-3). This delayed reaction is not dependent on a serum antibody but rather on a cell-mediated immune reaction involving sensitized T-lymphocytes. Microscopic examination of a cutaneous biopsy

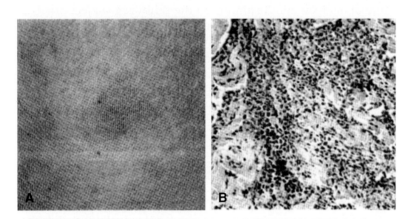

**Figure 1-3.** Clinical and histologic appearance of delayed (tuberculin)-type hypersensitivity. *A,* The erythema and induration of the skin is maximal 48 to 72 hours after intradermal injection of antigen. *B,* Histologically, the delayed hypersensitivity skin reaction appears as a dense dermal infiltrate of mononuclear cells, including small lymphocytes and macrophages. (Reproduced with permission from Roitt et al., 1995.)

of delayed hypersensitivity skin reaction reveals moderate mononuclear cellular infiltrate, consisting primarily of small lymphocytes. These different IgE- and T-cell–mediated cutaneous manifestations are not mutually exclusive and may be elicited in the same host, depending on the variables listed previously.

## GELL AND COOMBS CLASSIFICATION SCHEMA

To better comprehend the concepts of allergy, including the cutaneous immediate and delayed hypersensitivity reactions, Gell and Coombs proposed a classification of the immunopathologic mechanisms.[2] They separated the reactions by which a specific antigen can induce cellular and tissue injury into four groups: Type I (immediate or anaphylactic), Type II (cytotoxic or cytolytic), Type III (antigen-antibody complex), and Type IV (delayed or cell mediated) (Fig. 1-4). These four reactions patterns are not mutually exclusive; often, more than one of them occurs in the same patient. Hence, some immunologists do not accept or utilize this schema.[8] For example, there may be several allergic immune reactions to penicillin. Urticaria may develop, representing a Type I response involving IgE. In other patients, a hemolytic anemia can result from the formation of an immune complex composed of penicillin, IgG antibody, and complement (Type III). Further, contact dermatitis, mediated by sensitized T-lymphocytes reacting to the penicillin (Type IV), may also arise. Appreciating that these inconsistencies exist, the authors feel that this classification is helpful for the clinician in understanding the pathogenesis of allergic and immunologic diseases.

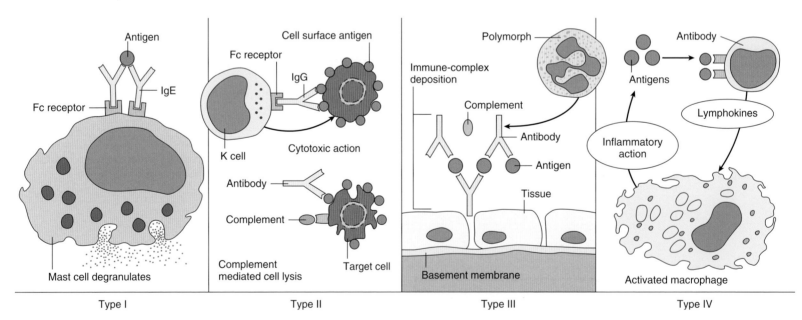

**Figure 1-4.** Summary of the four types of hypersensitivity reactions. Type I: Mast cells bind immunoglobulin E (IgE) via Fc receptors. On encountering antigen, the IgE becomes cross-linked, inducing degranulation and release of mediators. Type II: Antibodies are directed against antigens on an individual's own cells (target cells). This may lead to complement-mediated lysis or cytotoxic action by killer cells. Type III: Immune complexes are deposited in the tissues, complement is activated, and polymorphs are attracted to the site of antigen deposition, causing local damage. Type IV: Antigen-sensitized T-cells release lymphokines following a secondary contact with the same antigen. Lymphokines induce inflammatory reactions, activating and attracting macrophages, which release mediators. IgG, immunoglobulin G.

## Type I Reaction

The Type I reaction of Gell and Coombs is referred to as the immediate, anaphylactic, or homocytotopic antibody reaction. This reaction might also be called an atopic phenomenon, and it is responsible for many of the common allergic diseases. Clinical examples include asthma, hay fever, urticaria, angioedema, and anaphylaxis.

In the Type I reaction, mast cells or peripheral blood basophil leukocytes are passively sensitized by homocytotropic IgE antibodies, which are synthesized by plasma cells on stimulation by appropriate allergens. The binding of IgE to the mast cells involves the Fc portion of the IgE molecule and a receptor on the cell surface. During this initial sensitization phase, there is no overt deleterious host reaction. On subsequent challenge, however, this same allergen combines with its specific IgE antibody at the cell membrane of the sensitized mast cell and/or the blood basophil. This combination of allergen and antibody results in a sequence of energy-dependent enzyme reactions, with alteration of the cell membrane that initiates the synthesis and release of the specific pharmacologic mediators of the Type I immediate hypersensitivity reaction.[9] These mediators may be preformed and stored in the mast cell granules or generated from phospholipids of the mast cell or basophil membrane. The preformed mediators include histamine and eosinophil chemotactic factor (ECF-A). The newly synthesized mediators of anaphylaxis include metabolites of arachidonic acid, especially including the prostaglandins, which are products of the cyclo-oxygenase pathway, and the leukotrienes, which are the result of the lipoxygenase pathway.

The Type I reaction usually occurs within minutes of exposure to an appropriate antigen but may be sustained for 2 to 6 hours without additional antigen contact as a late-phase IgE reaction. After the mast cells and basophils have been through a refractory period of several hours, they resynthesize the pharmacologic mediators of hypersensitivity and once again become capable of responding to a specific allergen.

The specific intracellular biochemical events that occur during the Type I response are not entirely understood on a molecular level, but in vitro studies suggest that mediator release is promoted by those processes that decrease intracellular cyclic adenosine monophosphate (cAMP). It has been noted that adrenergic agents, especially the more selective beta-adrenergic agents, increase intracellular cyclic adenosine monophosphate and thereby inhibit histamine release. Cyclic adenosine monophosphate is normally catabolized by phosphodiesterase; if phosphodiesterase is inhibited by a phosphodiesterase inhibitor, intracellular cyclic adenosine monophosphate is increased, and less histamine and other mediators may be released. Theophylline, a methylxanthine derivative, is a phosphodiesterase inhibitor. Calcium and magnesium appear to be essential to the release of histamine from sensitized mast cells and basophils in vitro.[10]

Interaction of IgE antibodies and an allergen at the mast cell membrane does not appear to be capable of activating the complement sequence by the classic pathway; however, complement activation by the alternative pathway may occur.[11] In most situations, the immunologic effectors of the Type I immediate hypersensitivity allergic reaction have been shown to be IgE antibodies; it should be emphasized, however, that it is the inflammatory mediators (e.g., histamine, prostaglandins, and leukotrienes) that are responsible for the pathophysiologic changes observed in the patient.

## Type II Reaction

The Type II reaction as described by Gell and Coombs is referred to as the cytotoxic or cytolytic reaction. In this allergic situation, circulating IgG and IgM antibodies react with antigens that may actually be portions of cells, such as erythrocytes and their membranes, or with an unrelated antigen, such as a drug that has become associated with these cells. The fact that the antigen is a cell or a cell constituent indicates that this reaction may be expressed as a form of autoimmunization or isoimmunization in clinical situations. In most cases, both IgM and IgG are involved in this reaction, as is the complement system. The complement-activated mediators are responsible for an inflammatory reaction. The cell that functions as the antigen or carries the appropriate antigenic determinant is usually destroyed or altered; there may be injury to erythrocytes, leukocytes, and platelets, and other cytotoxic reactions may be involved in this mechanism. Clinical examples of Type II reactions include autoimmune hemolytic anemia; transfusion reactions; hemolytic disease of the newborn; Goodpasture's syndrome; and drug-induced, antibody-dependent hemolytic anemia, leucopenia, and thrombocytopenia. It is the destruction or alteration of a target cell that differentiates this type of immunologic injury.

## Type III Reaction

The Type III reaction is referred to as immune-complex injury or tissue damage. In this immunopathologic reaction, serum IgG antibodies interact with an antigen but not necessarily at a cell surface or membrane. Antigen–antibody complexes are formed, usually in moderate antigen excess, when antigen and antibody concentrations are appropriate. These microprecipitates or complexes aggregate in and near blood vessels. They induce inflammation in the tissues in which they are deposited, which leads to vascular damage and thrombosis.[12] Frequently, these antigen–antibody complexes are formed in areas of high blood flow, with deposition occurring in such tissues as the kidneys, lungs, and walls of small blood vessels.[12]

The antigen–antibody complexes activate the complement system, and components C5, C6, and C7 attract polymorphonuclear leukocytes to the reaction site. Phagocytosis of the complexes by these leukocytes, as well as other macrophages, result in the release of enzymes, cytokines, and other mediators responsible for the observed inflammation and tissue destruction. Clinical examples of this Type III reaction include serum sickness syndrome, acute poststreptococcal glomerulonephritis, and certain collagen vascular diseases, especially systemic lupus erythematosus.

## Type IV Reaction

The Type IV reaction of Gell and Coombs is the T-cell–mediated immune response or delayed hypersensitivity reaction (Fig. 1-3). The immunopathologic response in the Type IV reaction appears to be dependent on sensitized small T-lymphocytes and their cytokines; serum antibodies to the appropriate antigens have not been implicated in the pathogenesis of this immune reaction. Many of these cytokines are identified as interleukins. There is no apparent interaction of the antigen with humoral antibodies, either at the cell membranes or in tissues, and it has been proposed that the antigens react directly with the sensitized lymphocytes.

After challenge with an antigen, the cell-mediated immune reaction results in the accumulation of mononuclear cells at the site of tissue inflammation within 24 to 48 hours. Activation of dendritic cells, local proliferation of lymphocytes, and additional release of cytokines are important in the development of the delayed hypersensitivity, cell-mediated immune reaction. These cytokines are the mediators of the cell-mediated delayed hypersensitivity reaction and will be discussed in greater detail later in this chapter. Complement does not appear to be involved in this reaction. Cell-mediated delayed hypersensitivity represents the pathophysiologic basis for contact dermatitis, as well as for many aspects of organ transplant and skin graft rejection phenomena. In certain pulmonary diseases (e.g., tuberculosis, fungal diseases, and sarcoidosis), the observed tissue damage and inflammation appear to be due to cell-mediated, delayed hypersensitivity responses of the host to various antigens.

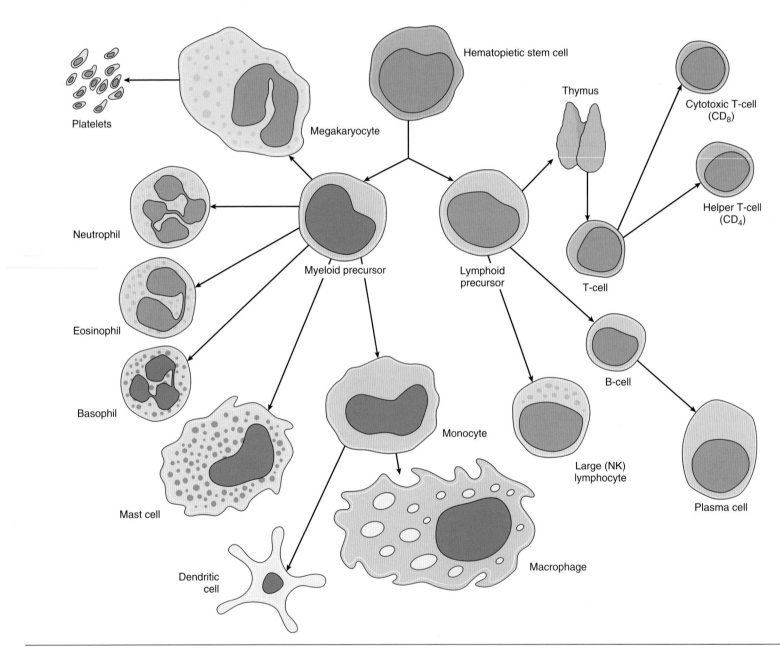

**Figure 1-5.** Ontogeny of the cells participating in the immune allergic response. All of these cells differentiate from pluripotent hematopietic stem cells that develop into the two distinct progenitor lineages: one for lymphoid and the other for myeloid cells. From the progenitor lymphoid cells, the T cells develop under the environmental influences of the thymus. They then differentiate into the various T-cell subpopulations, including helper (CD4) and cytotoxic T cells (CD8). Other lymphoid progenitor cells develop into B cells, which further differentiate into immunoglobulin-secreting plasma cells. Lymphoid cells also develop into the large, granular lymphocytes; i.e., natural killer (NK) cells. The myeloid cells differentiate into the neutrophils, eosinophils, basophils, mast cells, and monocytes. Monocytes are precursors to either macrophages or dendritic cells that are also known as type 1 dendritic cells. Dendritic cells can also arise from lymphoid progenitor cells and then are called type 2 dendritic cells (not depicted in this figure). (Modified with permission from Roitt et al., 1995.)

# CELLS INVOLVED IN IMMUNE REACTIONS

The human immune system consists of several lymphoid organs, including the lymph nodes, spleen, thymus, and other lymphoid tissues sites in the bone marrow, respiratory tract, and intestinal tract. These lymphoid tissues contain a number of different cells that respond in various ways on exposure to an antigen. All of the cells of the immune system are derived from pluripotent hematologic stem cells, which probably arise in the primordial liver and then traffic to the thymus and bone marrow. These cells differentiate via two major pathways into either progenitor lymphoid or progenitor myeloid cells (Fig. 1-5). This cell differentiation is influenced by several cell-derived substances described as cytokines. Some cytokines, which promote intercellular communication as well as cellular proliferation and growth, are referred to as interleukins and are discussed later in this chapter. These lymphoid cells are heterogenous, both morphologically and functionally.

## *LYMPHOCYTES*

Lymphocytes are key players in acquired immunity. They circulate in blood and enter peripheral lymphoid tissues, where they scan antigen-presenting cells for foreign antigens. Once they recognize foreign antigens, they become activated and exert both regulatory and effector functions. T-lymphocytes play a pivotal role in cellular immunity; whereas in humoral immunity, B-lymphocytes give rise to plasma cells that produce antibodies (Fig. 1-6A). T cells make up about 65% of the peripheral blood lymphocytes, and they mature in the thymus. On the other hand, B cells make up 5% to 15% of the peripheral blood lymphocytes, and they mature in bone marrow. NK cells comprise the remaining peripheral blood lymphocytes, are larger than T- and B-lymphocytes, and contain granules in their cytoplasm (Fig. 1-6B). NK cells are early responders to infection and as such belong to the innate immune system.

## T-Lymphocytes

The developmental pathway of the T-lymphocytes from the bone marrow via the thymus is illustrated in Figure 1-7. They are grouped in two major subclasses based on their receptors.[13] CD8 T-lymphocytes are also called cytotoxic T cells because of their ability to kill cells that contain intracellular pathogens. They are able to recognize foreign antigen when these cells present antigen in conjunction with major histocompatibility complex (MHC) type 1 molecule. CD derives its name from monoclonal antibodies (clusters of differentiation) that identify the same cell surface molecules. The cell surface molecule is designated CD followed by a number. There are more than 200 known CD molecules. CD4 T-lymphocytes recognize foreign antigen when co-expressed with MHC class 2 molecules on antigen-presenting cells, and their function is to regulate the responses of other cells; thus, they are called helper T cells (Fig. 1-8).

The CD4 subclass of helper T cells is further divided into Th1 and Th2 subsets (Fig. 1-9). The Th1 subset primarily secretes interferon gamma (IFN-$\gamma$) and tumor necrosis factor beta (TNF-$\beta$).[14] These cytokines serve to activate macrophages, and they suppress Th2 cytokines. Unlike the Th1 subset, Th2 lymphocytes primarily secrete interleukin (IL)-4, IL-5, and IL-13. These cytokines suppress Th1 type cytokines and stimulate B-cell differentiation into plasma cells, which secrete antibodies. (Detailed cytokine functions are discussed later.) Therefore, these Th subsets influence each other, and predominance of either one has been associated with pathologic states. For example, Crohn's disease is characterized by Th1 polarization, while asthma is known for Th2 predominance.[15,16] Lately, new evidence has emerged to reveal another subset called regulatory, or Tr-, lymphocytes that control Th1 and Th2 responses and play a pivotal role in preventing autoimmune and allergic disorders. Two types of regulatory T-lymphocytes have been proposed: natural and adaptive (Fig. 1-10).[17] Natural regulatory T-lymphocytes are thymus-derived CD4 CD25 lymphocytes that block immune cells through physical contact. Adaptive regulatory T cells are induced in the periphery and block immune cells through production of cytokines.

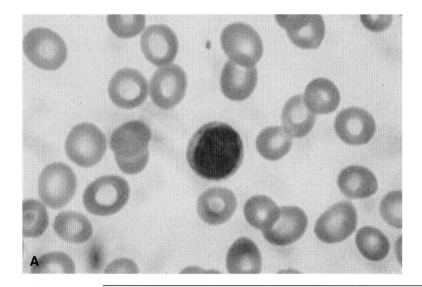
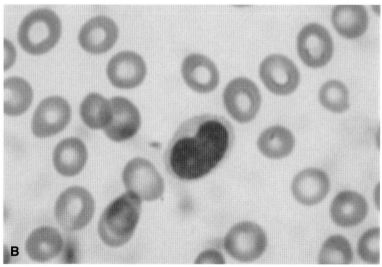

**Figure 1-6.** *A,* Light micrograph of a small lymphocyte. The cell shows a prominent nucleus, very little cytoplasm, and only a few granules. *B,* The large granular lymphocyte (the natural killer cell) contains more cytoplasm and more azurophilic granules. Both specimens were prepared with Wright's stain and magnified ×6000. (Courtesy of Dr. Lila Penchansky, Children's Hospital of Pittsburgh.)

## B-lymphocytes

The B-lymphocytes are defined by the presence of endogenously produced immunoglobulins; these molecules become associated with the B-cell surface membrane and then function as specific antigen receptors. These membrane markers can be detected by staining the B-lymphocytes with anti-human immunoglobulins (Fig. 1-11). Most of the peripheral blood B cells express surface IgM and IgD antibodies, with a few having IgG, IgA, or IgE markers.

After initial development in the liver, the B cell matures in the bone marrow. During this maturation in the bone marrow, a series of antigen-independent DNA rearrangements of Ig heavy-chain genes and light-chain genes occur enabling production of membrane immunoglobulin and secreted immunoglobulin molecules. Differentiation of mature B cells in peripheral blood or tissues is antigen driven, and at this stage, its main function is antigen recognition with subsequent plasma cell differentiation (Fig. 1-12). Two types of mature B cells can be recognized on the basis of their B-cell receptors (BCR); naïve B cells, which co-express B-cell receptors of IgM and IgD isotypes, and memory B-cells, which express a single-isotype B-cell receptor (i.e., IgG, IgE, IgA, or IgM). Upon antigen stimulation, these naïve B cells proliferate and differentiate into plasma cells that produce antibodies of IgM isotype. With recall contact with the same antigen, many B cells undergo class switching to produce antibodies of IgG isotype or into memory B cells expressing a B-cell receptor of a single different isotype.[18] The plasma cells contain intracytoplasmic immunoglobulin and are typically found in the germinal follicles of lymphoid tissue (Fig. 1-13). They synthesize and secrete the immunoglobulins. A single plasma cell appears to be capable of producing only one immunoglobulin isotype.

## Natural Killer Cells

Natural killer cells were initially described on the basis of their "natural" capacity to kill certain tumor cells in vitro, a process known as "natural killing." NK cells are large, granular lymphocytes (see Fig. 1-6*B*). They do not express the T-cell receptor or B-cell receptor; they instead express three types of receptors:

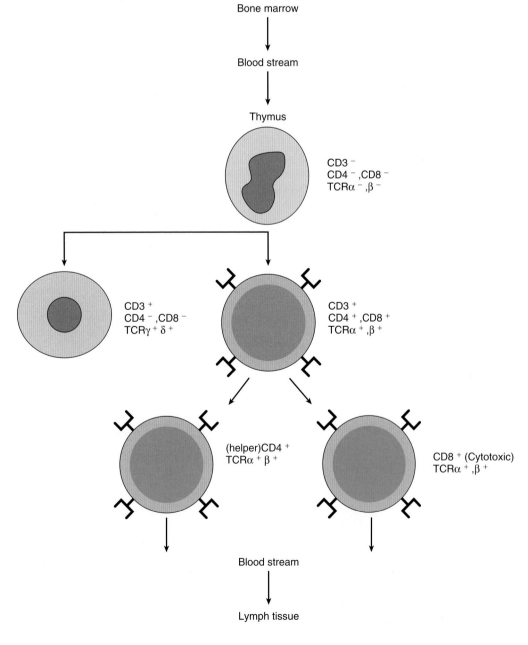

Bone marrow

Blood stream

Thymus

CD3 $^-$
CD4 $^-$,CD8 $^-$
TCRα $^-$,β $^-$

CD3 $^+$
CD4 $^-$,CD8 $^-$
TCRγ $^+$δ $^+$

CD3 $^+$
CD4 $^+$,CD8 $^+$
TCRα $^+$,β $^+$

(helper)CD4 $^+$
TCRα $^+$β $^+$

CD8 $^+$ (Cytotoxic)
TCRα $^+$,β $^+$

Blood stream

Lymph tissue

**Figure 1-7.** Initially, the intrathymic T cells do not manifest any cell surface markers and are called "double-negative" thymocytes. With maturation, two different lineages arise: CD3 + αβ T-cell receptor cells (majority) and CD3 + γd T-cell receptor cells (minority). CD3 + αβ T-cell receptor cells also acquire initially both CD4 and CD8 receptors and they are called "double positive" thymocytes. Subsequently, they divide into CD4 or CD8 lymphocytes and leave thymus for peripheral blood and tissues. (Modified from Shearer WT, Fleisher TA: The immune system. In Adkinson NF Jr, Yunginger JW, Busse WW, et al (eds): Middleton's Allergy Principles and Practice, 6th ed. St. Louis, C.V. Mosby, 2003, p 3.)

activating, inhibitory, and co-stimulatory. The susceptibility of tumor targets to natural killing is inversely related to target-cell expression of MHC class I molecules. NK cells survey tissues for expression of these molecules. In the absence of otherwise ubiquitously expressed MHC class I molecules, NK cells are released from the negative influence of these molecules and kill the target. It is believed that defects in NK cell development might lead to malignant transformation and cancer formation in humans. NK cells are also crucial for innate host defense against pathogens, particularly against viral infections. Importantly, NK cells use the same mechanisms to resist tumors and infections. Finally, in human NK cells, there seems to be a "division of labor," with one subset of NK cells having a cytolitic (killing) capacity and the other performing a regulatory function through the production of cytokines such as IFN-γ, TNF, lymphotoxin (LT-β), granulocyte-macrophage colony-stimulating factor (GM-CSF), IL-10, and IL-13.[19]

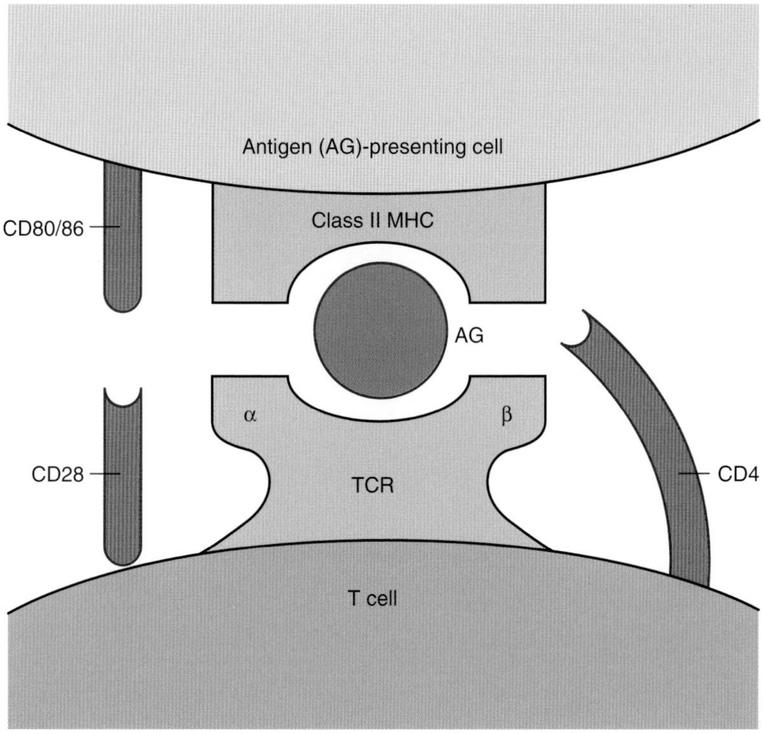

## MACROPHAGES

Macrophages were discovered and named by the Russian immunologist Elie Mechnikoff in 1892. The definition of macrophage in Greek is "big eater" because of macrophages' ability to ingest foreign substances and microbes. Macrophages derive from bone marrow and differentiate into varied morphologic types (Fig. 1-14). They reside both in tissues and in blood, where they are called monocytes. Monocytes are the largest normal blood cells and constitute 8% to 10% of normal leukocyte blood cells (Fig. 1-15). Tissue macrophages derive from monocytes, and they are distributed throughout the body. Monocytes and tissue macrophages form the mononuclear phagocyte system (a.k.a. reticuloendothelial system). Macrophages play a role in innate and specific acquired immunity. In natural immunity, the macrophages function as the principle scavenger cells in tissues, along with the polymorphonuclear leukocytes. They phagocytose microbes and foreign substances as well as injured or dead red blood cells, leukocytes, and other tissues. In addition, these cells secrete enzymes, nitric oxide, and lipid-derived mediators, such as prostaglandins, which control the spread of infection but also contribute to inflammation and injury. The macrophages also produce cytokines (IL-1, TNF-α, IL-6, IL-8, IL-12) and growth factors, which also participate in inflammation.

Mononuclear phagocytes function as both antigen-presenting cells and effector cells of the adaptive immune response.[20] As antigen-presenting cells, the macrophages express on their surface proteins that promote T-cell activation. In return, T-lymphocytes (especially Th1 lymphocytes) activate macrophages, making them effector cells of cellular immunity. They are more efficient in phagocytosis than the prior nonstimulated macrophages. Because the macrophages also express surface receptors for antibodies and

**Figure 1-8.** Activation of CD4+ T cells, with binding of T-cell receptor (TCR) to class II major histocompatibility complex (MHC)-antigen complex on antigen-presenting cell and accessory molecules CD28 to CD80/86. TCR consists of two different polypeptide chains termed *TCRα* and *TCRβ* chains. (Modified from Shearer WT, Fleisher TA: The immune system. In Adkinson NF Jr, Yunginger JW, Busse WW, et al (eds): Middleton's Allergy Principles and Practice, 6th ed. St. Louis, C.V. Mosby, 2003, p 5.)

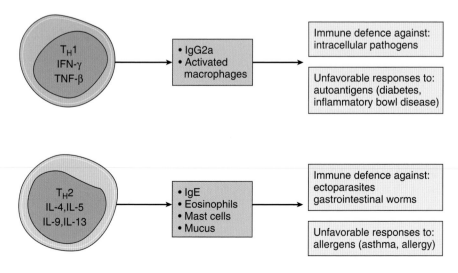

**Figure 1-9.** Functions of T-helper 1 cell ($T_H1$) and T-helper 2 cell ($T_H2$) and their cytokines. IFN-γ, interferon gamma; Ig, immunoglobulin; IL, interleukin; TNF-β, tumor necrosis factor beta. (Modified from Herrick CA, Bottomly K: To respond or not to respond: T-cells in allergic asthma. Nature Rev Immunol 2003;3:405–412.)

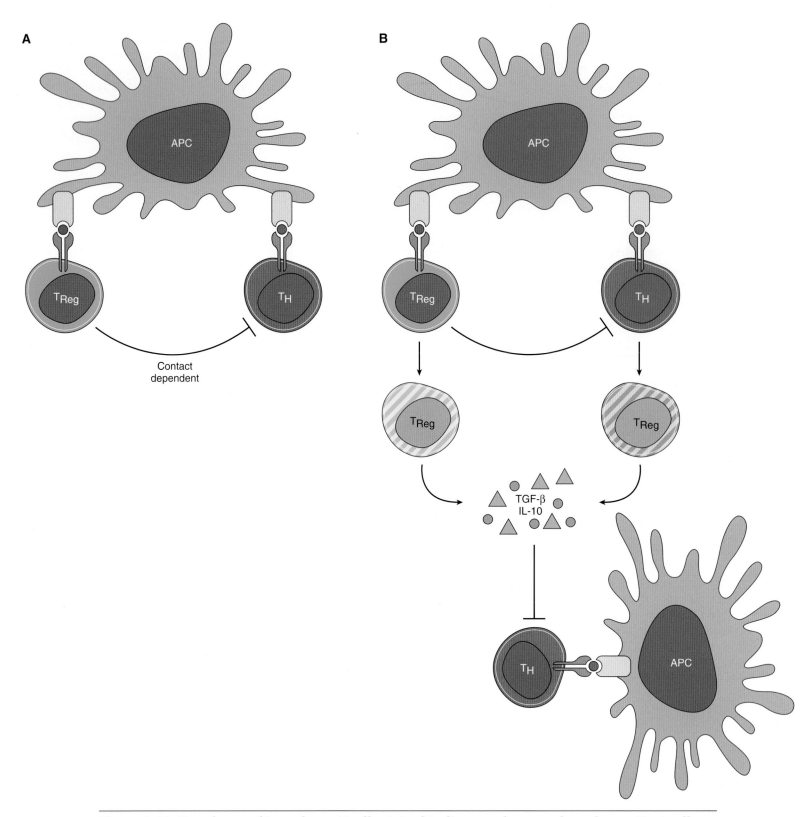

**Figure 1-10.** Two classes of irregulatory T cells. *A,* In this diagram, the natural regulatory (T$_{Reg}$) cells *(blue)* suppress immune responses in a contact-dependent manner and function in general homeostasis to block the actions of autoimmune T cells *(red)* in noninflammatory settings. *B,* The adaptive T$_{Reg}$ cells suppress immune response through secretion of cytokines in the inflammatory setting. Importantly, adaptive T$_{Reg}$ cells can develop either from natural T$_{Reg}$ cells *(blue striped)* or by altering the activity of helper T cells *(red striped;* T$_H$). APC, antigen-presenting cell; IL-10, interleukin-10; TGF-β, transforming growth factor beta. (Modified from Bluestone, JA, Abbas AK: Natural versus adaptive regulatory T-cells. Nature Rev Immunol 2003;3:253–257.)

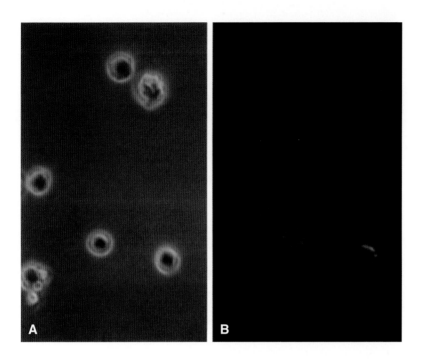

**Figure 1-11.** *A,* B cells stained for surface immunoglobulins. Human peripheral blood B cells stained with fluorescent anti-human immunoglobulin M (IgM) antiserum show a patchy surface fluorescence when viewed under ultraviolet light. *B,* Phase-contrast light microscopy reveals that only two of the six cells in this field are actually B-lymphocytes. (Reproduced with permission from Roitt et al., 1995.)

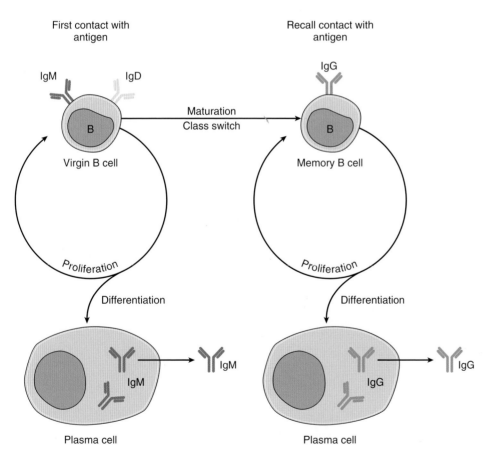

**Figure 1-12.** Virgin B cells recognize antigen through their B-cell receptors, typically of immunoglobulin (Ig) M and IgD isotypes. The cells proliferate heavily in the germinal centers, and part of the cells differentiate into plasma cells producing IgM antibodies, whereas others undergo class switching and mature into memory B cells expressing B-cell receptors of a different isotype (e.g., IgG) and higher affinity for the antigen that induced the process. When B cells differentiate into plasma cells, their function changes from antigen capture/recognition (through the B-cell receptors) to the production of antibodies. (Holgate ST, Church MK, Lichtenstein LM (eds): Allergy, 2nd ed. St. Louis, C.V. Mosby, 2001.)

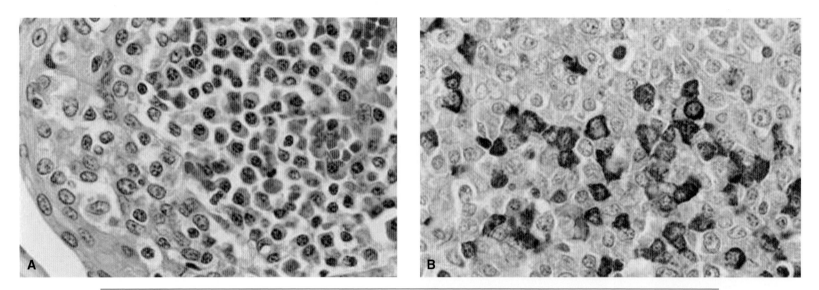

**Figure 1-13.** *A,* Photomicrograph showing abundant plasma cells beneath the squamous epithelium of the tonsil. The plasma cells have eccentric oval nuclei with clocklike condensation of the chromatin, and amphophilic *(blue)* cytoplasm with a paranuclear clearing. The specimen was stained with hematoxylin and eosin and magnified ×75. *B,* Histochemical staining of intracytoplasmic immunoglobulin in plasma cells. Human plasma cells treated with immunoperoxide-conjugated antihuman immunoglobulin G (IgG; heavy chain) show considerable intracytoplasmic staining. The specimen was magnified ×210. (Courtesy of Dr. Ronald Jaffe, Children's Hospital of Pittsburgh.)

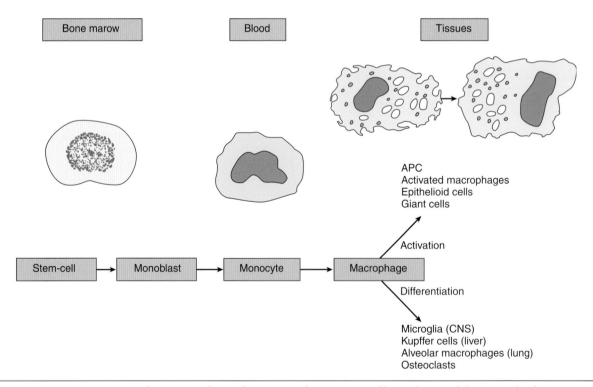

**Figure 1-14.** Maturation of mononuclear phagocytes from stem cells and monoblasts in the bone marrow to monocytes in the peripheral blood to macrophages in tissues. Macrophages are found in all organs and connective tissues. In specific locations, these macrophages are differentiated by pathologists as microglia cells in the central nervous system (CNS), Kupffer cells that line the sinusoids of the liver, alveolar macrophages in the pulmonary airways, and osteoclasts in bone tissue. Activation of macrophages promotes both the natural and specific immune reactions. They function as accessory cells with antigen presentation and promote lymphocyte activation. The antigen-presenting cells (APCs), when activated, may change their histologic appearance into epitheliod and giant cells.

complement proteins, they can bind and phagocytose antibody-coated particles much more avidly than nonantibody complexed substances. In this manner, the macrophages also participate in the humoral immune response. The ability of macrophages and lymphocytes to stimulate each other presents an important amplification mechanism for immunity.

## DENDRITIC CELLS

Dendritic cells (DCs) comprise two major groups of cells. One is bone marrow derived and specialized for the uptake, transport, processing, and presentation of antigens to T-lymphocytes. Another population that maintains immunologic memory is follicular DCs of nonhematopoietic stromal cell origin. DCs are present in many locations throughout the body. In the skin epidermis they were originally named Langerhans' cells. DCs can be found in the submucosal tissue of respiratory and gastrointestinal tracts and the interstitium of the heart, lungs, liver, and other organs. DCs are also present in the lymph nodes and the thymus.[21]

Dendritic cells are adept at capturing antigens because of their stellate morphology and multiple cytoplasmic processes, which provide greater surface area. DCs go through various stages of activation when they encounter antigen. Prior to encountering antigen, DCs are called immature and do not express co-stimulatory molecules. After capturing antigens, DCs become activated and migrate into the lymphoid organs, where they initiate activation of those T-lymphocytes that are specific for these antigens (Fig. 1-16). (See also T-Lymphocyte Activation.) Once activated, DCs are no longer able to capture antigens, but they express co-stimulatory molecules on their surface that are necessary for T-cell activation. Finally, DCs can also be quiescent when they are sufficiently mature to express moderate levels of co-stimulatory molecules, but they are not fully activated, and their role might be

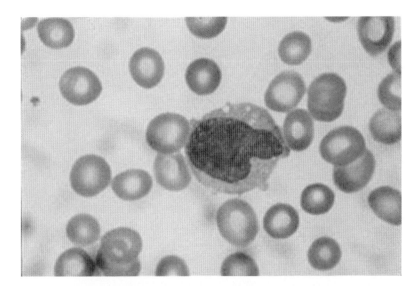

**Figure 1-15.** Morphology of the monocyte. Peripheral blood monocytes have typical horseshoe-shaped nuclei. They are larger than most peripheral blood lymphocytes. This cell can function as a phagocytic macrophage and as an antigen-presenting cell. The specimen was prepared with Wright's stain and magnified ×4500. (Courtesy of Dr. Lila Penchansky, Children's Hospital of Pittsburgh.)

in mediating T-lymphocyte tolerance (Fig. 1-17).[22] Follicular DCs are an exception to this group because they are believed to retain immune complexes and have a role in maintaining B-lymphocyte memory and regulating germinal centers in the lymph nodes.[23]

In conclusion, DCs act as the gatekeepers of the immune system by capturing antigens. They are instrumental in stimulating the response of the immune system against microbes and neoplastic cells and in inducing tolerance to many allergens and self-antigens. From a clinical standpoint, therapeutic manipulation of dendritic cells and their cytokines has become the main focus of research in allergic and infectious diseases, autoimmunity, oncology, and organ transplantation. It is anticipated that a better understanding of the functional capacity of DCs will be forthcoming in the future.

## GRANULOCYTES

The myeloid precursor cells can also differentiate into polymorphonuclear granulocytes under the influence of GM-CSF, which is also produced by stimulated T cells. These granulocytes represent 60% to 70% of the peripheral blood leukocytes and have a relatively short lifespan: about 2 or 3 days. In contrast, monocytes, macrophages, and T cells may circulate for months or years. On the basis of the histologic staining of their cytoplasmic granules, the granulocytes are characterized as neutrophils, eosinophils, or basophils.

### Neutrophils

Neutrophils represent 80% to 90% of the granulocytes in the peripheral blood (Fig. 1-18). Their primary role is phagocytosis and the killing of ingested organisms that are critical components of natural innate immunity. These cells have no apparent immunologic specificity but are very important in acute and chronic inflammation. IL-1 enhances the accumulation as well as release of neutrophils from the bone marrow, and IL-6 influences the maturation of neutrophils.

Neutrophils, as well as other cells that participate in the immune response, use adhesion molecules to migrate to the site of inflammation. Adhesion molecules are divided into three groups: the selectins, the integrins, and the proteins of the immunoglobulin superfamily.[24] Selectins are located on the surface of activated endothelial cells, and they facilitate initial binding of neutrophils to endothelial cells. Subsequently, stronger interaction occurs between the integrins that are present on neutrophils and molecules of the immunoglobulin superfamily (intercellular adhesion molecules and vascular cell adhesion molecule [VCAM]) that are present on activated endothelial cells. The resultant tight binding of neutrophils to endothelial cells allows the neutrophils to leave the blood circulation by squeezing between the endothelial cells and extravasate into the tissues.

### Eosinophils

The eosinophils (Fig. 1-19) make up 2% to 5% of peripheral blood leukocytes in normal healthy individuals. They participate in the inflammatory process, and their numbers are increased in the tissues, secretions, and peripheral blood (>600/mm³) of many patients with allergic disease. Eosinophil levels are also elevated in parasitic disease. IL-5 and GM-CSF promote the differentiation and proliferation of eosinophils. Like neutrophils, eosinophils are also capable of phagocytosis and the killing of ingested organisms, especially parasites, but this is not their only or primary function with regard to allergic diseases. They are attracted to sites of inflammation by chemotactic factors released by T cells, basophils, and mast cells. Upon degranulation, they release several toxic proteins, identified as major basic protein (MBP), eosinophil cationic protein (ECP), and eosinophil-derived neurotoxin, as well as histaminase, eosinophil proxidase, and aryl sulfatase.

Eosinophils are also a major source of cysteinyl leukotriene C4 (LTC4) and its active metabolites LTD4 and LTE4. Eosinophils, along with mast cells and basophils, are the principal LTC4 synthase-producing cell in asthmatic bronchial mucosa. Eosinophils are capable of producing a number of cytokines, including IL-1, TGF-β, IL-3, IL-4, IL-5, IL-8, and TNF-α.[25] However, eosinophils produce lower amounts of cytokines than do other inflammatory cells such as T cells.

## Basophils

Basophils are derived from CD34+ hematopoietic progenitor cells and mature in the bone marrow and then circulate in the peripheral blood (Fig. 1-20). Basophils are the least frequent of the granulocytes, accounting for less than 0.5% of circulating leukocytes. Basophils have a short lifespan of several days. IL-3 promotes the production and survival of basophils in vitro and induce basophilia in vivo.

Mediators stored in the cytoplasmic granules include chondroitin sulphates, proteases, and histamine. Basophils are the source of most of the histamine found in the blood. It was also

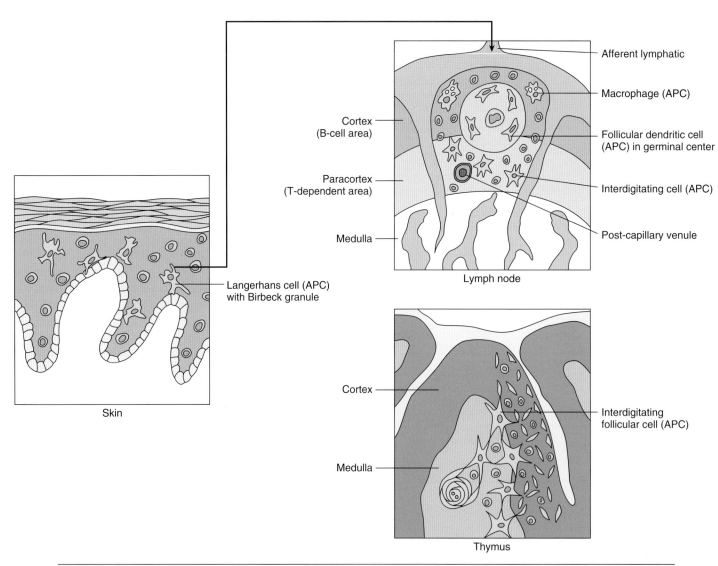

**Figure 1-16.** Antigen-presenting cells (APCs), which are bone marrow–derived cells found in large numbers in the skin, lymphoid tissue, and other organs. In the skin, APCs are identified as dendritic Langerhans' cells, which are found in the epidermis. Their cytoplasm contains Birbeck granules, the function of which is unknown. Histocompatibility locus antigen (HLA-DR) determinants are present on the APCs' cellular membranes. After processing antigens, these dendritic cells migrate via the afferent lymphatics into regional lymph nodes, where they interact and interdigitate with lymphocytes. Macrophages found in the paracortex of the lymph nodes also function as APCs. (Adapted with permission from Roitt et al., 1995.)

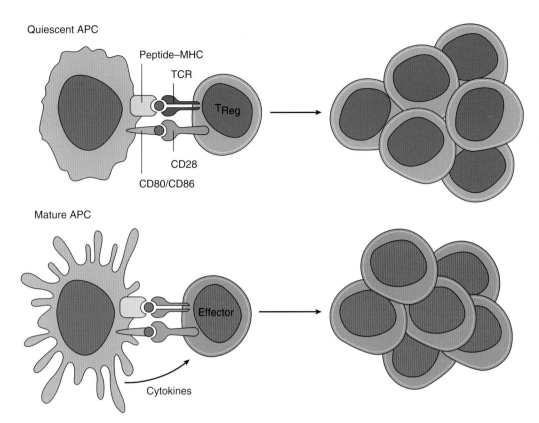

**Figure 1-17.** Model of two pathways of T-cell activation. Quiescent dendritic cells present antigen in a setting without cytokines produced by the innate immune system or perhaps without effective presentation of peptide major histocompatibility complex (MHC). Under these noninflammatory conditions, the natural regulatory ($T_{Reg}$) cell subset is induced (*blue*), and CD28 co-stimulation acts de facto to promote suppression. By contrast, effector T cells (*red*) are generated in a similar CD28-dependent manner but under inflammatory conditions associated with mature dendritic cells, leading to the development of immune response. APC, antigen-presenting cell; TCR, T-cell receptor. (Modified from Bluestone JA, Abbas AK: Natural versus adaptive regulatory T-cells. Nature Rev Immunol 2003;3:253–257.)

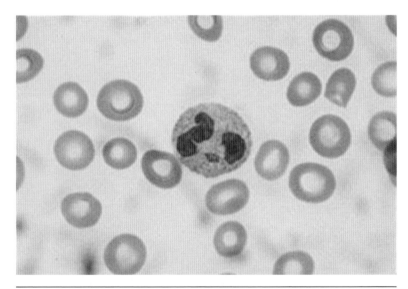

**Figure 1-18.** Morphology of the neutrophils. This photomicrograph of a peripheral blood smear stained with hematoxylin and eosin shows the polymorphonuclear shape and neutrophilic cytoplasm typical of neutrophils. (Courtesy of Dr. Lila Penchansky, Children's Hospital of Pittsburgh.)

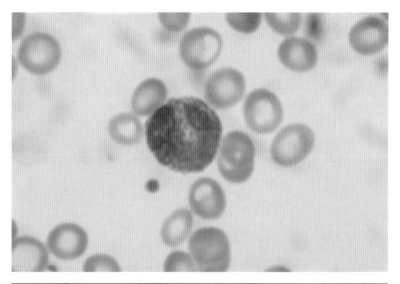

**Figure 1-19.** Morphology of the eosinophil. This photomicrograph of a blood smear shows an eosinophil with its multi-lobe lobe nucleus and reddish-stained cytoplasmic granules. The specimen was prepared with Wright's stain, and magnified ×4500. (Courtesy of Dr. Lila Penchansky, Children's Hospital of Pittsburgh.)

shown that activation of basophils can induce the production and secretion of leukotriene C4 and the release of IL-4 and IL-13.[26]

Basophils of normal individuals express basophil marker Bsp-1, while they do not express surface kit or cell-associated tryptase, chymas, or carboxypeptidase. However, in individuals with asthma or allergies, basophils were found to express all these markers.

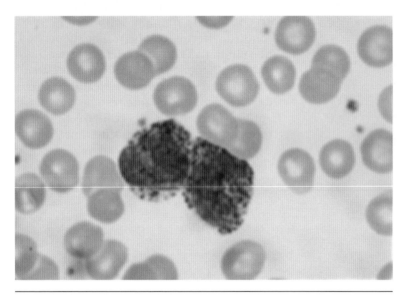

**Figure 1-20.** Morphology of the basophil. This photomicrograph of a peripheral blood smear shows a typical basophil with its dark violet-blue granules. The specimen was stained with Wright's, and magnified ×4500. (Courtesy of Dr. Lila Penchansky, Children's Hospital of Pittsburgh.)

## MAST CELLS

Mast cells are derived from CD34+ hematopoietic progenitor cells but ordinarily do not circulate in the blood. They are very long lived and can retain the ability to proliferate under certain conditions. They are found around blood vessels and peripheral nerves and beneath the epithelial surface of the respiratory tract, gastrointestinal tract, and skin (Fig. 1-21). Their development and survival are regulated by multiple cytokines and growth factors, including stem cell factor, IL-3, IL-4, IL-9, and IL-10.[27]

Mast cells granules contain proteoglycans, proteases, and histamine. Chondroitin sulfate and heparin are proteoglycans that bind proteases and histamine and contribute to the packaging of these molecules. Heparin is unique to mast cells, a feature that distinguishes them from basophils. Mast cell neutral proteases include chymase, typtase, carboxypeptidase, and cathepsin G. Mast cells also secrete lipid mediators that are cyclo-oxygenase and lipoxygenase metabolites of arachidonic acid. The major cyclo-oxygenase product of mast cells is PGD2, and the major lipoxygenase product is LTC4 and its derivates LTD4 and LTE4. Mast cells produce in smaller quantities LTB4 and platelet activation factor (PAF). Mast cells also represent a source of a vast array of cytokines: IL-1, IL-2, IL-3, IL-4, IL-5, IL-6, IL-8, IL-13, IL-16, GM-CSF, TNF-$\alpha$, TGF-$\beta$, and several chemokines.[27] Some mast cells contain pools of stored TNF-$\alpha$ that are available for immediate release.

Human mast cells are heterogenous with two phenotypes distinguishable by their neural proteinase content. The $MC_T$ phenotype contains only tryptase, and the $MC_{TC}$ phenotype contains both tryptase and chymase.[28] Although initially thought to be distinguished as to location in mucosal or connective tissue, variable amounts of each type are found in any given tissue. It has been suggested that the $MC_T$ phenotype appears to be

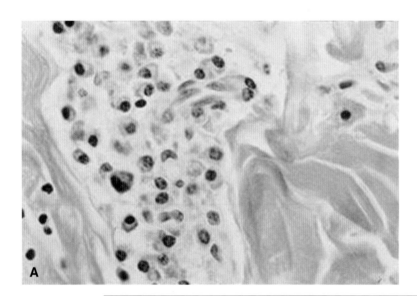

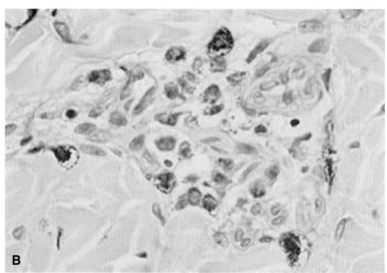

**Figure 1-21.** *A,* Histology of the dermis. Inflammatory cells, predominantly plasma cells, surround a small vessel in the dermis. A mast cell is present. Note that the nucleus of the mature mast cell is smaller and rounder than that of the plasma cell, and in the hematoxylin and eosin stain, the cytoplasmic granules of the mast cell are barely visible (magnification ×210). *B,* A perivascular dermal space, similar to that shown in *part A.* Giemsa stain reveals the mast cells by staining the granules intensely metachromatic (*purple*). There are at least five mast cells in this field, which is magnified ×210. (Courtesy of Dr. Ronald Jaffe, Children's Hospital of Pittsburgh.)

immune-system related, whereas the $MC_{TC}$ phenoptype appears to be nonimmune related, with function in angiogenesis and tissue remodeling rather than immunologic protection (Table 1-1).

## CELLULAR INTERACTION AND IMMUNE REGULATION

### CYTOKINES

Cytokines are low-molecular-weight proteins produced by a variety of cells that affect the behavior of other cells. Cytokines are involved in almost every aspect of immunity and inflammation, from innate acute phase responses to all components of acquired immunity. They usually act in an autocrine (on the cell that produced them), paracrine (on cells close by), or endocrine (distal cell) manner (Fig. 1-22). After binding to specific cell surface receptors at the cell membrane, cytokines initiate a cascade that leads to induction, enhancement, or inhibition of a number of cytokine-regulated genes and, ultimately, to altered cell behavior (Fig. 1-23). A detailed and complete description of cytokine signaling pathways is beyond the scope of this book.

Cytokines have a wide variety of names. ILs, IFNs, CSFs, TNFs, growth factors, chemokines, and many other proteins with the word *factor* in their name can all be considered cytokines. The cytokines and their receptors are divided into four groups based on their three-dimensional protein structure (Box 1-4).

The type I, or hematopoietic family, cytokines have a similar four-helix bundle motif, and each receptor has a single trans-

membrane segment with its N-terminus outside and C-terminus inside. The cytokine-receptor complexes of this family modulate a wide variety of immune inflammatory and hormonal responses. IL-4 is essential for Th2 lymphocyte differentiation and is an inducer of IgE production.[29] IL-5 promotes the production and

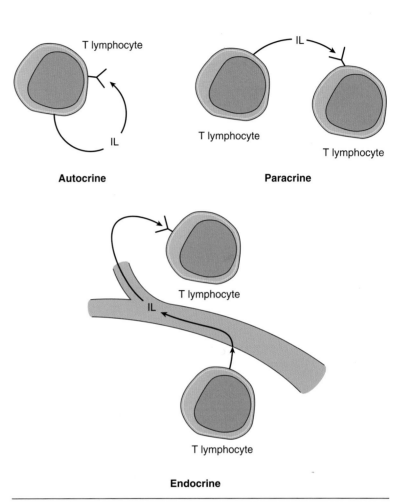

**Figure 1-22.** Model of actions of cytokines. Cytokines may function in an autocrine manner to act on the cell producing the cytokine. Alternatively, cytokines may act in a paracrine manner on the cells in the vicinity of the cell producing the cytokine. Finally, some cytokines are secreted in much higher concentrations and are designed to act on distal cells in a hormonal fashion. IL, interleukin. (Modified from Borish L, Rosenwasser LJ: Cytokines in allergic inflammation. In Adkinson NF Jr, Yunginger JW, Busse WW, et al (eds): Middleton's Allergy Principles and Practice, 6th ed. St. Louis Mosby, 2003, p 136.)

---

**TABLE 1-1**
**Characteristics of the Two Types of Mast Cells**

| $MC_T$ | $MC_{TC}$ |
| --- | --- |
| Immune system–associated MC | Non–immune system–associated MC |
| Proteases<br>Tryptase | Proteases<br>Tryptase<br>Chymase<br>Carboxypeptidase<br>Cathepsin G |
| Characteristics<br>Increased around sites of helper T-cell activation | Characteristics<br>Increased in fibrotic disease |
| Increased in allergic and parasitic diseases | Unchanged in allergic and parasitic diseases |
| Decreased in AIDS and chronic immunodeficiency diseases | Unchanged in AIDS and chronic immuno-deficiency diseases |

The characteristics of the two types of mast cell (MC). $MC_T$ cells appear to be immune system–related mast cells, whereas $MC_{TC}$ cells are non–immune system related. (Holgate ST, Church MK, Lichtenstein LM (eds): Allergy, 2nd ed. St. Louis, C.V. Mosby, 2001.)

---

**BOX 1-4**
**Cytokines**

Type 1 or hematopoietic family
Type 2 family
Tumor necrosis factor family (TNF)
Chemokines

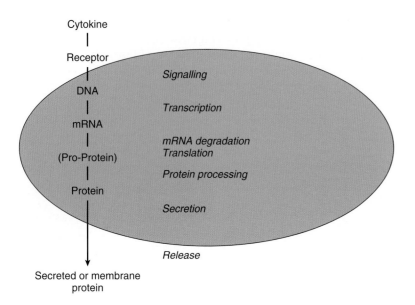

**Figure 1-23.** Mechanism of cytokine action on the cell. Shown are the main levels of regulation from the initial cytokine-receptor interaction to synthesis of the protein that changes the cell behavior. (Modified from Kelso A: Cytokines: Principles and prospects. Immunol Cell Biol 1998;76(4):300–317.)

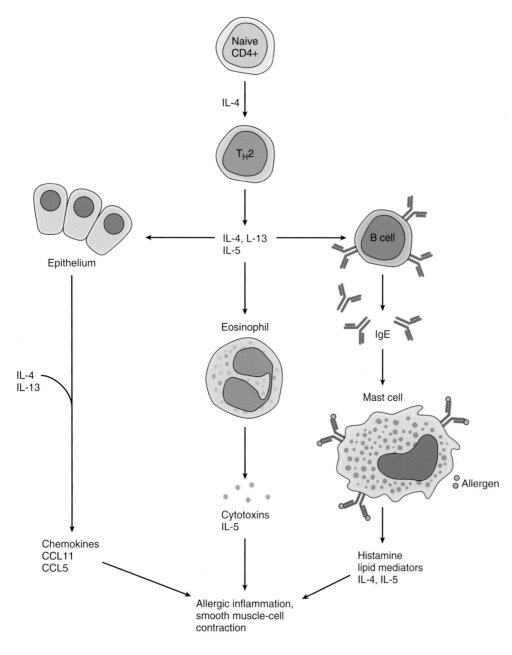

**Figure 1-24.** Immune pathways of allergic inflammation. Interleukin (IL)-4 is a key player in the pathogenesis of atopic disorders. IL-4 promotes T-helper 2 (TH2) cell development. Subsequently, TH2 cytokines promote allergic diseases by several mechanisms. IL-4 and IL-13 induce B-cell isotype switching and immunoglobulin E production and also induce the expression of chemokines by epithelial cells and other cell types. IL-5 promotes eosinophil production and the secretion of cytotoxins. TH2 cytokines also directly affect smooth muscle cells. Mast cells secrete inflammatory mediators after allergen encounters immunoglobulin E (IgE) bound on mast cell membrane. (Modified from Li-Weber M, Krammer PH: Regulation of IL-4 gene expression by T cells and therapeutic perspectives. Nature Rev Immunol 2003;3:534–543.)

survival of eosinophils. IL-4, IL-5, and IL-13 mediate allergic inflammation, including allergen-induced asthma, allergic rhinitis, and anaphylaxis (Fig. 1-24). IL-12 is produced by dendritic cells and phagocytes in response to microbes during infection. It stimulates the production of IFN-γ, stimulates innate immune response, and favors the differentiation of Th1 lymphocyte response.[30]

The type II family cytokines and their receptors are characterized by a common structure. Despite their structural similarities, the actions of class II cytokines are divergent. The best illustration of these different, and sometimes antagonistic, activities can be seen by comparing IL-10 and IFN-γ. IFN-γ is a major pro-inflammatory cytokine because of its ability to activate macrophages and endothelial cells. By contrast, IL-10 downregulates the production of inflammatory cytokines by macrophages. Therefore, a balance in the production of IFN-γ and IL-10 is required to maintain the homeostasis of inflammatory processes.[31] More recently, CD4 regulatory T-lymphocytes that produce high levels of IL-10 have been described and were indicated to have an essential role in tolerance to self-antigens and allergens. In addition, IFN-γ from Th1 cells promotes the development of cell-mediated immunity of the acquired immune system. Interferons are the oldest known cytokines, first described in 1957 by Isaacs and Lindenmann. IFN-α is preferentially expressed by cells of a lymphoid origin, and IFN-β is expressed virtually on all cells. They are crucial cytokines in orchestrating antiviral responses. An additional role of IFN-α is in therapy for cancers, because it suppresses cell growth. IFN-γ has anti-inflammatory activity that

has been shown in patients with multiple sclerosis, in which IFN-γ reduces the number of IFN-γ–secreting cells, as well as the frequency of relapses. Additionally, newly discovered IL-28A, IL-28B, and IL-29 were shown to have antiviral activity and are also known as IFNλ-2, IFNλ-1, and IFNλ-3.[31]

Another large group of cytokines and receptors belongs to the TNF family. At present, 19 different TNF cytokines have been identified. TNF cytokines are mostly transmembrane proteins. They act through 29 TNF receptors. After binding to the receptor, members of the TNF superfamily mediate apoptosis (programmed cell death), survival, differentiation, or proliferation. Research during the past two decades has shown that TNF and its superfamily members have both beneficial and harmful activities. Although TNF and its superfamily members are essential for hematopoiesis, protection from bacterial infection, immune surveillance, and tumor regression, their disregulation contributes to many diseases (Fig. 1-25). On the other hand, knowledge of TNF and its superfamily members and their mechanisms of action led to discovery of monoclonal antibody medications such as infliximab and etanercept, which are being used for treatment of Crohn's disease and rheumatoid arthritis, respectively.[32]

Chemokines are the largest mammalian cytokine family. They have distinct molecular structures and are unique among the cytokines in their chemotactic properties and ability to stimulate the migration and activation of cells, especially in inflammatory responses. Compared with many other cytokines, chemokines are relatively small (7 to 10 kDa) comprising 70 to 80 amino acids.

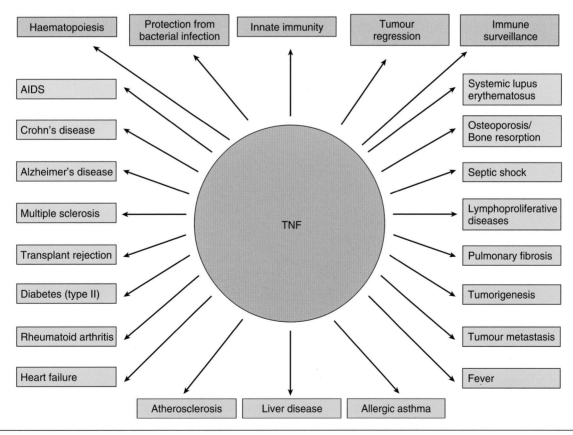

**Figure 1-25.** The main physiologic and pathologic effects linked to members of the tumor necrosis factor (TNF) family. Different studies indicate that although TNF and its family members are essential for hemotopoiesis, protection from bacterial infection, immune surveillance, and tumor regression (*green*); its dysregulation leads to various diseases (*blue*). (Modified from Aggarwal BB: Signalling pathways of the TNF superfamily: A double-edged sword. Nat Rev Immunol 2003;3:745–756.)

The chemokines can be subdivided into four classes: the C-C, C-X-C, C, and C-X3-C chemokines, depending on the location of the first two cysteines in their protein sequence. So far, 24 human C-C chemokines (CC1–CC28), 15 C-X-C chemokines (CXC1–CXC15), and one of each of CX3X and C chemokines subclasses have been identified.[33]

Chemokines regulate transport of inflammatory cells (dendritic cells, leukocytes, lymphocytes, NK cells) into tissues by mediating adhesion of cells to endothelial cells, initiation of transendothelial migration, and tissue invasion. For example, CC chemokines act through their receptors to recruit the leukocytes that mediate chronic inflammation, such as eosinophils and T cells in asthma and monocytes/macrophages and T cells in autoimmune diseases such as multiple sclerosis (Fig. 1-26). In addition to immune response, chemokines function as growth factors for certain tumors. (CXC8, also called IL-8, acts as a direct autocrine growth factor for malignant melanoma, liver, pancreatic, and colon tumors.) IL-8 was also shown to induce the activity of enzymes, such as matrix metalloproteinases, facilitating transmigration through basement membranes and leading to enhanced metastasis. Some other chemokines act as angiogenic factors, stimulating activation and proliferation of endothelial factors, which leads to tumor growth. Other studies indicate that certain chemokines,

such as CXC4 (platelet l factor 4), CXC9, and CXC10 can inhibit tumor growth by interfering with angiogenesis.[34] Manipulation of chemokines represents a new therapeutic tool in experimental immunotherapy of cancers and other diseases that involve the immune system.

## ACTIVATION OF MAST CELLS AND BASOPHILS

Mast cells and basophils share the ability to bind IgE antibodies to Fc epsilon RI, the high-affinity receptor for IgE. Antigen cross-linking of IgE induces degranulation and the release of preformed mediators and also induces the de novo synthesis and secretion of lipid mediators and cytokines (Fig. 1-27). The mast cells with high levels of Fc expression are able to secrete more cytokines and growth factors than cells with low expression. The Fc epsilon RI expression is regulated by levels of IgE. The mast cells and basophils in subjects with high levels of IgE (as in allergic patients) have an enhanced ability to secrete cytokines. The mast cells have been classically associated with early and late phases of acquired IgE-mediated allergic inflammation. In addition, they participate in innate immunity against bacterial infections, as well as acquired immunity against parasites, asthma remodeling, and chronic

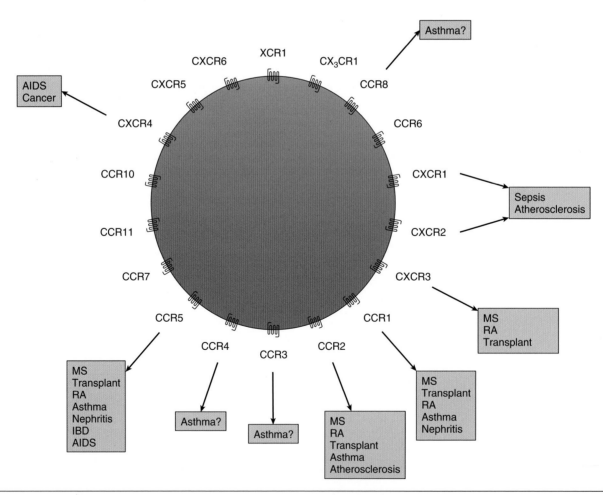

**Figure 1-26.** The chemokine receptors in pathological conditions. Chemokines and their receptors play a significant role in pathophysiology in many diseases. For example, CXCR4 is, along with CD4 receptor, one of the main receptors for HIV entry into CD4 cell. IBD, inflammatory bowel disease; MS, multiple sclerosis; RA, rheumatoid arthritis. (Modified from Proudfoot AEI: Chemokine receptors: Multifaceted therapeutic targets. Nat Rev Immunol 2002;2:106–115.)

allergic inflammation.[35] Therefore, these cells can also participate in non–IgE-mediated inflammation. The granules of mast cells contain mediators of inflammation, especially histamine, as well as enzymes such as tryptase. Other mediators, including prostaglandins and leukotrienes, are generated from the phospholipid membranes of these cells during inflammation (Fig. 1-28). These mediators promote the pathophysiologic changes responsible for many of the allergic patient's symptoms.

## T-LYMPHOCYTE ACTIVATION

To perform its functions, the naïve T cell needs to be activated. The lymphocyte activation occurs through two signals: Signal 1 occurs when a specific antigen is recognized by lymphocytes and is provided by the interaction of the peptide-antigen-MHC with the T-cell receptor. Signal 2 is delivered to T cells by co-stimulatory cell surface molecules expressed on antigen-presenting cells.

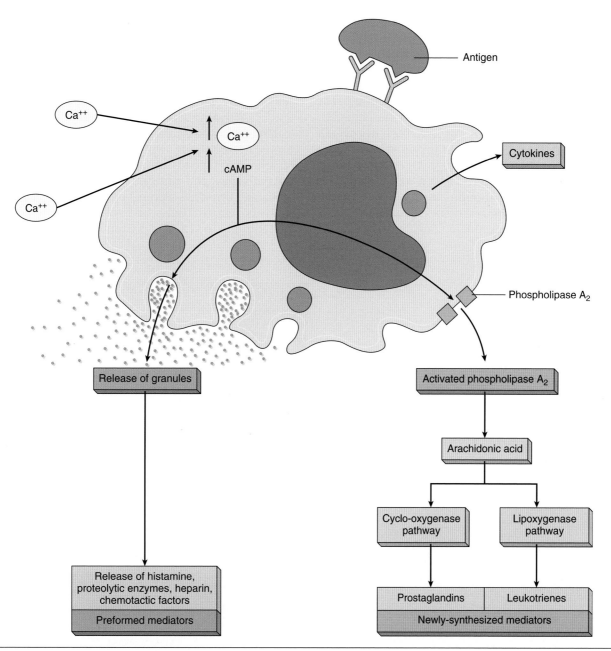

**Figure 1-27.** Mast cell activation. Immunologic triggers (antigen or immunoglobulin E [IgE]) perturb the mast cell membrane, causing a calcium ion ($Ca^{++}$) influx, which is essential to degranulation. Microtubule formation and movement of granules to the cell membrane lead to a fusion of the granules with the plasma membrane. In this way, the granule-associated mediators are released into the intercellular space. Plasma membrane activation allows phospholipase A2 to release arachidonic acid, which is then metabolized by either lipoxygenase or cyclo-oxygenase enzymes, depending on the mast cell type. The end products of these two distinct pathways include prostaglandins and thromboxane (cyclo-oxygenase pathway) and leukotrienes (lipoxygenase pathway). Cytokines including interleukin (IL)-1, 2, 3, 4, 5, 6, 8, 13, 16, granulocyte-macrophage colony-stimulating factor (GM-CSF), tumor necrosis factor (TNF)-α, and TNF-β are also synthesized after activation. cAMP, cyclic adenosine monophosphate. (Reproduced with permission from Roitt et al., 1995.)

Without co-stimulation, T cells will become anergic, that is, rendered unresponsive to antigenic stimulation. Of note, initial binding of dendritic cell to T cell is mediated by adhesion molecules (see "Neutrophils" section). For example, intercellular adhesion molecule 3 on a naïve T cell binds to a C-type lectin DC-SIGN on a dendritic cell.[36]

The B7-1/B7-2-CD28/CTLA-4 pathway is the best-characterized T-cell co-stimulatory pathway.[37] B7-1 and B7-2 molecules are located on antigen-presenting cells and provide important co-stimulatory signals to augment and sustain T-cell activation through an interaction with CD28. On the other hand, B7-1 and B7-2 molecules also engage CTLA-4 molecule present on T cells, which inhibits T-cell receptor– and CD28-mediated signaling (Fig. 1-29). Once a naïve T cell is activated, it expresses CD40 ligand, which binds CD40 on antigen-presenting cells. Binding of CD40 ligand to CD40 stimulates the antigen-presenting cells to express B7 molecules, thus augmenting T-cell proliferation. Additionally, new co-stimulatory pathways have been discovered (ICOS/ICOS ligand, PD-1/PD-1 ligand), and they may have more of a regulatory role in the immune response. Once the T cell is activated, it secretes IL-2 in autocrine fashion and upregulates the IL-2 receptor. IL-2 provides a stimulus for the T cell to start proliferating and migrating to peripheral tissues, where it exerts its effector functions. Once a T cell has differentiated into an effector cell, encounters with its specific antigen result in immune attack without the need for co-stimulation.[36]

In conclusion, the outcome of an immune response involves a balance between CD28-mediated T-cell activation and CTLA-4–mediated inhibition. The balance of stimulatory and inhibitory signals has pivotal importance in maximizing protective immune responses while maintaining immunologic tolerance and preventing autoimmunity.

## T-LYMPHOCYTE DIFFERENTIATION

Th1, Th2, and regulatory T-cell responses arise in a complex interplay between antigens and innate and adaptive immune responses. In case of infection, immature dendritic cells become activated by PAMPs through their pathogen-recognition receptors.[6,38] Activated dendritic cells present antigens to T-lymphocyte leading to activation and differentiation of T-lymphocyte. Whether naïve T-lymphocyte will become Th1, Th2, or regulatory T-lymphocyte depends on several factors: the type of PAMPs on the pathogens and pathogen-recognition receptors that recognize them, and cytokines secreted by inflammatory cells (dendritic cells, NK cells, macrophages, and so forth) (Fig. 1-30). For example, if IFN-γ and IL-12 are predominant cytokines (e.g., viral and

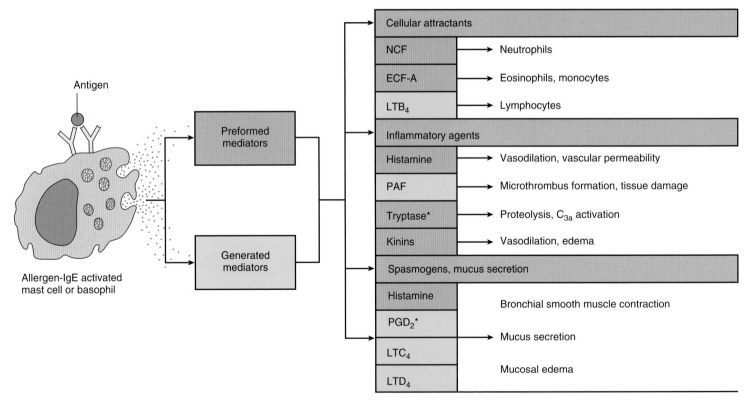

*Tryptase and PGD$_2$ produced mostly by mast cells

**Figure 1-28.** Pathophysiologic and inflammatory effects of mediators derived from mast cells and basophils. The preformed (granule-associated) mediators and those generated from the phospholipids cell membranes via the arachidonic acid cascade have multiple activities. The cellular attractants draw a variety of cells, including neutrophils, eosinophils, monocytes, and lymphocytes, to the site of allergic reaction. These mediators also promote inflammation by direct action on tissues, causing vasodilation, edema, smooth muscle contraction, and mucous secretion. ECF, eosinophil chemotactic factor; IgE, immunoglobulin E; LT, leukotriene; NCF, neutrophil chemotactic factor; PAF, platelet activation factor; PG, prostaglandin. (Adapted with permission from Roitt et al., 1995.)

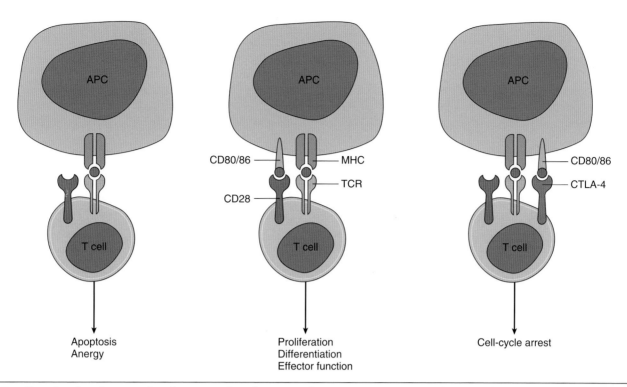

**Figure 1-29.** T-cell activation by co-stimulatory molecules. Simultaneous recognition of a specific major histocompatibility complex (MHC)–peptide complex by the T-cell receptor (TCR) and of CD80 or CD86 by the co-stimulatory receptor CD28 results in T-cell activation and cytokine production, proliferation, and differentiation. In the absence of CD28 ligation, T cells undergo apoptosis or become anergic. After T-cell activation and upregulation of cytotoxic T-lymphocyte antigen 4 (CTLA-4), co-ligation of the TCR and CTLA-4 results in cell-cycle arrest and termination of T-cell activation. APC, antigen-presenting cell. (Modified from Alegre ML, Frauwirth KA, Thompson CB: T-cell regulation by CD28 and CTLA-4. Nat Rev Immunol 2001;1:220–228.)

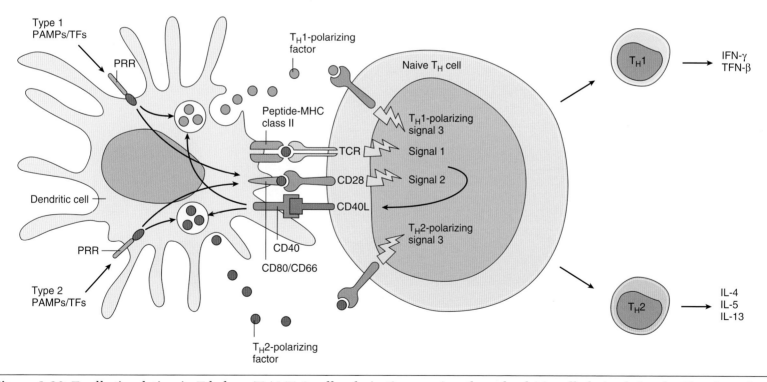

**Figure 1-30.** T-cell stimulation in T-helper (T$_H$)1/T$_H$2-cell polarization requires three dendritic cell–derived signals. Signal one is the antigen-specific signal that is mediated through T-cell receptor (TCR) triggering by major histocompatibility complex (MHC) class 2–associated peptides processed from pathogens after internalization through specialized pattern recognition receptors (PRRs). Signal two is the co-stimulatory signal, mainly mediated by triggering of CD28 by CD80 and CD86, which are expressed by dendritic cells after ligation of PRRs, such as Toll-like receptors that are specialized to sense infection through recognition of pathogen-associated molecular patterns (PAMPs) or inflammatory tissue factors (TFs). Signal three is the polarizing signal that is mediated by various soluble or membrane-bound factors such as interleukin (IL)-12 and IL-4 that promote the development of T$_H$1 or T$_H$2 cells, respectively. IFN-γ, interferon gamma; L, ligand; TNF-β, tumor necrosis factor beta. (Modified from Kapsenberg ML: Dendritic cell control of pathogen-driven T-cell polarization. Nat Rev Immunol 2003;3:984–993.)

bacterial infections) a Th1 response will ensue. A Th2 response develops if IL-4 is the predominant cytokine, as is the case with exposure to helminthes and certain allergens. IL-10 was traditionally part of Th2 response, although it is now thought that it regulates the expansion of regulatory T-lymphocytes.[16] Regulatory T-lymphocytes have been implicated as key cells that prevent allergic and autoimmune diseases. For example, the "Hygiene Theory" maintains that recurrent infections are protective in early childhood because they stimulate the development of regulatory T-lymphocytes that limit unwanted immune responses.[16] Thus, in the setting of infrequent infections and exposure to allergen, regulatory T-lymphocytes fail to develop, with subsequent uncontrolled activation of Th2 lymphocytes (Fig. 1-31) as well as consequences of allergic IgE-mediated inflammation.

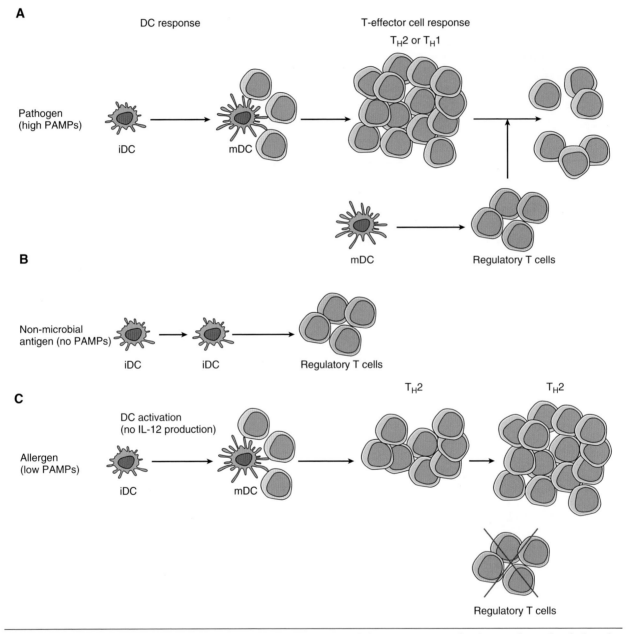

**Figure 1-31.** Types of immune responses. *A,* In the first model, strong, microbial signaling (high-level exposure to pathogen-associated molecular patterns [PAMPs]) leads to both effector CD4+ T-cell responses (helper T [T$_H$] 1 or T$_H$2) and induction of regulatory T cells. This is believed to be part of a natural homeostatic mechanism that regulates the level of immune responses. *B,* In the second model, exposure to antigen in the absence of PAMPs fails to generate effector T cells but leads to induction of regulatory T cells. In this case, the lack of dendritic cell (DC) activation has been implicated in regulatory T-cell generation. *C,* In the third model, in the setting of low or infrequent infections, allergens seem to generate effector T$_H$2 cells without induction of regulatory T cells. IDC, immature dendritic cell; IL, interleukin; mDC, mature dendritic cell. (Modified from Kapsenberg ML: Dendritic cell control of pathogen-driven T-cell polarization. Nat Rev Immunol 2003;3:984–993.)

# IMMUNOGLOBULINS AND ANTIBODIES

The lymphoid system and its cellular components are essential to the synthesis of the antibodies involved in the allergic reaction. After being processed by antigen-presenting cells and presented to the lymphoid system, the allergen's antigenic determinants activate the T-lymphocytes. These activated helper CD4 T-lymphocytes, via cell-to-cell interaction and the elaboration of cytokines, assist the bone marrow–derived B-lymphocytes in initiating antibody synthesis. The B-lymphocytes mature and differentiate into plasma cells that synthesize and secrete the specific immunoglobulin antibodies (Fig. 1-32). After sensitization, T- and B-lymphocytes continue to cooperate to upregulate and

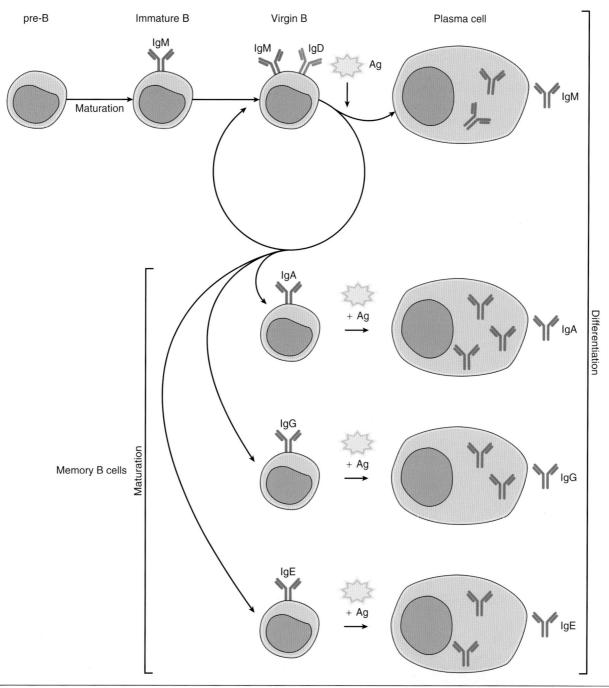

**Figure 1-32.** B-lymphocyte development with maturation and differentiation into plasma cells that secrete the specific immunoglobulins. Pre–B cells found in the bone marrow mature from an immunoglobulin (Ig) M expressing immature B cell into a mature B cell, which can be found in the peripheral blood and co-expresses IgM and IgD. These virgin B cells, on interaction with antigen (Ag), differentiate into IgM-producing plasma cells or further mature on antigen exposure into memory B cells that have undergone class switch to IgG, IgA, or IgE synthesis. (Modified from Holgate ST, Church MK, Lichtenstein LM (eds): Allergy, 2nd ed. St. Louis, C.V. Mosby, 2001.)

downregulate immunoglobulin synthesis.[39] Without this capacity to reduce antibody production, the normal patient would end up with excessive immunoglobulin levels, as can be seen in some proliferative diseases, such as multiple myeloma or Waldenström's macroglobulinemia.

## STRUCTURAL CHARACTERISTICS OF IMMUNOGLOBULINS

The immunoglobulins are a group of glycoproteins present in the serum and tissue. All humans, except those few patients who manifest an immunoglobulin deficiency syndrome (see Chapter 20) produce immunoglobulin molecules capable of antibody activity. The immunoglobulin molecule is constructed in a manner that serves its two primary antibody functions. One region of the molecule confers the capacity to recognize and bind to an enormous number of antigenic determinants from bacteria, viruses, fungi, plants, and animals. The normal human can synthesize approximately $10^7$ antibody molecules with different antigen-binding specificities. A different region of the molecule is involved in mediating the biologic effects of the antigen–antibody reactions through specific interaction with the host's proteins and inflammatory cells. Immunoglobulins exist in a membrane-bound form that serves as the B-lymphocyte antigen receptor and also in a secreted soluble form in the vascular and interstitial fluid, where they mediate the humoral antibody responses.

### Immunoglobulin Isotypes

Five distinct classes (isotypes) of immunoglobulins—IgG, IgA, IgM, IgD, and IgE—are recognized in most higher mammals. They differ from one another in size, charge, and chemical composition. Yet they share the basic four-chain polypeptide structure shown in Figure 1-33. The four polypeptides—two light and two heavy chains—are linked by disulfide bonds plus intermolecular forces. If treated with the enzyme papain, the molecule cleaves into three fragments: two identical Fab fragments, consisting of the amino terminal ends of the heavy chains with light chains attached, and one Fc fragment, consistent of the carboxy terminal ends of the heavy chains. The designation *Fab* refers to the antigen-binding fragments of the immunoglobulin antibody, which are uniquely adapted to combine with one and only one antigenic or closely similar determinant. The variable regions of the heavy ($V_H$) and light ($V_L$) chains show marked variation in amino acid sequence and composition in different antibody molecules. These amino acid sequences determine the specificity of the antigen-binding sites of the Fab fragment. The Fc fragment of the molecule contains the site that determines the deposition of antigens that bind the Fab portion of the molecule. The Fc fragment bears the site for interaction with the complement system components and for binding to various cells, including neutrophils, monocytes, and macrophages.[40]

### Heavy and Light Chains

The five immunoglobulin isotypes—IgG, IgA, IgM, IgD, and IgE—differ from one another in the structure of their respective heavy (H) chains, which are designated by the corresponding Greek letters γ, α, μ, δ, and ε, respectively. There are two types of light (L) chains, designated λ and κ. Of IgG molecules, 65% have two κL chains and two γH chains, and 35% have two λL chains and two γH chains. A similar distribution is found for IgA and IgM molecules.

The differences among the various immunoglobulins are shown in Figure 1-33. IgG and IgE are present in the serum as monomeric structures with molecular weights of 150,000 and 180,000, respectively, while serum IgM is a pentamer with a molecular weight of 900,000. IgA is present in the serum but also is the predominant secretory immunoglobulin in the nasal, salivary, bronchial, optic, and intestinal exocrine secretions. The secretory IgA exists as a dimeric form in which two IgA monomers are joined together by another protein synthesized in the epithelial cells and called the secretory, or transport, piece. IgA is normally present in the serum as either a monomer or a polymer. IgE has also been detected in secretions, but secretory IgE, unlike secretory IgA, appears to be physiochemically similar to serum IgE and does not contain a secretory piece. IgG comprises four subclasses designated as subtypes 1, 2, 3, and 4 (Table 1-2). IgA has two subtypes, whereas IgM, IgD, and IgE have one subtype. The properties of these different subclasses are determined by differences in the L chains.

Genetic markers have been discovered on the class-specific H and L chains of the immunoglobulins, permitting classification of individuals according to these differences.[41] For IgG, these markers are called Gm allotypes, and almost 30 have been identified. It has been shown that injection of IgG of one Gm allotype results in the formation of antibodies against the injected IgG. Antibody

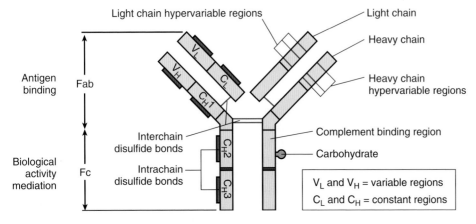

**Figure 1-33.** Structural characteristics of the immunoglobulins. All immunoglobulins manifest a basic chain polypeptide structure with two light (L) chains and two heavy (H) chains linked by disulfide bonds. Enzymatic treatment with papain produces three peptides: two identical Fab fragments, which contain the L chains and the posterior portions of the H chains, and a single Fc fragment, which contains the carboxyl terminal ends of the H chains.

molecules can be distinguished by antigenic determinants expressed on the variable regions of the molecule. These determinants are referred to as idiotopes, and a set of idiotopes are referred to as idiotypes. Because the number of variable regions an individual expresses is large, many more idiotypes exist than allotypes or isotypes. Clinical studies suggest a role for autologous anti-idiotypic antibodies in several autoimmune disorders.

## Immunoglobulin Concentrations (Normal and Abnormal Levels)

Immunoglobulin G accounts for most of the immunoglobulins found in normal human serum (70% to 80%). There are smaller amounts of IgA (10% to 15%) and IgM (5% to 10%) and minute amounts of IgE (<1%) and IgD (<0.1%) (Fig. 1-34). The immunoglobulins have differences in electrophoretic mobility, but these differences are not clinically useful in specifically quantifying the serum levels of each isotype. IgE levels are best measured in serum by sensitive radioimmunoassay or enzyme-linked immunosorbent assay procedures; the nephelometry or agar precipitation techniques, such as those used for the measurement of IgG, IgA, and IgM, are not sufficiently sensitive.

The normal adult serum level for IgG is 10 mg/mL. For IgA, it is 2.0 mg/mL; for IgM, it is 1.5 mg/mL; and for IgE, it is 0.0002 mg/mL. The serum concentration of each immunoglobulin is determined by its synthetic and catabolic rate. The normal biologic half-life of IgG is 23 days, which is the longest of the five immunoglobulins. IgE has the shortest half-life (i.e., 2.3 days). IgG, IgA, and IgE are distributed almost equally between the intravascular and extravascular compartments, whereas IgM and IgD are found primarily in the intravascular compartment.

Statistically higher mean serum IgE concentrations are present in patients with allergic diseases, such as asthma and allergic rhinitis, but not all patients with allergic disease have elevated serum IgE (Fig. 1-35). Marked elevation of serum IgE may be seen in patients with atopic dermatitis, bronchopulmonary aspergillosis, and helminthic parasitic infections. Higher mean serum IgG concentrations are found in many patients with rheumatoid disease

or other chronic illnesses that manifest inflammation. Low serum levels of the several immunoglobulins are found in patients with various immunodeficiency diseases (see Chapter 20).

## Immunoglobulins and Fetal Development

B-lymphocytes with cell membrane receptors for IgM, IgE, IgA, IgG, and IgD are demonstrable in the fetus between the 10th and 12th weeks of gestation and may reach adult levels by the end of the second trimester. However, synthesis of the corresponding quantities of serum immunoglobulins does not generally begin until after birth, unless the fetus is infected or antigens gain access to fetal tissues. In these cases, serum immunoglobulins (usually IgM and IgA) may be synthesized in appreciable amounts prior to birth.

Unlike maternal IgG, maternal IgE, IgM, and IgA do not traverse the placenta. Consequently, the mother who is allergic cannot passively sensitize her fetus; the fetus is, in a sense,

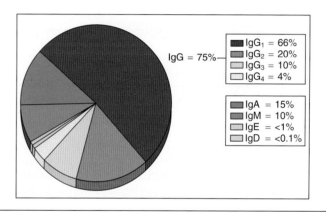

**Figure 1-34.** The relative adult concentrations of the various serum immunoglobulins (Igs). Serum IgG accounts for 75% of the serum immunoglobulins, whereas IgE accounts for less than 1% of normal adult serum levels. Of the IgG subclasses, subclass 1 comprises 66% of the total IgG concentration.

**TABLE 1-2**
**Structural and Metabolic Properties of Immunoglobulins**

| | Immunoglobulins | | | | | | | | |
| | IgG Subclasses | | | | | | | | |
| | IgG$_1$ | IgG$_2$ | IgG$_3$ | IgG$_4$ | IgM | IgA$_1$** | IgA$_2$** | sIgA* | IgE |
|---|---|---|---|---|---|---|---|---|---|
| Heavy chain | $\gamma_1$ | $\gamma_2$ | $\gamma_3$ | $\gamma_4$ | $\mu$ | $\alpha_1$ | $\alpha_2$ | $\alpha_1, \alpha_2$ | $\varepsilon$ |
| Adult mean serum level (mg/ml) | 6 | 3 | 1 | 0.5 | 1.5 | 3.0 | 0.5 | 0.05 | $5 \times 10^{-5}$ |
| Molecular weight | $1.5 \times 10^5$ | $1.5 \times 10^5$ | $1.7 \times 10^5$ | $1.5 \times 10^5$ | $1 \times 10^6$ | $1.6 \times 10^5$ | $1.6 \times 10^5$ | $3.8 \times 10^5$ | $1.9 \times 10^5$ |
| Placental transfer | + | + | + | + | − | − | − | − | − |
| Complement fixation | ++ | + | +++ | − | +++ | − | − | − | − |
| In secretions | − | − | − | − | − | − | − | ++ | + |

*Secretory IgA; **IgA subclasses.

protected from the mother's allergic antibodies. Thus, with the exception of IgG, which comes from the mother, the infant is deficient in the other immunoglobulins at birth. As maternal IgG is catabolized, the infant's total serum IgG decreases from birth until 3 to 6 months of age, when synthesis of the child's own IgG increases. Endogenous IgG, along with IgM, IgA, and IgE, gradually increases during the first year of life, but adult concentrations are not reached until 3 to 6 years of age. Serum IgE increases above adult levels before and during adolescence, stabilizes during the middle years, and gradually decreases in old age.

## FUNCTIONAL ASPECTS OF IMMUNOGLOBULINS

### Biologic Activity of the Isotypes

The function of the humoral immune system is to make harmful foreign substances and microbes harmless to the host. The humoral immune system must also differentiate self-antigens from foreign antigens and be able to recognize a large variety of antigenic determinants. As mentioned earlier, antibody activity has been demonstrated in all the immunoglobulin isotypes except IgD (Table 1-3). There are differences in biologic activity among antibodies developed in the different immunoglobulin isotypes. These differences reside in the variable portion of the heavy chains that are unique for each immunoglobulin. Serum IgG, serum IgM, and secretory IgA are capable of viral neutralization, but serum IgE and IgA are not. Toxin neturalization is carried out by serum IgG but not serum IgM or IgE. Bactericidal activity against Gram-negative organisms is carried out for the most part by IgM, with minor involvement of IgG. IgG subtype 1 contains most of the IgG antibodies to protein antigens, such as tetanus toxin; IgG subtype 2 contains antibodies to the capsular polysaccharide antigens of *Streptococcus pneumoniae* and *Haemophilus influenzae*. IgG subtypes 3 and 4 antibodies are ill defined. However, foreign antigens are primarily inactivated through the additional interaction of host proteins and cells with antigen-specific antibody. Activation of complement, neutrophils, monocytes, platelets, and lymphocytes is the major mechanism through which specific antibody can clear foreign antigens. Interaction of allergen with IgE on mast cells or basophils is the central event of immediate-type hypersensitivity.

The usual evolution of an antibody immune response involves the initial production of specific IgM followed by a switch to specific IgG (or IgA or IgE). Cytokines regulate class switching primarily through the induction or suppression of germline transcriptions, along with T-cell and B-cell collaboration through CD40

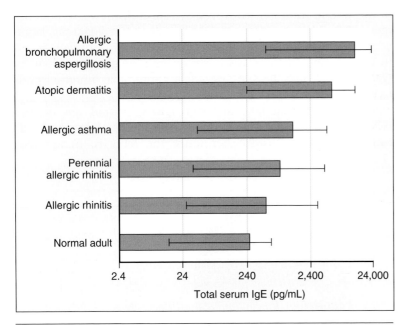

**Figure 1-35.** Serum immunoglobulin E (IgE) levels (expressed in pg/mL) are increased in approximately 33% of adult patients with either seasonal or perennial allergic rhinitis and in about 66% of adult patients with allergic asthma. Though mean serum IgE concentrations of both groups are statistically higher than normal, one third of patients with allergic asthma and two thirds of those with allergic rhinitis have normal IgE levels. Approximately 90% of atopic dermatitis patients and 99% of allergic bronchopulmonary aspergillosis patients have elevated serum IgE levels.

**TABLE 1-3**
**Antibody Activities of the Immunoglobulins**

| | Immunoglobulins | | | | | | | |
| | IgG Subclasses | | | | | | | |
| | IgG$_1$ | IgG$_2$ | IgG$_3$ | IgG$_4$ | IgM | IgA | sIgA* | IgE |
|---|---|---|---|---|---|---|---|---|
| Antibody activity | + | + | + | + | + | + | + | + |
| Viral neutralization | + | + | + | ± | + | − | + | − |
| Toxin neutralization | + | ? | ? | ? | − | ? | ? | − |
| Bactericidal activity (Gram-negative) | − | − | − | − | + | − | − | − |
| Antibody to polysaccharide antigen | ± | ++ | − | − | − | − | − | − |
| Wheal-and-flare reactivity | − | − | − | ± | − | − | − | ++ |

*Secretory IgA.

signaling.[42] Normal B-cell isotype switching requires two signals: (1) an activation signal provided through CD40 binding on B-cell surface with the CD40 ligand on T-cells and (2) regulatory signal provided by cytokines. The cytokines IL-4 and IL-13 can direct switching to IgE, and IFN-γ inhibits switching to IgE.[43] TGF-β directs switching to IgA. Sequential switching can also take place from IgM to IgG to IgE from all of the IgG subclasses. Patients with hyper–IgM immunodeficiency lack expression of CD40 ligand and are unable to accomplish normal isotype switching from IgM to IgG (see Chapter 20).

One of the identifying characteristics of the sensitized allergic individual is the presence, in the serum and tissues, of an antibody that is capable of eliciting a wheal-and-flare reaction within 20 minutes of a cutaneous allergen challenge. Initially, the synthesis of skin-sensitizing antibody, primarily but not exclusively IgE, was thought to be a phenomenon limited to individuals with a so-called atopic constitution. However, it is now accepted that production of IgE can be induced in virtually all humans by an appropriate allergen stimulation or immunization. In addition to IgE production, a variety of immune responses occur in allergic patients after natural exposure to or intentional immunization with a given allergen. These responses include the development of sensitized T-lymphocytes responsible for cell-mediated immune responses and the production of a spectrum of antibodies that may be associated with the IgG, IgA, IgM, and IgE immunoglobulins.

Although IgE antibodies have been shown to be synthesized in response to a variety of antigens, including parasites, bacteria, and other infectious agents, they generally have no neutralizing, bactericidal, or opsonizing activities. The antibody activities of secretory IgE appear to be similar to those of IgE in serum or in tissues. In contrast, secretory IgA shows antiviral capacities, whereas serum IgA does not.

## Antigen Binding

Antigen binding occurs via the B-cell antigen receptor. The B-cell antigen receptor is composed of a molecular complex containing membrane immunoglobulin and a disulfide-linked heterodimer (Fig. 1-36). Antigen binding to membrane immunoglobulin results in the cross-linking of antigen receptors and activation of tyrosine kinases of the src, syk, or Jak family. As shown in Figure 1-36, activation of tyrosine kinases leads ultimately to transcriptional activation of the B cell. Genetic defects in tyrosine kinases can result in altered B-cell development and immunodeficiency syndrome (see Chapter 20).

An IgG antibody is divalent, and an antigen molecule binds to two molecules of IgG via the Fab portion of the antibody molecules. IgE and IgA are also divalent, and IgM may have as many as 10 antigen-binding sites. The Fc peptide of IgE reacts with high-affinity receptors on the membranes of mast cells and peripheral and blood basophils and represents the means by which IgE is able to bind to tissue sites. Fc fragments can block the passive sensitization of skin by IgE antibodies in the Prausnitz-Kustner test. If the Fc fragment of IgE is treated with mercaptoethanol, which disrupts disulfide bonds, it loses its ability to attach to the mast cell or basophil receptors.

## Immunoglobulin–Mast Cell Interactions

Although there is a relatively low concentration of IgE in the serum, IgE has an extremely high affinity for the mast cells and

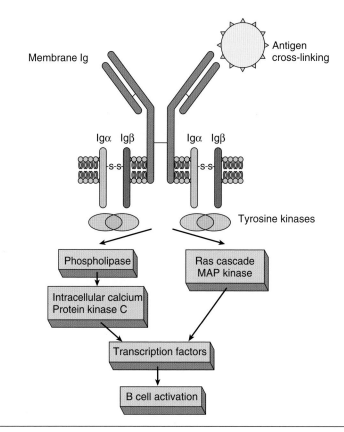

**Figure 1-36.** Diagram of the B-cell antigen receptor which consists of membrane immunoglobulin (Ig) in association with Igα disulfide–linked Igβ heterodimers. Antigen cross-linking of the B-cell antigen receptor results in activation of tyrosine kinases followed by several intermediary enzymatic sequences. These lead to induction of transcription factors and B-cell activation.

blood basophils.[43] The IgE affinity for basophils was calculated at $10^9$ per mole, as compared with $10^5$ per mole for IgG. Although cutaneous sensitization with IgE antibody may persist for weeks, the half-life of IgE in circulation is only 2.3 days, as compared with 3 to 4 weeks for IgG.

Generally, there are between 10,000 and 30,000 IgE molecules on the surface of a blood basophil, and full saturation may indicate that there are as many as 100,000 IgE receptor sites on that cell. The affinity of IgE for the mast cells or basophils appears to be the same in allergic and nonallergic individuals. Owing to an increased IgE synthesis, the basophil or mast cell receptors of allergic individuals are likely to be more highly saturated than those in normal subjects. Thus, normal individuals have more unoccupied IgE receptors on their tissue mast cells or basophils.

# COMPLEMENT

Normal serum contains a series of proteins—the complement components—which interact with each other in a cascade-like sequence so as to mediate a variety of host immune responses of both the innate and adaptive immune reactions. These proteins are synthesized in large part by the liver. This system of proteins, many of which are enzymes, nonspecifically implements the innate immune system. In addition, several peptides generated during the complement cascade have multiple effects in activating inflammation and cellular phenomena that play roles in both host defense and collagen-vascular rheumatic disorders (Fig. 1-37).

Proteins of the complement system form three interrelated enzyme cascades, termed the *classical*, the *mannose binding (lectin)*, and the *alternative* pathways, which provide three routes to the cleavage of C3, the central player in the complement system (Fig. 1-38). Each enzyme precursor is activated by the previous complement component or complex, which often has proteinase activity.[44,45] This converts the enzyme precursor into its catalytically active form. During this limited proteolysis, a peptide fragment is cleaved and a membrane-binding site is exposed, resulting in initiation of the next complement sequence. Because each enzyme can amplify several enzyme precursors, the system can amplify this cascade of events.

## COMPLEMENT PROTEINS

The classical complement components are numbered C1 to C9, but the sequence of their activation does not follow the numeric order (see Fig. 1-38). Rather, they interact in the following sequence: C1, C4, C2, C3, C5, C6, C7, C8, and C9. The C1 complex is composed of C1q, C1r, and C1s. There is one proteinase inhibitor in the classical pathway, which is specific to C1, a serine proteinase. This C1 inhibitor is discussed later, in the context of protein deficiency in hereditary angioedema (see Chapter 18). The alternative pathway involves several additional serum proteins, factors B, D, and H and properdin. The alternate pathway bypasses activation of C1, C4, and C2. The mannose-binding (lectin) pathway also bypasses activation of C1, C4, and C2. The mannose-binding

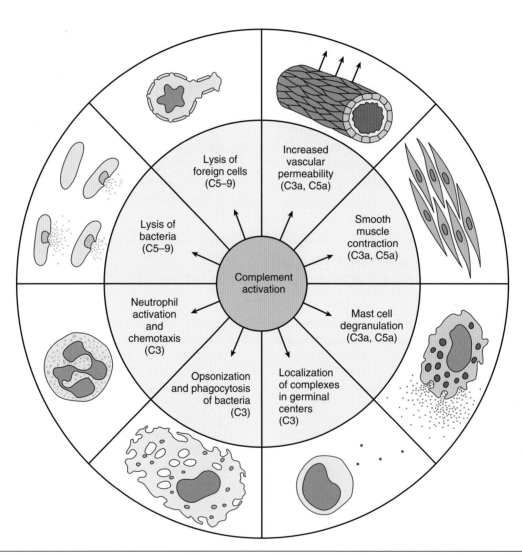

**Figure 1-37.** The multiple effects of complement activation. Complement components participate in various aspects of inflammation. After the complement reaction is initiated, the generation of C3a and C5a increases vascular permeability, causing smooth muscle contraction and mast cell degranulation. C3 facilitates the action of immune complexes and the opsonization and phagocytosis of bacteria. C3 and C5 activate neutrophils, attracting them by chemotaxis to phagocytize the opsonized bacteria. Components C5 to C9 bind to cell membranes, resulting in lysis of bacteria, red blood cells, or foreign cells. (Adapted with permission from Roitt et al., 1995.)

pathway is amplified by two proteins, the mannose-binding–associated proteins (MASP1 and MASP2). A primary or secondary deficiency of complement components is an important consideration in evaluating patients with undue susceptibility to infection (see Chapter 20) and rheumatologic diseases (see Chapter 19).

## COMPLEMENT ACTIVATION

IgG and IgM, but not IgA and IgE, have the capacity to activate the classic complement sequence. Because complement activation is important for bacterial phagocytosis or lysis, IgG and IgM play a major role in adaptive immunity to infectious diseases. The recognition unit of the complement system is the C1 complex, and the process begins when the C1q component binds to immunoglobulin. Only certain IgG subclasses (IgG1 and IgG2), as well as IgM, can fix C1. When C1q, C1r, and C1s interact, C1 esterase is generated. The C1s splits the peptide C4a, leaving C4b, which reacts with C2b to form the enzyme C14b,2b. This enzyme splits the C3 anaphylatoxin (C3a) from C3. The remainder, C3b, acts on C5 to form C5a. The C5b becomes fixed to a cell membrane, and this is followed by the sequential interaction of C6, C7, C8, and C9 to form the C5b,6,7,8 complex, which disrupts the cell membrane and causes cytolysis. The alternate pathway and the mannose-binding (lectin) pathway bypass C1, C4, and C2 and directly activate C3 and initiate the complement cascade. The alternate and mannose-binding (lectin) pathways are important aspects of innate immunity.

## BIOLOGIC EFFECTS OF C3a AND C5a

Anaphylatoxins C3a and C5a can mimic the IgE-mediated reaction. It is important for the allergist and clinical immunologist to appreciate that complement activation can provoke what appears to be an IgE-mediated syndrome. For example, C3a causes smooth muscle contraction (i.e., bronchospasm) and reacts with mast cells to cause the release of histamine and other mediators. It also enhances vascular permeability, with resultant urticaria or angioedema. C5a is 10 to 20 times more active than C3a, with wider biologic activity. However, it may be present in lower concentrations. It also causes smooth muscle contraction and mast cell degranulation and increases vascular permeability. C5a is a major chemotactic factor for neutrophils, and it also initiates the bactericidal activity of these cells. C5a switches on neutrophil production of leukotriene B4. The alternate pathway can also be initiated in the absence of antibody–antigen interaction. What's more, this pathway results in the activation of C3a, which binds to factor B. In the presence of properdin, the alternative pathway is potentiated and prolonged. Activated C3 and C5 also are important in clearance of immune complexes, which along with the other complement-generated biologic activities, are important in the pathogenesis of rheumatologic diseases.

# IMMUNOGENETIC ASPECTS OF ALLERGIC (ATOPIC) REACTIONS

The familial nature of allergic diseases has been recognized for years, and a positive family history of atopic disease has been reported in approximately 75% of allergic patients. Though the tendency for developing allergic disease is clearly familial, the specific clinical allergic reaction is not directly inherited, since the host response is dependent on the appropriate environmental exposure. If there is no exposure to the allergen, there is no allergic disease, regardless of familial predisposition. Family studies comparing the allergic high-IgE phenotype to the nonallergic low-IgE phenotype suggest a recessive inheritance for high-IgE levels. However, studies of IgE levels in monozygotic and dizygotic twins were not conclusive. Although a major portion of the variation in IgE levels is genetic, other environmental factors are likely to be involved.

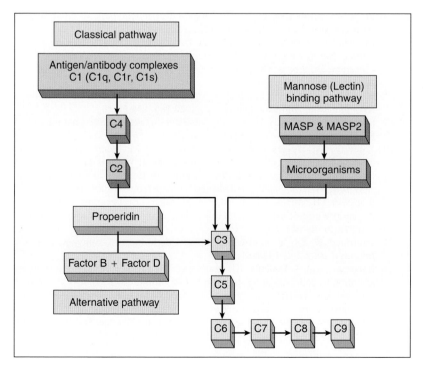

**Figure 1-38.** Activation of the three complement pathways. Activation of the classical pathway is initiated when the antigen–antibody complexes act on the C1 complex. The activated Cqrs acts on C4, which activates C2. This, in turn, cleaves C3. The mannose-binding (lectin) pathway is amplified by two factors (MASP and MASP2), whose enzymatic activity amplifies the relationship to bacteria by which direct cleavage of C3 attacks the microbe's cell membrane. The alternative pathway, usually initiated by nonimmune factors, including properidin, involves direct cleavage of C3, bypassing C1, C4, and C2. Thereafter, C3 activation of C5 initiates the next sequence—C5 acting on C6, C7, C8, and C9 to form the C5–C9 membrane attack complex.

Investigations of inbred animals suggested that specific antibody synthesis to a well-characterized antigen is controlled, in part, by immune response (Ir) genes linked to the major tissue histocompatibility locus antigen (HLA). Analogous Ir genes linked to HLA have been described in humans. Ragweed hay fever symptoms and a positive skin test for the purified ragweed antigen E correlated highly with a particular HLA haplotype in successive generations of allergic families. The observed haplotype varied from family to family, suggesting that the Ir genes for this response were linked to (not associated with) HLA. The responses to complex multiple allergens, such as those used in clinical practice, may be dominated by the general level of IgE production rather than by the presence of specific HLA-linked Ir genes. Recently, a dominant autosomal trait was uncovered in allergic families, through use of restrictive enzymes, and the IgE immune response gene has been linked to chromosome 11. However, these results were not universal in other populations, and other studies suggest the gene is located on chromosome 5. In the past 10 years, there have been other linkage and association studies examining genetic susceptibility to allergic disease. A multifactorial mode of inheritance also has been proposed, and many investigators feel that several loci are involved in the expression of allergic disease; interaction with environmental exposures is also important.[46]

Parents often become concerned with the risk of having allergic children if one or both of them have allergic problems or if they already have an affected child. Retrospective family studies suggest that when both parents are affected, allergic disease is present in about 60% of the offspring, and when only one parent is affected, about 30% of the children are allergic (Fig. 1-39). When environmental exposure is probably the same for siblings in a given family, the risk of developing allergic disease is probably the same for each pregnancy, unless the family initiates preventive tactics to reduce antigen exposure. Many clinicians suggest breast-feeding during the first year of life to reduce the possibility of cow's milk allergy. It remains to be proven that avoidance of inhalant allergens during infancy reduces the incidence of respiratory allergy.

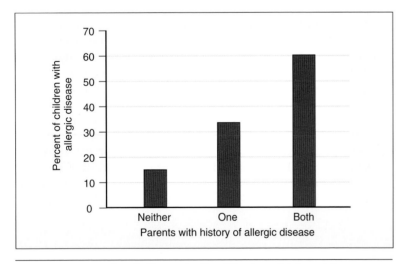

**Figure 1-39.** Risk of allergy in families in which neither, one, or both of the parents have a history of allergic disease. The greater the parental history of allergic disease, the greater the risk of atopy in the offspring.

# CONCLUSIONS

The advances in immunology of the past several decades have enhanced our understanding of allergic and immunologic diseases. Immunology has provided the clinician with a rational mechanism for many of the accepted diagnostic and therapeutic measures. It is anticipated that immunology will be the basis for new and better understanding of diagnosis and therapy of these diseases in the future. Subsequent chapters of this book further define and describe the major allergic and clinical immunologic diseases and the immunologic mechanisms underlying them.

# REFERENCES

1. vonPirquet C: Allergie. Munch Med Woch 1906;53:1457.
2. Gell PGH, Coombs RRA (eds): Clinical Aspects of Immunology. Philadelphia, F.A. Davis, 1963.
3. Coca AF, Cooke RA: On the classification of the phenomenon of hypersensitiveness. J Immunol 1923;8:163.
4. Ishizaka K: Cellular events in the IgE antibody response. Adv Immunol 1976; 23:1–75.
5. Medzhitov R, Janeway CA Jr: Innate immunity: The virtues of a nonclonal system of recognition. Cell 1997;91:295–298.
6. Hemmi H, Takeuchi O, Kawai T, et al: A toll-like receptor recognizes bacterial DNA. Nature 2000;408(6813):740–745.
7. Chaplin DD: Overview of the immune response. J Allergy Clin Immunol 2003;111(2):S442–S459.
8. Sell S: Immunopathology. In Rich RR, Fleisher TA, Schwartz BD, et al (eds): Clinical Immunology: Principles and Practice. St. Louis, Mosby, 1996, pp 449–477.
9. Schwartz LB: Mast cells and basophils. Clin Allergy Immunol 2002;16:3–42.
10. Bochner BS, Schleimer RP: Mast cells, basophils and eosinophils: Distinct but overlapping pathways for recruitment. Immunol Rev 2001;179:5–15.
11. Frank MM, Fries LF: The role of complement in inflammation and phagocytosis. Immunol Today 1991;12(9):322–326.
12. Danning CL, Illei GG, Boumpas DT: Vasculitis associated with primary rheumatologic diseases. Curr Opin Rheumatol 1998;19(1):58–65.
13. Janeway CA, Trevers P, Walport M, Shlomchik M: Antigen recognition by T-cells. In Janeway C, Trevers P, Walport M, Shlomchik M (eds): Immunobiology: The Immune System in Health And Disease, 5th ed. New York, Garland Science Publishing/Taylor & Francis, 2001, pp 105–121.
14. Murphy KM, Reiner SL: The lineage decisions of helper T-cells. Nat Rev Immunol 2002;2(12):933–944.
15. Bouma G, Strober W: The immunological and genetic basis of inflammatory bowel disease. Nat Rev Immunol 2003;3(7):521–533.
16. Herrick CA, Bottomly K: To respond or not to respond: T-cells in allergic asthma. Nat Rev Immunol 2003;3(5):405–412.
17. Bluestone JA, Abbas AK: Natural versus adaptive regulatory T-cells. Nat Rev Immunol 2003;3(3):253–257.
18. Honjo T, Kinoshita K, Muramatsu M: Molecular mechanism of class switch recombination. Ann Rev Immunol 2002;20:165–196.
19. Colucci F, Caligiuri MA, DiSanto JP: What does it take to make a natural killer? Nat Rev Immunol 2003;3(5):413–425.
20. Janeway CA, Trevers P, Walport M, Shlomchik M: Macrophage activation by armed CD4 Th1 cells. In Janeway C, Trevers P, Walport M, Shlomchik M (eds): Immunobiology: The Immune System in Health and Disease, 5th ed. New York, Garland Science Publishing/Taylor & Francis, 2001, pp 333–338.
21. Stockwin LH, McGonagle D, Martin IG, Blair EG: Dendritic cells: Immunological sentinels with a central role in health and disease. Immunol Cell Biol 2000;78(2):91–102.
22. Shortman K, Liu Y: Mouse and human dendritic cell subtypes. Nat Rev Immunol 2002;2(3):151–161.
23. Haberman AM, Shlomchik MJ: Reassessing the function of immune-complex retention by follicular dendritic cells. Nat Rev Immunol 2003;3(9):757–764.
24. Janeway CA, Trevers P, Walport M, Shlomchik M: Induced innate responses to infection. In Janeway C, Trevers P, Walport M, Shlomchik M (eds): Immunobiology: The Immune System in Health and Disease, 5th ed. New York, Garland Science Publishing/Taylor & Francis, 2001, pp 69–87.

25. Kita H, Adolphson CR, Gleich GJ: Biology of eosinophils. In Middleton E, Adkinson NF Jr, Yunginger JW, et al (eds): Allergy: Principles and Practice, 6th ed. St. Louis, C.V. Mosby, 2003.

26. Schroeder JT, Lichtenstein LM: Biology of basophils. In Middleton E, Adkinson NF Jr, Yunginger JW, et al (eds): Allergy: Principles and Practice, 6th ed. St. Louis, C.V. Mosby, 2003.

27. Ryan JJ, Huff TF: Biology of mast cells. In Middleton E, Adkinson NF Jr, Yunginger JW, et al (eds): Allergy: Principles and Practice, 6th ed. St. Louis, C.V. Mosby, 2003.

28. Metcalfe DD, Baram D, Mekori YA: Mast cells. Physiol Rev 2002;77:1033–1079.

29. Li-Weber M, Krammer PH: Regulation of IL4 gene expression by T-cells and therapeutic perspectives. Nat Rev Immunol 2003;3(7):534–543.

30. Trinchieri G: Interleukin-12 and the regulation of innate resistance and adaptive immunity. Nat Rev Immunol 2003;3(2):133–156.

31. Renauld JC: Class II cytokine receptors and their ligands: Key antiviral and inflammatory modulators. Nat Rev Immunol 2003;3(8):667–676.

32. Aggarwal BB: Signalling pathways of the TNF superfamily: A double-edged sword. Nat Rev Immunol 2003;3(9):745–756.

33. Proudfoot AEI: Chemokine receptors: Multifaceted therapeutic targets. Nat Rev Immunol 2002;2(2):106–115.

34. Homey B, Miller A, Zlotnik A: Chemokines: Agents for the immunotherapy of cancer? Nat Rev Immunol 2002;2(3):175–184.

35. McLachlan JB, Hart JP, Pizzo SV, et al: Mast cell-derived tumor necrosis factor induces hypertrophy of draining lymph nodes during infection. Nat Immunol 2003;4(12):1199–1205.

36. Janeway CA, Trevers P, Walport M, Schlomchik M: The production of armed effector T cells. In Janeway CA, Trevers P, Walport M, Schlomchik M (eds): Immunobiology: The Immune System in Health and Disease, 5th ed. New York, Garland Science Publishing/Taylor & Francis, 2001, pp 297–319.

37. Sharpe AH, Freeman GJ: The B7-CD28 superfamily. Nat Rev Immunol 2002;2(2):116–126.

38. Kapsenberg ML: Dendritic-cell control of pathogen-driven T-cell polarization. Nat Rev Immunol 2003;3(12):984–993.

39. Hawke NA, Yoder JA, Litman GW: Expanding our understanding of immunoglobulin, T-cell antigen receptor, and novel immune-type receptor genes: A subset of the immunoglobulin gene superfamily. Immunogenetics 1999;50:124–133.

40. Flesch BK, Neppert J: Functions of the Fc receptors for immunoglobulin G. J Clin Lab Anal 2000;14:141–156.

41. Pallares N, Lefebre S, Contet V, et al: The human immunoglobulin heavy diversity (IGHD) and joining (IGHJ) segments. Exp Clin Immunogenet 1999;16(3):173–184.

42. Lorenz M, Jung S, Radbruch A: Switch transcripts in immunoglobulin class switching. Science 1995;267:1825–1828.

43. Kinet JP: The high affinity IgE receptor (Fc epsilon RI): From physiology to pathology. Annu Rev Immunol 1999;17:931–972.

44. Walport MJ: Complement, Part I. N Engl J Med 2001;344:1058–1066.

45. Walport MJ: Complement, Part II. N Engl J Med 2001;344:1140–1144.

46. Holloway JW, Cakebread JA, Holgate ST: Genetics of allergic disease and asthma. In Middleton E, Leung DYM (eds): Pediatric Allergy: Principles and Practice, 5th ed. St. Louis, C.V. Mosby, 2003, pp 23–38.

*Philip Fireman*

# *2* Allergens

Allergens are those antigens responsible for clinical allergic diseases. They are usually proteins or glycoproteins capable of inducing synthesis of immunoglobulin (Ig) E antibodies, thereby sensitizing the potentially allergic person. Upon reexposure to the same allergen, the previously sensitized patient manifests the signs and symptoms of allergy, as the allergen reacts with cell-related IgE tissue antibody, and the cells generate the mediators of inflammation. It is imperative that the clinician links the circumstances of allergic disease to allergen exposure, as allergens represent important etiologic factors in the pathogenesis of allergy.

As shown in Box 2-1, allergens can be classified on the basis of the nature or manner in which the patient is exposed. Those allergens responsible for allergic respiratory diseases, including allergic asthma and allergic rhinitis, are principally inhalants. These aeroallergens, which can be present outdoors or indoors, are responsible for the majority of all allergic diseases. Foods and other ingestants, including drugs, are also important, especially for allergic gastrointestinal and skin diseases. The contactants are principally responsible for allergic contact dermatitis. In addition to drugs, the injectant group includes the venom and saliva of insects. This chapter is limited to a discussion of the inhalant allergens, as the other allergens are described in the separate chapters on food allergy, drug allergy, contact dermatitis, and anaphylaxis.

The inhalant allergens can be grouped as outlined in Box 2-2. Pollens were the earliest known causes of allergic respiratory diseases, being identified as such in the 19th century. They remain the most commonly recognized today. The spores of fungi, often referred to as molds by clinicians, are especially important when airborne in those environments in which the humidity supports their growth. Animal products, both mammalian and arthropod, have been increasingly recognized during the 20th century as being causative factors in allergic diseases, as have other organic and inorganic dusts to which sufferers are exposed in the home and workplace. Algae are relatively uncommon inhalant allergens.

## ALLERGEN DETECTION

The detection and quantification of aero-allergens have provided the clinician with the basis for understanding the etiology of allergic respiratory illnesses.[1] The methods of aeroallergen detection and measurement are listed in Table 2-1. An environmental survey based on the history given by the patient or visual inspection of the environment provides valuable information regarding potential aeroallergen sources and can provide clues as to the source of the allergen. Direct microscopic examination is the most widely employed means of detecting and counting pollen and fungal spores.[2] The quantification of pollens has been traditionally performed by collecting the pollen grains onto greased microscope slides using the Durham gravity system.

Only during the past two to three decades have impact samplers (Rotorod) and suction samplers (Burkard, Kramer-Collins

---

**BOX 2-1**

**Classification of Allergens According to the Route Through Which They Enter the Body**

Inhalants
   Outdoor
   Indoor
Ingestants
Contactants
Injectants

---

**BOX 2-2**

**Classification of Inhalant Allergens**

Pollens
Fungi (molds)
Animal products
   Mammalian
   Arthropod
Dusts
Algae

and Andersen) been used, providing truly quantitative ways of measuring these allergens (Table 2-2). As described later, the pollen grains have unique microscopic characteristics that are identifiable, making them countable when stained and examined under a microscope. Airborne pollen grains range in size from 5 to 60 μm. They are principally deposited in the upper airway and, because of their relative size, cannot reach the bronchi. Recently, immunochemical techniques have been developed that can identify the soluble allergen constituents of ragweed pollen, as well as other allergens such as dust mites. Using aerodynamic air samplers, ragweed allergenic particulates smaller than the intact ragweed pollen have been identified, not only during the ragweed pollen seasons, but before and after as well.[3] Such observations indicate that these smaller ragweed allergen particles, which cannot be identified microscopically, could penetrate both the upper respiratory tract and the bronchi and bronchioles. These types of studies have become very important in finding other amorphous airborne allergens that cannot be identified using microscopy. Propagation

of viable micro-organisms in culture media can be used depending on the material under study and the type of data desired.

# ALLERGEN NOMENCLATURE

Utilizing molecular biologic technology, many of the clinically important inhalant allergens have been isolated and sequenced and their structure defined.[4] The Allergen Nomenclature Committee of the International Union of Immunological Societies (IUIS) has devised a unified nomenclature system for purified allergens.[5] Allergens are phenotypically designated by the first three letters of the genus followed by a space, the first letter of the species, another space, and finally, an Arabic number; occasionally an additional letter must be added to either the genus or the species designation. Allergens are genotypically designated with italics; for example, the two genes encoding the two polypeptide chains of the major house cat (*Felis domesticus*) allergen *Fel d 1* are

---

**TABLE 2-1**
**Aeroallergen Detection and Measurement**

| Methods | Application |
|---|---|
| Visual inspection or retrospective | Clinical environment survey (no sampling device) |
| Microscopic analysis | Identification and enumeration of pollen grains and fungal spores |
| Immunoassay | Specific allergen detection and measurement |
| Propagation (culture) | Identification of viable micro-organisms |

---

**TABLE 2-2**
**Quantitative Measurement of Allergens**

| Apparatus | Description | Advantages | Disadvantages |
|---|---|---|---|
| Durham sampler | Passive deposition of airborne particles on adhesive-coated microscope slide | Simple, low cost, durability | Cannot provide volumetric data |
| Rotorod sampler | Rotating impactor: Captures particles onto adhesive-coated rods | Provides volumetric data; unaffected by wind speed | Misses episodic showers of airborne particulates |
| Burkard trap | Suction sampler: Deposits particles onto slowly moving tape | Efficient; provides volumetric data; no particle overloading | Expensive |
| Kramer-Collins trap | Suction sampler: Deposits particles onto rotating drum | Efficient; provides volumetric data; moderate cost; wind oriented | Misses episodic showers of airborne particulates |
| Andersen sampler | Suction sampler: Deposits viable particles onto culture plates | Efficient; identifies fungal spores hard to identify visually | Expensive |

designated *Fel d 1A* and *Fel d 1B*. A complete and updated Internet-based listing of purified allergens is maintained by the IUIS.[6]

# POLLENS

Pollens are the viable male germinal cells that are essential for the reproduction of most seed plants. The sources of pollens include trees, grasses, and weeds (Box 2-3). Because pollen production is related to the life cycle of a given plant, the pollens usually have a seasonal or cyclic occurrence in the atmosphere. Because of this seasonal variation in atmospheric pollen, the patient who develops pollen allergy manifests a seasonal symptomatology, such as seasonal allergic rhinitis. In some tropical and subtropical regions of the world, however, climatic conditions show little annual variation, and pollen prevalence may be perennial with a resultant perennial allergic rhinitis. Guidelines for the characterization of those pollens that can become potent allergens were initially postulated by Thommen in 1931 (Box 2-4). In general, pollens that are wind-borne (anemophilous) are of greater clinical relevance than those carried by insects (entomophilous). Thus, the pollens of attractive, brightly colored flowering plants are infrequently the cause of allergic diseases. These insect-borne pollens tend to be heavy, sticky, and less numerous. For example, the pollens of roses and goldenrod are often incorrectly incriminated as important inhalant allergens, since their flowers bloom in temperate climates at the height of the grass pollen and ragweed pollen seasons, respectively. However, florists, landscapers, hobbyists, and others whose occupational or recreational pursuits increase their exposure do become sensitized to the pollens of flowering plants.

The buoyancy, relative size, and density of a pollen can contribute to its dispersion. Ragweed pollen has a long wind-borne range and has been detected many miles offshore of lakes and oceans. Certain plants are widely distributed and produce large amounts of pollen—a single ragweed plant may release a million pollen grains in one day. Trees, especially conifers such as pine, may release clouds of pollen (Fig. 2-1), but these are generally less allergenic than ragweed.

Typically, the onset of pollination for many pollens is predictable to within a margin of a week or less, a characteristic that is important for clinical diagnosis. However, global warming and recent El Niño events may change patterns of pollination. The seasonal patterns for the presence of airborne individual pollens are discussed later; clinicians should know the most prevalent pollen allergens in their area of the world, as well as their seasonal occurrence.[7-9] The worldwide distributions of many of the common pollens are shown in Figures 2-2, 2-3, and 2-4.

Even though the seasonal appearance of the pollen is predictable, the amount produced in a given season varies, depending on climatic conditions. Extended dry periods during plant development and growth reduce the eventual pollen production. Also, a rainy day during the pollen season reduces the amount of airborne pollen on that day, whereas a dry, windy day increases the airborne concentration.

In addition to allergen exposure, the allergenicity of the pollen is another important factor. It is not known what accounts for certain pollens being more potent-sensitizing allergens than others. As discussed in other chapters, only a subset (10% to 20%) of the population become sensitized and show allergic symptoms, even though the entire community is exposed to the allergens.

# WEEDS

Weeds are commonly defined as those annual plants that grow wildly and have little decorative or agricultural value (Table 2-3). The pollens of weeds are common causes of seasonal allergic rhinitis. The worldwide distributions of the weed pollens are shown in Figures 2-2, 2-3, and 2-4, respectively. The most notorious in North America is ragweed and is most prevalent in the midwestern and northeastern areas of North America, where it is widespread. The most prevalent allergenic ragweeds are the short (*Ambrosia artemisiifolia*) and giant ragweeds (*Ambrosia trifida*); the latter can reach a stately 12 feet (3.7 m) in height (Fig. 2-5), and the former, shown in Figure 2-6, is now found across all of

---

**BOX 2-3**
## The Three Main Sources of Allergenic Pollens

Trees
Grasses
Weeds

---

**BOX 2-4**
## Factors That Contribute to the Allergenicity of Pollens

Wind borne (anemophilous)
Buoyant (of small particle size)
Produced in large quantity
Potent antigen

---

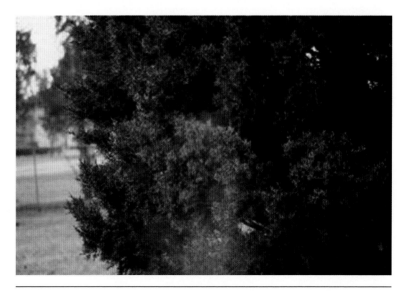

**Figure 2-1.** Cloud of pollen released from a juniper tree.

North America. Its pollen is released in temperate areas as the days become shorter, with peak pollen counts in the northeastern and midwestern areas of the United States from mid-August to mid-September. In the southern and southwestern states, ragweed pollen (see Fig. 2-7) can be airborne throughout the spring, summer, and fall. Although ragweed was ecologically native to North America, it has spread as an alien species to other parts of the world, especially Europe and Japan, probably due to international travel.

Botanically, ragweed is a member of the same *Asteraclae* composite family as many flowering plants, including chrysanthemums, marigolds, asters, some daisies, and sunflowers. These others, however, are only bothersome to those such as florists or gardeners who handle them regularly. Pyrethrum is an insecticide made form the flower heads of certain chrysanthemums, and inhalation of this compound can provoke symptoms in ragweed-allergic patients. The major allergens of ragweed have been isolated and characterized as *Amb a I* (antigen E) and *Amb a II* (antigen K).

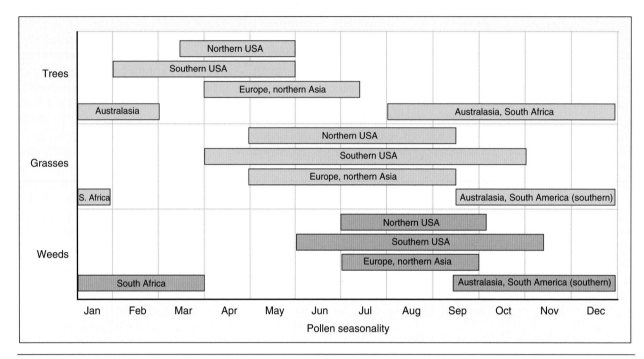

**Figure 2-2.** Pollen seasons in the Northern Hemisphere (United States, Europe, and Northern Asia) and Southern Hemisphere (Australasia, South Africa, southern South America). (Adapted from Sicherer SH, Eggelston PA: Environmental allergens. In Liebermann P, Anderson J (eds): Allergic Diseases: Diagnosis and Treatment. Totowa, New Jersey, Humana Press, 2000.)

**TABLE 2-3**
**Selected Common Allergenic Weeds**

| Family | Genus/Species | Common Name |
|---|---|---|
| Asteraceae | Ambrosia trifida | Giant ragweed |
| | Ambrosia artemisiifalia | Short ragweed |
| | Ambrosia trifida | Sagabrush |
| | Ambrosia vulgaris | Mugwort |
| | Xanthium strumarium | Cocklebur |
| | Kochia scoparia | Burning bush |
| Amaranthaceae | Amaranthors retroflyus | Pigweed |
| (Chenopodideae) | Chenopidium album | Lamb's quarter |
| | Salsola kali | Russian thistle |
| Plantaginaceae | Plantago lanceoleta | English plantain |
| Polygonaceae | Rumex acetabella | Red sorrel |
| Urticaceae | Urtica dioica | Neetle |

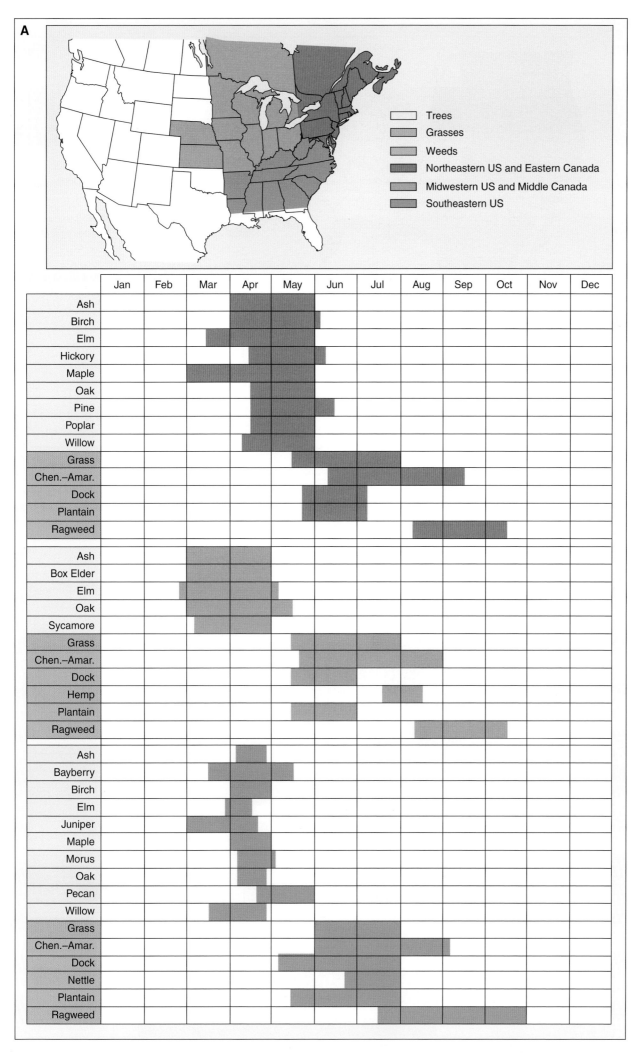

**Figure 2-3.** Geographic distribution of common allergenic pollens in the various regions of North America over the course of 1 year.

*Continued*

**Figure 2-3—cont'd**

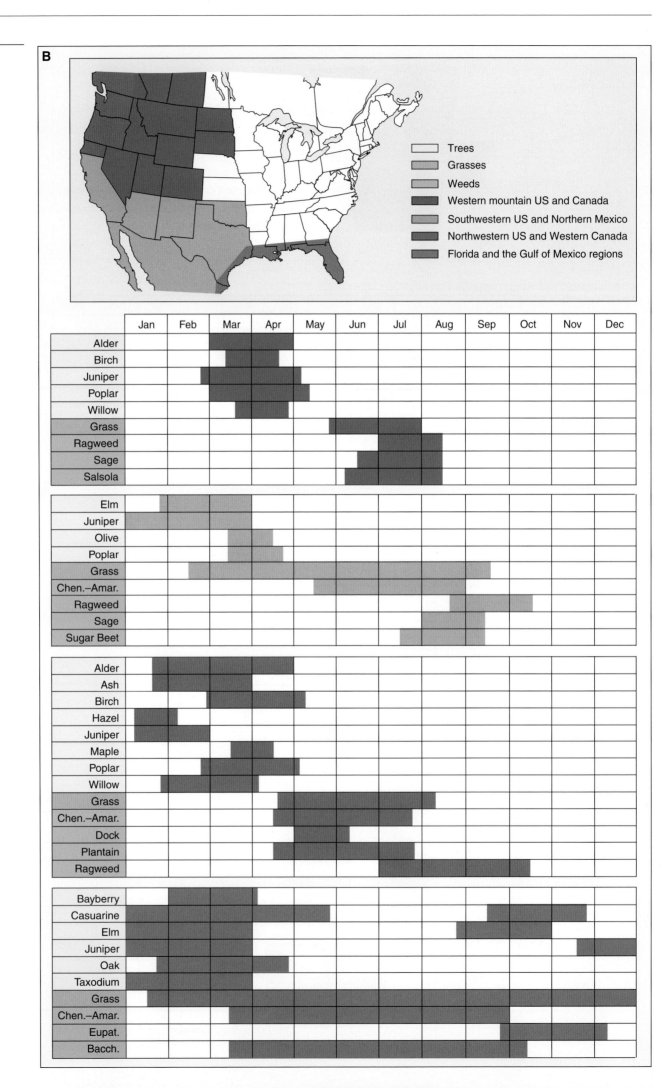

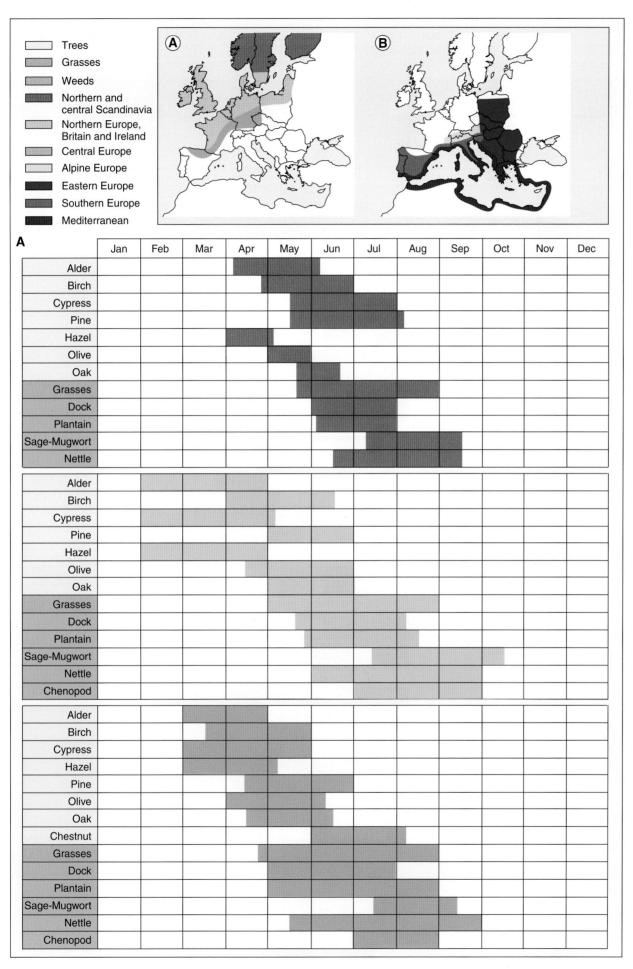

**Figure 2-4.** Seasonal pollen distribution in Europe.

*Continued*

**Figure 2-4.—cont'd**

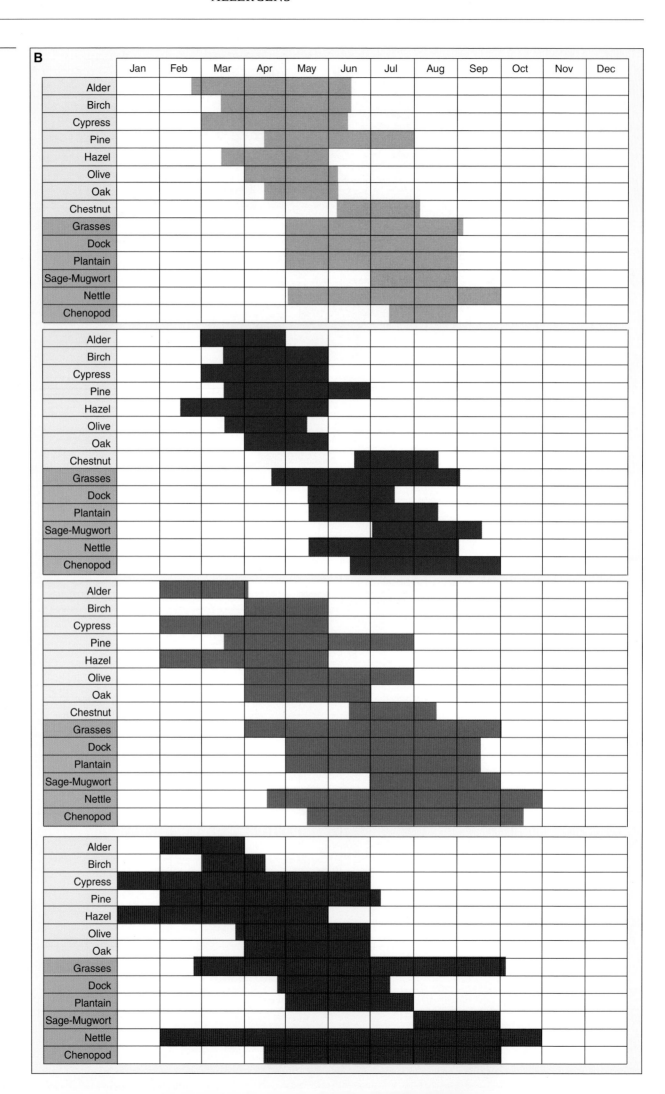

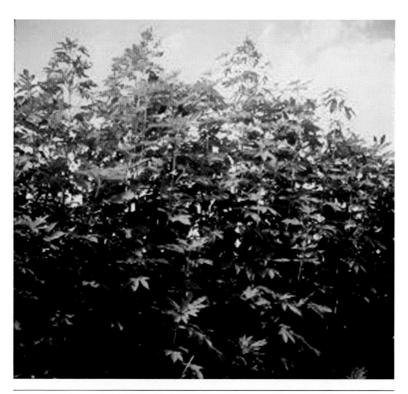

**Figure 2-5.** Giant ragweed (*Ambrosia trifida*). One of the two common forms of ragweed in North America, this plant can reach heights of up to 12 ft (3.7 m).

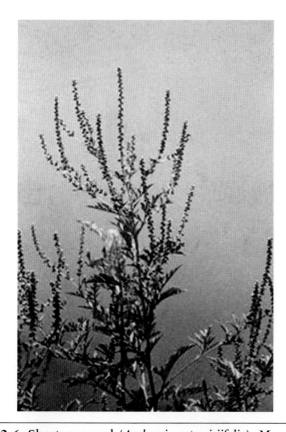

**Figure 2-6.** Short ragweed (*Ambrosia artemisiifolia*). More widespread than giant ragweed, this plant is now found in much of North America, as well as other parts of the world, proliferating in more temperate climates. The pollen may be airborne throughout the year in some regions; peak counts generally occur during August and September in the temperate Northern Hemisphere.

Commercial extracts of ragweed pollen used in clinical allergy testing and immunotherapy are now required by the U.S. Food and Drug Administration (FDA) to be standardized to *Amb a 1* content.[10]

Depending on geographic locale, other weeds can be important allergens as well. English plantain (Fig. 2-8) can provoke significant allergic rhinitis, which can be confused with grass pollen allergy because English plantain (ribgrass) pollinates in May, June, and July—the same season during which grasses pollinate in the United States and the Canadian northeast and midwest. Sagebush (Fig. 2-9) is found in the southwestern United States and northern Mexico and is related to ragweed, with which it sometimes cross-reacts. Prevalent also in this region are the pollens of Russian thistle and burning bush (Fig. 2-10). Other cross-reactive allergenic weeds include lamb's quarter and pigweed (Fig. 2-11), whose pollens are microscopically similar and therefore grouped together by the family name, chenopod-amaranth, a combination of two families that have pollens that look alike and cross-react strongly.

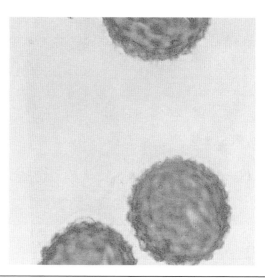

**Figure 2-7.** Ragweed pollen grains. Oil emersion photomicrograph, 450×. (Courtesy of Greer Laboratories.)

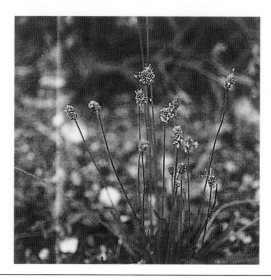

**Figure 2-8.** English plantain. This plant pollinates during the same season as the grasses. It can trigger allergic rhinitis in some individuals, which may be confused with an allergic response to grass pollens.

Except for ragweed, the most common weeds throughout the world are similar to those found in North America. These include nettle, plantain, dock, sage, mugwort, lamb's quarter, and pigweed. Depending on the climate and the local geography, the pollination of weeds frequently coincides with that of grasses in many temperate areas of the world.

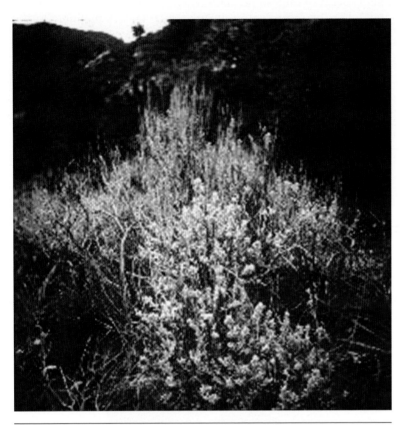

**Figure 2-9.** Sagebrush. This is another of the common allergenic plants in the western regions of North America. (Courtesy of Greer Laboratories.)

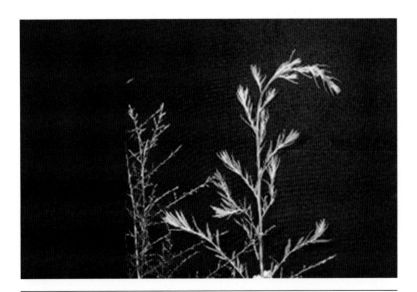

**Figure 2-10.** Burning bush, also known as Mexican fireweed (*left, foreground*), and Russian thistle. These are common, often cross-reactive allergenic plants in the prairie and western North America.

# GRASSES

In Europe, South America, Asia, and Africa grasses are the most important causes of pollen allergy; grasses also provoke significant allergic disease in North America (Table 2-4). Allergic rhinitis was described initially in England in 1889 by Blackley as *hay fever* because of the association of nasal symptoms with the harvesting of the forage grass, timothy, which is used to make hay (Fig. 2-12). Most of the grasses are cultivated either agriculturally or ornamentally and are prevalent where people live. The considerable production of pollen by these widespread plants contributes to the frequency of symptoms associated with grasses. The pollens of the different grasses vary in size from 20 to 40 μm, and they all have a single germinal pore, which makes them difficult to distinguish microscopically (see Fig. 2-12*C*).

Only about a dozen of the more than 5000 species of grass are important allergens, as many of the grasses do not produce abundant pollen. The bulk of the airborne grass pollen in the

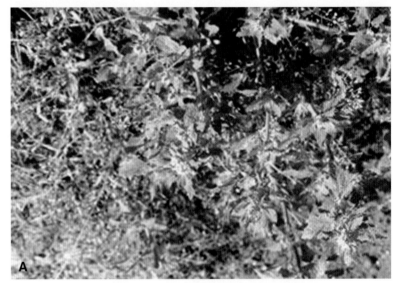

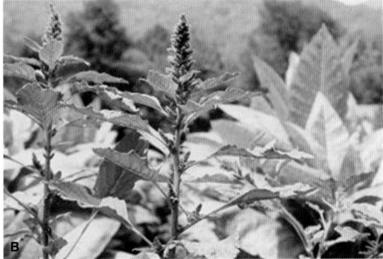

**Figure 2-11.** Lamb's quarter (*Chenopodium album; A*) and pigweed (*Amaranthus retroflexus; B*). The microscopic similarity between the pollen grains of these two plants has led to their classification under a combined family name of chenopod-amaranth.

**TABLE 2-4**
Selected Allergenic Grasses (Family *Poaceeae*)

| Sub-Family | Genus/Species | Common Name |
|---|---|---|
| Pooideae | Phleum pretense | Timothy grass |
| | Dactylis glomerata | Orchard grass |
| | Festica pratensis | Meadow fescue |
| | Lilium perenne | Rye grass, perennial |
| | Poa protensis | Kentucky bluegrass |
| | Agrostis gigantean | Redtop |
| | Anthoxanthum odoratum | Sweet vernal grass |
| Cloridorideae | Cynadon dactylin | Bermuda grass |
| Panicoideae | Paspalum notatum | Bahia grass |
| | Sorgham halepense | Johnson grass |

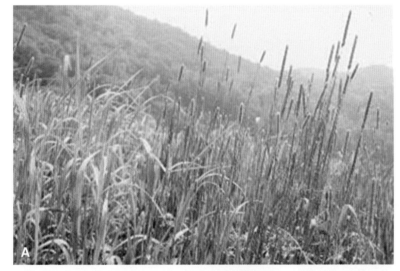

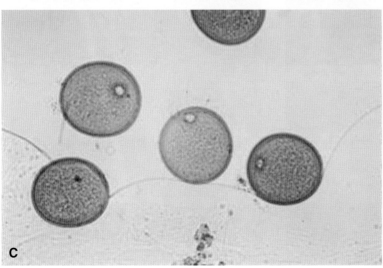

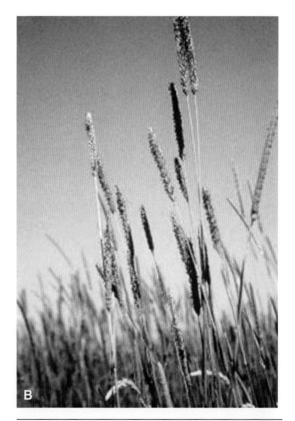

**Figure 2-12.** *A,* Timothy grass as it appears in the field. *B,* Closer view showing detail of the timothy grass plant, which is widely cultivated as hay. (Courtesy of Hollister-Stier Laboratories.) *C,* Timothy grass pollen. Oil emersion photomicrograph, 450×. (Courtesy of Greer Laboratories.)

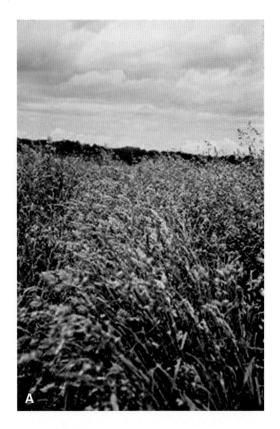

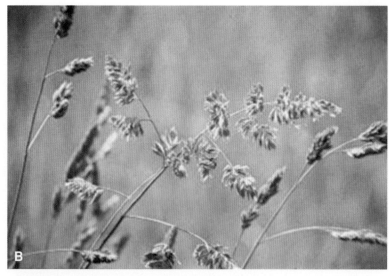

**Figure 2-13.** Orchard grass *(A)* in the field and *(B)* close up. The allergenic pollen of this grass reaches peak levels in the early summer. (Courtesy Hollister-Stier Laboratories.)

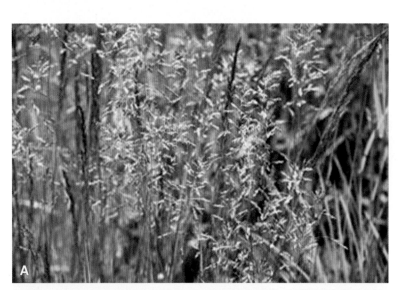

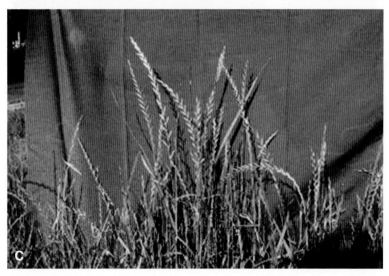

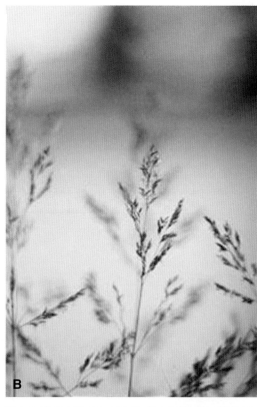

**Figure 2-14.** Bluegrass *(A)*, Redtop grass *(B)*, and perennial ryegrass *(C)*. Though allergenically distinct, these three grasses show considerable cross-reactivity. (*A* and *B,* courtesy of Greer Laboratories.)

Northern Hemisphere, United States, Canada, Europe, and northern Asia is present in the late spring and early summer—from May to July. Whereas in the Southern Hemisphere, including Australia, South America, southern Asia, and South Africa, the seasons are reversed (see Figs. 2-2, 2-3, and 2-4). The important early grasses include sweet, vernal, and orchard (Fig. 2-13), which are followed by timothy, bluegrass, fescue, redtop, and perennial ryegrass (Figs. 2-14*A* and *C*). All of these grasses show considerable allergen cross-reactivity, but they are allergenically distinct from the southern grasses. In the subtropical and tropical areas of the world, including the southern United States, Bermuda grass is found nearly all year round, and Johnson and salt grasses also have long seasons (Figs. 2-15*A* and *C*). In southern Europe and the Mediterranean areas, grasses may pollinate from February to October.

# TREES

Tree pollens are prevalent worldwide, but because of a shorter pollen season in most countries, they do not produce as much allergic disease as do the grasses and weeds (Table 2-5). The fruit-bearing trees, such as apple, pear, and peach, are insect pollinated, and their entomophilian pollens are not relevant in most clinical allergy. Still, trees should not be ignored. In much of North America, Europe, and temperate areas of the world, the pollen seasons for trees typically precede those of the weeds and grasses, sometimes making these early-onset symptoms easy to relate to the tree pollens. There is less antigenic cross-reactivity among the tree pollens than among the grass pollens.

In the Mediterranean region and southern Europe, cypress and hazel tree pollens can appear as early as January, whereas in the northeastern forests of North America and Europe, the earliest tree pollens appear in March and April, with the release of pollen from birch, elm, maple, ash, alder, and hazel trees (Figs. 2-16*A* and *D*). Birch is a major allergen in Scandinavian countries. Oak trees (Figs. 2-17*A* and *C*) shed more pollen than many other plants and are present in all of Europe and North America except Alaska, Hawaii, and other hot, tropical, or very cold climates. In the Northern Hemisphere, airborne oak pollens are present in April and May, whereas in the Southern Hemisphere, these and others can initially appear during August and September. In general, conifer (pine) trees produce large amounts of pollen but cause modest allergic symptoms, with the exception of the mountain cedar (Fig. 2-18) in Texas and the Japanese cedar in California, Japan, and other parts of Asia.

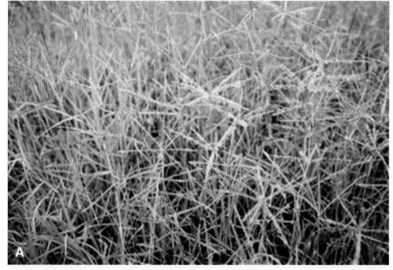

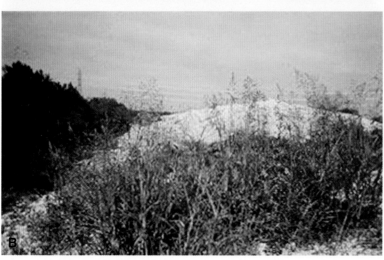

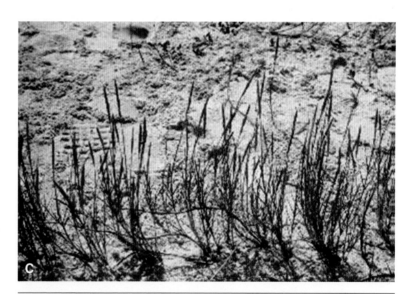

**Figure 2-15.** Bermuda *(A)*, Johnson *(B)*, and salt grasses *(C)*. These three plants have long seasons in the sub-tropic regions and tropical regions of the world. (*A* and *B*, courtesy of Hollister-Stier Laboratories.)

| Family | Genus/Species | Common Name |
|---|---|---|
| *Aceraceae* | *Acer saccharum* | Sugar maple |
| *Betalaceae* | *Betula populifolia* | White birch |
| *Cupressaceae* | *Juniperus oshei* | Mountain cedar |
| *Hamamelidaceae* | *Liquidambar styraciflue* | Sweet gum |
| *Fagaceae* | *Quercus alba* | White oak |
| | *Quercus velutina* | Black oak |
| *Oleaceae* | *Olea europaea* | Olive |
| | *Fraxinus Pennsylvania* | Ash |
| *Plantanaceae* | *Platanus accidentelis* | Sycamore |
| *Salicaceae* | *Populus deltoids* | Eastern cottonwood |
| | *Populus alba* | White poplar |
| | *Salix migra* | Black willow |
| *Ulmaceae* | *Ulmus americaria* | Elm |
| *Juglandaceae* | *Juglaus nigra* | Walnut |
| | *Carya alba* | Hickory |

**TABLE 2-5**
Selected Common Allergenic Tree Pollens

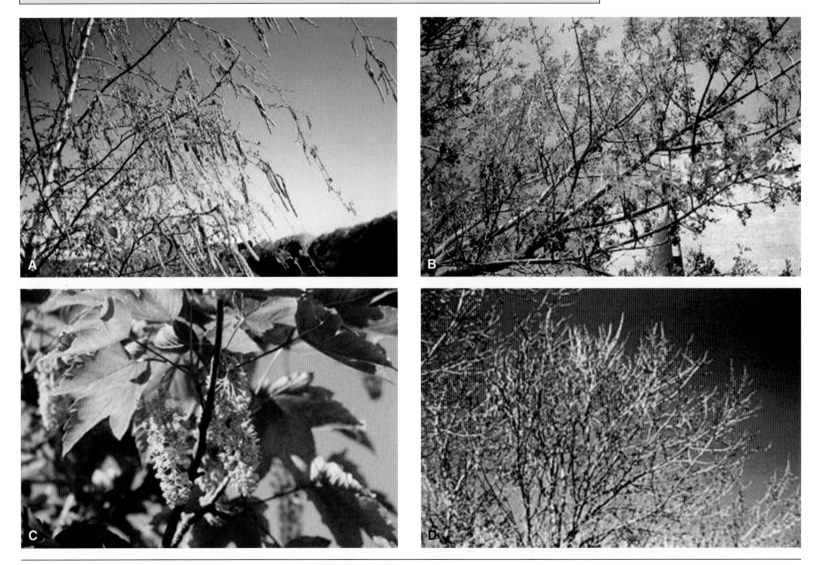

**Figure 2-16.** Birch *(A)*, ash *(B)*, maple *(C)*, and red maple *(D)* trees in spring bloom in the Northern Hemisphere. Pollens from these trees begin to reach peak levels in the very early spring. (Courtesy of Hollister-Stier Laboratories.)

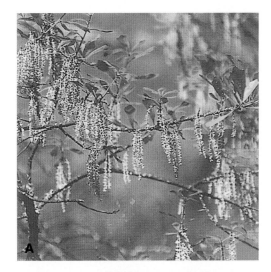

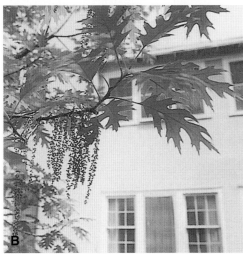

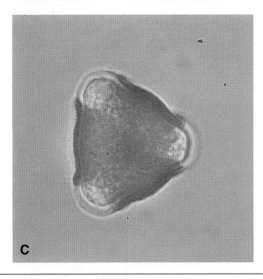

**Figure 2-17.** White oak *(A)* and Black oak *(B)* as they appear in the spring. *C,* Oil emersion photomicrograph of oak pollen, 450×. (Courtesy of Greer Laboratories.)

# FUNGI (MOLDS)

Fungi are saprophytic organisms that are present throughout most of the world. Most fungi produce airborne spores that can become important inhalant allergens. As allergens, fungi can be detected both outdoors and indoors and may show seasonal or perennial presence.[11] Many clinicians and patients refer to *fungi* as *molds,* and the terms are interchangeable. It is helpful in clinical practice to group the mold spores based on the history of environmental exposure, that is, out of doors (seasonal) or indoors (perennial), even though this classification may not be precise because indoor fungi are acquired from outside sources (Table 2-6). Like the pollens, some of the fungi can be collected and identified microscopically by outdoor air samplers, and they tend to show seasonal patterns in temperate climates.[12] Their numbers increase in the air during the warm months and decrease when hard frost prevents growth, and they are absent when the ground is snow covered. In those areas of the world without a winter season, outdoor fungi spores can be perennial aero-allergens. *Alternaria* and *Cladosporium (Hormodendrum)* species (Fig. 2-19) are the most numerous in late summer and early fall in the Northern Hemisphere. These molds are saprophytic fungi and grow on decaying leaves and dead plants. They are often increased atmospherically in the daytime. Some, such as *Drechslera (Helminthosporium),* grow abundantly on grasses and cereal crops and in the soil and are more numerous in subtropical climates.

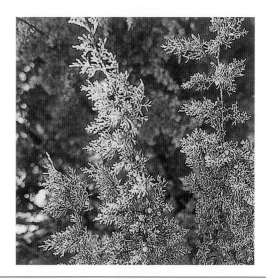

**Figure 2-18. Mountain cedar. This is one of the conifers that causes allergic responses in sensitive people. (Courtesy of Hollister-Stier Laboratories.)**

**TABLE 2-6**
**Classification of Common Allergenic Fungal (Mold) Spores**

| Outdoor (Seasonal) | Indoor (Perennial) |
|---|---|
| *Alternaria* | *Aspergillus* |
| *Cladosporium (Hormodendrum)* | *Penicillium* |
| *Helminthosporium (Drechslera)* | *Epicoccum* |

Water (humidity) is the primary controlling factor for fungal growth, both outdoors and indoors. Different fungi colonize susceptible indoor materials under different moisture conditions.[13] In cool weather, warmer moist indoor air diffuses through walls and on contact with cold vapor barriers forms condensation with growth of fungi. In this fashion, molds such as *Aspergillus*, *Penicillium*

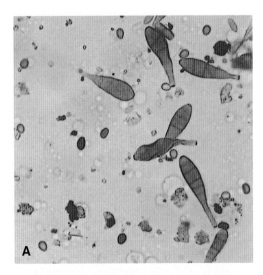

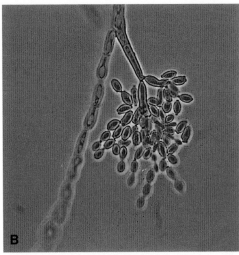

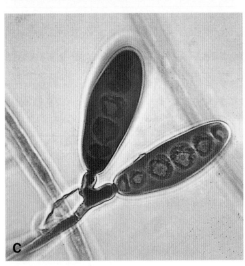

**Figure 2-19.** Photomicrograph of spores of *Alternaria (A)* (courtesy of Dr. William Solomon), *Cladosporium (B)*, and *Drechslera (Helminthosporium; C)*. (*B* and *C*, courtesy of Greer Laboratories.)

(Fig. 2-20), and *Stachybotrys* can grow indoors with a humidity lower than 85%. These are the organisms most typically found in sheds, barns, and homes, especially in basements and crawlspaces. *Aspergillus* is also commonly found in barns associated with stored grains or vegetables. *Penicillium* is the green "mildew" seen typically on items stored in damp basements. *Stachybotrys* is often referred to as the "black mold." *Epicoccum* can be found both in storage areas and outdoors as a seasonal aero-allergen. Fungi can also often be found in damp bathrooms and on houseplants. Vaporizers, humidifiers, and air conditioners that have water storage units can be contaminated with fungi and then become a source of aerosolized mold spores. The potential of fungal allergy should not be ignored, as recent studies have indicated that many asthmatics in large cities had positive immediate skin tests to *Alternaria* and *Penicillin*.[13]

The detection of storage fungi in an indoor environment can be accomplished by placing uncovered plates of growth media, such as Sabouraud's, in the suspected room or area for 10 minutes. After incubating the plates, the growing fungal colonies are

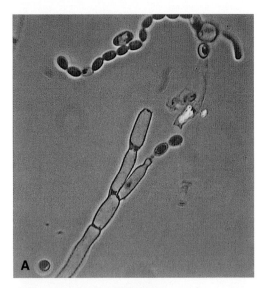

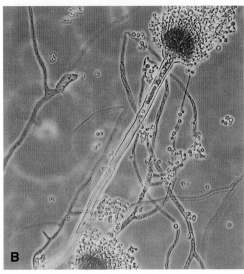

**Figure 2-20.** Photomicrographs of penicillium spores *(A)* and *Aspergillus flavus* spores *(B)*. Both of these common storage molds can grow in low-moisture conditions. They tend to be found in sheds, barns, and basements. (Courtesy of Greer Laboratories.)

identified and enumerated. Aerodynamic air sampling can be used to inoculate culture plates, and immunochemical detection of fungal allergens has been employed recently to detect mold allergens in office buildings with mold-contaminated air conditioning or ventilation systems. Unfortunately, there are no generally accepted standards for interpretation of fungal levels in indoor or outdoor air.[14] At present, the best approach to indoor fungal control is moisture control in the indoor environment.

# INDOOR ALLERGENS

Airborne indoor allergens are important causes of clinical allergy.[15] It has been known for years that indoor exposure to dusts, either through household or occupational exposure, can provoke respiratory allergy (Box 2-5). For years, the source of the allergen in house dust was debated, but in 1967, its principal allergenic component was shown to be a mite.[16] House dust or mattress mites (*Dermatophygoides*), as well as other mite species, are found

worldwide (Fig. 2-21). *D. pteronyssius* is more common in Europe, along with *Euroglyphus maynei*, *D. farinae*, and *D. pteronyssius*, which are both found in the United States and Japan.

The tropical mite *Blomia tropicalis* has been detected in Brazil, Venezuela, Puerto Rico, and Florida and is probably present in many tropical areas. These eight-legged, sightless arthropods cannot be observed without magnification, but they can be identified microscopically with lower-power lenses (Fig. 2-22). They feed on human or animal epithelium and other high-protein debris found in human environmental dusts. The highest concentrations of mites have been found in mattresses, pillows, rugs, upholstered furniture, and vacuum sweepings. Mites do not search for or drink water but absorb water from ambient humidity. For optimal propagation, mites require temperatures of 25°C to 30°C and humidity greater than 50%. In temperate climates, they attain their maximal numbers in early fall, but they can survive for many months at lower temperatures and humidity as well. Temperatures greater than 130°F (54°C) or less than 32°F (0°C) can kill the mites. They are rarely found in arid or arctic climates or at high altitudes.

The major mite allergen has been found in the spherical mite fecal particles. Their shape and size (10 to 35 μm in diameter) make these particles comparable to many pollens. Moderate amounts of mite allergen are found in the body cuticle. The two major allergens in dust mites have been purified and are identified as *D. pteronyssius* allergen I (*Der p 1*) and *Der p 2* and *D. farinae* (*Der f 1*) and *Der f 2*).[17] These purified *Der p 1* allergens have homology with cysteine proteinases with enzyme activity and are cross-reacting allergens with *Der f 1*. However, these purified *Der p* and *Der f* allergens only partially cross-react with the tropical dust mite (*B. tropicalis*). In the United States and England, 10% of the population and 80% to 90% of allergic asthmatics have positive immediate skin tests to the purified dust mite allergen. Reductions in mite exposure by reducing the environment concentration of mites lead to lower levels of specific IgE antibody and fewer allergic symptoms. About 10% of allergic patients who are symptomatic indoors in the United States do not react to skin testing

---

**BOX 2-5**
**Selected Indoor Allergens**

**Acarids**
Dust mites

**Mammals**
Cat, dog, rabbit, ferret, guinea pig, gerbil, mouse, rat

**Insects**
Cockroach

**Fungi**
Aspergillus, epicoccum

---

Worldwide Distribution of Dust Mite

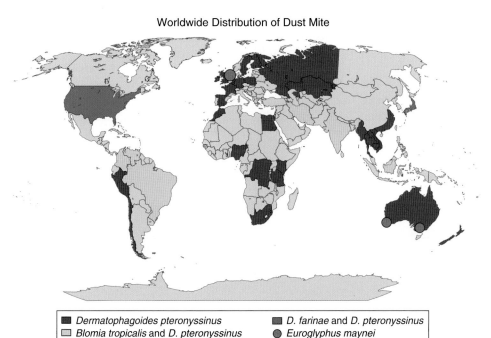

■ *Dermatophagoides pteronyssinus*　　■ *D. farinae* and *D. pteronyssinus*
□ *Blomia tropicalis* and *D. pteronyssinus*　　● *Euroglyphus maynei*

**Figure 2-21.** Worldwide distribution of the dust mite. (From Holgate, Church, Lichtenstein. Allergy, second edition.)

with dust mites; they are reactive to another allergenic constituent in their environmental house dust.

Another important indoor aeroallergen is the cockroach, which can introduce important aeroallergens into the household dusts of certain environments. The several species of cockroach associated with allergic respiratory diseases are listed in Box 2-6. Studies comparing air samples in crowded New York tenements versus suburban middle-class homes showed comparable concentrations of house dust mite allergen but remarkably higher levels of German cockroach allergen in the older urban apartments, with a significant association of cockroach IgE antibodies with asthma.[18] As with the dust mite, the major cockroach allergens are related to the gastrointestinal tract or the feces and are greater than 10 μm in size; however, more studies are needed. Another arthropod, the mayfly, can be an outdoor inhalant allergen during the summer months along the Great Lakes. The major allergen of the mayfly is thought to be in its body, which becomes airborne during flight.

# MAMMALIAN ANIMAL ALLERGENS

Domestic pets are a very common source of indoor inhalant allergens that provoke significant respiratory complaints and disease in many patients with asthma and allergic rhinitis.[19] More than 50% of households in the United States have indoor domestic pets. Allergic symptoms can occur not only in owners, family, and friends of dogs, cats, or other pets but also in veterinarians and farmers, as well as laboratory workers exposed to horses, cattle, sheep, and rodents, including rabbits, rats, mice, and guinea

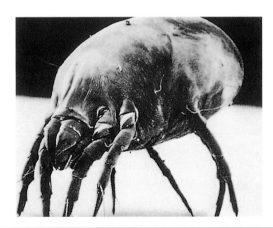

**Figure 2-22.** House dust mite (*Dermatophygoides farinae*). This and other species of mites compose the principal allergenic component of common house dust.

pigs. The hair or fur of these animals was initially incriminated as allergenic, but in truth, hair is neither buoyant nor of a suitable size to become an inhalant allergen. It has subsequently been shown that the desquamated epithelium, also known as dander, that is attached to the hair becomes aerosolized and is the potent allergen. Epithelial desquamation is a constant process in mammals and is a continual source of aerosolized, highly allergenic proteins, as well as body excretions (Table 2-7).

It is common for animal-allergic individuals to develop urticaria at sites where they have been licked by a cat or dog or scratched by its claws or teeth. Among the house pets, cats seem to cause the more prominent symptoms. However, dogs do spend more time out of doors and are less frequently kept in bedrooms or beds and may be groomed more frequently than cats. Recent studies have shown that cat allergens are found in the skin, saliva, and sebaceous glands of the skin. It has also been suggested that cat urine can become aerosolized from litter pans, and urinary proteins can act as allergens. Dog allergens have been shown on fur and in dander, saliva, and serum proteins. It has been suggested that some breeds of dog are less allergenic than others, but this may be more quantitative than qualitative and related to frequency of grooming.

The main cat allergen, *Fel d 1*, has been purified from both cat washing solutions and pelt. The allergens prepared from pelt extracts are thought to be less representative of natural exposure because they contain a relatively large concentration of cat tissue proteins (e.g., albumin). When cats are washed repeatedly, the allergen recovered decreases progressively. These observations lead to the clinical recommendation that washing cats is a method of reducing exposure to allergen in cat-allergic patients. However, not all cats tolerate washing, and this effect is short lived—less than a week. To be effective, washing of cats or dogs needs to be repeated frequently, at least once a week. The major dog allergen (*Can f 1*) has also been purified. Identification of the major cat and dog allergens has enabled specific environmental immunoassays. Using these assays, significant levels of both cat and dog allergens have been documented, not only in homes of pet owners but also in dust from schools.[20] Recent reports suggest that persistent daily exposure to the allergens from dogs or cats from early infancy may result in statistically less allergic inhalant symptoms than intermittent or daily exposure as an older child or adult.[21] These observations need to be confirmed and may provide future means to induce immune tolerance to animal allergens.

Rodent inhalant allergens cause illness in about 20% of exposed laboratory animal workers. It is the urinary proteins of mice, rats, and guinea pigs, as well as their dander, that can be allergenic. Remarkable levels of mouse and rat aeroallergens have been found in older New York City tenements, as compared

---

**BOX 2-6**
**Species of Cockroach**

*Blattella germanica* (German)
*Periplaneta americana* (American)
*Blatta orientalis* (Oriental)

---

**TABLE 2-7**
**Common Inhalant Allergens from Animal Sources**

| Epidermal | Excretions |
|---|---|
| Dander (desquamated epithelium) | Saliva |
| Cuticle (body) | Urine |
| | Feces |

with newer suburban middle- and upper-class homes.[22] Feathers of pet birds, chickens, ducks, and geese, have been found to be a significant source of inhalant allergens, as are feathers used in pillows, bedding, and garments. It is unclear whether it is the pulverized feather or another associated protein that becomes the aerosolized allergen.

# OTHER ENVIRONMENTAL DUSTS

A variety of inhalant airborne allergens have been defined for various occupations—these are described in detail in Chapter 6. They include organic dusts, such as baker's flour, grain mill dust, and enzymes used in laundry detergents, as well as trimellitic anhydride, plicatic acid from wood dust, toluene di-isocyanate, and the salts of nickel, chrome, and platinum. Kapok, a plant fiber from the Kapok tree, is very resilient and has been used in pillows and upholstered furniture. It is impervious to water, making it a useful material for boat cushions and life jackets. When pulverized and airborne, kapok is a potent allergen. It is being replaced by various synthetic polymers in pillows and cushions.

Occasionally, foods become aerosolized allergens during cooking. If inhaled by a sensitive person, certain food allergens may provoke severe respiratory allergy. However, most food-allergic individuals manifest their reactions, which can include respiratory symptoms, after ingestion of the specific food (see Chapter 13).

Many clinicians feel that respiratory complaints related to our environment have increased in the past several decades. Terms such as *sick building syndrome* have been coined to describe allergies that might be related to exposure to inhaled substances from closed environments with inadequate ventilation. Some of these complaints may be related to specific inhalant allergens, such as molds. However, in evaluating such patients, the clinician must be careful not to label chemical or physical irritants as allergens, even if these inhalants provoke symptoms of asthma and rhinitis. Such nonantigenic irritants, which can exacerbate allergic respiratory disease, include sulfur dioxide, cigarette smoke, cold air, auto exhaust fumes, hairsprays, perfumed aerosols, and solvent vapors. These substances may directly provoke the activation of mediators of inflammation, such as histamine or leukotrienes, which then cause respiratory symptoms without any mediation by an IgE antibody and allergen reaction. If combined with exposure to an allergen such as dust mites or fungi, these nonallergic irritants can potentiate or exacerbate an allergic respiratory disease. Therefore, exposure to these toxic factors should not be ignored, and avoidance precautions should be recommended. However, to be identified and incriminated as an allergen, these inhalants must induce an IgE-mediated immune response as well as provoke respiratory symptoms.

# REFERENCES

1. Muilenberg ML: Aeroallergen assessment by microscopy and culture. Immunol Allerg Clin North Am 1989;9:245–268.
2. Aalberse RC: Structural biology of allergens. J Allergy Clin Immunol 2000; 106(2):228–238.
3. Agarwal MK, Swanson MC, Reed CE, Yuninger JW: Airborne ragweed allergens: Association with various particle sizes and short ragweed plant parts. J Allergy Clin Immunol 1984;74(5):687–693.
4. Solomon WR, Platts-Mills TA: Aerobiology and inhalant allergens. In Middleton E, Reed CE, Ellis EF (eds): Allergy: Principles and Practice, 5th ed. St. Louis, C.V. Mosby, 1998, pp 367–403.
5. King TP, Hoffman D, Lowenstein H, et al: Allergen nomenclature. J Allergy Clin Immunol 1995;96:5–14.
6. Allergen nomenclature, International Union of Immunological Societies Allergen Nomenclature Sub-Committee, www.allergen.org/list.htm, 2002.
7. Lewis WH, Vinay P, Zenger VE: Airborne and Allergenic Pollen of North America. Baltimore, Johns Hopkins Press, 1983.
8. D'Amato G, Spieksma FT, Liccardi G, et al: Pollen-related allergy in Europe. Allergy 1998;53(6):567–578.
9. Roth A: Allergy in the World: A Guide for Physicians and Travelers. University of Hawaii Press, Honolulu, 1978.
10. Esch RE, Bush RK: Aerobiology of outdoor allergens. In Middleton E, Adkinson NF Jr, Yuninger JW, et al (eds): Allergy: Principles and Practice, 6th ed. St. Louis, C.V. Mosby, 2003.
11. Nolles G, Hockstra MO, Schouten JP, et al: Prevalence of immunoglobulin E for fungi in atopic children. Clin Exp Allergy 2001;31(10):1564–1570.
12. Horner WE, Helbling A, Salvaggio JE, Lehrer SB: Fungal allergens. Clin Microbiol Rev 1995;8(2):161–179.
13. Licorish K, Novey HS, Kozak P, et al: Role of alternaria and penicillium spores in the pathogenesis of asthma. J Allergy Clin Immunol 1985;76(6):819–825.
14. Burge H: An update on pollen and fungal spore aerobiology. J Allergy Clin Immunol 2002;110(4):544–552.
15. Platts-Mills TA: Indoor allergen. In Middleton E, Adkinson NF Jr, Yuninger JW, et al (eds): Allergy: Principles and Practice, 6th ed. St. Louis, C.V. Mosby, 2003.
16. Voorhorst R, Spieksma FTM, Vanekamp MJ, et al: The house dust mite (*Dermatophagoides pteronyssinus*) and the allergens it produces. Identity with the house dust allergen. J Allergy 1967;39:325–328.
17. Lind P: Purification and partial characterization of two major allergens from the house dust mite *Dermatophagoides pteronyssinus*. J Allergy Clin Immunol 1985;76(5):753–761.
18. Eggleston PA, Rosenstreich D, Lynn H, et al: Relationship of indoor allergen exposure to skin test sensitivity in inner-city children with asthma. J Allergy Clin Immunol 1998;102(4):563–570.
19. Ingram JM, Sporik R, Rose G, et al: Quantitative assessment of exposure to dog (*Can f 1*) and cat (*Fel d 1*) allergens: Relation to sensitization and asthma among children living in Los Alamos, New Mexico. J Allergy Clin Immunol 1995; 96(4):449–456.
20. Patchett K, Lewis S, Crane J, Fitzharris P: Cat allergen (*Fel d 1*) levels on school children's clothing and in primary school classrooms in Wellington, New Zealand. J Allergy Clin Immunol 1997;100(6 Pt 1):755–759.
21. Hesselmar B, Aberg N, Aberg B, et al: Does early exposure to cat or dog protect against later allergy development? Clin Exp Allergy 1999;29(5):611–617.
22. Phipatanakul W, Eggleston PA, Wright EC, Wood RA: National Cooperative Inner-City Asthma Study. Mouse allergen II. The relationship of mouse allergen exposure to mouse sensitization and asthma morbidity in inner-city children with asthma. J Allergy Clin Immunol 2000;106(6):1075–1080.

*Deborah A. Gentile*

# *3* Diagnostic Tests in Allergy

The diagnosis of allergic diseases should always begin with the procurement of a careful patient history and an appropriate physical examination. When an allergic disorder is suspected on the basis of clinical grounds, a variety of procedures can be used to confirm the diagnosis. Diagnostic tests can also be helpful in ruling out allergic disorders and clarifying the specific responsible antigens or allergens.

## SKIN TESTS

Skin testing is the tool used most widely to diagnose clinical allergies.[1] The basic procedure involves delivering an aqueous solution of antigen beneath the stratum corneum and barrier zone of the epidermis. As the antigen combines with immunoglobulin (Ig) E antibody fixed to mast cells, mediator substances, particularly histamine, are released from the mast cells. The mediators cause local vasodilation and increased capillary permeability. Wheal-and-flare reactions appear within 15 to 20 minutes (Figs. 3-1 and 3-2).[2] A typical scoring system is listed in Table 3-1.[3] The immediate wheal-and-flare reactions are often followed by late-phase reactions. There is evidence that if high enough concentrations of antigens are presented, 100% of immediate reactions will go on to late phases. These late-phase reactions in the skin are also manifested in the nasal mucosa and bronchi (see Fig. 3-11).

There are two types of skin tests—the epicutaneous, also referred to as scratch, puncture, and prick technique (Fig. 3-3), and the intracutaneous, or intradermal, test.

### *EPICUTANEOUS SKIN TESTS*

The epicutaneous method has many advantages. It is easy and safe to perform and causes little discomfort. It is inexpensive, and test solutions are stable because they are suspended in 50% glycerine. Positive epicutaneous tests correlate well with clinical symptoms (Table 3-2). One possible disadvantage to this method is that it can result in false-negative reactions due to a lack of sensitivity (Table 3-3).

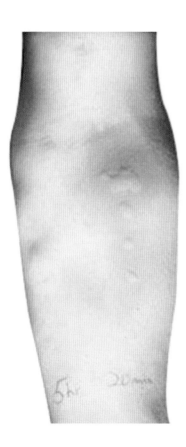

**Figure 3-1.** Skin prick tests with grass-pollen allergen in a patient with typical summer hay fever. Skin tests were performed 5 hours *(left)* and 20 minutes *(right)* before the photograph was taken. The tests on the right show a typical end-point titration of a Type I immediate wheal-and-flare reaction. The late-phase skin reaction *(left)* can be clearly seen at 5 hours, especially where a large immediate response has preceded it. Figures for allergen dilution are given. (Reproduced with permission from Roitt et al., 2001.)

**TABLE 3-1**
**Commonly Used Scoring System for Grading the Response to Hypersensitivity Skin Testing**

| Grade | Wheal | Erythema |
|---|---|---|
| 0(–) | <3 mm | 0–5 mm |
| 1+ | 3–5 mm | 0–10 mm |
| 2+ | 5–10 mm | 5–10 mm |
| 3+ | 10–15 mm | >10 mm |
| 4+ | >15 mm or with pseudopods | >20 mm |

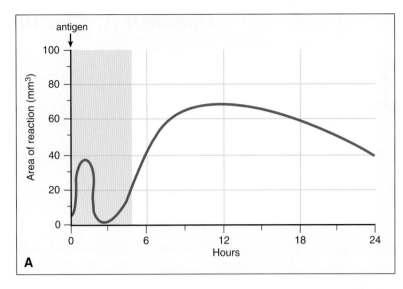

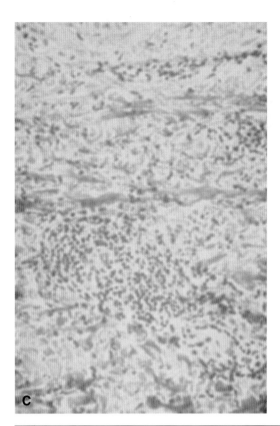

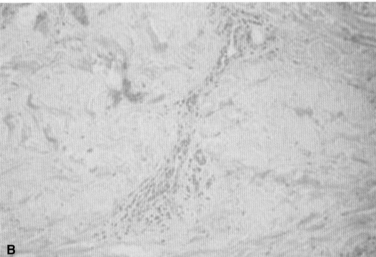

**Figure 3-2.** Immediate and late-phase skin reactions. Using the intradermal method of skin testing, an immediate wheal-and-flare reaction is often followed by a late-phase reaction. *A,* This late phase may last for 24 hours, and the reaction is larger and generally more edematous than the immediate response. *B,* The immediate type of reaction (here exemplified by a biopsy of chronic urticaria) has a sparse cellular infiltrate around the dermal vessels, consisting primarily of neutrophils. *C,* The late reaction has a dense infiltrate with many basophils. The late-phase reaction can be seen following challenge of the skin, nasal mucosa, and bronchi and may be particularly important in the development of chronic asthma. (Reproduced with permission from Roitt et al., 2001.)

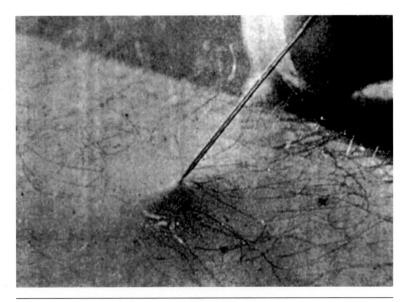

**Figure 3-3.** A needle used to lift and break the skin in the epicutaneous skin test technique.

## INTRACUTANEOUS SKIN TESTS

Intracutaneous skin tests are more reproducible than epicutaneous tests and are 100 to 1000 times more sensitive. Thus, they are associated with fewer false-negative reactions. The drawbacks to intradermal tests are that they are time consuming and tedious to perform and are often associated with discomfort and an increased risk of systemic reactions. Even more important, they are more likely to produce false-positive results because of their increased sensitivity. Mildly positive intradermal reactions are not considered clinically relevant.

A disposable multitest applicator has recently gained popularity because of its convenience and the reproducibility of results that it offers (Fig. 3-4); eight epicutaneous tests can be applied at one time (Fig. 3-5). Results compare favorably with those that are obtained by intracutaneous tests.

## TEST RESULTS

The value of skin tests, like that of any diagnostic procedure, depends on the knowledge of their interpreter. To be informative, the tests must be related to the clinical context of the patient's history and physical examination. The selection of antigens and the administration of tests require experience and knowledge. The physician must be aware of the many reasons for false-positive and false-negative reactions to properly interpret test results.

### False-Negative Results

Several circumstances may account for negative skin test results in a patient who truly has an IgE-mediated allergic disease (Box 3-1). The antigen in solution—a protein—if improperly stored may lose potency with time or exposure to heat, thereby causing a

**TABLE 3-2**
**Advantages of Epicutaneous Versus Intracutaneous Skin Tests**

| Epicutaneous | Intracutaneous |
|---|---|
| Easy to perform | More reproducible |
| Safe | More sensitive |
| Little discomfort | |
| Inexpensive | |
| Stable test solutions | |
| Correlates well with symptoms | |

**TABLE 3-3**
**Disadvantages of Epicutaneous Versus Intracutaneous Skin Tissue**

| Epicutaneous | Intracutaneous |
|---|---|
| Less sensitive | More time consuming |
| | More difficult to perform |
| | More discomfort |
| | Increased risk of systemic reaction |
| | More false-positive results |

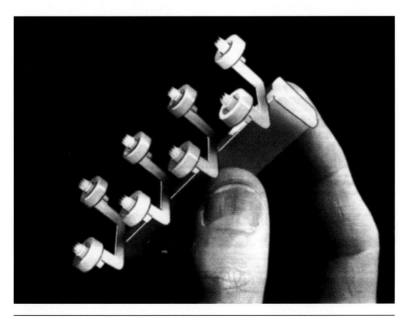

**Figure 3-4.** The multitest applicator. (Courtesy of Lincoln Diagnostics, Inc., Decatur, IL.)

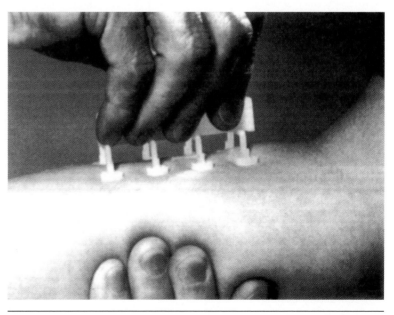

**Figure 3-5.** A multitest applicator delivers eight antigens at once, simplifying epicutaneous testing. (Courtesy of Lincoln Diagnostics Inc., Decatur, IL.)

false-negative result. Antigen solutions must be refrigerated and replaced at appropriate intervals.

A false-negative result may also occur due to the improper administration of a test. Too superficial a scratch or prick of the skin or too deep an intracutaneous injection will prevent the allergen solution to reach the skin area in which mast cells are located.

The patient's age must also be considered when a skin test result is negative. In general, the skin of infants and elderly persons is less reactive than that of other age groups. In the same individual, the skin on the forearm is less reactive than the skin on the back, and responsiveness is lower in the early morning than later in the day.

The refractory period of a test may also contribute to a false-negative result. Soon after a systemic reaction to an allergen, such as insect venom, penicillin, or food, the patient enters a refractory period during which a skin test reaction to that substance may be negative. The reason is that specific IgE is consumed by the severe allergic reaction, so a 3- to 4-week period is needed for the allergic antibody to build back up to its prereaction levels. Therefore, if a patient has a systemic reaction to an allergen, it is best to wait a full 4 weeks before performing skin tests.

Finally, a number of drugs, particularly antihistamines, may inhibit skin reactivity and therefore should be discontinued at least 72 hours before skin testing. Whenever a skin test is performed, histamine should be included as a positive control. If the histamine skin test is negative, further testing should be deferred. A more complete list of drugs that can inhibit immediate skin reactivity is provided in Box 3-2. Corticosteroids, theophylline, cromolyn, leukotriene modifiers, beta agonists, and decongestants are not presently known to be inhibitory.

## False-Positive Results

When a skin test is positive in the face of a negative clinical picture, several explanations may be offered (Box 3-3). Many factors contribute to the production of nonspecifically irritating skin test solutions. Deviation from a physiologic pH or from the correct osmolarity may cause a false-positive skin test result. Extracts may contain low-molecular-weight irritants, and it is necessary to dialyze these materials before utilizing them as skin testing agents. Glycerine, commonly used as a preservative in allergy extracts,

causes nonspecific irritation at a concentration of 6% if injected intradermally. Injecting too large a volume of extract intradermally may also cause false-positive reactions. The optimal injection volume is 0.02 mL.

Materials that are urticariogenic may cause a wheal and erythema skin test response in all subjects on a non–IgE-mediated basis. Examples are morphine and codeine. Some food extracts, particularly those from cheese, have a high histamine content and may cause false-positive reactions.

Dermographism also may be responsible for a false-positive test result. It is present in 5% to 20% of the population, depending on the degree of pressure applied. Skin testing should also include a negative saline control to ensure that the patient is not dermographic. A positive response to saline obviously makes other positive skin test reactions suspect.

Positive skin test reactivity may persist in an individual whose clinical sensitivity has disappeared either spontaneously or through the use of immunotherapy. Additionally, false-positive results are often harbingers of future sensitivity. The onset of clinical symptoms of allergic rhinitis is generally preceded by a positive pollen prick test. The development of hay fever in college seniors who, as freshmen, had no clinical manifestations of allergies is more than 10 times higher in students with initial positive pollen scratch tests than in students with no positive pollen scratch tests.[4] Thus, the risk of developing an allergic condition is

---

**BOX 3-2**
**Drugs That May Inhibit Immediate Skin Test Reactivity**

All $H_1$-blocking antihistamines
  Variable: Hydroxyzine, high; cyproheptadine, low
Ranitidine
Amitriptyline
Desipramine
Nortriptyline
Imipramine
Protriptyline
Trimipramine
Triavil

---

**BOX 3-1**
**Reasons for False-Negative Skin Test Results**

Improper storage of antigens
Improper administration
Inherent host factors
  Age
  Skin area
  Time of day
  Skin temperature
Refractory period
Inhibiting drugs

---

**BOX 3-3**
**Reasons for False-Positive Skin Test Results**

Improper preparation and administration of allergen solution
Nonspecific histamine release
Dermographism
Remnant of past sensitivity
Harbinger of future sensitivity
Disparity with clinical sensitivity

considerably greater for individuals with positive skin test results (Table 3-4).[1]

Perhaps the most important reason for the false-positive skin test reaction is the physician's failure to recognize that a positive skin test is not necessarily an indicator of clinical sensitivity. In any group of tested persons, there are a certain number of positive responses that are better classified as clinically insignificant than false positive. Several studies have pointed out the high incidence of immediate skin test reactivity in a normal adult population (Table 3-5).

# ENZYME-LINKED IMMUNOSORBENT ASSAY

## TOTAL SERUM IMMUNOGLOBULIN E DETERMINATION

The discovery of IgE as the antibody responsible for allergic reactions in humans has led to the development of sophisticated techniques for IgE measurement. The two most commonly employed methods for the measurement of IgE are radioimmunoassay (RIA) and enzyme-linked immunosassay (EIA). EIA has largely supplanted radioimmunoassay because it is nonisotopic, the reagents have long shelf lives, and there are no waste disposal problems (Fig. 3-6). This is a competition type of assay.

Immunoglobulin E levels are often elevated in cases of allergic disease, but these levels cannot be considered pathognomonic signs of allergy. IgE levels vary widely, both in allergic and non-allergic individuals. A normal IgE level does not exclude allergy (Fig. 3-7), while definitely elevated levels may be seen in non-atopic people.[2,5]

## ALLERGEN-SPECIFIC IMMUNOGLOBULIN E ANTIBODY DETERMINATION

Sandwich EIAs are routinely used to quantify the amount of IgE antibody that is directed to a specific allergen (Fig. 3-8).[2,6,7] The EIA has replaced the RAST (radioallergosorbent test), the original allergen-specific IgE test. In the EIA technique, an allergen is bound to a cellulose derivative on a surface. The patient's serum is added, and any IgE in the serum that is specific for that allergen adheres on the surface. Enzyme-labeled antibody to IgE is then added. Thus, the specific IgE antibody in the serum combines with it specific allergen that is fixed to the cellulose surface and then acts as antigen to the enzyme-labeled anti-IgE antibody. The amount of enzyme activity generated is then measured and therefore is directly related to the amount of specific IgE antibody present in the serum. This test has high speed, precision, and reproducibility, which contribute to high levels of sensitivity and specificity. This technique has significantly increased diagnostic efficacy as compared with previously available methods.

## SERUM-SPECIFIC IMMUNOGLOBULIN E ANTIBODY LEVELS VERSUS SKIN TESTS

Disagreement exists as to the precise role of serum specific IgE antibody levels in everyday allergy practice.[8] There is no question that the former is more expensive to administer than the latter, but proponents of serum-specific IgE antibody measurements maintain that this technique offers several advantages over skin tests. These include greater safety, better quantitative results, protection from drug interference, greater allergen stability, preference in problem patients, and fewer injections. Table 3-6 lists these proposed advantages with appropriate rebuttals.

**TABLE 3-4**
**Predictive Value of Immediate Skin Tests**

| Epicutaneous Skin Tests | Incidence of Allergic Rhinitis 3 yr Later |
| --- | --- |
| Negative | 1.7% |
| Positive | 18.2% (*P* value 0.01) |

**TABLE 3-5**
**Frequency of Positive Skin Tests in Asymptomatic Patients**

| Study | Method | Allergen | Allergen, % |
| --- | --- | --- | --- |
| 1 | ID | House dust—concentrate | 50 |
| 2 | ID | House dust—1:100 | 4 |
| 3 | ID | Various | 9 |
| 4 | EC | Various | 4 |
|  | ID | Grass | 6 |
|  | EC | Various | 12 |

EC, epicutaneous; ID, intradermal.

# PROVOCATIVE CHALLENGE TESTING

The skin test and measurement of total serum IgE and specific IgE antibody levels in the serum are indirect assays of an allergic state. Direct challenge, either by inhaling or ingesting antigens, may be of greater diagnostic use.[9] In addition to the antigen challenge, the general hyperresponsive state of the airway associated with asthma may be evaluated by exercise or by inhalation of chemical substances to which asthmatic individuals are more sensitive than are nonasthmatics (Table 3-7).

## NONSPECIFIC TESTS

### Exercise

Physical exercise is a major precipitant of bronchial asthma. The diagnosis of asthma can usually be made after 6 to 8 minutes of exercise and pre- and postpulmonary function testing (Fig. 3-9). Initially, the patient exhibits a bronchodilation effect, along with an increase in the forced expiratory volume in one second ($FEV_1$). In the patient with exercise-induced bronchoconstriction, 6 to 8 minutes of exercise is generally followed by a 20% or greater fall in $FEV_1$.[10]

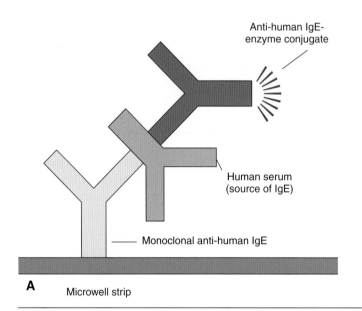

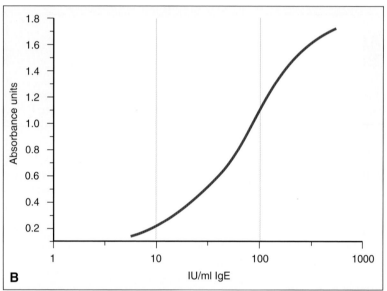

**Figure 3-6.** *A,* The enzyme-linked immunoassay. In this assay, microwell strips are coated with monoclonal anti-human immunoglobulin (Ig) E antibody. Test serum is added, and IgE is captured. After washing to remove unbound proteins, anti-human IgE peroxidase conjugate (or another suitable enzyme) is added to the well. The bound enzyme-linked antibody is quantitated by adding a substrate solution that changes color when hydrolyzed by the enzyme. Therefore, the higher the level of IgE, the more enzyme-linked anti-IgE is bound and the more intense the color that develops, which can be analyzed in a spectrophotometer. *B,* The typical normal IgE standard curve.

**Figure 3-7.** Immunoglobulin (Ig) E levels in allergic patients. Each point in this chart represents the serum IgE level of a patient. IgE levels vary over a wide range, but the levels in atopic patients are generally elevated above the levels in normal subjects of the same age. For many atopic individuals with less severe diseases, the serum IgE levels fall within the normal range. IgE titers are usually expressed in international units per milliliter, by reference to standard sera, where 1 IU = 2.4 ng. The normal range of IgE in nonatopic subjects is *shaded.* (Adapted with permission from Roitt et al., 2001.)

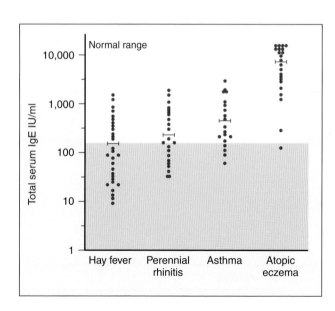

## Bronchial Challenges

Asthma is characterized by enhanced bronchial hyperreactivity. This hyperreactivity can be manifested clinically by the asthmatic's adverse response to cold air, cigarette smoke, fumes, weather changes, and other stimuli that have little or no effect on a non-asthmatic patient. In the doctor's office setting, hyperreactivity can be demonstrated by the patient's response to a bronchial challenge, such as the inhalation of methacholine or histamine (Fig. 3-10). A greater than 20% fall in $FEV_1$ after the inhalation of a methacholine solution at a concentration of less than 25 mg/mL is indicative of a positive response.[10]

## SPECIFIC TESTS

### Bronchial Challenges

Specific airway reactivity can be assessed by measuring the patient's bronchial response to the inhalation of certain allergen

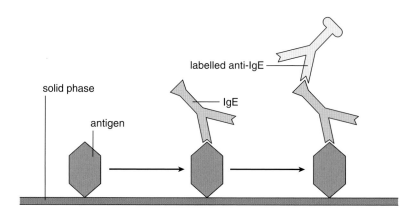

1. add antigen (allergen)    2. add IgE (test serum)    3. add anti-IgE (ligand)

block disc    wash    wash and count

**Figure 3-8.** The sandwich enzyme immunoassay (EIA). This test measures antigen-specific IgE in an EIA where the ligand is an enzyme-labeled anti-IgE antibody. The antigen (allergen) is covalently bound to a cellulose surface. Having much more antigen available on the surface permits the high sensitivity necessary to bind the small quantities of IgE present in the test serum. (Adapted with permission from Roitt et al., 2001.)

---

**TABLE 3-6**
**EIA Versus Skin Tests**

| EIA Advantages | Rebuttals |
|---|---|
| Greater safety | There is virtually no risk to a carefully performed and administered epicutaneous skin test. |
| Quantitative results | Though it provides quantitative results, EIA is fraught with technical problems. Studies have shown tremendous variability in results from one laboratory to another. |
| Not influenced by drugs | Stopping antihistamines 72 hr before skin testing obviates any interference by medications in that technique. |
| Greater allergen stability | Epicutaneous extracts stored in glycerine are as stable as EIA allergens. |
| Preferable for children | There is actually less physical and emotional trauma to small children in epicutaneous skin testing. |
| Preferable for patients with dermographism | Dermographism can be overcome with the use of appropriate antihistamines and lesser downward pressure when epicutaneous skin testing is performed. |
| Preferable for patients with widespread dermatitis | It is rare to find a skin condition so severe that a small patch of normal skin cannot be found for skin tests. |
| Fewer immunotherapy injections | EIA proponents claim that a modification of the EIA makes it possible to place patients in different clinical classes so that immunotherapy can start at higher concentrations, thereby decreasing the total number of injections. A recent, well-controlled study showed that in 98% of allergic patients, the starting dose was the same as the one "conventional" allergists used. |

EIA, enzyme-linked immunoassay.

solutions. There is evidence that skin test results generally correlate well with bronchial-provocation test results. Therefore, bronchial-challenge testing with specific allergens is generally not necessary in everyday practice. There may be special instances, however, such as with occupational asthma (see Chapter 6), or in investigative work when specific bronchial-challenge testing is indicated. Several bronchial responses have been documented after the inhalation of antigen solutions. Figure 3-11 illustrates the immediate, dual, and late-phase responses that are seen. The "classic" asthmatic response to inhaled allergens had been thought to be immediate, occurring in all cases within minutes, but it is now estimated that approximately 50% of allergic asthmatics demonstrate a dual immediate and late-phase response. An isolated late-phase bronchial response is seen largely in instances of occupational asthma. Pretreatment with different medications may alter the bronchial responses to antigen inhalation. Beta agonists block the late reaction but have no effect on the immediate response, and pretreatment with cromolyn inhibits both bronchial responses.

## Nasal Challenges

Inhaled antigen solutions can also be used to challenge the nasal mucosa, to diagnose allergic rhinitis. The response can be gauged by the measurement of nasal airway resistance through anterior or posterior rhinomanometry or by changes in the cellular or mediator content of the nasal mucus. The nasal challenge technique is useful in studying the pathophysiology of the nose, the action of drugs, and instances of occupational rhinitis (see Chapter 6).

## Oral Challenges

In instances when a suspected allergen is ingested, an oral challenge can be performed. The challenge can be open, in which case both the physician and the patient know the content of the substance ingested; single blind, with only the doctor knowing the content; or double blind, with neither the patient nor the physician knowing the content of the challenge. The food or drug

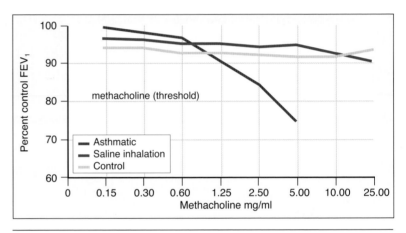

**Figure 3-10.** The effect of methacholine inhalation on an asthmatic patient. The asthmatic subject shows a greater than 20% fall in $FEV_1$ after inhalation of methacholine 5 mg/mL. Saline inhalation results in no change in $FEV_1$. A control patient inhales methacholine through a concentration of 25 mg/mL and shows no change in $FEV_1$.

| TABLE 3-7 | |
|---|---|
| **Provocative Challenge Tests** | |
| **Nonspecific** | **Specific (Antigen)** |
| Exercise | Bronchial |
| Assessment of airway reactivity | Nasal |
|    Histamine | |
|    Methacholine | Oral |
|    Cold air | Injection |
| |    Local anesthetics |
| |    Stinging insects |

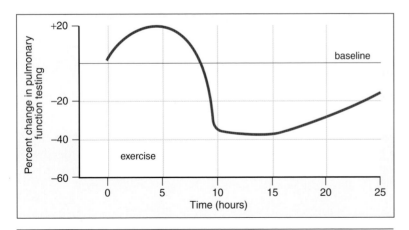

**Figure 3-9.** A classic response in exercise-induced asthma.

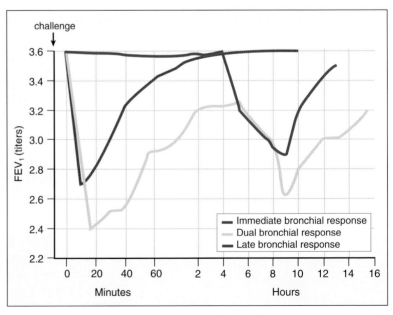

**Figure 3-11.** The different patterns of bronchial response after a bronchial challenge.

can be administered either whole or in a lyophilized preparation contained in an opaque capsule.

Oral challenges serve several purposes. First, double-blind, placebo-controlled food challenges have proven useful in discerning IgE-mediated food sensitivities (see Chapter 13). Second, oral challenges can also help diagnose sensitivity to ingested substances, such as aspirin or sulfites, in which the sensitivity is not on an IgE basis (Fig. 3-12). In such instances, skin testing or measurement of serum specific IgE levels would be of no use.

## Injections

When an antigen causing an IgE-mediated allergic response is delivered by the injected route, skin testing or measurement of serum-specific IgE levels serves as an adequate diagnostic procedure. Examples of injected-route allergies are naturally occurring phenomena, such as insect stings (see Chapter 4), or the iatrogenic administration of penicillin subcutaneously or intramuscularly (see Chapter 17).

As with oral challenges, some substances that are injected may cause reactions that are not IgE mediated. Local anesthetics are examples of agents for which skin testing or measurement of serum-specific IgE levels are of little use in detecting sensitivity. In these instances, a graduated type of challenge up to the full therapeutic dose may be utilized (Table 3-8).

A naturally occurring injection in the form of a *Hymenoptera* family insect sting has been carried out at some medical centers. This has been performed to determine whether a preceding course of immunotherapy with venom of that particular insect had been successful. At present, this is an experimental technique that should only be performed under the most carefully controlled conditions.

# UNPROVEN DIAGNOSTIC TECHNIQUES AND THEORIES

In this chapter, we have thus far discussed diagnostic techniques that have scientific validity and have been subjected to careful evaluation. A group of practitioners who often refer to their medical practice as "clinical ecology" offer allergic patients alternative ways to diagnose allergies; these have no scientific basis and have not been subjected to careful controlled scrutiny.[11] Table 3-9 lists several diagnostic techniques and theories that are unproven and in some instances have been shown to be invalid.

The cytotoxic test is based on the unproven theory that food allergy alters the morphology of leukocytes. Several blind studies have shown the test to be totally invalid. In the provocation-neutralization technique, increasing doses of a substance are

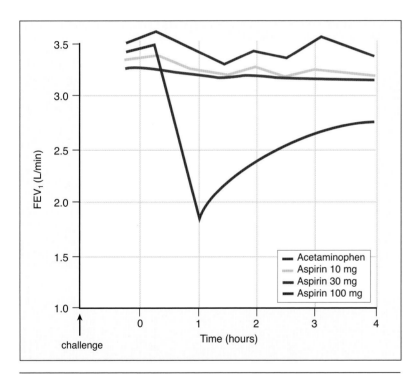

**Figure 3-12.** An aspirin challenge in an aspirin-sensitive asthmatic. A graduated increase in aspirin dosage results in a significant fall in FEV$_1$ 1 hour after ingesting 100 mg. An acetaminophen challenge is negative.

**TABLE 3-8**
**Suggested Schedule for Local Anesthetic Challenge**

| Technique | Dose |
| --- | --- |
| Puncture | Full strength |
| Intradermal | 0.02 mL diluted 1:100 |
| Inradermal | 0.02 mL full strength |
| Subcutaneous | 0.10 mL full strength |
| Subcutaneous | 0.50 mL full strength |

**TABLE 3-9**
Unproven Diagnostic Techniques and Theories

| Unproven Diagnostic Techniques | Unproven Theories |
| --- | --- |
| Cytotoxic tests | Multiple chemical sensitivity |
| Provocation–neutralization | *Candida* hypersensitivity syndrome |
| Applied kinesiology | |
| IgG or immune complexes to foods | |

IgG, immunoglobulin G.

administered subcutaneously or sublingually until the patient experiences a "sensation." Further concentrations are then given until the patient reports the absence of symptoms. A double-blind placebo-controlled study demonstrated no difference between the test substance and the placebo. Applied kinesiology is based on a claim that allergy impairs the strength of skeletal muscle. There is no scientific basis for this, and there are no clinical studies of efficacy. Laboratory tests can, indeed, detect both IgG antibodies and immune complexes to food, but there is simply no proof that they are responsible for IgE-mediated allergic disease. For example, antigluten IgG antibodies are present in certain patients who have gluten (wheat)-provoked celiac disease.

Multiple-chemical sensitivity embodies the concept that a whole host of symptoms may be caused by exposure to ordinary quantities of synthetic chemicals in our environment. The syndrome is characterized by subjective symptoms only; there are no physical findings, and there is no pathology. There is no scientific evidence that such an entity exists, but the number of patients claiming such sensitivity continues to rise.

*Candida* hypersensitivity is the concept that the normal presence of *Candida albicans* in the body can cause multisystem, polysymptomatic subjective illness. Patients are advised to follow a strict diet and take antifungal drugs. A well-controlled study demonstrated that antifungal agents had no more effect than placebo, and such therapy is inappropriate.

# FUTURE DEVELOPMENTS

In this chapter, we have reviewed diagnostic tests in allergy and attempted to put the various techniques presently in use into their proper clinical contexts. It is anticipated that investigative work being performed currently will result in more accurate diagnoses of allergic diseases in the future. In particular, new immunochemical procedures for purifying antigens hold great promise. With better-defined, -characterized, and -standardized antigens that can be used for both in vitro and in vivo testing, diagnostic capabilities will be markedly enhanced. Other exciting advances include the measurement of exhaled nitric oxide and other inflammatory mediators to potentially aid in the diagnosis and management of patients with asthma and allergic disorders.[12,13]

# REFERENCES

1. Demoly P, Michel F-B, Bousquet J: In vivo methods for study of allergy: Skin tests, techniques and interpretation. In Middleton E Jr, Reed CE, Ellis EF, et al (eds): Allergy: Principles and Practice, 5th ed. St Louis, C.V. Mosby, 1998, pp 430–439.
2. Roitt IM, Brostoff J, Male DK: Immunology, 5th ed. London, Mosby, 2001, pp 19.1–19.7.
3. Gentile DA, Michaels MG, Skoner DP: Allergy and immunology. In Zitelli BJ, Davis HW (eds): Atlas of Pediatric Physical Diagnosis, 4th ed. London, Gower Medical Publishing, 2002, pp 87–126.
4. Hagy GW, Settipane GA: Prognosis of positive allergy skin tests in an asymptomatic population. J Allergy Clin Immunol 1971;48:200–211.
5. Ownby DR: Clinical significance of IgE. In Middleton E Jr, Reed CE, Ellis EF, et al (eds): Allergy: Principles and Practice, 5th ed. St Louis, C.V. Mosby, 1998.
6. Leimgruber A, Mosimann B, Clacys M, Seppey M, Jacard Y: Clinical evaluation of a new in-vitro assay for specific IgE, the immune CAP system. Clin Exp Allergy 1991; 21:127–131.
7. Homburger HA: Methods in laboratory immunology. In Middleton E Jr, Reed CE, Ellis EF, et al (eds): Allergy: Principles and Practice, 5th ed. St Louis, C.V. Mosby, 1998, pp 417–429.
8. Hamilton RG, Adkinson NF: Clinical laboratory assessment of IgE-dependent hypersensitivity. J Allergy Clin Immunol 2003;111:S687–S701.
9. Naclerio RM, Norman PS: In vivo methods for study of allergic rhinitis: Mucosal tests, techniques and interpretation. In Middleton E Jr, Reed CE, Ellis EF, et al (eds): Allergy: Principles and Practice, 5th ed. St Louis, C.V. Mosby, 1998, pp 440–453.
10. Fish JE, Peters SP: Bronchial challenge testing. In Middleton E Jr, Reed CE, Ellis EF, et al (eds): Allergy: Principles and Practice, 5th ed. St Louis, C.V. Mosby, 1998, pp 454–464.
11. Terr AI: Unconventional theories and unproven methods in allergy. In Middleton E Jr, Reed CE, Ellis EF, et al (eds): Allergy: Principles and Practice, 5th ed. St Louis, C.V. Mosby, 1998, pp 1235–1249.
12. Kharitonov SA, Donnelly LE, Montuschi P, et al: Dose-dependent onset and cessation of action of inhaled budesonide on exhaled nitric oxide and symptoms in mild asthma. Thorax 2002;57:889–896.
13. Csoma Z, Kharitonov SA, Balint B, et al: Increased leukotrienes in exhaled breath condensate in childhood asthma. Am J Respir Crit Care Med 2002; 166:1345–1349.

*Gilbert A. Friday, Jr. and Philip Fireman*

# *4* Anaphylaxis and Insect Allergy

The term *anaphylaxis* has been used to define the allergic adverse reaction characterized by systemic clinical manifestations that occur in an individual who had been primarily sensitized to a foreign substance on subsequent reexposure by any route, whether inhalation, oral, or injection, of the same material. A potentially life-threatening clinical syndrome, anaphylaxis was initially defined in 1902 by Portier and Richet as a fatal reaction to injection of a previously tolerated foreign protein during prophylaxis antisera treatment in dogs. The term *anaphylaxis* was derived from the Greek words *a*- (against) and -*phylaxis* (immunity, protection).[1] Approximately 4500 years earlier, the Egyptians described fatal reactions to *Hymenoptera* insect stings, which probably represented anaphylaxis.

Over the years, anaphylaxis has gradually come to mean the acute life-threatening syndrome that results from the rapid release of large amounts of chemical mediators of inflammation from mast cells and basophils in response to a specific allergen in a previously sensitized host. The allergens responsible for reactions can be protein, hapten-protein conjugates, lipoproteins, or polysaccharides.

The clinical features of anaphylaxis are produced typically by immunologic mechanisms, but nonimmunologic-mediated reactions also occur. Immune-provoked anaphylaxis is mediated by immunoglobulin (Ig) E antibody or immune antigen–antibody complexes. Perhaps the most common causes of anaphylaxis today are adverse drug reactions, especially to penicillin. Nonimmune anaphylaxis occurs in relation to direct mast cell degranulating agents, such as opiates, radiocontrast media, and nonsteroidal anti-inflammatory agents. Idiopathic anaphylaxis may also occur.

The terms *anaphylactic* and *anaphylactoid* refer to similar if not identical syndromes but have been utilized in the past by some clinicians as meaning IgE-mediated or non–IgE-mediated systemic reactions, respectively. Detailed clinical examples of immune and nonimmune types of anaphylaxis provoked by drug reactions, insect stings, and exercise are presented later in this chapter.

## EPIDEMIOLOGY

Data on the overall incidence of anaphylaxis are unavailable, as it is not a reportable disease in the United States. The estimated risk of anaphylaxis in the United States is 1% to 3%.[2,3] Anaphylactic reactions have been described at approximately 2.5 per 1000 (0.25%) for allergen injections administered in aeroallergen immunotherapy of respiratory allergic disease.[4] Fatal anaphylaxis due to penicillin allergy has been reported at a rate of 0.002% for parenteral injections and is much less frequent for oral penicillin therapy.[5] Antibiotics in general may account for one death in 50,000 to 100,000 courses. The incidence of anaphylaxis in the perioperative period is estimated at 1:5000 cases, with 3% to 4% deaths. Hymenoptera insect sting anaphylaxis probably accounts for 50 deaths per year.[6] An estimated 150 fatalities from food-induced anaphylaxis occur each year in the United States.[7]

## ETIOLOGY

### *IMMUNE MECHANISMS*

#### IgE-Mediated Reactions

A wide variety of agents are potentially responsible for IgE-mediated anaphylaxis; a partial list of the most common is provided in Box 4-1. Antibiotics, such as the penicillins and cephalosporins, cause anaphylactic reactions through a hapten-protein–initiated IgE antibody–mediated mechanism. Proteins—including insulin, chymotrypsin, and venoms—as well as therapeutic agents—such as allergy vaccines and various other vaccines—can also be responsible. Foods are a significant source of IgE-mediated anaphylaxis, reactions most commonly occurring with eggs, shellfish, and nuts.[7]

#### Non–IgE-Mediated Mechanisms

Anaphylaxis may occur during the administration of blood and blood products through a non-IgE immune complex (probably IgG) mechanism. These reactions are provoked by the development of antibodies to the red blood cell antigen or plasma protein (such as immunoglobulin), are presumed to be mediated by activation of complement, and can also induce anaphylaxis via fixation of complement. However, administration of blood products containing IgA to selective IgA-deficient patients may induce the development of IgE antibodies to IgA, which could mediate an anaphylactic reaction.

## NONIMMUNE MECHANISMS

Box 4-2 lists agents that cause anaphylaxis via nonimmune mechanisms. Direct mast cell degranulating agents, such as opiates, curare muscle relaxants, plasma expander polysaccharides (dextran), certain antibiotics, and iodinated radiocontrast media, have been noted to release histamine from basophils and mast cells. Aspirin is also known to cause anaphylaxis through uncertain mechanisms. Aspirin-sensitive patients may also show intolerance to other nonsteroidal anti-inflammatory agents, including ibuprofen, indomethacin, and tolmetin. The role of tartrazine and other dyes in producing anaphylaxis is a matter of controversy. Patients with systemic mastocytosis can also manifest reactions resembling anaphylaxis due to release of histamine and other mediators from the abundant and excessive mast cells without an overt immune mechanism.

## IDIOPATHIC ANAPHYLAXIS

A number of patients are also recognized as having idiopathic anaphylaxis, during which symptoms occur in the absence of any identifiable inciting agent.[8] It is thought that this type of reaction may represent the most severe form of a spectrum of immediate-type reactions due to abnormal and inappropriate mast cell or basophil activation. Exercise-induced anaphylaxis may be included in this category. These individuals have been described as developing anaphylaxis more readily after eating certain foods, such as celery, just prior to exercise. Another subgroup of patients with idiopathic anaphylaxis has been classified as having an undifferentiated somatoform disorder, because the patient history mimics idiopathic anaphylaxis but lacks correlating objective physical findings and has no response to appropriate therapy.[9]

## CLINICAL PRESENTATION

Systemic anaphylaxis frequently involves multiple organ systems of the body, including the skin and the respiratory, gastrointestinal, genital, cardiac, and neural systems. The clinical manifestations are outlined in Box 4-3. The most important and life-threatening features are those involving the cardiovascular system and respiratory tract. Individuals vary greatly in their manifestations of anaphylaxis, especially in the manner of onset and course. It may develop rapidly, reaching peak severity within 5 to 30 minutes. Late-phase reactions may occur 6 to 12 hours later and may last 5 to 30 hours, despite treatment. The typical patient develops generalized itching followed by cutaneous flushing, urticaria, a fullness in the throat, a feeling of "anxiety," then tightness in the chest, faintness, and, finally, loss of consciousness.

Austen described the clinical and postmortem findings in six cases of fatal human anaphylaxis, calling attention to the fact that the interval between parenteral administration of an allergen and death ranged from a brief 16 minutes to 2 hours.[10]

### CUTANEOUS AND RESPIRATORY SYMPTOMS

Skin manifestations, including pruritus, angioedema, and urticaria, can predominate (Fig. 4-1A). Acute swelling, as seen following a bee sting in Figure 4-1B, may be followed by upper airway swelling and respiratory failure. Involvement of the eyes, nose, and mouth, with tearing, redness of the eyes, runny nose, stuffiness, and sneezing may be accompanied by or seen in concert with upper respiratory signs and symptoms of hoarseness or a sensation of narrowing in the throat, with stridor, edema of the uvula, and, eventually, in some instances, complete laryngeal obstruction. Lower respiratory symptoms may involve hyperventilation,

---

**BOX 4-1**
**Examples of Agents Causing Anaphylaxis via Immune Mechanisms**

**IgE Mediated**
1. **Antimicrobial agents (haptens)**
   Penicillin, cephalosporin, tetracycline, aminoglycoside, streptomycin, amphotericin-B, nitrofurantoin, sulfamethoxazole

2. **Hormones**
   Insulin, TSH, corticotrophin, progesterone, ACTH

3. **Enzymes**
   Streptokinase, penicillinase, chymotrypsin, trypsin

4. **Antiserum**
   Tetanus, diphtheria, antitoxins, antithymocyte, antilymphocyte globulin

5. **Venoms (and saliva)**
   *Hymenoptera* (bee, vespid and wasp, fire ant), *Chrysops* (deer fly), triatoma (kissing bug)

6. **Vaccines**
   Tetanus, egg-containing vaccines (influenza), allergen vaccines

7. **Foods**
   Milk, egg, wheat, fish and shellfish, legumes (peanuts), nuts (tree); exercise with foods

8. **Miscellaneous**
   Latex, seminal fluid; animal or human proteins; polysaccharides

**Complement Mediated**
1. Transfusion reaction associated with IgA deficiency
2. Cytotoxic (cell-fixed antigen, transfusion reactions to cellular elements, IgG, IgM)
3. Aggregate (intravenous immunoglobulins)

ACTH, adrenocorticotropic hormone; Ig, immunoglobulin; TSH, thyroid-stimulating hormone.

wheezing associated with bronchospasm and asthma, decreased air exchange, use of accessory muscles, and, finally, apnea with respiratory arrest. The more rapid the onset of the signs and symptoms of anaphylaxis after exposure to an offending stimulus, the more likely the reaction will be severe and life threatening.

## CARDIOVASCULAR AND NEUROLOGIC SYMPTOMS

Cardiovascular signs are very frequent in anaphylaxis and may vary from marked tachycardia to bradycardia or dysrhythmias. Table 4-1 lists electrocardiographic changes in 186 patients with cardiovascular collapse due to clinical anaphylaxis. Hypotension may eventually lead to cardiac arrest. Myocardial infarction has been reported to complicate anaphylaxis. Chemical mediators of anaphylaxis appear to affect the myocardium directly. Histamine receptor type 1 ($H_1$) mediates coronary vasoconstriction and increases vascular permeability, whereas $H_2$ increases atrial and ventricular contractile forces, atrial rate, and coronary artery vasodilation. The interaction of $H_1$ and $H_2$ stimulation appears to mediate decreased diastolic pressure and increased pulse pressure. There may be a modulatory role for $H_3$. Echocardiography, nuclear imaging, and hemodynamic measurements confirm the presence of myocardial function.

Increased vascular permeability during anaphylaxis can result in a transfer of 50% of the intravascular fluid into the extravascular space within 10 minutes.[11] This shift in effective blood volume activates the renin-angiotension-aldosterone system and

---

**BOX 4-2**
**Examples of Nonimmune Mechanisms or Conditions Causing Anaphylaxis (Immunoglobulin E Independent)**

1. **Direct histamine-releasing agents**
   Muscle relaxants, ciproflaxin, vancomycin, pentamidine, radiocontrast media, angiotensin-converting enzyme inhibitor, opioids, plasma expander polysaccharides (Dextran)

2. **Arachidonate mediated**
   Aspirin and nonsteroidal anti-inflammatory drugs

3. **Physical**
   Exercise, temperature (cold, heat)

4. **Idiopathic**

5. **Undifferentiated somatoform idiopathic anaphylaxis**
   Nonorganic symptoms mimicking anaphylaxis

---

**BOX 4-3**
**Clinical Manifestations of Anaphylaxis**

1. **Cutaneous**
   Pruritus, erythema, urticaria, angioedema

2. **Respiratory**
   Sneezing, rhinorrhea, hoarseness, dysphonia, lump in throat, edema of upper airway (tongue, uvula, vocal cords), tachypnea, bronchospasm (wheezing, decreased breath sounds), apnea, asphyxia

3. **Cardiovascular**
   Tachycardia, arrhythmia, vascular collapse, cardiac arrest (myocardial infarction)

4. **Gastrointestinal**
   Nausea, vomiting, cramps, pain, watery or bloody stools

5. **Genital**
   Uterine cramps

6. **Neuropsychiatric**
   Seizures, feelings of "impending doom," unconsciousness

---

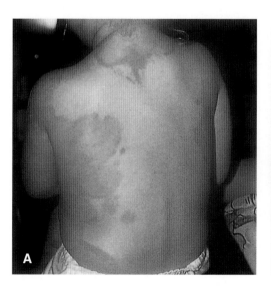
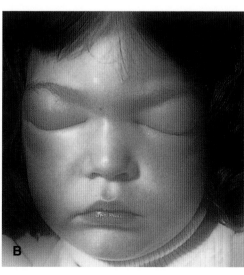

**Figure 4-1.** *A,* Acute urticaria associated with anaphylaxis. *B,* Facial swelling (angioedema), following a hymenoptera sting, associated with systemic anaphylaxis.

| ECG Changes | Patients, *n* |
|---|---|
| Supraventricular tachycardia | 153 |
| Supraventricular tachycardia with sinus tachycardia elevation | 8 |
| Supraventricular tachycardia with ventricular fibrillation | 4 |
| Supraventricular tachycardia following transient sinus bradycardia | 6 |
| Sinus bradycardia in presence of beta-blockers | 4 |
| Bradycardia and asystole | 2 |
| Rapid atrial fibrillation | 4 |
| Other | 5 |

**TABLE 4-1**

Electrocardiographic Changes in 186 Patients with Cardiovascular Collapse Due to Clinical Anaphylaxis

Reproduced with permission from Fisher M: Anaphylaxis. Disease-a-Month 1987;33:433.

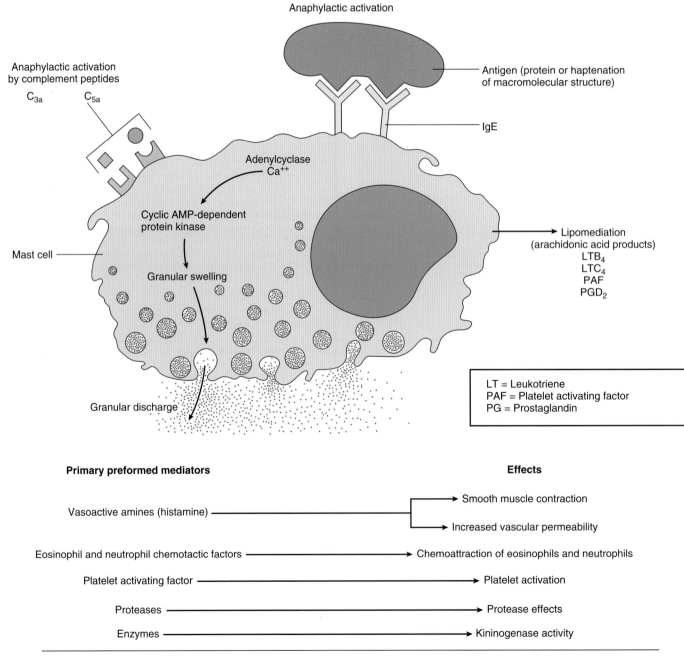

**Figure 4-2.** Activation of the mast cell. Ca++, calcium ion; IgE, immunoglobulin E.

causes compensatory catecholamine release, both of which have variable clinical effects from a cardiovascular standpoint. Because antibodies attached to mast cell receptors can trigger degranulation, this could cause vasospasm. It has been hypothesized that any allergic reaction may potentially facilitate coronary artery plaque disruption, which, in association with vasospasm, may cause myocardial infarction.

Neurologic symptoms may be secondary to hypoxia and include dizziness, weakness, seizures, and even the sensation of "impending doom."

# PATHOGENESIS

## IMMUNOGLOBULIN E MEDIATION

Immunoglobulin E mediation has been considered responsible for anaphylaxis caused by antibiotics, foreign proteins, foods, drugs, preservatives, and venoms. Anaphylaxis mediated by IgE may occur in both atopic and nonatopic patients, indicating that a prior history of allergic rhinitis, atopic dermatitis, and asthma does not necessarily define an IgE-mediated mechanism as being operative in a particular anaphylactic situation. In fact, anaphylaxis is rarely a consequence of the natural exposure of an atopic individual to an allergen. IgE antibodies on the surface of mast cells mediate anaphylaxis by binding to complete antigens or to antigen determinants formed by the covalent attachment of haptens (incomplete antigens) to large molecules such as albumin (Fig. 4-2). This interaction leads to the release of several preformed mast cell mediators, which are listed in Box 4-4. In addition, this IgE immune response initiates a group of phospholipid-derived mediators whose synthetic pathways are diagrammed in Figure 4-3. These include platelet-activating factor and the arachidonic acid–derived mediators, leukotrienes (LTs), prostaglandins, lipoxins, and thromboxanes.

## MEDIATOR RELEASE

The mast cell mediator identified most commonly in anaphylaxis is histamine, and tissues rich in mast cells are the primary target tissues in anaphylaxis. Figure 4-4 relates plasma histamine levels with some symptoms and manifestation of anaphylaxis.[12] Histamine activates $H_1$ and $H_2$ receptors. Pruritus, rhinorrhea, tachycardia, and bronchospasm are caused by activation of $H_1$, whereas both $H_1$ and $H_2$ mediate headache, flushing, and hypotension. $H_3$ has been implicated in the canine model of anaphylaxis.[13] Potential implications for $H_3$ for human subjects and anaphylaxis have not been studied.

Tryptases are concentrated in the secretory granules of human mast cells, and release correlates with clinical severity. β-Tryptase is stored in mast cell secretory granules, and its release may be more specific for activation than that of α-protryptase, which appears to be secreted constitutively.[14]

---

**BOX 4-4**
**Classes of Preformed Human Mast-Cell Mediators**

1. Biogenic amines (histamine)
2. Neutral proteases (tryptase, chymase, carboxypeptidase)
3. Acid hydrolases (arysulfatase)
4. Oxidative enzymes (superoxide, peroxidase)
5. Chemotactic factors (eosinophil, neutrophil)
6. Proteoglycans (heparin)
7. Histamine-releasing factor

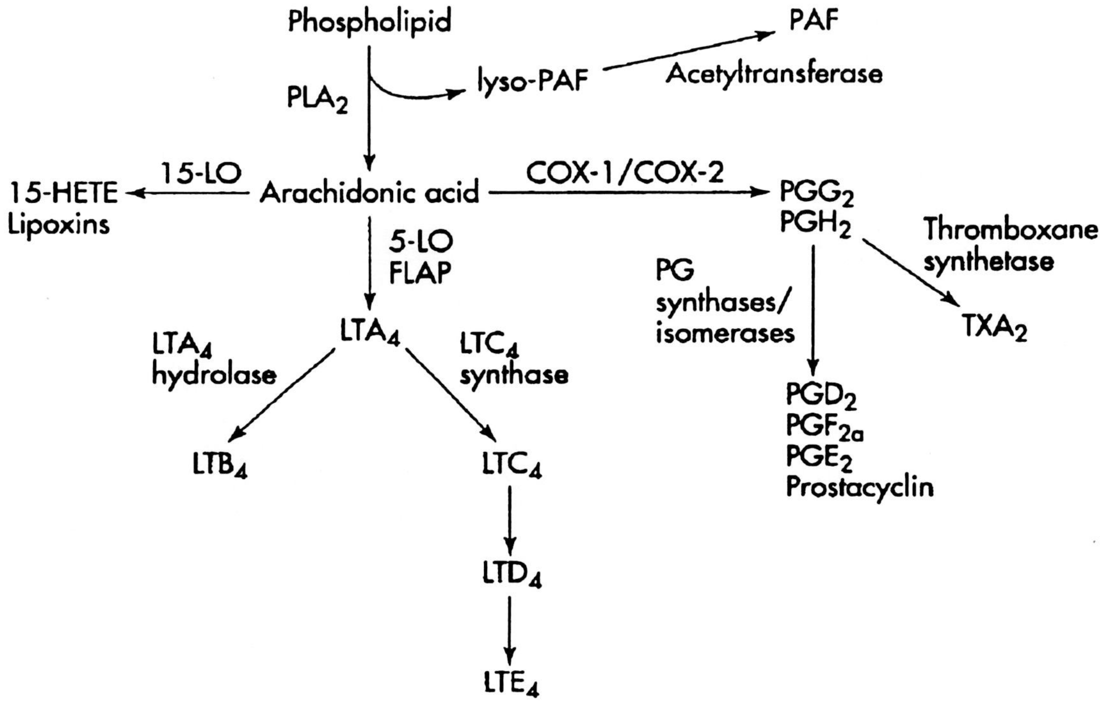

---

Figure 4-3. Lipid mediator synthetic pathways. COX, cyclo-oxygenase; FLAP, 5-lipoxygenase activating protein; HETE, hydroxyeicosatetraenoic acid; LO, lipoxygenase; LT, leukotriene; PAF, platelet-activating factor; PG, prostaglandin; $PLA_2$, phospholipase $A_2$; $TXA_2$, thromboxane $A_2$.

Other pathogenetic factors that must be considered include nitric oxide, a potent autacoid vasodilator, as well as metabolites of arachidonic acid, the LTs, and prostaglandins, which are products of the lipoxygenase and cyclo-oxgenase pathways. $LTB_4$ might contribute to the late phase of anaphylaxis and to protracted reactions.

Anaphylaxis can also follow the release of mediators following massive complement activation, which generates anaphylatoxins $C_{3a}$ and $C_{5a}$ (see Fig. 4-2). These anaphylatoxins bind to mast cell receptors, alter the cell membrane, and initiate mast cell degranulation. The mechanisms by which acetylsalicylic acid and other structurally unrelated nonsteroidal anti-inflammatory agents that cause anaphylaxis are not fully understood. When aspirin is introduced, cyclo-oxygenase-1 is inhibited in all cells of the body, and LTs and prostaglandin $E_2$ is rapidly depleted. Without prostaglandin $E_2$, 5-lipoxygenase rapidly synthesizes more LTs, producing the adverse respiratory reactions seen when the entire body is affected. An alternative theory is that cyclo-oxygenase-2 is altered by aspirin and synthesizes a new metabolite, 15-hydroxy-eicosatetraenoic acid, that is converted by leukocyte 5-lipoxygenase to 15 epilipoxin, one of a newly discovered class of mediators that modulate inflammation by decreasing leukocyte activity.[15] Their ability to induce anaphylaxis may possibly be related to their potency in inhibiting prostaglandin synthesis by shifting arachidonic acid metabolism to lipoxygenase-dependent pathways or by activating platelets. Disorders of hemostasis have been observed during anaphylaxis, possibly related to release of heparin from mast cells or alteration of platelets or other components of hemostasis and coagulant. The role of specific mediators in the pathogenesis of anaphylaxis remains speculative. One can presume that a diverse number of mediators act in concert to produce the clinical pathologic findings.

## PATHOLOGY

The principle anatomic and microscopic findings in fatal anaphylaxis include pulmonary emphysema (Fig. 4-5), laryngeal edema (Fig. 4-6), visceral congestion, pulmonary edema, intra-alveolar hemorrhage, urticaria, and angioedema. These findings result from hypoxia and hypovolemia. Autopsy findings may be complicated by therapeutic measures (iatrogenic procedures).

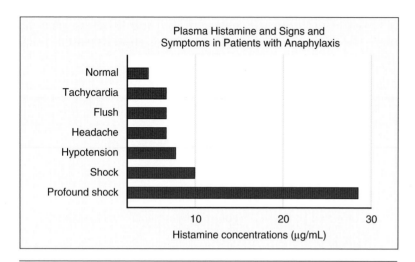

**Figure 4-4.** Symptoms and signs associated with plasma histamine levels in normal subjects and patients experiencing anaphylaxis with varying degrees of severity. (Modified with permission from Fisher M: Anaphylaxis. Disease-a-Month 1987;33:433.)

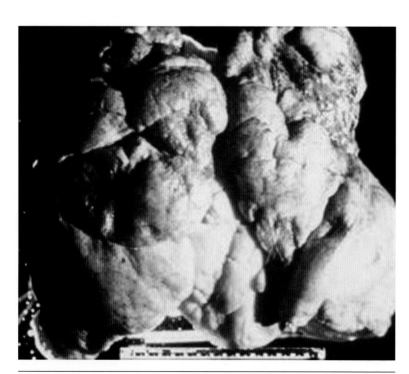

**Figure 4-5.** Pulmonary emphysema.

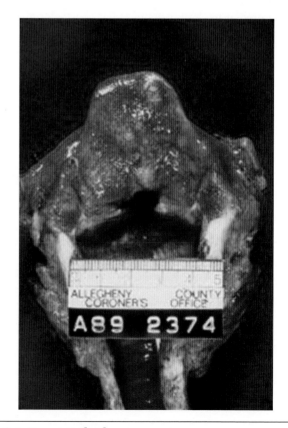

**Figure 4-6.** Laryngeal edema.

Microscopic evidence (Fig. 4-7) that suggests myocardial infarction, pulmonary hemorrhage, edema, increased bronchial secretions, peribronchial vascular congestion, and eosinophilic infiltration of the bronchial walls can be found. There is accumulation of thin noninflammatory fluid in the lamina propria of the hypopharynx, epiglottis, and larynx in as many as two thirds of fatal cases. Other less-specific findings associated with systemic anaphylaxis include liver, spleen, and other abdominal visceral congestion, with an increased number of eosinophils in the red pulp of the spleen. Hemorrhagic gastritis also may be seen.

# DIAGNOSIS

## PHYSICAL EVALUATION

The diagnosis of systemic anaphylaxis has been based on recognition of the clinical features. It is generally, but not always readily, apparent. Urticaria and angioedema are the most common manifestations of anaphylaxis, followed by respiratory tract symptoms, dizziness, syncope, and gastrointestinal symptoms. The more rapidly anaphylaxis occurs after exposure to an offending stimulus, the more likely the reaction is severe and potentially life threatening.

The patient with vasovagal collapse (a neuropsychological reaction) can be confused with anaphylaxis. This typically occurs during stressful circumstances, such as during venipuncture or injection. The patient appears pale, complains of nausea, sweats, has bradycardia, and generally maintains a normal blood pressure. There is no pruritus, urticaria, tachycardia, or angioedema. If laryngeal edema is present during anaphylaxis, hoarseness or aphonia develops. Globus hystericus, the disturbing subjective sensation of a lump in the throat seen in hysteria conversion/ behavior disorders, may be considered. However, it is usually milder, nonprogressive, and without any signs of anatomic changes in the pharynx or hypopharnyx. Other medical conditions that are occasionally confused with anaphylaxis are listed in Box 4-5.

This differential diagnosis includes cardiac dysrhythmias, pulmonary embolism, seizures, strokes, hyperventilation, hereditary angioedema, and hypoglycemia.

# LABORATORY EVALUATION

Laboratory evaluation of the patient with anaphylactic hypersenstivity is performed to identify the potential causative antigens or agents. It can best be performed by in vivo skin tests for certain agents and in vitro tests for others. IgE antibody to insect venoms or penicillin can be detected by the more-sensitive epicutaneous (prick modification of the scratch) skin test, using appropriate precautions. Although less sensitive, it may be safer to initially perform in vitro serum tests for IgE antibodies to suspected anaphylaxis-provoking allergens, such as foods, which are less well characterized. Such tests, including radioallergosorbent (RAST) or enzyme-linked immunosorbent assay (ELISA), eliminate the risk of inducing anaphylaxis by introducing allergen onto or into the skin. Serum histamine release from leukocytes of sensitive individuals on in vitro challenge is not yet suitable for clinical practice and is limited to research studies at this time. Complement consumption in vitro has not been utilized to define anaphylactic mechanisms, although its absence in vivo has been noted in exercise-induced anaphylaxis. Serum histamine levels have been measured and correlated with symptoms of anaphylaxis but are not yet practical in the clinical management of anaphylaxis because of its rapid catabolism. Urine histamine levels may be elevated but are rarely clinically useful. However, serum tryptase levels should be used as an indicator of anaphylaxis. Elevated serum tryptase levels may persist as long as 18 hours after the event.

Oral provocative challenge studies with various foods, chemicals, and drugs can be performed but may be hazardous if previous experience has been life threatening. However, sensitivity to aspirin and other nonsteroidal anti-inflammatory agents may be confirmed by carefully graded oral challenge with close monitoring, observation, and measurement of pulmonary function and blood pressure.

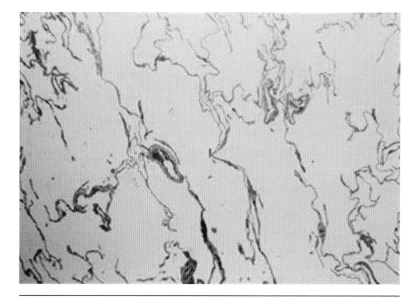

**Figure 4-7.** Microscopic changes: lung.

---

**BOX 4-5**
**Disorders Confused with Anaphylaxis**

1. **Cardiac conditions**
   Dysrhythmias, myocardial infarction, arrest

2. **Endocrine problems**
   Carcinoid tumor, pheochromocytoma, hypoglycemia

3. **Pulmonary embolus**
   Pneumothorax, hyperventilation, severe asthma, tracheal foreign body (food, etc.)

4. **Neurologic conditions**
   Head injury, epilepsy, cerebrovascular accident

5. **Other problems**
   Hereditary angioedema, drug/alcohol reactions, factitious stridor, cold urticaria

# TREATMENT OF ANAPHYLAXIS

The treatment of anaphylaxis can be life saving. Prompt recognition is essential, as death may occur within minutes. Therapy, as outlined in Box 4-6, must be initiated even if there is doubt about the diagnosis, such as in the instance of vasovagal neurogenic reactions following parenteral administration of a vaccine or allergen extract.[2,16,17] Anoxia is life threatening, and an adequate airway with supplements of oxygen when available is essential. Equipment helpful in this emergency situation is shown in Figure 4-8.

## MEDICAL TREATMENT

The initial treatment of anaphylaxis with epinephrine is crucial in

- Supporting blood pressure
- Decreasing bronchospasm, which helps maintain an effective airway

- Decreasing laryngeal edema, especially when given as a racemic epinephrine aerosol
- Slowing the absorption of injected agents if promptly used to infiltrate the site of injection

A tourniquet can also be applied above the injection site, because this can reduce and compress venous return at the site of an injection and decrease systemic absorption of antigen. It should be released for 1 of every 3 minutes.

It is essential to move the patient as soon as possible to an emergency room or intensive care hospital facility that can manage major complications, such as cardiac arrhythmias, cardiorespiratory arrest, seizures, myocardial infarction, hypovolemia, and obstruction of the airway. Antihistamines ($H_1$ and $H_2$ blockers) are suggested and may decrease the potential for cardiac arrhythmias and peripheral vasodilation, as well as possibly urticaria/angioedema and gastrointestinal symptoms. Corticosteroids, although requiring several hours to exert beneficial effects, are indicated and may prevent late-phase reactions. Recurrent or biphasic anaphylaxis occurs 8 to 12 hours after the initial attack in as many as 20% of subjects who experience anaphylaxis.

If a patient who is on therapy with a beta-adrenergic–blocking agent, such as propranolol for hypertension, vascular headaches, mitral valve prolapse, or cardiac arrhythmias, develops anaphylaxis, the management may be compromised by the propranolol. Treatment may require massive infusing of fluid (saline or colloid solutions) to support the circulation compromised by the decreased peripheral resistance. In addition, judicious administration of epinephrine for alpha-adrenergic activity and isoproterenol to attempt to overcome the beta blockade may be indicated. Glucagon 1 to 5 mg (20–30 µg/kg [maximum, 1 mg] in children) administered intravenously over 5 minutes, followed by an infusion of 5 to 15 µg/minute may be used when beta-blocker therapy complicates treatment.

Cardiopulmonary arrest occurring during anaphylaxis may require a high dose of epinephrine administered intravenously

---

**BOX 4-6**
**Physician-Supervised Management of Anaphylaxis**

1. Assess rapidly (airway, breathing, circulation, and adequacy of mentation).

2. Place in recumbent position and elevate lower extremities.

3. Discontinue inciting agent or allergen.

4. Inject epinephrine 1:1000, 0.01 mL/kg (max 0.3–0.5 mL) intramuscularly, preferably into the anterolateral thigh or arm (deltoid). Repeat every 5 min as necessary to control symptoms and blood pressure. Epinephrine 1:10,000 dilution may be utilized intravenously in moribund subjects.

5. Establish and maintain airway. May need racemic epinephrine by nebulizer into a tracheal tube.

6. Provide supplement oxygen if needed (6–8 L/min)

7. Establish IV to maintain blood pressure with IV fluids (saline or volume expanders), pressors (dopamine hydrochloride 2–10 µg/kg/min or norepinephrine bitartrate 2–4 µg/min).

8. Give diphenhydramine 1.25 mg/kg (max. 50 mg) IV over 3–5 min.

9. Ranitidine, 50 mg (1 mg/kg in children), may be diluted in 5% dextrose to a total of 20 mL and injected intravenously over 3–5 min. Inhaled β-agonists (albuterol or levalbuterol) or aminophylline 5 mg/kg over 30 min (may be helpful for severe bronchospasm 0.5–1.0 mg/kg/hr).

10. Provide hydrocortisone 5 mg/kg (max. 100 mg) IV q 6 hr or methylprednisolone 1–2 mg/kg per 24 hr.

---

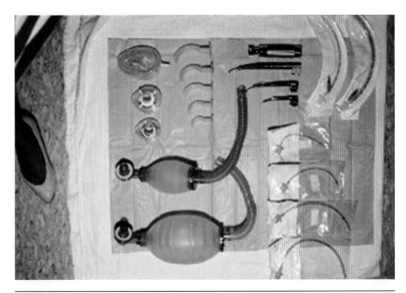

**Figure 4-8.** *A* and *B,* Equipment to maintain airway in case of anaphylaxis.

(1:10,000 dilution). Rapid volume expansion is also mandatory, as is the use of atropine and transcutaneous pacing.

## PREVENTION

The avoidance of potential and future anaphylaxis is of great importance. Steps should be taken to limit exposure to agents known to precipitate and aggravate anaphylaxis (Box 4-7). In general, agents given by the oral route, instead of parenterally, provoke anaphylaxis much less frequently. This is especially true for penicillin and other antimicrobials, due to the decreased rate of absorption when given orally. If the parenteral route is chosen, the patient should be observed for 20 to 30 minutes after the injections.

If a drug known to have caused anaphylaxis in the past is urgently needed to treat a life-threatening disease, desensitization can be performed to minimize the severity of the expected reaction. This procedure is described later. Patients should carry on their person medical information regarding known anaphylactic sensitivity and wear a bracelet. Administration of pretreatment corticosteroids and antihistamines ($H_1$ and $H_2$) to prevent anaphylaxis in selected situations, such as known sensitivity to radiocontrast media, is recommended. Alternative medication, especially antibiotics, should be utilized. It is also now possible to substitute a nonionic radiocontrast agent to lessen the possibility of anaphylactic reactions to radiocontrast media in susceptible patients.

Avoid using beta-adrenergic–blocking agents in patients with a history of anaphylaxis. Caution and judgment must be exercised when skin testing allergic patients who are being treated with beta-blockers for any of a variety of illnesses, such as hypertension, migraine, and glaucoma. Immunotherapy for patients taking the beta-blocker drugs should be avoided until alternative drug regimens for the beta-blocker can be instituted. Other risk factors for anaphylaxis related to immunotherapy include co-existing or exacerbated asthma and increasing allergen dose concentration in patients with high allergen sensitivity during a high allergen exposure in their active allergy season.

# SELECTED EXAMPLES OF ANAPHYLAXIS

## IMMUNOLOGICALLY MEDIATED ANAPHYLAXIS

### Stinging Hymenoptera Insect Venom Anaphylaxis

Generalized systemic reactions to stinging hymenopteras have been recognized as potentially life-threatening phenomena related to the IgE antibodies to the various components of venom from the honeybee, yellow jacket, white-faced hornet, yellow hornet, and wasp (Figs. 4-9 to 4-11). Imported fire ants now infest large areas of southern United States. Fire ants are classified in the order of *Hymenoptera* (Fig. 4-12). Fire ants can produce anaphylaxis as well as large local skin reactions. Most fatal reactions to insect venom occur in adults, as noted in Table 4-2. The diagnosis of IgE hypersensitivity to insect venom is best determined by skin testing. For appropriate diagnosis and therapy, it is important to define the specific insect venom responsible for the reaction.

Because local reactions without systemic anaphylaxis do not warrant allergy testing, it is important to establish a definitive history of anaphylaxis prior to diagnostic testing. Specific venoms are used as skin test reagents for the diagnosis of honeybee, wasp, hornet, and yellow jacket. Whole-body extract is used as a skin test reagent for the diagnosis of fire ant allergy.

Table 4-3 lists the several clinical indications for the selection of patients for venom skin testing, as well as indications for immunotherapy. If skin testing is not available, serologic IgE antibody testing can be used for diagnosis.

Children 16 years or younger who have experienced only non–life-threatening cutaneous manifestations with their allergic reactions (i.e., generalized urticaria) do not warrant routine venom immunotherapy, even in the presence of positive IgE antibodies.

---

**BOX 4-7**
**Prevention of Anaphylaxis**

1. Avoid exposure to agents known to cause anaphylaxis.

2. Use oral rather than parenteral medication.

3. Have patients carry information on person concerning anaphylactic sensitivity.

4. Avoid beta-adrenergic–blocking agents in anaphylaxis-prone patients.

5. Pretreat with steroids and antihistamines if patient requires procedure (radiocontrast media) or must have medications.

---

**TABLE 4-2**
**Insect Sting Deaths in the United States**

| Age (yr) | 1979 | 1983 | 1998 |
|---|---|---|---|
| 0–9 | 1 | 2 | 1 |
| 10–19 | 1 | 3 | 0 |
| 20–29 | 1 | 9 | 4 |
| 30–39 | 4 | 8 | 4 |
| 40–49 | 10 | 9 | 13 |
| 50–59 | 7 | 9 | 13 |
| 60–69 | 13 | 10 | 4 |
| 70+ | 1 | 8 | 8 |
| Total | 38 | 58 | 47 |

From the National Center for Health Statistics, Atlanta, 2000.

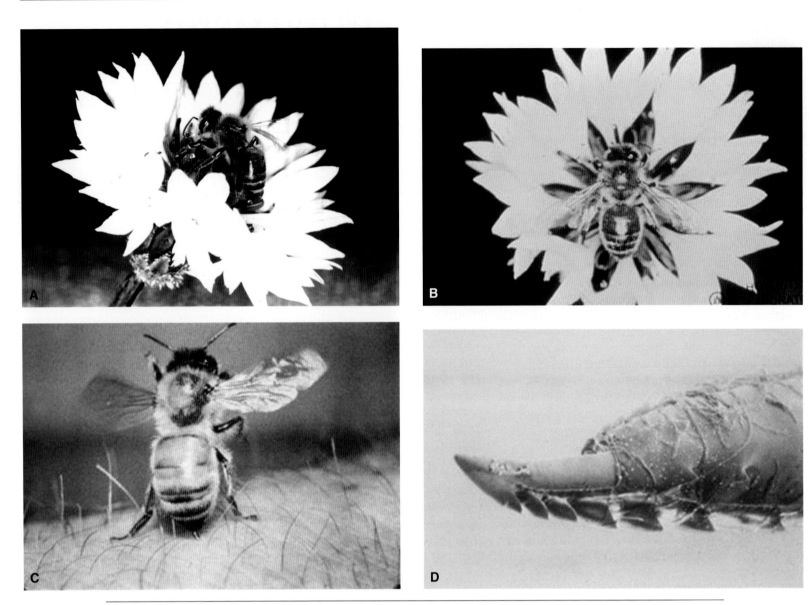

**Figure 4-9.** *Hymenoptera* (honeybee). *A,* Lateral view. *B,* Dorsal view. *C,* Stinging with barbed stinger. *D,* Barbed stinger left in skin after sting.

**TABLE 4-3**

Selection of Patients for Venom Skin Testing and Immunotherapy

| Classification of Sting Reaction by History | Venom Skin Test | Venom Immunotherapy |
|---|---|---|
| Local | +/− | No |
| Large local | +/− | No |
| Systemic | | |
| Life threatening | + | Yes |
| Non–life threatening | | |
| Adult | + | Yes |
| Children (<16 yr) | + | No |
| Toxic | +/− | No |
| Delayed (>24 hr) | +/− | No |

Adults with life-threatening as well as non–life-threatening anaphylaxis who have positive IgE antibody skin tests should be treated with venom immunotherapy.

If the decision is made to provide venom immunotherapy, a schedule should be followed, such as that illustrated in Figure 4-13. Because purified venom is not available for fire ant immunotherapy, the treatment employs whole-body extracts using weight-to-volume concentration.

Virtually 100% of patients can be protected after increasing the dose of venom to 100 µg, which is approximately equivalent to the amount of venom in two stings. The interval of immunotherapy injections after reaching the maintenance dose is between 4 and 8 weeks. The duration of the immunotherapy should be at least 5 years. Some clinicians suggest longer periods of therapy, perhaps even for a lifetime, in those who have had severe reactions, but this is not definitely established at this time. There are no definitive tests to help the clinician decide when to discontinue venom immunotherapy. Protection is probably related to the loss of IgE allergic reactivity, which may be manifested as negative allergy skin tests, but this has not been established for

clinical practice. After 3 months of venom immunotherapy, patients are protected but still would have positive venom skin tests. After 5 years of venom immunotherapy, less than 50% of patients have developed negative venom skin tests. Even so, most of them can discontinue venom immunotherapy and can tolerate subsequent stings without developing anaphylaxis.[18]

## Immune-Mediated Penicillin Anaphylaxis

Drug hapten-protein hypersensitivity can be best illustrated by penicillin allergy. Penicillin anaphylaxis has been estimated to account for 200 to 500 deaths per year in the United States, or 97% of drug anaphylaxis deaths.[19]

The history of a pruritic macular- or urticarial-type eruption while taking penicillin is suggestive of allergy. However, the rash may be associated with the infection for which the penicillin is prescribed and not caused by penicillin allergy. A history of life-threatening anaphylaxis with penicillin in a patient who requires penicillin treatment is a serious consideration. The antigenic determinant for most penicillin allergy is the penicilloyl

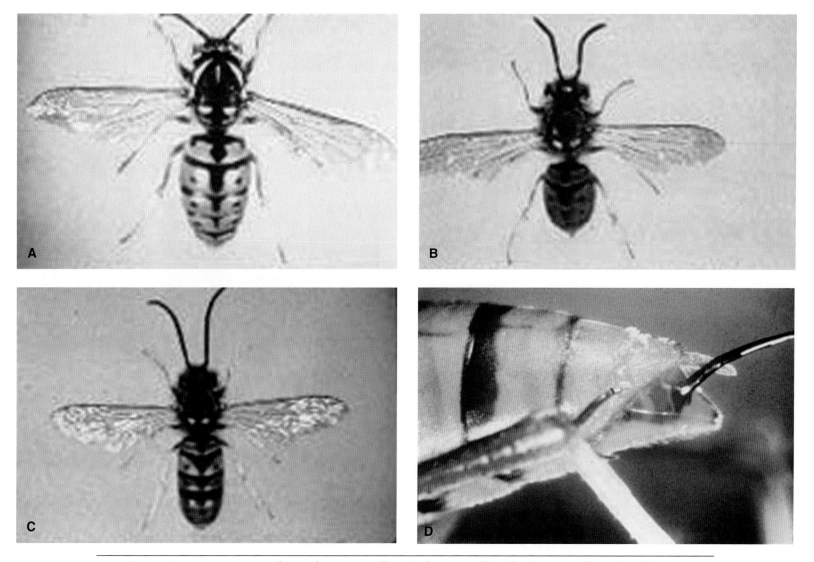

**Figure 4-10.** *Hymenoptera* (honeybee). *A,* Yellow jacket. *B,* Yellow hornet. *C,* White-faced hornet.

metabolic byproduct of penicillin metabolism. Skin testing with benzylpenicilloylpolylysine, the penicilloyl synthetic polypeptide conjugate (Pre-Pen), and freshly prepared aqueous penicillin is used to document specific IgE-mediated allergy (Table 4-4). If no reaction to skin testing with these reagents occurs, then penicillin can be cautiously administered. If skin tests are positive, then desensitization of a proven allergic individual may be performed orally, subcutaneously, intramuscularly, or intravenously (Table 4-5). During these procedures, personal physician observation and availability of medications and equipment for treatment of anaphylaxis are mandatory (see Fig. 4-8 and Box 4-6).

Sensitivities to other hapten-protein antigens, including anesthetic agents, cephalosporin, and insulin, can be similarly evaluated and tested. No skin testing procedures are available for macrolides, sulfas, tetracyclines, or fluoroquinolones. Provocative challenges with antibiotics, especially parenteral preparations, may be dangerous and should be avoided or performed under constant medical supervision. Failure to react to the skin tests for penicillin allergy guarantees safety from significant anaphylaxis in 98% of patients but does not rule out late-phase allergic reactions.

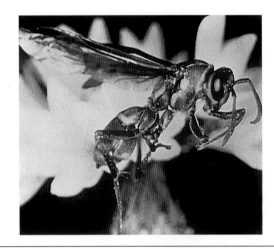

**Figure 4-11.** *Hymenoptera:* wasp.

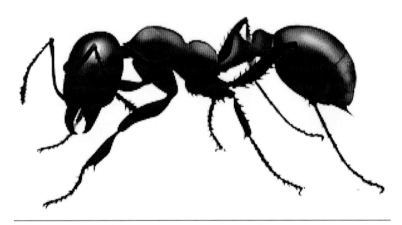

**Figure 4-12.** *Hymenoptera:* fire ant.

**Dosage Regimen for Venom Immunotherapy**

| Week no. | Vial concentration (ug/ml) | Volume (ml/cm³) |
|---|---|---|
| 1 | 1 | 0.05 |
| 2 | 1 | 0.10 |
| 3 | 1 | 0.20 |
| 4 | 1 | 0.40 |
| 5 | 10 | 0.05 |
| 6 | 10 | 0.10 |
| 7 | 10 | 0.20 |
| 8 | 10 | 0.40 |
| 9 | 100 | 0.05 |
| 10 | 100 | 0.10 |
| 11 | 100 | 0.20 |
| 12 | 100 | 0.40 |
| 13 | 100 | 0.60 |
| 14 | 100 | 0.80 |
| 15 | 100 | 1 cm³ |
| 16 | 100 | 1 cm³ |
| 17 | no injection | |
| 18 | 100 | 1 cm³ |
| 19 | no injection | |
| 20 | no injection | |
| 21 | 100 | 1 cm³ |
| Begin maintenance q 4 weeks | | |
| 25 | 100 | 1 cm³ |
| Continue maintenance q 4 weeks until the end of the first year (52 weeks), | | |
| then q 6 weeks (if anti-venom IgG level is >3 ($\mu$g/mL) | 100 | 1 cm³ |

**A**

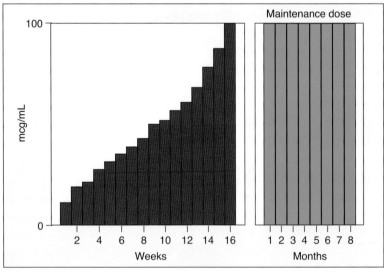

**B**

**Figure 4-13.** *A,* Dosage regimen for bee, wasp, hornet, or yellow jacket venom immunotherapy. *B,* Treatment schedule.

# NON–IMMUNE-MEDIATED ANAPHYLAXIS

## Radiocontrast Media

An example of non–immune-mediated anaphylaxis is that which manifests with administration of ionic iodinated contrast media (sodium meglumine salts of ionic acids). The reported incidence of such severe reactions is 1 in 1000 uses of the contrast media; the reported incidence of deaths is 1 in 1200 to 1 in 75,000 contrast studies.[20] This reaction can be primarily cutaneous, manifesting as pruritus or urticaria, or it can be systemic, with upper airway edema and smooth muscle contraction. Dyspnea due to bronchospasm or shock due to capillary dilation and increased permeability may occur and, if not reversed, can be fatal.

No diagnostic laboratory tests are available. The history of a previous anaphylactic reaction is the important criteria for prophylactic treatment if the patient requires future diagnostic imaging with contrast media. This can be in the form of pretreating with $H_1$- and $H_2$-blocking antihistamines (diphenhydramine and cimetadine), corticosteroids (prednisone or methylprednisolone), and, less commonly, beta-adrenergic agents (ephedrine). The use of $H_1$- and $H_2$-blocking antihistamines may reduce the potential for cardiac arrhythmias and peripheral vasolidation. Corticosteroids can prevent potential late-phase reactions. Box 4-8 outlines options for the prevention of this potential anaphylactic reaction.[21]

The recent introduction of non-ionic, low-osmolar contrast media (iodixanol, iohexol, iopamidol, iopromide, ioversol, ioxaglate, ioxilan, sodium iothalamate, and sodium mitrizoate) has greatly reduced the risk of serious anaphylactic reactions to iodinated contrast media. The substitution of these agents for the ionic iodinated, relatively high-osmolar contrast media must still be preceded by prophylactic medications as noted previously if the patient has a history of anaphylaxis to ionic contrast media.

## Exercise-Induced Anaphylaxis

Another example of non–immune-mediated anaphylaxis occurs uncommonly in a few individuals who manifest a tendency to develop anaphylaxis during exercise. Signs and symptoms begin with generalized itching followed by flushing, urticaria, angioedema, collapse, choking with respiratory distress, abdominal cramps, and headache. In rare instances, exercise is preceded by the ingestion of specific foods, such as celery, fish, or shellfish, within 2 to 4 hours or even as many as 12 hours preceding exercise. Stopping exercise at the first sign of impending anaphylaxis, such as itching, is advisable. Once the reaction is under way, the usual treatment for anaphylaxis is indicated as outlined previously. Prophylactic antihistamine treatment has not been preventive, but antihistamines can be helpful in ameliorating the cutaneous manifestations.[22]

---

**BOX 4-8**

**Medication Options for Prevention of Radiocontrast Media Anaphylaxis**

1. **Corticosteroids**
   Prednisone 50 mg PO 13, 7, and 1 hr before procedure

2. **$H_1$-blocking antihistamine**
   Diphenhydramine PO 1 hr before procedure

3. **$H_2$-blocking antihistamine**
   Cimetidine 5 mg/kg (max. 300 mg)

   Ranitidine 1 mg/kg (max. 50 mg) PO or IV q 6 hr, 18–24 hr or immediately before procedure

4. **Beta-adrenergic agents**
   Ephedrine 0.5 mg/kg (max. 25 mg) PO 1 hr before procedure, unless contraindicated by angina, hypertension, or arrhythmias

---

**TABLE 4-4**
Prototype Penicillin Allergy Skin Testing Chart

| Puncture | Size of Wheal and Flare | Intradermal | Size of Wheal and Flare |
|---|---|---|---|
| Pre-Pen® (benzylpenicilloyl-polylysine) | | Pre-Pen® (benzylpenicilloyl-polylysine) | |
| Aq. Pen-G<br>100 U<br>1000 U<br>10,000 U | | Aq. Pen-G<br>100 U<br>1000 U<br>10,000 U | |
| Diluent control | | Diluent control | |
| Histamine control 1:1000 | | Histamine control 1:10,000 | |

**TABLE 4-5**
Oral Desensitization Protocol*

### Desensitization Protocols for Penicillin

| Step[†] | Penicillin, mg/mL | Amount, mL | Dose Given, mg | Cumulative Dose, mg |
|---|---|---|---|---|
| 1 | 0.5 | 0.1 | 0.05 | 0.05 |
| 2 | 0.5 | 0.2 | 0.1 | 0.15 |
| 3 | 0.5 | 0.4 | 0.2 | 0.35 |
| 4 | 0.5 | 0.8 | 0.4 | 0.75 |
| 5 | 0.5 | 1.6 | 0.8 | 1.55 |
| 6 | 0.5 | 3.2 | 1.6 | 3.15 |
| 7 | 0.5 | 6.4 | 3.2 | 6.35 |
| 8 | 5 | 1.2 | 6 | 12.35 |
| 9 | 5 | 2.4 | 12 | 24.35 |
| 10 | 5 | 5 | 25 | 49.35 |
| 11 | 50 | 1 | 50 | 100 |
| 12 | 50 | 2 | 100 | 200 |
| 13 | 50 | 4 | 200 | 400 |
| 14 | 50 | 8 | 400 | 800 |

### Intravenous Desensitization Protocol with Drug Added by Piggyback Infusion*

| Step[†] | Penicillin, mg/mL | Amount, mL | Dose Given, mg | Cumulative Dose, mg |
|---|---|---|---|---|
| 1 | 0.1 | 0.1 | 0.1 | 0.01 |
| 2 | 0.1 | 0.2 | 0.2 | 0.03 |
| 3 | 0.1 | 0.4 | 0.4 | 0.07 |
| 4 | 0.1 | 0.8 | 0.8 | 0.15 |
| 5 | 0.1 | 1.6 | 0.16 | 0.31 |
| 6 | 1 | 0.32 | 0.32 | 0.63 |
| 7 | 1 | 0.64 | 0.64 | 1.27 |
| 8 | 1 | 1.2 | 1.2 | 2.47 |
| 9 | 10 | 0.24 | 2.4 | 4.87 |
| 10 | 10 | 0.48 | 4.8 | 10 |
| 11 | 10 | 1 | 10 | 20 |
| 12 | 10 | 2 | 20 | 40 |
| 13 | 100 | 0.4 | 40 | 80 |
| 14 | 100 | 0.8 | 80 | 160 |
| 15 | 100 | 1.6 | 160 | 320 |
| 16 | 1000 | 0.32 | 320 | 640 |
| 17 | 1000 | 0.64 | 640 | 1280 |

*Observe patient for 30 min, then give full therapeutic dose by the desired route.
[†]Interval between doses is 15 min.
Adapted from Sullivan TJ: Drug allergy. In Middleton E, Reed CE, Ellis EF, et al (eds): Allergy: Principles and Practice, 4th ed. St. Louis, C.V. Mosby, 1993, pp 1726–1746; with permission.

# REFERENCES

1. Cohen SG: Portier, Richet and the discovery of anaphylaxis: A centennial. J Allergy Clin Immunol 2002;110:331–336.
2. Kemp SF: Current concepts in pathophysiology, diagnosis, and management of anaphylaxis. Immunol Allergy Clin North Am 2001;21(4):612–613.
3. Yocum MW, Butterfield JH, Klein JS, et al: Epidemiology of anaphylaxis in Olmsted County: A population-based study. J Allergy Clin Immunol 1999; 104:452–456.
4. Kemp SF: Adverse effects of allergen immunotherapy: Assessment and treatment. Immunol Allergy Clin North Am 2000;20:571–591.
5. Valentine M, Frank M, Friedland L, et al: Allergic emergencies. In Drause RM (ed): Asthma and Other Allergic Diseases. NIAID Task Force Report, Bethesda, MD. National Institutes of Health, 1979.
6. Graft DF, Schuberth KC, Kagey-Sobotka A, et al: A prospective study of the natural history of large local reactions after *Hymenoptera* stings in children. J Pediatr 1984;104:664–668.
7. Bock SA, Munoz-Furlong A, Sampson HA: Fatalities due to anaphylactic reactions to foods. J Allergy Clin Immunol 2001;107:191–193.
8. Ditto AM, Harris KE, Krasnick J, et al: Idiopathic anaphylaxis: A series of 335 cases. Ann Allergy Asthma Immunol 1996;77:285–291.
9. Choy AC, Patterson R, Patterson DR, et al: Undifferentiated somatoform idiopathic anaphylaxis: Nonorganic symptoms mimicking idiopathic anaphylaxis. J Allergy Clin Immunol 1995;96:893–900.
10. Austen KF: Systemic anaphylaxis in the human being. N Engl J Med 1974; 291:661–664.
11. Fisher MM: Clinical observation on the pathophysiology and treatment of anaphylactic cardiovascular collapse. Anaesth Intensive Care 1986;14:17.
12. Fisher M: Anaphylaxis. Disease-a-Month 1987;33:433–479.
13. Chrusch D, Sharma S, Unruh H, et al: Histamine H3 receptor blockade improves cardiac function in canine anaphylaxis. Am J Respir Crit Care Med 1999;160:1142–1149.
14. Kanthawanta S, Carias K, Arnaout R: The potential clinical utility of serum alpha-protryptase levels. J Allergy Clin Immunol 1999;103:1092–1099.
15. Stevenson DD: Anaphylactic and anaphylactoid reactions to aspirin and other non-steroidal anti-inflammatory drugs. Immunol Allergy Clin North Am 2001;21(4):745–768.
16. Simons FER, Roberts JR, Gu X: Epinephrine absorption in children with a history of anaphylaxis. J Allergy Clin Immunol 1998;101:33–37.
17. Simons FER, Gu X, Simons KJ: Epinephrine absorption in adults: Intramuscular versus subcutaneous injection. J Allergy Clin Immunol 2001; 108:871–873.
18. Graft DF, Golden DBK, Reisman RE, et al: Position statement: The discontinuation of *Hymenoptera* venom immunotherapy. JACI 1998;101:573.
19. Solensky R, Mendelson LM: Systemic reactions to antibiotics. Immunol Allergy Clin North Am 2001;21(4):679–697.
20. Hong SJ, Wong JT, Bloch KJ: Reactions to radiocontrast media. Allergy and Asthma Proc 2002;223:347–351.
21. Greenberger PA, Patterson R: The prevention of immediate generalized reaction to radiocontrast media in high-risk patients. J Allergy Clin Immunol 1991;87:867–872.
22. Horan RF, Dubuske LM, Sheffer AL: Exercise-induced anaphylaxis. Immunol Allergy Clin North Am 2001;21(4):769–782.

*David P. Skoner*

# 5 Asthma

Asthma, a lower airways disease characterized by enhanced responsiveness to a variety of stimuli and manifested by airways obstruction that changes spontaneously or therapeutically, is a common illness in both the pediatric and adult populations.[1–5] The most widely accepted definition of asthma includes the following characteristics (Fig. 5-1):

- Lower airway obstruction that is partially or fully reversible, either spontaneously or with bronchodilator or anti-inflammatory treatments.
- The presence of chronic airway inflammation.
- Increased lower airway responsiveness to several stimuli, such as cold air or exercise in the natural environment and inhaled methacholine or histamine in a laboratory environment, with recurrent episodes of wheezing, coughing, and shortness of breath.

Increasingly, asthma is being recognized as a clinical syndrome, or a set of diseases, all of which share a common clinical presentation (symptoms of episodic airflow limitation) and underlying etiology (airway inflammation) but have multiple pathogenic pathways (i.e., different types and causes of inflammation). An appropriate genetic background, along with certain environmental exposures (viruses, allergens) at critical developmental ages, appears to form the foundation for the development of this disease (Fig. 5-2). Also, asthma is increasingly recognized as a progressive disease[6,7] in which airway inflammation leads to a remodeling of the airway and structural changes that may result in a time-dependent loss of lung function and reversibility. This chapter reviews our current understanding of the etiology, natural history, symptomatology, identification, and outpatient and inpatient treatment of asthma.

## EPIDEMIOLOGY

The burden of asthma has been increasing worldwide, with regard to prevalence, cost, morbidity, and mortality.[8] Approximately 26 million individuals in the United States have received a diagnosis of asthma sometime during their lifetime, 8.6 million of which were younger than 18 years. Prevalence by age group is illustrated in (Fig. 5-3). The onset of asthma in children is before the age of 2 years in 50% and before the age of 5 years in 80%. Asthma is now the most common chronic illness of childhood and is a leading cause of school absenteeism. Prevalence has been increasing worldwide, as illustrated in (Fig. 5-4) and is as high as 32% in some countries. In particular, the prevalence increased in U.S. children between 1982 and 1992. According to the widely accepted hygiene hypothesis, westernization and cleaner living have caused the immune system to develop in a fashion that promotes the increased expression of allergic and asthmatic disease. Thus, environmental changes appear to be the predominant force driving at least some of the observed epidemiologic changes.

Hospitalizations increased 17.2% between 1980 and 1999. The largest increase occurred in the preschool-age group. In children alone, asthma was associated with more than 3.5 million physician visits, over 650,000 emergency department visits, and 190,000 hospitalizations in 1999. The rise in asthma admissions at Children's Hospital of Pittsburgh is illustrated in (Fig. 5-5).

Unfortunately, mortality associated with asthma has also been increasing, especially in children (Fig. 5-6). Surprisingly, approximately one third of asthma-related deaths occur in children with mild disease. Moreover, the underdiagnosis of asthma is a major problem, because 10% to 15% of schoolchildren have undiagnosed asthma. Asthma kills approximately 5000 people each year in the United States. Most asthma-related hospitalizations and deaths are preventable with appropriate attention to disease severity, trigger factors, and treatment.

Many of the epidemiologic trends are disproportionately expressed in African American children. Possible explanations for this include the lack of access to appropriate medical care and

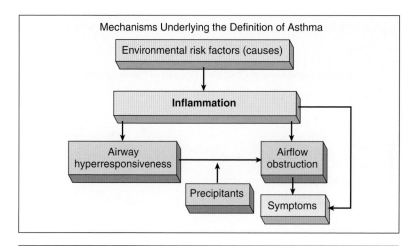

**Figure 5-1.** Mechanisms underlying the definition of asthma.

**Figure 5-2.** Origins and natural history of asthma. Asthma symptoms can begin in childhood or as an adult. Affected children can have apparent remissions, with possible relapse later, or can experience disease progression (loss of lung function and reversibility). Viruses, allergens, and genes appear to be involved in the development of asthma. hx, history.

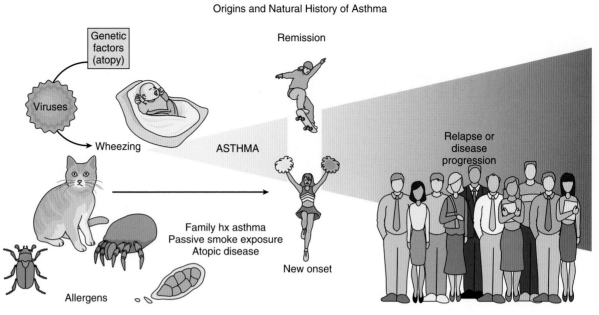

Origins and Natural History of Asthma

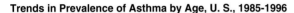

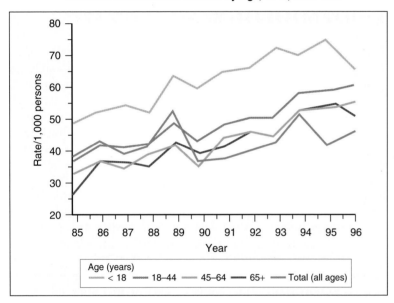

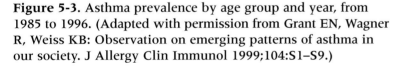

**Figure 5-3.** Asthma prevalence by age group and year, from 1985 to 1996. (Adapted with permission from Grant EN, Wagner R, Weiss KB: Observation on emerging patterns of asthma in our society. J Allergy Clin Immunol 1999;104:S1–S9.)

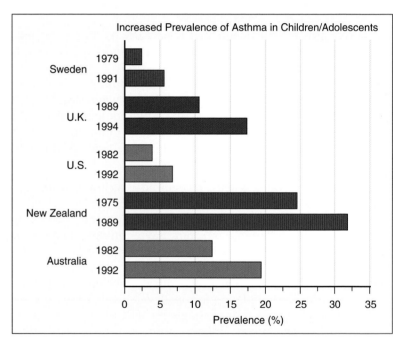

**Figure 5-4.** Time-dependent increases in asthma prevalence internationally from 1979 to 1992 (GINA). (Adapted from GINA teaching slide set, www.ginasthma.com, slide 21.)

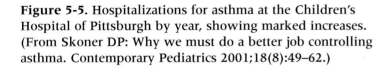

**Figure 5-5.** Hospitalizations for asthma at the Children's Hospital of Pittsburgh by year, showing marked increases. (From Skoner DP: Why we must do a better job controlling asthma. Contemporary Pediatrics 2001;18(8):49–62.)

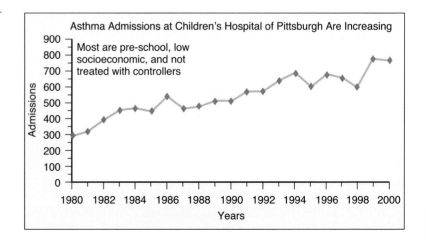

poverty, as often exists in inner cities, as well as a sedentary lifestyle and intense exposure to tobacco smoke and allergens such as cockroaches. A major factor is underuse of appropriate controller medications.

Wheezing is very common in young children and is only sometimes caused by asthma. Some birth cohort studies have reported that as many as 50% of all children experience a wheezing episode in the first few years of life.[9] However, at 6 years of age, only about 40% of these children have persistent wheezing and

asthma, whereas the remainder have a condition termed *transient, benign wheezing of infancy* (Fig. 5-7). Factors linked to the former, but not the latter group, include early allergen sensitization and wheezing outside of colds. The infants with transient, benign wheezing appear to be born with small airways that predispose them to wheeze when they have viral infections. As their airways grow in size, their symptoms subside. In contrast, those with persistent wheezing and asthma are born with normal lung function, but, consistent with the hypothesis that asthma is a progressive disease, they already have developed abnormal lung function by the age of 6 years. Also consistent with that hypothesis, large epidemiologic studies have documented a progressive loss of lung function with time in asthmatics[10] (Fig. 5-8). This collection of studies has led to the widely promoted concept that an early intervention window may allow for the prevention of such progression.

In childhood, boys are affected 30% more often than girls and tend to have more severe disease. Beyond puberty, the sex distribution is equal, and female patients predominate in some studies.

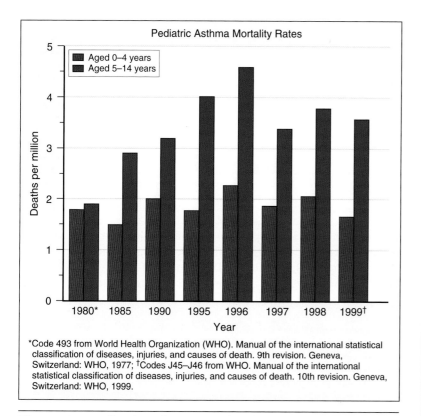

**Figure 5-6.** Pediatric asthma mortality by year, illustrating that asthma deaths more than doubled for children 0 to 14 years of age between 1980 and 1999. (Adapted from Centers for Disease Control and Prevention MMWR 1998;47(SS-1):1–26.)

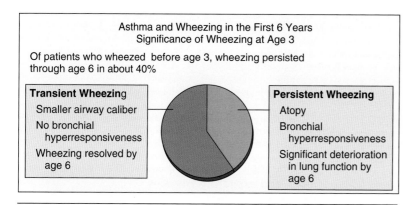

**Figure 5-7.** Asthma and wheezing in the first 6 years of life. Of children who wheezed before the age of 3 years, most had a transient condition that cleared up by 6 years of age, while approximately 40% had persistent wheezing suggesting asthma. The characteristics of those two groups are illustrated. (From Martinez FD, Wright AL, Taussig LM, et al: Asthma and wheezing in the first six years of life. N Engl J Med 1995;332:133–138.)

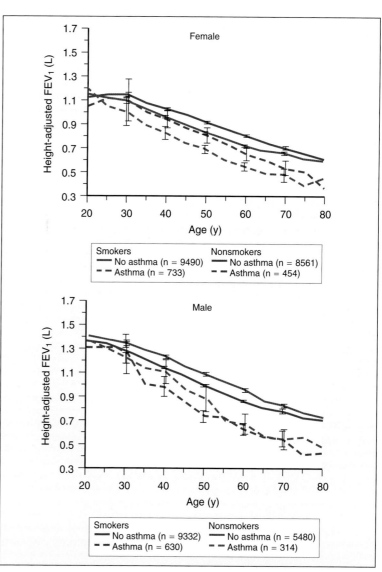

**Figure 5-8.** Changes with age in the height-adjusted forced expiratory volume in 1 second (FEV$_1$) according to sex, smoking status, and the presence or absence of asthma. (Lange P, Parner J, Vestbo J, et al.: A 15-year follow-up study of ventilatory function in adults with asthma. N Engl J Med, 1998;339(17):1197.)

Asthma is considered a component of the atopic march, whereby genetically predisposed infants typically develop eczema (often with food allergies) shortly after birth, which often subsides as they develop inhalant allergen sensitivities and allergic rhinitis during the 2nd to 4th years of life and, very often, symptoms of asthma.

The term *intrinsic asthma* has been applied to those in whom immunoglobuin (Ig) E antibody was not detectable by skin testing. However, one study documented increased serum IgE levels in a large asthmatic cohort (Fig. 5-9), indicating that asthma prevalence is associated with IgE levels.[11] In certain patients, however, the specific IgE antibody involved is not detectable using conventional methodologies, such as skin or serum IgE antibody testing (thus, *intrinsic* asthma). Consequently, the use of the terms *extrinsic* (involving IgE) and *intrinsic* to characterize asthma has been discontinued.

Viral infections that are clinically detectable only in the upper respiratory tract can be associated with bronchial hyperreactivity and small airway dysfunction. Viral infections account for as many as 80% of wheezing episodes in young children during the fall and winter seasons.[12] Typically, respiratory syncytial virus predomintes in children younger than 2 years, whereas rhinovirus predominates in those older than 2 years (Fig. 5-10). *Mycoplasma pneumoniae* may cause more than 50% of wheezing episodes in adolescents. Respiratory syncytial virus is the main cause of infantile bronchiolitis, which generally manifests as wheezing in small babies and, at times, must be differentiated from asthma (Table 5-1). Virtually all children develop an infection with respiratory syncytial virus during the first 2 years of life, but only some develop bronchiolitis. Indeed, involvement of the lower respiratory tract during such an infection appears to be a strong risk factor for persistent wheezing and the later diagnosis of asthma.

As many as 50% of children with asthma, especially those with milder levels of severity, have a clinical remission and become asymptomatic during the 10- to 20-year follow-up period. However, in these people, airway biopsy studies have documented

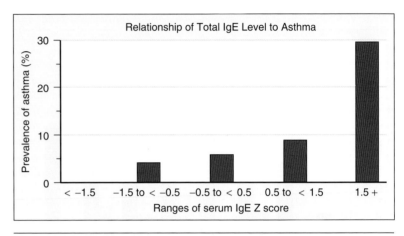

**Figure 5-9.** Relationship of total immunoglobulin (Ig) E level to the prevalence of asthma. Note the strong relationship. (From Burrows B, Martinez FD, Haloren M, et al.: Association of asthma with serum IgE levels and skin-test reactivity to allergens. N Engl J Med 1989;320:271–277.)

**TABLE 5-1**

**Differentiating Features of Asthma and Bronchiolitis in Children**

| | **Asthma** | **Bronchiolitis** |
|---|---|---|
| Primary cause of symptoms | Viruses, allergens, exercise, etc. | Respiratory syncytial virus, metapneumovirus |
| Age of onset | 50% by 2 yr<br>80% by 5 yr | <24 mo |
| Recurrent wheezing | Yes (characteristic) | 70% (two episodes)<br>30% progress to asthma (three episodes) |
| Onset of wheezing | Acute if allergic or exercise induced | Insidious |
| Concomitant symptoms of upper respiratory infection | Yes, if infectious | Yes |
| Family history of allergy and asthma | Frequent | Infrequent in children with two episodes |
| Nasal eosinophilia | With allergic rhinitis | Absent |
| Chest auscultation | If viral, as in bronchiolitis<br>Nonviral: high-pitched expiratory wheezes | Fine, sibilant rales, and coarse inspiratory and expiratory wheezes |
| Concomitant allergic manifestations | If allergic asthma | Usually absent |
| IgE level | Elevated | Normal |
| Responsive to bronchodilator | Yes (characteristic) | Unresponsive or partially responsive |

Ig, immunoglobulin.

ongoing airway inflammation and remodeling, and many experience a recrudescence of symptoms during years of follow-up. At minimum, this requires careful vigilance and monitoring if daily controller treatment is discontinued. However, this observation, along with the evidence that asthma is a progressive disease, has prompted most clinicians to recommend long-term, seamless treatment with daily, anti-inflammatory controller medications.

# PATHOPHYSIOLOGY

## GENERAL PATHOPHYSIOLOGY

Although the underlying pathology in asthma is airway inflammation, clinical manifestations of asthma are related to the periodic development of airway obstruction (Fig. 5-11). When evaluated, patients with mild intermittent or persistent asthma may have no detectable evidence of airflow obstruction on routine pulmonary function testing. However, those with moderate and severe persistent asthma may have abnormalities detectable both on physical examination and in pulmonary function testing (office-based spirometry or home-based peak expiratory flow measurements).

Despite the variability in the presence and degree of airflow obstruction during sequential office-based evaluations, the history usually reveals that asthma patients develop clinical symptoms (and thus, airflow limitation) after exposure to allergens, environmental irritants, viral infections, exercise, and cold air[1] (Table 5-2). This propensity to develop airway obstruction in response to normally innocuous environmental agents is known as airway hyperreactivity. Its presence can be documented in the clinical pulmonary function laboratory using bronchoprovocation testing, in which pulmonary function is monitored while patients inhale increased concentrations of methacholine or histamine to establish the provocative concentration that causes a 20% fall in forced expiratory volume in 1 second ($FEV_1$). Virtually all patients with asthma have airway hyperreactivity, although patients with other disorders such as cystic fibrosis can be affected to a lesser extent.

Other stimuli that can be used to measure the degree of airway hyperreactivity include nonpharmacologic agents such as hyperventilation with cold, dry air, and with exercise. Indeed, the clinical severity of asthma—and thus, medication requirements—tends to parallel the degree of airway hyperreactivity. Severe airway hyperreactivity results in a considerable degree of bronchial lability in asthmatics, such that decreases in airway flow rates can develop precipitously and unexpectedly.

One of the signs of airway hyperreactivity in patients with asthma is an exaggerated fluctuation in morning and evening peak expiratory flow rates (Fig. 5-12). This assessment has been incorporated into the asthma guidelines in the classification of asthma severity. The normal diurnal variability in airflow in nonasthmatics is approximately 10% or less, but the variability may increase dramatically in patients with high degrees of airway hyperreactivity and severe asthma.

Postulated mechanisms for the development of airway hyperreactivity include airway inflammation, abnormalities in bronchial epithelial integrity, changes in intrinsic bronchial smooth muscle function, changes in autonomic neural control of airways (decreased beta-adrenergic and enhanced alpha-adrenergic and cholinergic responses), and the degree of baseline airflow obstruction.

One of the primary mechanisms responsible for the development of airway hyperreactivity is airway inflammation, which has now been documented directly using mucosal biopsies[13] (Fig. 5-13). The airway inflammation is complex and variable but is present in all persistent asthma severity levels and very early in the course of disease in adults and children. Th-2 lymphocytes, mast cells,

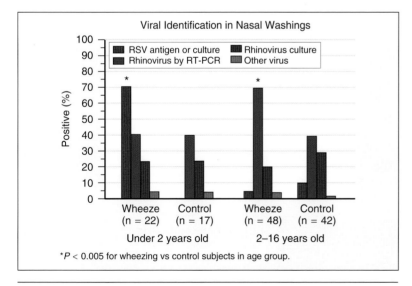

**Figure 5-10.** Viral identification in nasal washings of wheezing and control children based on age. RSV, respiratory syncytial virus; RT-PCR, reverse transcriptase-polymerase-chain reaction. (From Rakes GP, Arruda E, Ingram JM, et al.: Rhinovirus and respiratory syncytial virus in wheezing children requiring emergency care. IgE and eosinophil analyses. Am J Respir Crit Care Med 1999;159(3):785–790.)

| **TABLE 5-2** Asthma Triggers | |
|---|---|
| 1. Infections | Viral<br>Bacterial sinusitis |
| 2. Allergens | Pollens<br>Animal products<br>Molds<br>Dusts<br>Cockroaches |
| 3. Airway factors | Cold air<br>Hyperventilation (e.g., crying, laughing)<br>Exercise |
| 4. Irritants | Noxious gases, odors<br>Cigarette smoke |
| 5. Pharmacologic | Aspirin |
| 6. Psychosocial | Emotions |

Pathological Changes in the Airways of Asthmatics

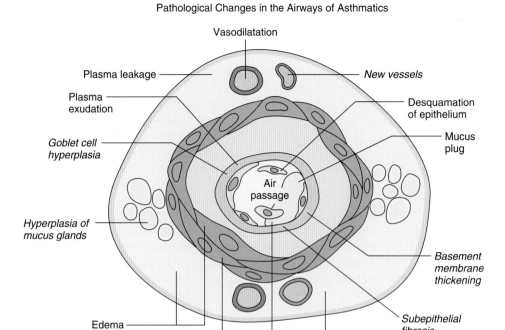

A

Chronic changes are identified in italics, the remainder are acute changes.

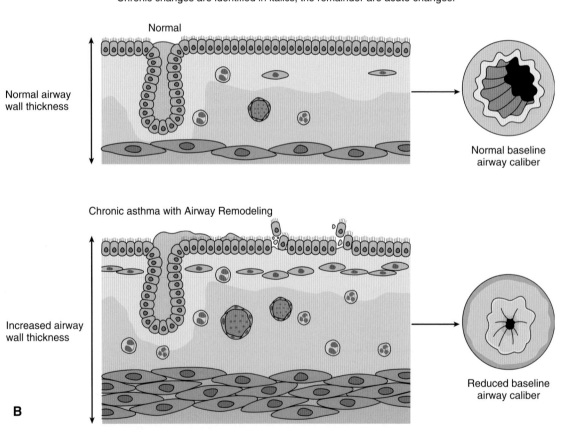

**Figure 5-11.** Pathologic changes in the airways of asthmatics (*A*) and the airway remodeling process in asthma (*B*).

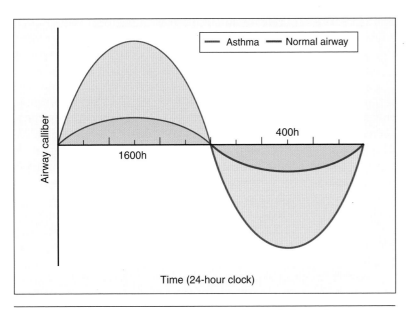

**Figure 5-12.** Illustration of the diurnal variability of airway caliber in asthma patients and normal individuals.

and eosinophils appear to be the main orchestrators of the inflammatory process, but neutrophils may be involved in more severe cases.[7,14] Eosinophils, whose tissue migration and activation may be directed by the secretory products of pulmonary mast cells, macrophages, and epithelial cells, have been linked to alterations in epithelial integrity, abnormalities in autonomic neural control of airway tone, and increased airway smooth muscle responsiveness. Another cell with a likely role in these events is the T-lymphocyte. Indeed, this cell, once activated by antigen, may orchestrate the development and maintenance of airway inflammation through the secretion of proinflammatory, soluble cytokines such as interleukin (IL)-4 and IL-5, which have the ability to influence the activation state of a variety of inflammatory cells in both autocrine and paracrine fashions.

Smoldering inflammation is also accompanied by a remodeling process, which includes epithelial disruption, edema, hypertrophied and hyperplastic smooth muscle bundles, increased vascularity, increased mucous secretion, and a remarkable thickening of the reticular basement membrane due to collagen deposition (see earlier figures). This remodeling may relate to the long-term decline in lung function and loss of reversibility observed in asthmatic patients.

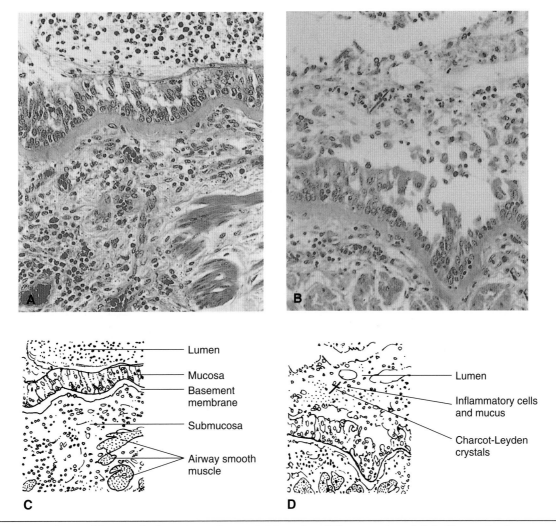

**Figure 5-13.** Airway histopathology in asthma. *A,* Note the diffuse eosinophil infiltrate in the submucosa and lumen, the intraluminal mucus, the smooth muscle hypertrophy, and the appearance of a thickened basement membrane, which may represent collagen deposited along the basement membrane. *B,* Note the red-staining, eosinophil-derived Charcot–Leyden crystal, surrounded by mucus and eosinophils in the airway lumen. *C,* Diagram of part *A* with tissue sites labeled. *D,* Diagram of part *B* with tissue sites labeled. (Courtesy of Dr Ronald Jaffe, Children's Hospital of Pittsburgh.)

Inflammatory mediators also play a major role in the pathogenesis of selected features of asthma, including the inflammation and remodeling processes (Fig. 5-14). These include the cysteinyl leukotrienes (Fig. 5-15). Some of the cells that release these potent mediators, including eosinophils, basophils, and mast cells, have an inherent enhanced degree of mediator releasability in asthma, thus providing a possible explanation for the observed elevations of plasma mediator levels during laboratory-provoked and naturally acquired acute asthma.

Genetics and environment both participate in the pathogenesis of asthma. Family history very often reveals affected siblings, parents, or other first-degree relatives. No specific asthma gene has yet been identified, but recent advances in molecular biology promise to better define the genetic basis for asthma (Fig. 5-16). Certain environmental factors may be prerequisite for its clinical presentation. For example, a propensity to develop airway hyperreactivity may be inherited, but appropriate exposure to certain allergens, respiratory viruses, chemicals, or psychosocial stimuli are associated as triggers for its clinical expression as asthma.

Laboratory experiments have demonstrated that inhalation of a relevant allergen by an allergic asthmatic patient results in the development of an acute decrease in $FEV_1$ and the onset of asthma symptoms within 30 minutes of exposure (Fig. 5-17). Such a trigger may cause bronchial mast cells, macrophages, and epithelial cells to release inflammatory mediators, which then trigger the bronchospasm. Over the ensuing hours, airway function returns to baseline in most patients. If their progress is monitored, approximately 50% of these patients then experience a second decline in $FEV_1$ approximately 4 to 8 hours after exposure, termed a *late-phase allergic reaction* (see Fig. 5-17). Importantly, the degree of bronchial hyperreactivity to nonspecific stimuli is increased in patients experiencing late-phase allergic reactions. This is believed to be related to the intense airway inflammation that develops in these patients, manifested by increased numbers of eosinophils in the airways, along with other cells. The migration of eosinophils into the airways and their activation may be directed by inflammatory mediators released earlier during the immediate allergic reaction. Indeed, patients who experience sequential late-phase bronchial reactions could thus experience progressively heightened levels of airway hyperreactivity, as seen in asthma.

Viral respiratory infections also play a role in the pathophysiology of asthma with the development of increased levels of airway hyperreactivity and an increased frequency of late-phase asthmatic reactions to allergen during acute infections. Indeed, the increases in airway hyperreactivity that follow a respiratory viral infection may persist for weeks beyond the infection. Possible contributors to these phenomena include direct epithelial damage, the production of virus-specific IgE antibodies, enhancement

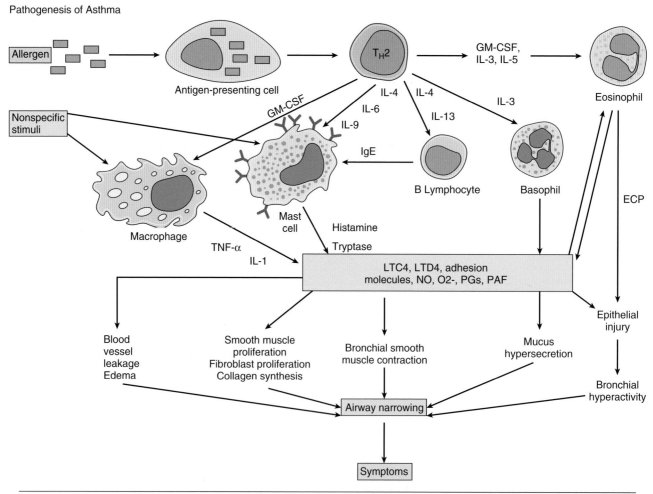

**Figure 5-14.** Cells and mediators interacting to result in asthma pathophysiology. ECP, eosinophil cationic protein; GM-CSF, granulocyte-macrophage colony-stimulating factor; IL, interleukin; LT, leukotriene; NO, nitric oxide; $O_2$., superoxide; PAF, platelet-activating factor; PGs, prostaglandins; $T_H$, helper T cell; TNF, tumor necrosis factor.

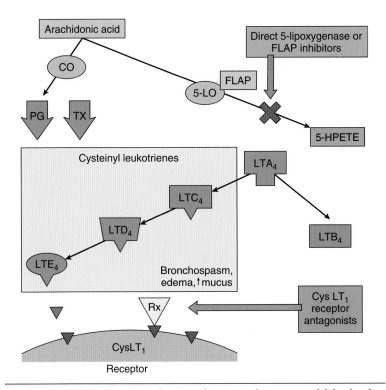

**Figure 5-15.** Leukotriene biosynthetic pathways and blockade. Note the interaction of the cysteinyl leukotrienes with the $CysLT_1$ (leukotriene) receptor and the role of receptor antagonists. Such a receptor is present on the surface of cells such as airway smooth muscle cells and eosinophils. $H_PETE$, hydroperoxy eicosatetraenoic acid; PG, prostaglandin; Rx, treatment; TX, thromboxane.

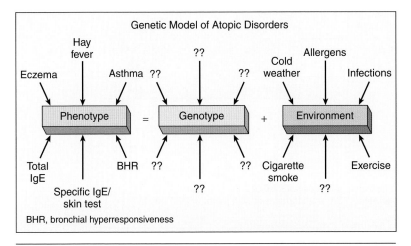

**Figure 5-16.** Genetic model of atopic disorders, whereby phenotype (disease expression) is determined by genotype and environmental exposure. Many of the genes are unknown, but some are being characterized. BHR, bronchial hyper-responsiveness; Ig, immunoglobulin.

of the production of IgE antibodies specific for other antigens, upregulation of neurogenic inflammatory pathways, and increases in the level of mediator release from inflammatory cells.

In addition to viruses and allergens, other environmental agents, including inhaled ozone, can induce airway inflammation and hyperreactivity. Once airway hyperreactivity is present, airway obstruction—and thus, the common asthma symptoms of wheezing and dyspnea—can be triggered by subthreshold levels of exposure to nonspecific environmental irritants, such as cigarette smoke and sulfur dioxide.

## PATHOPHYSIOLOGY OF ACUTE EXACERBATIONS OF ASTHMA

The development of the typical symptoms of acute asthma (progressive worsening of cough, breathlessness, wheezing, and chest tightness) is accompanied by decreases in expiratory airflow rates. Bronchial smooth-muscle contraction is one of the primary factors contributing to the airway obstruction. Other contributory factors include inflammation changes, such as mucosal edema and mucous plugging, which results in air trapping and hyperinflation. Physiologic changes that progress as the acute process worsens include both clinical and laboratory alterations. Clinically, patients with progressive airway obstruction use accessory muscles of respiration (sternocleidomastoid muscles) to maintain the state of hyperinflation. This, in turn, enables patients to maintain airway patency and thus, adequate gas exchange. Indeed, the use of accessory muscles to breathe correlates very well with the severity of an episode of acute asthma and is superior to dyspnea and wheezing as a sign of a severe episode.

The severity of acute asthma, however, is best assessed by pulmonary function testing. During acute asthma, progressive changes are noted in functional residual capacity (increased), $FEV_1$ (decreased), peak expiratory flow rate (decreased), and forced vital capacity (decreased or normal). The latter change correlates with the degree of hyperinflation. Blood gas assessment may reveal hypoxemia because of mismatching of ventilation and perfusion. Hypocapnia (reduced arterial carbon dioxide levels) and respiratory alkalosis (increased pH) are the usual manifestations of early acute asthma, because alveolar ventilation is maintained at this stage. However, with more severe obstruction, ventilation is compromised and arterial carbon dioxide levels rise (hypercapnia) with decreased pH and respiratory acidosis. The latter finding signals the development of acute respiratory insufficiency and the presence of an $FEV_1$ that is less than 25% of the predicted value.

Other physiologic changes that occur in acute asthma include increased pulmonary vascular resistance and an increased after-load on the left ventricle due to the high negative pleural pressures that result from lung hyperinflation. The clinical manifestation of these changes is the development of pulsus paradoxus, which is an exaggerated fall in systolic pressure during inspiration. Its presence correlates with an $FEV_1$ less than 50% of the predicted value for that patient.

## CLINICAL PRESENTATION AND DIFFERENTIAL DIAGNOSIS

Asthma can present in a number of different ways, ranging from a history of symptom association with upper respiratory infection or allergen exposure, isolated chronic cough, or exercise-induced wheezing to repeated episodes of wheezing, shortness of breath, and tachypnea of various levels of severity, requiring various levels of intervention (e.g., emergency department visit, hospitalization, intensive care unit stay). Clinically diagnosed asthma most likely represents a heterogeneous group of disorders with many possible underlying causes. This heterogeneity is probably responsible for the variability in presentation observed among different patients with asthma, as well as in the same individual at different times.

The diagnosis of asthma requires the documentation of episodic airway obstruction and the reversibility of that obstruction, preferably using spirometry in children older than 5 years and repeated clinical examinations in younger children, as well as the exclusion of alternative diagnoses. These alternative diagnoses can include disorders such as vocal cord dysfunction in the older patient and vascular ring in the younger child (Tables 5-3 and 5-4). The presence of recurrent cough or wheezing triggered at nighttime or by exercise or cold air exposures, especially in the context of a

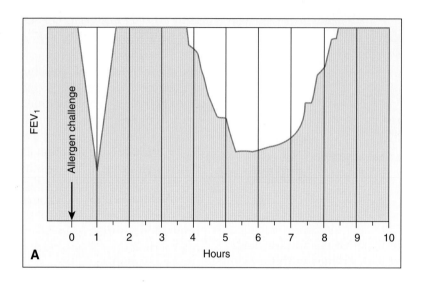

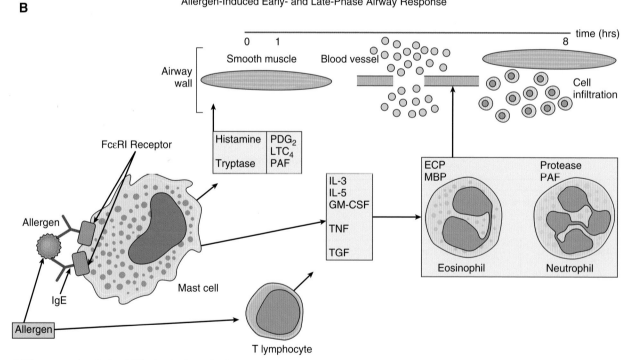

Allergen-Induced Early- and Late-Phase Airway Response

PGD$_2$, prostaglandin D$_2$; LTC$_4$, leukotriene C$_4$; PAF, platelet-activating factor; IL, interleukin; GM-CSF, granulocyte-macrophage colony-stimulating factor; TNF, tumor necrosis factor; TGF, transforming growth factor; ECP, eosinophil cationic protein; MBP, major basic protein.

**Figure 5-17.** *A,* Early and late asthmatic responses in FEV$_1$ (forced expiratory volume in 1 second) to inhaled allergen challenge. *B,* Allergen-induced early- and late-phase airway tissue responses. Notably, airway hyperreactivity increases after late-phase asthmatic responses. ECP, eosinophil cationic protein; FcεRI, Fcε receptor I; GM-CSF, granulocyte-macrophage colony-stimulating factor; Ig, immunoglobulin; IL, interleukin; LT, leukotriene; MBP, major basic protein; PAF, platelet-activating factor; PG, prostaglandin; TGF, transforming growth factor; TNF, tumor necrosis factor.

**TABLE 5-3**
**Differential Diagnosis of Wheezing (Causes Other Than Asthma)**

| Diagnostic Clues | Possible Cause |
| --- | --- |
| Sudden onset of wheezing, choking, or coughing; recurrent wheezing, persistent cough, or recurrent pneumonia | Foreign-body aspiration |
| Chronic wheezing that is not responsive to bronchodilators or corticosteroids; wheezing may increase with feeding, crying, positional changes, or flexion of the neck | Vascular rings |
| Persistent stridor and wheezing that have been present since birth | Laryngeal webs |
| Noisy breathing, especially on inspiration; noisy breathing and wheezing are intermittent and increase when the infant is supine; stridor present since birth; history of feeding difficulties | Laryngotracheobronchomalacia |
| Symptoms of upper respiratory tract infection (cough, fever, rhinitis); tachypnea, retractions, cyanosis | Bronchiolitis |
| Failure to thrive, fever, diarrhea, recurrent pneumonia | Cystic fibrosis |
| History of prematurity and intubation; increased airway hyperreactivity, severe respiratory distress | Bronchopulmonary dysplasia |
| Frequent emesis; irritability during feedings; recurrent wheezing | Gastroesophageal reflux |
| Recurrent wheezing and pneumonia; episodes of cough or cyanosis associated with feeding | Tracheoesophageal fistula |
| Recurrent sinusitis, otitis media, and pneumonia | Primary immunodeficiency |

From Fausnight TB, Gentile DA, Skoner DP: Determining the cause of recurrent wheezing in infants. J Respir Dis Pediatrician 2002;4:126–131.

**TABLE 5-4**
**Selected Diagnostic Tests for the Evaluation of Wheezing**

| Suspected Diagnosis | Selected Diagnostic Tests |
| --- | --- |
| Foreign body | Inspiratory and expiratory chest x-ray, bronchoscopy |
| Vascular rings | Barium esophagraphy |
| Laryngeal web | Direct laryngoscopy |
| Laryngotracheobronchomalacia | Direct laryngoscopy, airway fluoroscopy |
| Enlarged lymph nodes/tumors | Chest x-ray, CT scan, biopsy |
| Bronchiolitis | Nasal washing for presence of RSV |
| Cystic fibrosis | Sweat test, genetic tests |
| Gastroesophageal reflux | pH probe, endoscopy |
| Tracheoesophageal fistula | Barium esophagraphy and fluoroscopy |
| Primary immunodeficiency | CBC with differential, quantitative Ig levels |
| Asthma | Trial of bronchodilators and corticosteroids |
| Congenital Heart Disease | CXR, EKG, ECHO |

CBC, complete blood count; CT, computed tomography; CXR, chest x-ray; ECHO, echocardiogram; EKG, electrocardiogram; RSV, respiratory syncytial virus.
From Fausnight TB, Gentile DA, Skoner DP: Determining the cause of recurrent wheezing in infants. J Respir Dis Pediatrician 2002;4:126–131.

positive family history, is a particularly helpful clue in establishing the diagnosis of asthma.

Some patients present with cough as the sole manifestation of asthma. These patients typically have normal pulmonary function tests, with some improvement with the bronchodilator, and manifest airway hyperreactivity to provocative stimuli, such as methacholine, exercise, or cold air (see Chapter 3).

During the history and physical examination, particular attention should be focused on the growth pattern of children. Severe asthma can suppress the growth of young children,[15] but poor growth is a predominant feature of many of the masqueraders of asthma, such as cystic fibrosis. Also, the presence of upper respiratory findings compatible with allergic rhinitis (pale, boggy nasal turbinates, suborbital venous congestion—"shiners"—nasal crease, Denie's lines [see Chapter 9]), and skin manifestations of atopic dermatitis (see Chapter 15) should be noted. The examination should focus on the appearance of a hyperexpanded chest, presence of cyanosis, degree of respiratory distress, use of accessory muscles, wheezing, decreased inspiratory-to-expiratory ratio, rhonchi, and other findings on auscultation that might indicate pneumonia or atelectasis. The cardiac examination should be geared toward the identification of congenital heart disease in young children and congestive heart failure in adults.

Acute asthma symptoms usually consist of progressively increasing shortness of breath (dyspnea), cough and difficulty breathing with or without rhinorrhea, low-grade fever, and other manifestations of an upper respiratory infection. On auscultation, expiratory wheezing or a prolonged expiratory phase may be the only manifestation of mild asthma. However, as the obstructive process progresses, the expiratory phase becomes longer (Fig. 5-18) and the musical high-pitched rhonchi grow louder.

Without appropriate treatment and reversal, signs of hyperinflation (air trapping) develop, with depressed diaphragms, decreased excursions of the chest wall with respiration, and hyperresonance to percussion. Subjectively, the patient experiences chest tightness and anxiety and works harder to breath. Accessory muscle use (visible contractions of the scalene and/or sternocleidomastoid muscles) and retractions (visible depressions in the chest wall during inspiration) develop with or without a marked degree of wheezing on auscultation. The patient usually assumes an upright posture to maximize air exchange. As respiratory muscles tire, the patient becomes lethargic and cyanotic, even with supplemental oxygen.

Maximal effort to breathe produces feeble air exchange, manifested by decreased intensity and duration or lack of inspiratory breath sounds as air exchange decreases. Consequently, a patient with severe obstruction and impending respiratory failure may not have audible wheezing because too little air is being ventilated to create the sound. With extreme fatigue, respiratory muscles fail, retractions decrease, and respiratory failure is imminent unless appropriate therapy is promptly initiated.

Following the initial examination, serial assessment of the degree of respiratory distress, using a standardized clinical scoring system (Table 5-5), facilitates determination of response to therapy

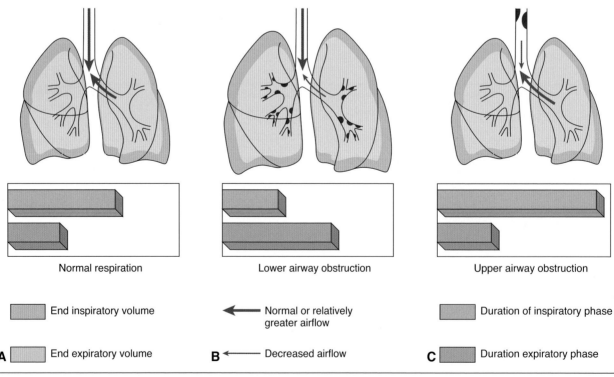

| | | |
|---|---|---|
| Normal respiration | Lower airway obstruction | Upper airway obstruction |

| End inspiratory volume | ← Normal or relatively greater airflow | Duration of inspiratory phase |
| **A** End expiratory volume | **B** ← Decreased airflow | **C** Duration expiratory phase |

**Figure 5-18.** Characteristic changes in lung volumes and duration of respiratory phases in upper and lower airway obstructive disorders. Normal respiration *(A)*. On auscultation, the expiratory phase is prolonged in lower airway disorders *(B)*, and the inspiratory phase is prolonged in upper airway disorders *(C)*. Note the increased lung volumes (hyperinflation) during both respiratory phases in lower airway disorders. (Adapted with permission from Skoner D, Stillwagon P, Friedman R, Fireman P: Pediatric Allergy and Immunology. In Davis H, Zitelli B (eds.): Atlas of Pediatric Physical Diagnosis. London, Gower Press, 1987.)

and ensures early detection of impending respiratory failure or other complications. Any change in sensorium requires a prompt evaluation for impending respiratory failure.

Between episodes of acute asthma, the physical findings vary with the chronicity of the disease process. In mild asthmatics, the examination is usually entirely normal, but wheezing may be elicited in children by gentle manual chest wall compression, which restricts chest expansion and increases the work of breathing. In contrast, severe asthmatics with a long history of airway obstruction that has not received appropriate therapy may have signs of chronic lung disease. These include a paucity of subcutaneous fatty tissue and a barrel-chest configuration (Fig. 5-19A). Adults with chronic asthma may produce copious amounts of sputum. Rales, wheezing, rhonchi, and decreased intensity and duration of the inspiratory phase of respiration are commonly found on auscultation. Chest radiography may show areas of atelectasis (Fig. 5-19B).

Asthma should be considered as part of the differential diagnosis in any patient with recurrent or chronic lower respiratory symptoms or signs of lower airway obstruction. Even though a high index of suspicion must be maintained, diagnoses may be excessive or erroneous if made hastily without the appropriate supportive evidence. Patients or their parents must be instructed that physician assessment is essential during suspected episodes of asthma so that wheezing or other signs of lower airway obstruction and reversibility, if present, can be documented.

Asthma is the most common cause of recurrent episodes of cough and wheezing in both adults and children. However, asthma is frequently misdiagnosed and underdiagnosed, especially in young children who wheeze only during respiratory infections and who are labeled as having bronchitis, bronchiolitis, or pneumonia. Nonetheless, the differential diagnosis of asthma includes a number of other disorders, depending on the age group under consideration (see earlier figures).

Any patient with acute asthma who develops symptoms of pleuritic chest pain, severe dyspnea, cyanosis, and tachypnea, as well as physical findings of unilaterally decreased or absent breath sounds, should be evaluated radiographically for pneumothorax (Fig. 5-20A). With tension pneumothorax, the trachea, mediastinum, and cardiac landmarks may be shifted to the opposite side (Fig. 5-20B). Pneumomediastinum and subcutaneous emphysema, usually involving the neck and supraclavicular areas, are more

**TABLE 5-5**
**Estimation of Severity of Acute Exacerbations of Asthma in Children***

| Sign/Symptom | Mild | Moderate | Severe |
|---|---|---|---|
| PEFR[†] | 70%–90% predicted or personal best | 50%–70% predicted or personal best | <50% predicted or personal best |
| Respiratory rate, resting or sleeping | Normal to 30% increase above the mean | 30%–50% increase above the mean | Increase over 50% above the mean |
| Alertness | Normal | Normal | May be decreased |
| Dyspnea[‡] | Absent or mild; speaks in complete sentences | Moderate; speaks in phrases or partial sentences; infant's cry softer and shorter; infant has difficulty suckling and feeding | Severe; speaks only in single words or short phrases; infant's cry softer and shorter; infant stops suckling and feeding |
| Pulsus paradoxicus[§] | <10 mm Hg | 10–20 mm Hg | 20–40 mm Hg |
| Accessory muscle use | No intercostal to mild retractions | Moderate intercostal retraction with tracheosternal retractions; use of sternocleidomastoid muscles; chest hyperinflation | Severe intercostal retractions, tracheosternal retractions with nasal flaring during inspiration; chest hyperinflation |
| Color | Good | Pale | Possibly cyanotic |
| Auscultation | End expiratory wheeze only | Wheeze during entire expiration and inspiration | Breath sounds becoming inaudible |
| Oxygen saturation | >95% | 90%–95% | <90% |
| $PCO_2$ | <35 | <40 | >40 |

*Within each category, the presence of several parameters, but not necessarily all, indicate the general classification of the exacerbation.
[†]For children 5 yr or older.
[‡]Parents' or physicians' impression of degree of child's breathlessness.
[§]Pulsus paradoxus does not correlate with phase of respiration in small children.
PEFR, peak expiratory flow rate.

common than pneumothorax. When mild, they may be asymptomatic and detected incidentally by radiography (Fig. 5-20C). With more extensive air dissection, the patient may complain of neck and chest pain, and the subcutaneous emphysema (see Fig. 5-20A) may be visibly evident as a soft tissue swelling of the neck and chest, which is crepitant (has a crunching sound) on palpation.

Cardiovascular manifestations can also be detected during acute asthma. Heart rate and blood pressure are frequently elevated. Pulsus paradoxus, an exaggerated decrease in systolic blood pressure during inspiration, can serve as an indicator of severity and a guide to therapy. Pulsus paradoxus and the patient's exaggerated use of accessory muscles both correlate highly with the degree of airway obstruction.

In patients who present with respiratory distress or wheezing for the first time, a complete differential diagnosis of all causes of upper and lower airway obstructive processes must be undertaken. In the older child or adult with mild, infrequent episodes of wheezing that respond to bronchodilator therapy, asthma is usually readily diagnosed. However, with daily wheezing, frequent exacerbations, lack of response to bronchodilators, or poor growth, other diagnoses must be considered. These include chronic obstructive pulmonary disease, cystic fibrosis, $\alpha_1$-antitrypsin deficiency, carcinoid syndrome, and an associated immunologic deficiency (see Chapter 20 and earlier tables).

Chronic obstructive pulmonary diseases, which include chronic bronchitis, emphysema, bronchiectasis, and bronchopulmonary dysplasia, are distinguished by their lack of significant reversibility with bronchodilator therapy. Cystic fibrosis, a multisystem disease, may present with chronic cough, wheezing, and recurrent infections, especially sinusitis. Additionally, malabsorption with bulky, foul-smelling stools, failure to thrive, and clubbing of the nail beds are common. Indeed, clubbing is a very rare sign of chronic asthma and, if present in a wheezing patient, suggests another chronic pulmonary disease. $\alpha_1$-Antitrypsin deficiency, an inherited autosomal-recessive disorder, is characterized by the onset of progressive emphysema in adults, especially those who smoke cigarettes, but may also manifest as hepatic disease in the neonate and young child.

In wheezing infants, the differential diagnosis includes disorders that are unique to that age group (see earlier tables), especially bronchiolitis. In many infants, bronchiolitis is the initial manifestation of asthma, and differentiation between the two is occasionally difficult. Even though these two diseases share common clinical manifestations, sequelae, and possible pathogeneses, the distinction between them remains clinically useful for the following reasons:

1. Many children with bronchiolitis do not develop asthma and may be inappropriately labeled as having asthma.
2. Children younger than 2 years frequently do not respond to inhaled or injected bronchodilators.

Even though acute management is the same, the clinician generally should attempt to differentiate on clinical grounds between virus- and non–virus-induced wheezing episodes. If wheezing due to allergen or other inhalant exposure is suspected historically, an appropriate evaluation for allergen IgE antibodies and the subsequent application of avoidance techniques to prevent future exacerbations should ensue.

Status asthmaticus, a complication of asthma, is diagnosed by failure to improve significantly after appropriate bronchodilator

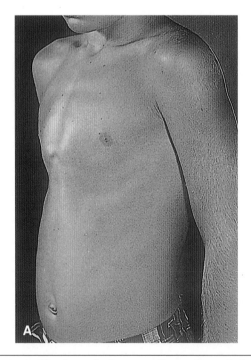
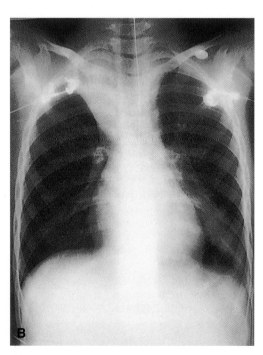

**Figure 5-19.** *A*, The barrel-chest configuration of chronic asthma. Physical findings include an increased anteroposterior diameter of the chest and decreased respiratory excursion of the chest wall. (Courtesy of Dr Meyer B. Marks and with permission from Skoner D, Stillwagon P, Friedman R, Fireman P: Pediatric Allergy and Immunology. In Davis H, Zitelli B (eds.): Atlas of Pediatric Physical Diagnosis. London, Gower Press, 1987.) *B*, Chest radiograph showing right upper lobe and left lower lobe atelectasis in a patient with acute asthma. (Courtesy of Dr. Beverly Newman, Children's Hospital of Pittsburgh.)

therapy and indicates a need for hospitalization. This is manifested by post-therapy wheezing, elevations in respiratory rate, and abnormalities in the inspiratory-to-expiratory ratio. Progressive deterioration of respiratory function in the context of maximal medical therapy for status asthmaticus indicates impending respiratory failure, which progresses to respiratory failure if untreated. The diagnosis of impending respiratory failure is based on arterial blood gas findings of $Pa_{O_2}$ of less than 70 in 40% $Fi_{O_2}$, and $Pa_{CO2}$ greater than 45 (or an increasing $Pa_{CO2}$ on serial blood gases) in the appropriate clinical setting.

In children older than 5 years, specific laboratory studies should be performed to document asthma or rule out disorders that mimic it. An algorithm for diagnosing asthma is shown in (Fig. 5-21). Pulmonary function tests in asthma show airway

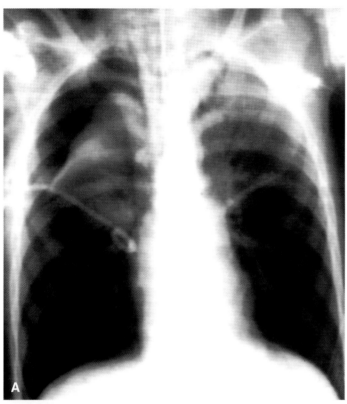

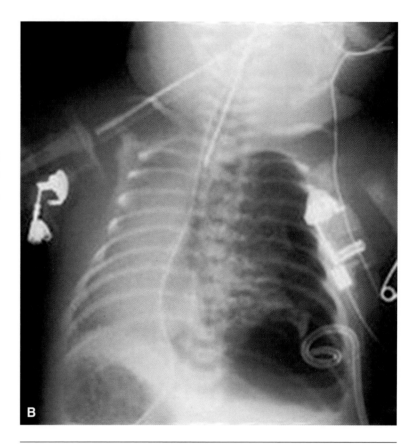

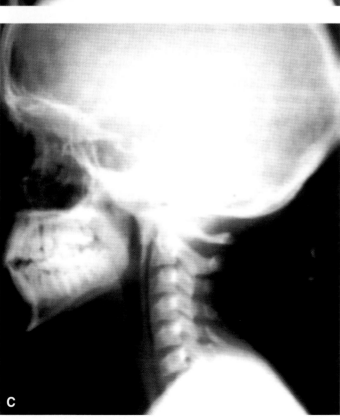

Figure 5-20. *A*, Chest radiograph showing right-sided pneumothorax in intubated patient with acute asthma and respiratory failure. Also note the marked hyperinflation of the lungs, which can result in cardiac compression (narrow cardiac shadow) and compromise of cardiac venous return, and the extensive right-sided subcutaneous emphysema. (Courtesy of Dr. Beverly Newman, Children's Hospital of Pittsburgh.) *B*, Chest radiograph showing right-sided tension pneumothorax. Note shifting of mediastinum to the left. *C*, Lateral neck radiograph showing spontaneous pneumomediastinum in a child with asthma. Note the dissection of air in soft tissues just anterior to the vertebrae. Clinical manifestations include dysphagia. (Courtesy of Dr. Beverly Newman, Children's Hospital of Pittsburgh.)

obstruction at baseline or after methacholine challenge and, further, document reversibility of airway obstruction after administration of an aerosolized bronchodilator. In children younger than 5 years or people such as the elderly in whom testing is unreliable, the diagnosis must be made solely on the basis of historical and physical findings, in conjunction with clinical response to bronchodilators. Lack of a prompt response to bronchodilators does not, however, eliminate asthma as a diagnostic consideration. In assessing preschool children with wheezing, which is only sometimes due to asthma, the risk of asthma is now assessable[16] (Fig. 5-22).

Patients who present with a history of isolated chronic cough or exercise-induced wheezing can be diagnosed by the reversibility of symptoms with a bronchodilator. When necessary, this impression can be confirmed by a positive pulmonary function or methacholine bronchoprovocation test. In patients who have sudden onset of wheezing and respiratory distress, the differential diagnosis for lower airway disorders includes respiratory infections, left ventricular failure, and foreign-body aspiration. Lower respiratory infections (pneumonia) generally produce fever and more localized findings of rales, decrease and change in quality of breath sounds, and egophony. A history of cardiac disease and auscultatory findings of diffuse crackles, basilar rales, and a third heart sound help to distinguish left ventricular failure with pulmonary edema from asthma.

In children, especially toddlers, aspiration of a foreign body that becomes lodged in a mainstem bronchus may produce wheezing that at times is partially responsive to bronchodilator

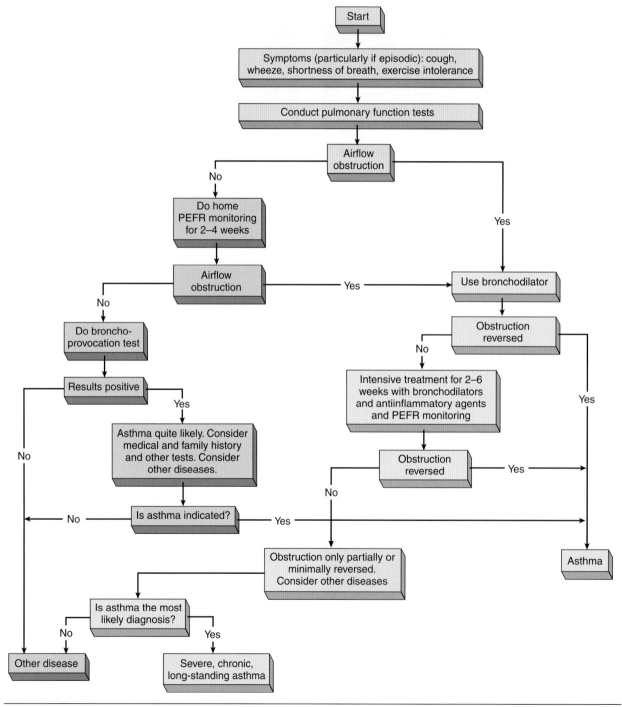

**Figure 5-21.** Algorithm for diagnosing asthma. PEFR, peak expiratory flow rates.

therapy (Fig. 5-23). The history of a choking episode and physical findings of unilateral wheezing and hyperresonance aid in distinguishing aspiration from asthma but do not confirm the diagnosis. Airway compression by anomalous vessels or mass lesions is often distinguishable from bronchiolitis by virtue of absence of signs of infection and from asthma by failure to respond to bronchodilators. Radiographic studies, such as barium swallow with fluoroscopy, can be very helpful in distinguishing between these entities (Fig. 5-24A). Gastroesophageal reflux can be associated with asthma and is diagnosed by pH-probe testing or radiography

(Fig. 5-24B). Cough secondary to drugs (e.g., angiotensin-converting enzyme [ACE] inhibitors) should be considered in patients presenting with cough as the primary manifestation. Patients in whom the diagnosis is unclear should be referred to an asthma care specialist.

Pulmonary function tests are important in confirming suspected asthma.[1] Between episodes of acute asthma, the findings depend on the chronicity and severity of the disease. Pulmonary function may be entirely normal in mild asthmatics, but acute airway obstruction can be induced by provocative methacholine inhalation. In contrast, marked reductions in expiratory flow rates may be present in severe asthmatics at baseline and are characteristically observed to a greater degree during acute asthma. However, a decreased expiratory flow rate due to asthma, an obstructive lung disease, must be differentiated from that due to restrictive lung diseases, such as cystic fibrosis (Fig. 5-25A).

Airway obstruction, when present, may or may not reverse with bronchodilators. If obstruction is detected, reversibility with bronchodilators, as illustrated conceptually in Figure 5-25B, should be determined and used to guide the formulation of a therapeutic regimen. Bronchodilator effectiveness may relate to the relative contribution of smooth muscle contraction versus inflammation as the cause of airway obstruction.

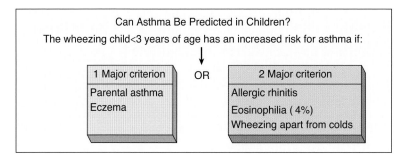

**Figure 5-22.** Criteria to determine if a wheezing child younger than 3 years has an increased risk for asthma. (From Castro-Rodriguez JA, Holberg CJ, Wright AL, Martinez FD: A clinical index to define risk of asthma in young children with recurrent wheezing. Am J Respir Crit Care Med 2000;162:1403–1406).

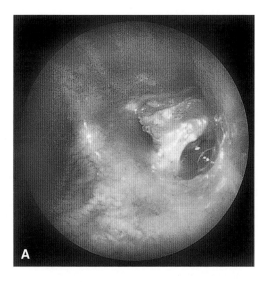

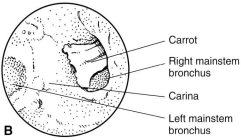

**Figure 5-23.** A, Piece of carrot lodged in right main-stem bronchus just below the carina, as visualized during bronchoscopy. Foreign bodies such as this can cause airway obstruction that is partially responsive to bronchodilators. B, Diagram of part A with tissue labeled. (Courtesy of Dr. Sylvan Stool, Children's Hospital of Pittsburgh.)

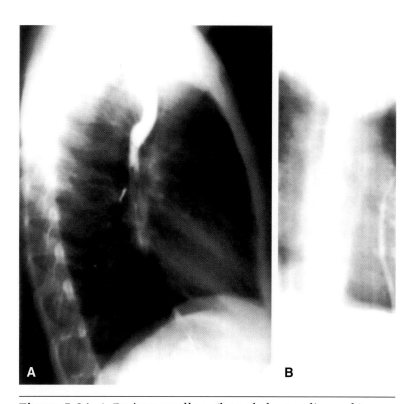

**Figure 5-24.** A, Barium swallow (lateral chest radiograph) demonstrating upper airway compression by right-sided aortic arch with aberrant left subclavian and diverticulum at the left subclavian origin. Note the round indentation on the posterior wall of the esophagus and the anterior displacement and compression of the trachea, which can cause wheezing and mimic asthma. B, Radiograph demonstrating gastroesophageal reflux. Note that the gastroesophageal sphincter is wide open, and the reflux of barium extends over the entire length of the esophagus. This can cause aspiration and wheezing, mimicking asthma. (Courtesy of Dr. Beverly Newman, Children's Hospital of Pittsburgh.)

The clinician conducting an outpatient laboratory evaluation for asthma should always consider an immunologic cause and include the appropriate allergy testing so that potential inciting agents can be avoided. The most economic and reliable method is allergy skin testing, with serum-specific IgE antibody tests serving as an alternative method when skin testing is contraindicated (see Chapter 3). IgE levels may be a useful adjunct in suggesting an allergic cause. Additionally, sinus radiographs may be indicated in selected patients, because chronic sinusitis can exacerbate asthma (see Chapter 10).

Peripheral blood and sputum eosinophilia are usually present during recurrent and chronic asthma. Some clinicians, particularly those caring for adults, use the eosinophil count in sputum or blood as a guide to therapy, as decreased counts generally accompany clinical improve-ment. The radiographic features of uncomplicated acute asthma include hyperinflation, peribronchial cuffing, and atelectasis. Arterial blood (Table 5-6) usually shows hypoxemia, hypocarbia, and respiratory alkalosis, due to hyperventilation during the early stages of acute asthma. However, as the degree of airway obstruction increases or respiratory muscles tire, hypoxemia persists

and carbon dioxide retention (hypercarbia) is detectable, resulting in a respiratory acidosis. This indicates impending respiratory failure.

Identification of a viral cause using fluorescent antibody tests or enzyme-linked immunosorbent assays (ELISA) has little impact on acute therapy due to the paucity of available antiviral

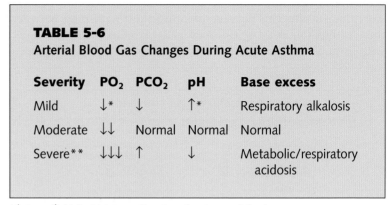

**TABLE 5-6**
**Arterial Blood Gas Changes During Acute Asthma**

| Severity | PO$_2$ | PCO$_2$ | pH | Base excess |
|---|---|---|---|---|
| Mild | ↓* | ↓ | ↑* | Respiratory alkalosis |
| Moderate | ↓↓ | Normal | Normal | Normal |
| Severe** | ↓↓↓ | ↑ | ↓ | Metabolic/respiratory acidosis |

*↓, Low; ↑, high; **status asthmaticus (respiratory failure).

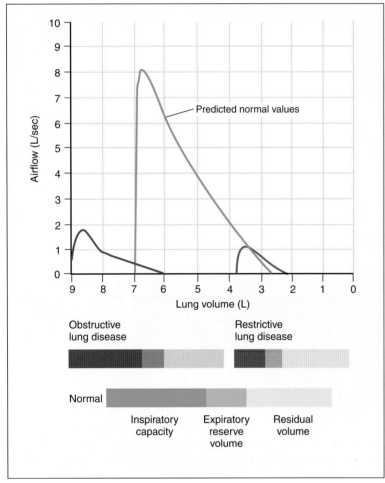

**A**

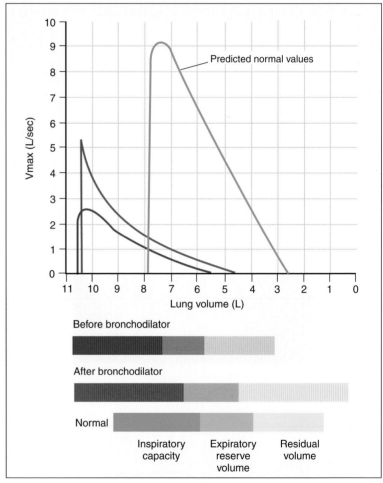

**B**

**Figure 5-25.** *A,* Maximal expiratory flow rates are reduced in both obstructive lung diseases, such as asthma, and restrictive lung diseases. However, in asthma, the airflow is limited at high lung volumes, in contrast to restrictive lung diseases, in which airflow is limited because the lung volume is decreased. (With permission from Cherniack, 1987, p. 91.) *B,* Bronchoconstriction characteristic of hyperreactive airways is generally reversible. Indices of expiratory airflow in asthmatic patients thus improve after inhalation of a nebulized bronchodilator (e.g., a beta-2–adrenergic agonist). (With permission from Cherniack, 1987.)

medications and should be limited to severely ill patients or the onset of an epidemic to document epidemiology.

# TREATMENT

Asthma therapy is administered in several different settings, including outpatient (home or office), emergency department, and inpatient (hospital) facilities.

## OUTPATIENT MANAGEMENT OF CHRONIC ASTHMA

The goals of effective outpatient asthma management are shown in (Box 5-1).[1,2] Several general principles should guide the clinician in providing asthma treatment. First, asthma is a chronic disease with periodic acute exacerbations. Second, treatment should be based on an understanding of the pathophysiology of asthma, highlighted by the prophylactic use of environmental control measures and anti-inflammatory agents to treat the underlying inflammation and the "as-needed" use of short-acting bronchodilator agents to treat the periodic acute bronchospasm. Recent guidelines have focused on four major components of outpatient asthma management: 1) assessment and monitoring; 2) control of factors contributing to asthma severity; 3) patient education for a partnership; and 4) pharmacologic therapy. Asthma is considered a very "care-responsive" disease.

### Assessment and Monitoring

The two main objective measures of lung function are office-based spirometry and home-based peak expiratory flow-rate

measurements. Pulmonary function studies by spirometry are essential in diagnosing asthma and in assessing asthma severity. The importance of obtaining these measurements is highlighted by the observation that the patient's symptoms and the physician's assessment of severity often do not correlate with the severity of airflow obstruction. Office-based spirometry should be conducted in the initial evaluation of all patients with suspected asthma and during subsequent evaluations on a periodic basis.

To assess the response to therapy in the office, emergency department, or hospital, either spirometry or peak expiratory flow-rate measurement can be used. Measurement of peak expiratory flow rate (PEFR) with a peak flow meter (Fig. 5-26) should

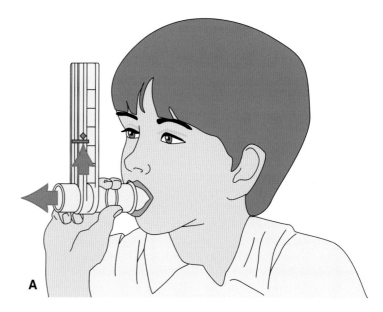

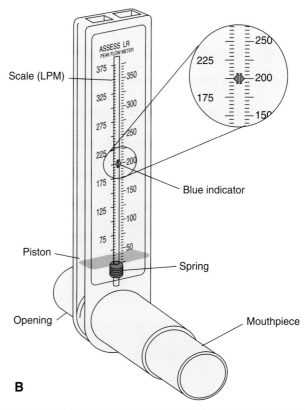

**Figure 5-26.** Example of *(A)* a patient using a peak flow meter, and *(B)* a typical peak flow meter used to monitor asthma severity.

---

**BOX 5-1**
**Goals of Asthma Care?**

- No chronic symptoms
- Normal or near-normal lung function
- Normal activity levels
- No recurrent exacerbations
- No missed school or work due to asthma
- No sleep disruption
- No (or minimal) need for emergency department visits or hospitalizations
- Optimal therapy with minimal adverse effects
- Fulfillment of patient and family expectations and satisfaction

From NAEPP. Guidelines for the Diagnosis and Management of Asthma. NIH publication 97-4051A, May, 1997, National Heart, Lung, and Blood Institute: Global Initiative for Asthma. November, 1998, NIH publication 96-3659B. American Academy of Allergy, Asthma, and Immunology: Pediatric Asthma: Promoting Best Practice: Guide for Managing Asthma in Children, Rochester, NY, Academic Services Consortium.

be used to monitor the course of persistent moderate to severe asthma at home and the response to therapy in patients 6 years of age or older. These values can provide valuable information to the managing clinician about asthma severity and the need to add or delete medications.

It is essential to provide teaching to patients for whom peak flow meters are prescribed, both on the proper use of the instrument and on the interpretation of values. For the latter, published predicted normal values for a given individual can be used. However, because the values for many patients are consistently higher or lower than predicted norms, establishing a "personal best" PEFR value is an acceptable alternative. The patient and clinician then use this value as a standard in evaluating subsequent measurements. Personal best PEFR values can be established by the performance of twice-daily PEFR measurements during a "well" period or during a period of maximal therapy. This value should be reestablished on a yearly basis. PEFR values should be recorded in the morning and evening, both before and after use of any inhaled medications. Highly stable asthmatics may not need to continuously monitor PEFR, although the ability to detect the early onset of obstruction may be compromised when not done daily during asymptomatic periods.

Through the use of predicted norm or personal best values, PEFR zones should be developed. Green zones (80% to 100% of predicted or personal best) indicate normal values. Yellow zones (50% to 80%) signal caution and a possible need for a temporary increase in medication. Alternatively, an increase in prophylactic therapy may be indicated. Finally, red zones (under 50%) indicate a medical emergency, whereby an inhaled bronchodilator should be used immediately and the clinician should be notified if the values do not increase into the yellow or green zones (Fig. 5-27). Transport to an emergency facility may be indicated if the response is inadequate. This also signals the need for a temporary increase in medication (such as systemic corticosteroids).

## Control of Factors Contributing to Asthma Severity

The identification of asthma triggers is essential in the management of asthma. An evaluation for the presence of allergen-specific IgE antibodies is warranted in any patient who has persistent asthma or who requires daily medications. This is usually accomplished with puncture skin testing (see Chapter 3). In vitro serum tests, which provide the same information as skin tests, may also be used. However, these tests are usually less sensitive and more expensive. Testing for IgE to a panel of inhalant allergens is indicated, but routine testing for food allergies is not indicated. One possible exception is the infant or young child with asthma, who may be allergic and wheeze in association with ingestion of milk, soy, or (rarely) other foods, such as peanut, egg, or wheat (see Chapter 13). Food allergens are uncommon triggers of asthma symptoms in older children and adults. Allergy skin testing should be conducted and supervised by the clinician, who interprets the results in the context of the medical history and physical examination and who recommends appropriate therapy. After identification of the offending allergens, thorough environmental control measures should be implemented in the patient's living and working environments. This may include measures to control outdoor allergen exposure, such as staying indoors with windows closed in an air-conditioned environment (especially during midday and afternoon, when pollen and mold counts may be high), and reduction of indoor allergen exposure to molds, dust mites, cockroaches, and pets. Indoor humidity levels should be maintained at 35% to 50%. Several other control measures may be particularly helpful, including air conditioning and the use of central indoor air-cleaning devices, such as mechanical filters (high-efficiency particulate air, or HEPA, filters) and electrical filters (electrostatic precipitator). Vacuum sweepers have a tendency to mobilize fine respirable allergens and provoke symptoms when

**Figure 5-27.** Typical peak flow meter diary. This patient dipped into the yellow zone on January 19th and recovered after use of a short-acting beta-2 agonist. The patient entered the red zone on January 22nd and gradually improved after beginning therapy with systemic corticosteroids. (National Asthma Education and Prevention Program: Practical Guide for the diagnosis and management of asthma. Bethesda, MD, National Heart, Lung, and Blood Institute; National Institutes of Health, 1997.)

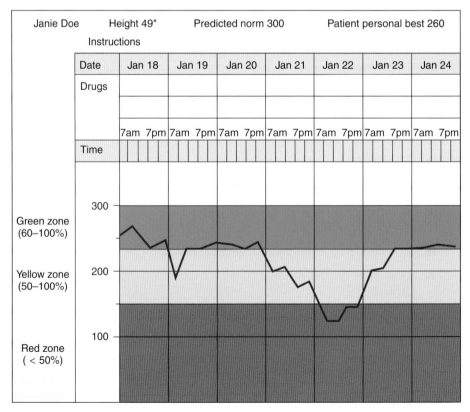

used by dust-allergic people, who should use a facemask, a central vacuum cleaner system with the collecting bag outside the home, or a cleaner fitted with a high-efficiency particulate air filter.

Additionally, nonallergen, indoor irritants, such as tobacco smoke, smoke from wood-burning heating stoves, strong odors and sprays, and chemical air pollutants, especially ozone and sulphur dioxide, may contribute to asthma exacerbations. Exposure to these irritants should also be reduced.

If allergen avoidance is not possible and the appropriate medications fail to control symptoms of allergic asthma, allergy immunotherapy may be considered.[17] Allergy immunotherapy has been shown to reduce the symptoms of asthma associated with a variety of allergens, including house dust, cat dander, grass pollen, and alternaria. More recent studies have documented that children with monosensitization are less likely to develop new allergen sensitivities and that children with allergic rhinitis alone are less likely to develop new asthma when treated with allergen immunotherapy. Specific details of allergen immunotherapy are presented in Chapter 22. Adverse reactions following allergen immunotherapy are higher in patients with asthma, so appropriate and additional vigilance and precautions are necessary to avoid asthma exacerbation.

Parents should also be queried about daycare attendance in infants and toddlers, since it may result in repeated exposure to respiratory viruses, which are a major trigger of wheezing in this age group. Reduction in the frequency of upper respiratory infections caused by such viruses may result in a significant clinical improvement.

## Patient Education for a Partnership

Asthma education and the formulation of a partnership between the patient, family, and physician are of paramount importance in managing asthma. Educational topics should include a definition of asthma, asthma triggers and how to avoid or control them, key points about signs and symptoms of asthma, characteristic changes in the airways of patients with asthma, the role of the different types of medications (anti-inflammatory, bronchodilator), treatment, and patient fears about medications. This should also include education on the correct use of inhalers, criteria for premedicating to prevent symptoms, the optimal use of home PEFR monitoring, and the provision of written plans on recommended treatments for daily therapy (maintenance plan) and episodic acute asthma exacerbations (action plan). Specific, individualized guidelines for seeking advice from the clinician or emergency department care should also be provided. Such asthma education has been shown to reduce the morbidity associated with asthma and to improve asthma control.

## Pharmacologic Therapy

### Goals of Therapy

In the past, emergency department visits, hospitalizations, and school or work absences were considered an unavoidable consequence of asthma. Recently published guidelines have established new standards that challenge the ability of the health care system to deliver the new therapeutic advances to affected individuals. As illustrated in Table 5-7, the general goals of therapy are to maximize exertion and lung function and minimize symptoms, exacerbations, and medication side effects. The tools and

knowledge needed to achieve such goals are currently available. Asthma is a very care-responsive disease, whereby a clinician can almost always have a significant impact on the patient's quality of life if the clinician invests time and has the appropriate knowledge base. However, it is also clear that inadequate attention to the details of asthma management can leave a patient with low quality of life and at risk of all of the known complications of poorly controlled airway inflammation. Unfortunately, these include growth suppression in children, permanent structural changes in the airways, and death. Inappropriate treatment is a major contributor to asthma morbidity and mortality. To maximize the fulfillment of goals, each patient should be provided with a written maintenance and action plan. The former summarizes daily medication use when asthma is controlled, and the latter illustrates the response when control is lessening or lost. The action plan should detail the patient's response to increased asthma symptoms or drops in peak expiratory flow rate and should include provisions for increasing albuterol use, possibly doubling the inhaled corticosteroid (ICS) dose for 1 to 2 weeks, the use of an oral corticosteroid (such as prednisone) burst (3 to 10 days, 2 mg/kg/day [maximum 60 mg/day] without tapering), and calling the physician's office.

### General Approach

*Starting Initial Therapy—Reliever/Rescue Therapy*

Every patient with asthma of any severity requires uninterrupted access to the as-needed use of a short-acting bronchodilator. As indicated in the "Rules of Two™" (Box 5-2), refill of such a "quick-relief inhaler" more than two times a year can serve as a useful indicator of patients whose disease is poorly controlled. Also, use of more than one canister in 1 month indicates inadequate control and the need for more anti-inflammatory therapy. Regularly scheduled, daily use of short-acting beta-2 agonists is generally not recommended, as these agents have no long-term anti-inflammatory activity. Albuterol is generally the drug of choice for relief of bronchospasm, even though it is composed of a 50/50 racemic mixture of two stereoisomers of albuterol. Levalbuterol, the stereoisomer that provides the therapeutic benefit, is available for use when the albuterol response is poor or includes side effects.

---

**BOX 5-2**
**Take Control of Your Asthma "Rules of Two™ Can Help"***

Do you take your quick-relief inhaler more than TWO TIMES A WEEK?

Do you awaken at night with asthma more than TWO TIMES A MONTH?

Do you refill your quick-relief inhaler more than TWO TIMES A YEAR?

If you can answer yes to any of these questions, ask your doctor or pharmacist about a long-term controller anti-inflammatory medication.

A long-term controller medication can help to improve breathing and prevent asthma emergencies!

*Rules of Two™ is a registered trademark of Baylor Health System, Houston, TX.

*Starting Initial Therapy—Controller Therapy*

**Define Severity Level:** Therapy should be considered immediately after diagnosis, because increasing disease severity has been linked to increasing duration of uncontrolled disease. The general approach to therapy emphasizes early and aggressive use of controller medications with anti-inflammatory activity for persistent asthma. After diagnosing asthma but before beginning therapy, the severity of a patient's asthma should be defined (Table 5-7). It is especially important to differentiate between intermittent and persistent asthma, as guidelines recommend a daily controller medication for the latter but not the former. Although each new set of international guidelines tends to reduce the severity threshold for defining persistence, current U.S. guidelines set the mark at daytime symptoms more than twice a week, nighttime symptoms more than twice a month, or a low $FEV_1$ on pulmonary function testing.[1,2] Pulmonary function testing is recommended, because individuals with minimal symptoms due to acclimation or poor perception can have very abnormal $FEV_1$ values. Importantly, the severity level assigned is based on the highest level achieved for any one of the parameters. For example, a patient who fulfilled the symptom criteria for mild persistent asthma would be assigned to the moderate persistent category if the $FEV_1$ were abnormal. Because pulmonary function testing is difficult in children younger than 6 years, only symptoms can be used to define severity in preschool asthma. Recently updated guidelines have made recommendations on the timing of initiation of controller therapy in preschool children with asthma (Box 5-3).

The severity level should decline after initiation of appropriate therapy. The patient's asthma can be reclassified after optimal therapy is attained according to the level of treatment required to maintain the control. These are as follows: (1) no daily controller needed for mild, intermittent; (2) one daily controller needed for mild, persistent; (3) inhaled corticosteroids (ICSs) with or without additional long-term control medications needed for moderate persistent; and (4) multiple, long-term control medications, including high-dose ICSs and possibly oral corticosteroids such as prednisone needed for severe persistent asthma.

There are several pitfalls to consider in assigning severity levels in patients with asthma. First, the severity of disease can change over time in either direction. Also, patients whose asthma is classified as "mild"—and indeed any patient with asthma—can have a severe exacerbation potentially resulting in death at any time. Finally, patients, particularly children, with viral-induced wheezing can have severe episodes with complete absence of symptoms for months in between the episodes.

**Tailor Therapy to Severity:** After assignment of a severity level, therapeutic options can be selected based on the severity classification (Fig. 5-28). For first-line therapy, the guidelines recommend no daily controller for intermittent asthma; daily inhaled corticosteroids (ICSs; Table 5-8) for mild (low dose), moderate (medium dose), and severe (high dose) persistent asthma; and consideration of several non-ICS alternatives, including leukotriene receptor antagonists, in children with mild persistent asthma.

There are two general approaches to therapy: step-up (start low and intensify if needed) and step-down (start high and taper). Starting therapy with a non-ICS alternative and then stepping up to an ICS if needed in a patient with mild persistent asthma is one example of the step-up approach. Another example is starting ICS therapy using a low dose and then stepping up to a medium dose if needed in a patient with moderate persistent asthma. In general, a step-down approach using corticosteroids and designed to gain the quickest control of inflammation is recommended. An example of this approach is starting the patient with moderate persistent asthma on one of the following regimens and then tapering to the lowest possible dose: a high-dose ICS or medium-dose ICS plus a short course of prednisone. To attain patient empowerment and the negotiation of adherence, it is important to mold guidelines to patients rather than patients to guidelines. Patient-specific factors such as age, ability to use inhalers, steroid phobia, and disease perception, as well as caregiver-specific factors, such as time available at the visit, should be considered. Proper inhaler use and airway delivery of the ICS depends on selection of the proper age-dependent delivery device (Fig. 5-29) and time spent educating the patient or parent.

The high incidence of mild persistent asthma and the unique allowance of nonsteroid alternatives as controller agents warrant special consideration for this severity category. Due to many factors, including guidelines, the U.S health care delivery system,

**TABLE 5-7**
Clinical Features of Asthma—Classification of Severity

| Classification | Days with Symptoms | Nights with Symptoms | For Children >5 yr Who Can Use a Spirometer or Peak Flow Meter | |
| --- | --- | --- | --- | --- |
| | | | FEV₁ or PEF (% Predicted Normal) | PEF Variability |
| Severe persistent | Continual | Frequent | ≤60% | >30% |
| Moderate persistent | Daily | ≥5/mo | >60%–<80% | >30% |
| Mild persistent | >2/week | 3–4/mo | ≥80% | 20%–30% |
| Mild intermittent | ≤2/week | ≤2/mo | ≥80% | <20% |

$FEV_1$, American Academy of Allergy, Asthma, and Immunology: Pediatric Asthma: Promoting Best Practice. Guide for Managing Asthma in Children. Rochester, NY, Academic Services Consortium 1999;1–139.

## BOX 5-3
## When to Initiate Daily Asthma Therapy for Infants and Children Younger Than 5 yr

- Three or more episodes/yr of wheezing lasting more than 1 day affecting sleep in a child with
   Atopic dermatitis and/or parental asthma
   Or two of the following—physician diagnosis of allergic rhinitis, peripheral eosinophils, wheezing apart from colds

- Symptomatic treatment more than two times a wk

- Two or more severe exacerbations less than 6 wk apart

Guideliness for Diagnosis and Management of Asthma—Update on Selected Topics 2002. Bethesda, MD, National Institutes of Health, National Heart, Lung, and Blood Institute. June 2002, Publication No. 02-5075.

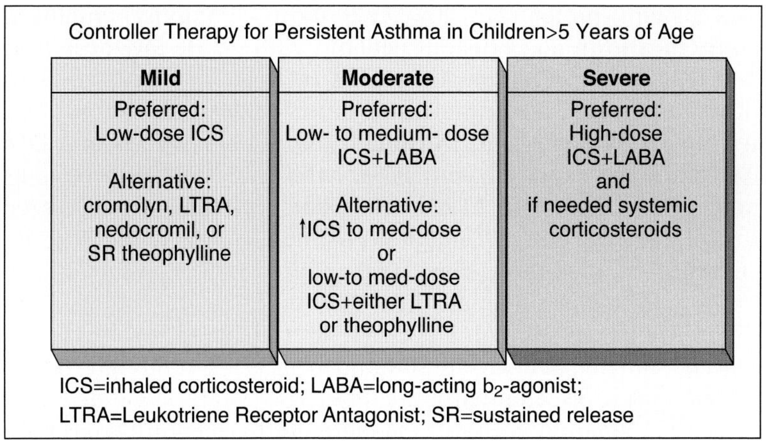

Controller Therapy for Persistent Asthma in Children>5 Years of Age

| Mild | Moderate | Severe |
|------|----------|--------|
| Preferred: Low-dose ICS | Preferred: Low- to medium- dose ICS+LABA | Preferred: High-dose ICS+LABA and if needed systemic corticosteroids |
| Alternative: cromolyn, LTRA, nedocromil, or SR theophylline | Alternative: ↑ICS to med-dose or low-to med-dose ICS+either LTRA or theophylline | |

ICS=inhaled corticosteroid; LABA=long-acting b₂-agonist;
LTRA=Leukotriene Receptor Antagonist; SR=sustained release

**Figure 5-28.** Controller therapy for persistent asthma in children older than 5 years. ICS, inhaled corticosteroid; LABA, long-acting beta-2 agonist; LTRA, leukotriene receptor antagonist. (From Executive Summary of the NAEPP Expert Panel Report: Guidelines for the diagnosis and management of asthma—update on selected topics 2002. National Institutes of Health; National Heart, Lung, and Blood Institute. Bethesda, MD, Publication No. 02-5075, June 2002.)

## TABLE 5-8
### Estimate Comparative Daily Dosages for Inhaled Corticosteroids

| Drug | Low Daily Dose | | Medium Daily Dose | | High Daily Dose | |
|------|-----------|---------|-----------|---------|-----------|---------|
| | Adult | Child* | Adult | Child* | Adult | Child* |
| Beclomethasone CFC 42 or 84 µg/puff | 168–504 µg | 84–336 µg | 504–840 µg | 336–672 µg | > 840 µg | >672 µg |
| Beclomethasone HFA 40 or 80 µg/puff | 80–240 µg | 80–160 µg | 240–480 µg | 160–320 µg | >480 µg | >320 µg |
| Budesonide DPI 200 µg/inhalation | 200–600 µg | 200–400 µg | 600–1200 µg | 400–800 µg | >1200 µg | >800 µg |
| Inhalation suspension for nebulization (child dose) | | 0.5 mg | | 1.0 mg | | 2.0 mg |
| Flunisolide 250 µg/puff | 500–1000 µg | 500–750 µg | 1000–2000 µg | 1000–1250 µg | >2000 µg | >1250 µg |
| Fluticasone MDI: 44, 110, or 220 µg/puff | 88–264 µg | 88–176 µg | 264–660 µg | 176–440 µg | >660 µg | >440 µg |
| DPI: 50, 100, or 250 µg/inhalation | 100–300 µg | 100–200 µg | 300–600 µg | 200–400 µg | >600 µg | >400 µg |
| Triamcinolone acetonide 100 µg/puff | 400–1000 µg | 400–800 µg | 1000–2000 µg | 800–1200 µg | >2000 µg | >1200 µg |

DPI, dry powder inhaler; MDI, metered-dose inhaler.
National Heart Lung and Blood Institute: The NAEPP Expert Panel Report: Guidelines for the Diagnosis and Management of Asthma—Update on Selected Topics 2002.
1. Medications. J Allergy Clin Immunol. 2002;110:S147–S193.

and patient preferences, the two most commonly employed controllers for mild persistent pediatric asthma are low-dose ICSs and leukotriene receptor antagonists (LTRAs). As discussed later, other controller medications have major limitations on their usefulness in this regard. Although the greatest effects and best outcomes are expected with ICSs,[18] the true long-term benefits and risks of ICSs and LTRAs have not been directly compared in children. The recent Childhood Asthma Management Program (CAMP)[19] studied more than 1000 children, 5 to 12 years of age, with mild-to-moderate asthma. The study results showed no difference in lung growth among children treated for 5 years with placebo, inhaled nedocromil sodium, or ICSs, even though clinical benefits were greater with the ICS. This study suggested that airways in children with asthma were not harmed in the absence

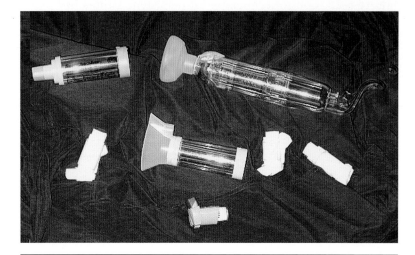

**Figure 5-29.** Age-dependent devices for delivery of inhaled medicine to children include holding chambers with or without face masks.

of ICSs. However, several of the desirable histologic and clinical benefits that have been shown almost exclusively for ICSs thus far are reductions in airway inflammation assessed by airway biopsy (Fig. 5-30) and a reduction in asthma mortality[20] (Fig. 5-31). Ultimately, the choice of a first-line controller is based on very unique aspects of each patient–clinician encounter.

Education should be provided to empower the patient or parent with sufficient knowledge to commit to and understand the needs as follows:

1. For the use of daily therapy (even if symptoms are minimal)
2. To continue using the drug even after symptoms improve
3. To not expect immediate benefit from a controller drug (in contrast to their reliever drug)
4. To maximize airway delivery of drug (if an inhaler or a nebulizer is chosen)
5. To understand possible medication side effects, expected benefits, and alternatives to treatment

The anticipated onset of action should be discussed so that the chances of premature and possibly harmful termination of therapy will be minimized. Although there is marked individual variability in responses, the onset of action of ICSs generally occurs over 7 to 10 days and, of LTRA, over 1 to 2 days.

**Reassessment After Starting Initial Therapy:** Reassessment should generally occur within 3 months of the initial visit, at which time disease control should be assessed as evidenced by minimal or no nighttime awakening and cough, exertional symptoms, rescue beta-agonist use, and normal pulmonary function testing or peak flow meter values.

If this assessment reveals adequate disease control and the initial therapy was an ICS, then a 25% to 50% dose reduction is recommended if tolerated. If the first-line controller provided incomplete or no control, additional considerations are warranted.

**Figure 5-30.** Asthmatic airway inflammation as assessed by biopsy. *A,* Before inhaled corticosteroids. *B,* After inhaled corticosteroids. BM, basement membrane; E, epithelium. (From Laitinen LA. J Allergy Clin Immunol. 1992 Jul;90(1):32–42.)

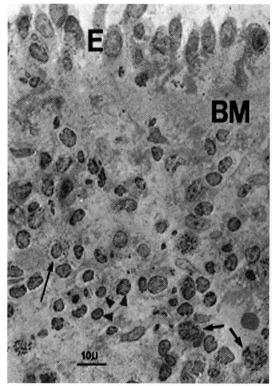
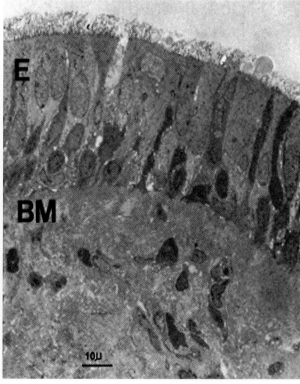

Alternative diagnoses should be considered and eliminated either clinically or in the laboratory. These include cystic fibrosis, immune deficiency, and congenital airway anomalies. Likewise, concomitant conditions that increase asthma severity, such as sinusitis and gastroesophageal reflux disease, should be considered and treated if present. Adherence and administration technique should also be evaluated. It is possible that patients who report adherence may not truly be adherent, which could be revealed during an examination of pharmacy prescription refills. Also, an excellent drug may be providing no benefit because of inadequate airway delivery secondary to poor technique or an improper delivery device. Environmental exposures to allergen or smoke could be driving disease severity, such that no medication or combination of medications will be able to provide complete disease control. If these considerations provide no cause for the lack of drug response, then a referral to an asthma specialist (allergist or pulmonologist) should be considered and drug therapy adjusted. Possibilities include a doubling of the dose of the ICS, or the addition of a second controller (such as an LTRA or a long-acting beta-2 agonist if the initial choice was an ICS), or replacement of the initial controller with a new controller (such as replacement of an LTRA with an ICS).

**Ongoing Reassessment:** After disease control is established, regularly scheduled office visits should occur roughly every 12 months for mild intermittent, every 6 months for mild persistent, every 3 months for moderate persistent, and every month for severe persistent asthma. Such regularly scheduled visits almost certainly and positively change the current practice where visits for acute asthma outnumber visits for "maintenance." Education about medication use and inhaler delivery should be reemphasized at each visit. Drug doses and the number of drugs should be adjusted, with the goal of using the minimum effective dose and minimal number of drugs. However, even subtle signs of poor disease control, such as occasional exertional symptoms, should be viewed as evidence against a reduction or elimination of therapy.

**Criteria for Possible Discontinuation of Controller Therapy:** Occasionally, patients with asthma become asymptomatic for long periods and warrant consideration for discontinuation of therapy. Some studies have detected ongoing airway inflammation and remodeling in these patients. There are no firm rules for making this decision, but one possible approach is as follows. Patients, especially children, who are on a low dose of a single drug, have been asymptomatic for at least 12 months (through all four major seasons of the year), and have a normal PEFR or FEV are the best candidates for discontinuation. Regular attention to dose reduction or elimination allows those who may have been mistakenly but inadvertently diagnosed with asthma to eventually discontinue nonessential drug therapy. Children in whom controller therapy is discontinued should be monitored carefully for evidence of recrudescence of disease activity, which has been reported within several months of discontinuation of long-term anti-inflammatory controller therapy.

**Exercise-Induced Bronchoconstriction:** Virtually every patient with typical, chronic asthma has exercise-induced bronchoconstriction (EIB) in varying degrees, but sometimes EIB can occur in isolation in the absence of any other evidence of chronic asthma. The treatment approach for the former type was summarized previously and includes daily controller therapy. However, even patients with well-controlled asthma may still have EIB. In general, most patients can prevent symptoms by use of a short-acting beta-2 agonist 15 minutes prior to exercise. However, albuterol is not always effective, and alternative medications should be considered. Inhaled cromolyn can prevent EIB and is free of the potential side effects of beta-2 agonists, such as tremor. For patients regularly active over an extended period, such as over 2 or more hours, a long-acting beta-2 agonist or LTRA can be considered because each has demonstrated a longer duration of effect and could be given at home. Finally, ICSs have been shown to reduce the severity of EIB and could be used daily to reduce the impact of EIB.

## Individual Drug Considerations

*Inhaled Corticosteroids*
Inhaled corticosteroids are the gold standard for the long-term management of asthma in adults and children because they have been shown to reduce asthma symptoms, rescue medication use, the markers of airway inflammation, and, uniquely, the risk of asthma mortality. Early intervention with ICSs may preserve pulmonary function and prevent irreversible airway obstruction, remodeling, and hyperresponsiveness. The benefits of early intervention with ICSs in milder cases with recent onset were recently documented.[21] These tremendous benefits must and can be balanced against small, well-defined, and manageable risks of potential systemic adverse effects, including growth suppression in children. Local airway effects, such as thrush and dysphonia, are rare when spacing devices and mouth-rinsing are utilized.

**Sources and Determinants of Systemic Bioavailability of Inhaled Corticosteroids:** Even though ICSs were developed to replace more highly bioavailable oral corticosteroids, they can nonetheless be absorbed into the systemic circulation. Ordinarily, approximately 20% of the dose of an ICS enters the airways, and the remainder (about 80%) is swallowed[15,22] (Fig. 5-32). ICSs can be absorbed from both the gastrointestinal system and the

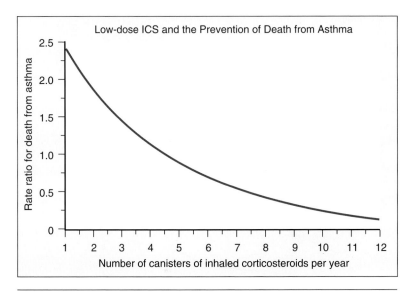

**Figure 5-31.** Low-dose inhaled corticosteroids and the prevention of death from asthma. (From Suissa S, Ernst P, Benayoun S, et al.: Low-dose inhaled corticosteroids and the prevention of death from asthma. N Engl J Med 2000;343:332–336.)

airway mucosa, but, especially for the newer ICSs, the majority of bioavailable drug originates from the airways. Thus, factors that increase the degree of airway delivery, while expected to enhance a drug's benefit, also generally increase the systemic bioavailability of a drug. Highly sensitive measurement techniques are required to detect the small effect that systemically bioavailable drugs can have on childhood growth.

**Inhaled Corticosteroids and Their Delivery Devices:** The swallowed fraction of the ICS dose is absorbed and metabolized "first-pass" in the liver. Fluticasone and mometasone are almost completely (approximately 99%) inactivated in the liver, and budesonide and triamcinolone, about 90% and about 80% to 90%, respectively, are also inactivated. Beclomethasone diproprionate, however, is largely metabolized to active metabolites and thus has the highest degree of gastrointestinal bioavailability. This difference likely provides the newer ICSs with a better safety profile compared with beclomethasone diproprionate.

Most of the drug in the blood, however, originates from the lower airways, where there is no local metabolism following absorption. Therefore, minimizing gastrointestinal bioavailability via the selection of newer ICSs or use of a spacing device will not necessarily eliminate the possibility of systemic bioavailability. Furthermore, factors that increase airway dose and delivery (i.e.,

increasing the microgram dose, use of spacers, formulation changes that result in smaller particle sizes [hydrofluroalkane-134a (HFA) versus chlorofluorocarbon (CFC) propellants], improved inhalation technique) may provide better benefit but may also increase the systemic bioavailability of the drug.

**Disease Severity Considerations:** In patients with mild asthma, airways are more patent than in those with more severe asthma. As a result, drug deposition and absorption, and thus systemic side effect risk, may be higher. Several studies and indirect lines of evidence support that possibility, and the growth effects of ICS generally have been greatest in those with the mildest severity (see later). ICS-induced adrenal axis suppression was directly related to airway function in one study of asthmatic individuals. Nonetheless, the results argue for the approach most often taken: using low-dose ICS for the mildest cases or considering nonsteroid alternatives.

**Growth Suppression:** Prior to examining the potential effects of ICS on growth, it is important to recognize that poorly controlled asthma and systemic corticosteroid bursts can adversely affect growth. The Food and Drug Administration recently issued new guidelines for the class labeling of all corticosteroids, both inhaled and nasal, to reflect the possibility of a small degree of growth

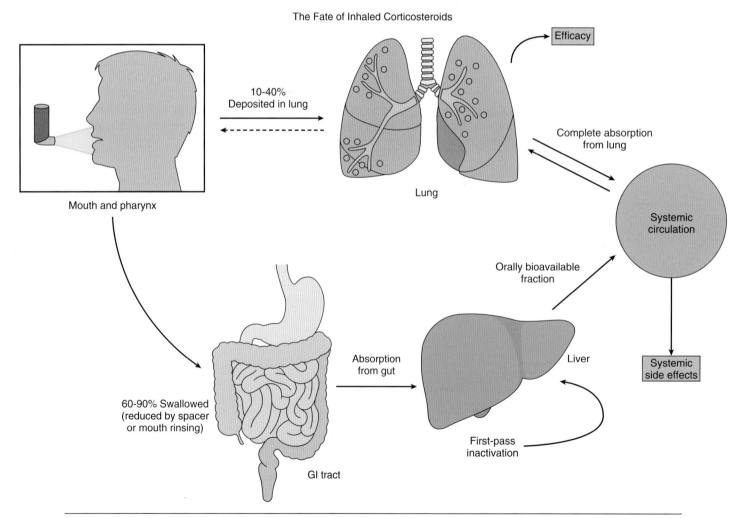

**Figure 5-32.** The fate of inhaled corticosteroids. Note that the major source of efficacy (lung delivery) is also the major source of systemic bioavailability and any safety concerns. GI, gastrointestinal.

suppression. Many factors likely influence this risk, including total dose, drug delivery device and technique, genetic predisposition, age, adherence, and asthma severity.

**Influence of Asthma Severity on Inhaled Corticosteroid–Induced Growth Suppression (Intermediate Term):** Three 1-year trials compared the growth of children from 6 months to 8 years of age treated with budesonide nebulizing suspension or conventional asthma therapy. In these trials, the group of children with the mildest severity manifested a small degree of growth suppression, while the two groups with higher severity levels showed no such evidence. Most of the earlier studies examining the growth effects of ICSs also enrolled children with milder degrees of disease severity because poorly controlled asthma and frequent prednisone bursts (in the more severe patients) can also have an adverse impact on growth.

**Long-Term Inhaled Corticosteroid Use:** Linear growth was examined in children with asthma in the Childhood Asthma Management Program (CAMP).[19] Compared with children receiving placebo or nedocromil sodium, the budesonide treatment group had a small reduction in growth velocity during the 1st year that was not sustained for the remainder of the 4- to 5-year study. This study was reassuring and suggested that the effect of ICSs on growth was transient and restricted to the 1st year of a 4- to 5-year course of continuous therapy. A second study, with a different design, produced similarly reassuring results. In that study, children treated with budesonide for an average of 9.2 years reached their calculated target adult height, based on parental height, compared with 18 control, ICS-naïve asthmatic patients and 51 healthy siblings.[23] This study showed that, even if the ICSs do suppress growth during the 1st year of therapy, "catch-up" growth likely occurs later.

**Risk Management: Strategies for Balancing Safety and Efficacy of Inhaled Corticosteroids:** The most obvious method is the step-down approach to ICS therapy, whereby the patient is started on a high dose to achieve quick control of airway inflammation and then gradually tapered to the minimum effective dose that would be continued to maintain long-term control and less likely to have any impact on susceptible processes such as growth. Determining and maintaining a "low" minimum effective dose could depend on attention to other aspects of asthma care, including rigorous smoke and allergen environmental controls, vaccination for influenza virus, the diagnosis and treatment of concomitant conditions that could worsen asthma (i.e., rhinitis, sinusitis, gastroesophageal reflux disease), and the appropriate use of add-on therapy.

The safety of ICSs can be further managed and optimized through attention to several other aspects of care. The time of day of ICS administration—morning or evening for those who are stable on once-daily dosing—may modify the risk for growth suppression. A 4-week study of children with asthma examined the growth-suppressing effects of budesonide (800 μg) administered under two different dosing strategies. During one period, it was given as a single dose in the morning; during the other period, it was given as two divided doses—400 μg in the morning and 400 μg in the evening. Lower leg growth rates were significantly lower in children receiving an evening dose than in children receiving only a morning dose. The results of this study suggest that for patients who are stable on once-daily dosing, the morning

is the safest time for administration. Because that administration time may not maximize adherence or efficacy, other factors must be considered in designing an individualized therapeutic strategy.

When the ICS fails to provide sufficient control, options include doubling the ICS dose or adding on a second nonsteroidal controller medication. The latter possibility was supported by a recent study showing that, in children treated with ICS, halving the ICS dose and adding a second nonsteroidal drug was associated with faster short-term lower leg growth with no loss of asthma control, versus maintaining the original higher ICS dose alone. This result supports the widely held recommendations to use the lowest effective dose and, in poorly controlled patients, to add non-ICS therapy rather than double the ICS dose.

Safety management should also incorporate the monitoring of growth every 3 to 6 months and interpreting the resultant measurement and changes. The mouth should be rinsed after ICS administration to minimize the swallowed portion of drug. Also, careful attention should be given to potency differences when dosing ICS, especially when changing from a lower-potency to a higher-potency ICS. For example, a clinically equivalent dose of fluticasone and beclomethasone diproprionate may differ by twofold—about 400 μg of beclomethasone diproprionate are equivalent to about 200 μg of fluticasone.

*Leukotriene Receptor Antagonists*

Leukotrienes promote smooth muscle constriction and inflammatory events. Not surprisingly, LTRAs can reduce markers of inflammation and smooth muscle contraction. Thus, pediatric asthma guidelines state that LTRAs may be an alternative to low-dose ICS therapy in mild persistent asthma and may be an effective add-on to ICS therapy in moderate persistent asthma.

Zafirlukast, the first LTRA approved in the United States, was shown to be effective in the management of mild-to-moderate asthma. It improved pulmonary function and reduced the clinical symptoms of asthma as well as the need for ICSs. Zafirlukast is indicated for twice-daily oral treatment for the management of asthma in children as young as 7 years. Because it can inhibit the CYP450 isoenzyme CYP3A4, it can increase concentrations of certain concomitant medications such as theophylline. Food can also reduce zafirlukast's bioavailability; therefore, according to its package insert, it should be taken 1 hour before or 2 hours after a meal.

Controlled clinical trials have shown that montelukast, another approved LTRA, is effective in the management of adult and pediatric asthma. Montelukast is indicated as once-daily therapy for the treatment of mild-to-moderate asthma in children as young as 12 months and does not have known drug interactions or food restrictions. Efficacy was initially demonstrated in adults and 6- to 14-year-old children[24] and, more recently, in younger children. Interestingly, montelukast provided beneficial effects on β-agonist use that were noted on the first day of use and provided the same improvement in pulmonary function, regardless of whether the patients were receiving ICS. A granule formulation of montelukast can be used to treat children as young as 1 year. Also, a recent controlled study showed that, in ICS-treated children with persistent asthma, the addition of montelukast improved pulmonary function and symptoms, with significant reduction in beta-2 agonist use.

*Chromones*

Cromolyn sodium has been used for more than 30 years as an inhaled mast cell stabilizer in the treatment of persistent asthma.

Efficacy has been demonstrated in adults and can be achieved in patients as young as 2 years using a nebulizer. Although patients taking cromolyn have experienced minor adverse effects such as cough, no serious adverse effects have been noted. The safety of this product has been the major driving force of usage over the years, even in the context of rather poor effectiveness. Controlled clinical trials in young children have shown that cromolyn is safe and efficacious as either monotherapy or in combination with beta-2 agonists. However, a randomized trial in more than 200 children 1 to 4 years of age with moderate asthma showed that cromolyn was not more effective than a placebo. Also, cromolyn added little or no benefit to ICS therapy, supporting current pediatric guidelines that do not recommend cromolyn as add-on therapy to ICSs. These results, combined with a requirement for frequent three- or four-times-a-day dosing and the need for metered dose inhaler (MDI)/spacer or nebulizer, have led to an overall decline in cromolyn use and a recommendation that cromolyn not be used as first-line preventive therapy.

Inhaled nedocromil sodium appears to have a similar mechanism of action and a similar clinical profile to cromolyn, with the major advantage of safety and major disadvantage of minimal efficacy. In addition, bitter taste is a frequent complaint of regular nedocromil users. In the CAMP study, nedocromil significantly reduced the number of urgent-care visits ($P = 0.02$) and courses of prednisone ($P = 0.01$) but was similar to placebo in all other endpoints, including airway hyperresponsiveness, pre- and post-bronchodilator $FEV_1$, rate of hospitalization, daily symptom score, and rescue bronchodilator use. One difference from cromolyn is that, added to ICS therapy, nedocromil was modestly beneficial in asthmatic adults. Because this efficacy was not demonstrated in children, pediatric asthma guidelines do not recommend the use of nedocromil as add-on therapy to ICSs.

### Methylxanthines

Theophylline has been used to treat asthma for more than 60 years. Theophylline is a phosphodiesterase inhibitor, relaxes airway smooth muscle (bronchodilation)—consequently improving airway function—and may have mild anti-inflammatory effects. However, its mechanism of action in asthma is not completely clear.

Theophylline was shown to be effective in treating mild-to-moderate asthma in children. Steroid-dependent children with asthma also demonstrated added benefit when theophylline was added to ICS therapy. These studies support the recommendation that theophylline can be used as add-on therapy to ICSs. Practically, it is usually the third drug added on after LTRAs and long-acting beta-agonists. Although it can be considered an alternative first-line therapy, it is not preferred for persistent asthma.

Theophylline use in children has been linked to changes in behavior and school performance. These adverse effects are more common when blood levels exceed the upper limits of the therapeutic range (10 µg/L to 20 µg/L in adults, 5 µg/L to 15 µg/L in children) but also can be seen at therapeutic concentrations. Adverse effects, such as headache and other effects on the central nervous system, tremor, nausea, vomiting, and gastric irritation, also have been reported frequently in patients taking theophylline. Theophylline has numerous drug interactions that alter plasma levels. As a result of these safety issues, as well as the need for plasma concentration monitoring, theophylline use has dramatically decreased recently despite relatively low cost.

### Long-Acting Beta-2 Agonists

Salmeterol is a long-acting inhaled beta-2 agonist indicated for long-term use and has been available as both an aerosol and a dry-powder inhaler. The latter is approved for children as young as 4 years. Salmeterol is not indicated for the treatment of acute symptoms or exacerbations, due to a slow onset of action. Thus, patient education about the role of this medication is essential. Salmeterol was more efficacious than short-acting beta-2 agonists and placebo in treating mild-to-moderate asthmatic children, with effects (bronchodilation) lasting up to 12 hours. Although long-term benefits are well established in adults, a recent review article raised questions about whether treated children experienced the same degree of benefit and whether they shared the same disease processes as adults.

Tolerance can develop with prolonged salmeterol use, which can result in decreased bronchoprotection against methacholine challenge and exercise-induced bronchoconstriction. Although salmeterol has a protective effect against exercise-induced asthma, the duration of this effect may wane even during regular once-daily salmeterol treatment, despite the reduced frequency of dosing and concomitant use of ICSs in children.

Current asthma guidelines recommend that long-acting beta-2 agonists should not replace anti-inflammatory therapy but should be considered as possible add-ons. For children with moderate-to- severe asthma, combining salmeterol with budesonide improved morning and evening PEFR and symptom-free days and reduced the use of rescue medications. Patients should be instructed not to stop anti-inflammatory therapy while taking salmeterol even though their symptoms may significantly improve. Also, salmeterol was recently reformulated to include fluticasone in a single inhaler. As such, the fluticasone/salmeterol dry-power inhaler may be a useful option for nonadherent patients or for those who require combination therapy, since it reduces the number of inhalations per day.

A second agent, formoterol, has been approved in the United States for use by adults and children older than 12 years. Formoterol has a quicker onset of action than salmeterol. The advantages and limitations of long-term asthma controllers, including long-acting beta-2 agonists, are summarized in Table 5-9.

### Oral Corticosteroids

Orally administered or injected corticosteroids are indicated for the acute, short-term therapy of severe asthma exacerbations. Systemic corticosteroid therapy is indicated in the management of acute asthma and is mandatory in the therapy of status asthmaticus. By appropriately timing the intervention with corticosteroids, the clinician may benefit the patient and reduce hospitalizations. Since the action of corticosteroids is dependent on cellular internalization, therapy should be instituted promptly once an indication for use is established.

Typically, patients begin oral prednisone (2 mg/kg/day or max. 60 mg/day) at the onset of an acute exacerbation and continue the treatment for 3 to 10 days. Oral preparations also can be used as alternate-day maintenance therapy for severe persistent asthma. Although high-dose, short-term corticosteroid therapy is relatively safe in severe life-threatening disorders, chronic systemic administration in patients with severe asthma carries a significant risk for adverse effects, including growth suppression, adrenal suppression, osteoporosis, fractures, cataracts and glaucoma, weight gain, and hypertension. Complications detectable on physical examination include weight gain, "moon-type" facies, hirsutism, polycythemia (red, ruddy complexion), and short stature (Fig. 5-33). Such side effects of excessive steroid therapy for chronic asthma should be avoidable complications, and oral corticosteroid exposure can be reduced by the use of inhaled corticosteroids.

*Anticholinergic Agents*
In the outpatient setting, anticholinergic agents such as ipratropium bromide can have possible additive benefit to inhaled beta-2 agonists for severe exacerbations and can be used as a possible alternative bronchodilator for children who do not tolerate inhaled beta-2 agonists.

*Anti-Immunoglobulin E Antibody*
Efficacy of a humanized monoclonal antibody against human IgE was recently demonstrated in patients with allergic asthma.[25,26] This antibody is administered by subcutaneous injection and dramatically reduces serum IgE levels. The drug improved a number of asthma outcomes but did not induce remission and also benefited patients with allergic rhinitis. Effects disappeared when the drug was discontinued. Likely positioning in the future will be in severe asthmatics who are using high-dose ICSs or maintenance oral corticosteroids and possibly in those who are nonadherent with daily controller therapy (because anti-IgE is given every several weeks). Cost will be an important consideration in its use.

*Allergen Immunotherapy*
Allergen immunotherapy has demonstrated efficacy in and is widely used to treat allergic rhinitis, even in patients with asthma. The role of allergen immunotherapy is less well defined in patients with asthma, and some studies have raised doubt about beneficial

effects in such cases. Safety concerns are also slightly higher in patients with asthma than in those with uncomplicated allergic rhinitis. When used properly by an asthma specialist, allergen immunotherapy may be a viable option for patients whose asthma is triggered by allergic triggers and whose condition cannot be controlled with pharmacologic therapy. The next decades are virtually certain to improve both the efficacy and safety of this therapeutic approach.

*Other Therapies*
Other therapies are available for patients who fail to respond adequately to the medications discussed here but will generally be used by asthma specialists due to issues regarding efficacy or safety. Most patients who are viable candidates for these therapies already failed therapy with high-dose ICSs and maintenance oral corticosteroids. These agents have immunosuppressive or anti-inflammatory effects and include methotrexate (an antimetabolite), cyclosporin A (an immunosuppressive fungal metabolite), gold, troleandomycin (a macrolide antibiotic), and cytokine-directed therapies. Annual influenza virus vaccination is recommended for adults and children with asthma severe enough to require regular medical follow-up or hospitalization.

## Adherence Issues in Asthma

Gaining adherence to a therapeutic strategy is one of the keys to successful asthma management, and barriers to adherence are similar to those encountered in the care of other chronic diseases such as hypertension and diabetes. In asthma, published adherence rates have generally been low. One of a clinician's goals is to select drugs that are proven efficacious by controlled trials and

**TABLE 5-9**
**Advantages and Limitations of Long-Term Asthma Controllers**

| Drug Class | Advantages | Limitations |
|---|---|---|
| Inhaled corticosteroids | • Reduce exacerbations<br>• Improve pulmonary function<br>• Reduce airway responsiveness<br>• Reduce airway inflammation | • Increased risk of systemic side effects with prolonged, high-dose therapy<br>• Limited information on long-term use in children<br>• Limited information on use in young children |
| Leukotriene antagonists | • Reduce symptoms<br>• Improve pulmonary function<br>• Reduce exercise-induced bronchospasm<br>• Prevent allergen-induced inflammation | • Limited information on reduction of airway inflammation<br>• No apparent effect on airway responsiveness<br>• No information about impact on natural history of asthma |
| Long-acting beta-2 agonists | • Reduce exacerbations<br>• Improve pulmonary function<br>• Reduce airway responsiveness<br>• Attenuate exercise-induced bronchospasm | • Reduced effect with long-term treatment<br>• No apparent effect on inflammation<br>• No information on use in young children |

National Heart, Lung, and Blood Institute: The NAEPP Expert Panel Report: Guidelines for the Diagnosis and Management of Asthma—Update on Selected Topics 2002.

gain effectiveness from them in the real-world practice setting. Such effectiveness is heavily influenced by patient adherence, which may be especially difficult to gain in patients with the mildest asthma, who clinically have the least disease burden. In controlled clinical trials and in contrast to the real world in which our patients live, adherence is carefully monitored and optimized with education. Adherence to the prescribed asthma regimen is influenced by numerous factors, including mode of administration, dosing frequency, onset of action, perceived efficacy, and anticipated adverse effects. One study showed a significant inverse relationship between asthma hospitalization rates and the ratio of ICS to beta-2 agonist use, illustrating the importance of adherence to and proper use of ICSs.

### Home/Emergency Department Management of Asthma Exacerbation

The guidelines for the management of asthma exacerbations at home, in the emergency department, and in the hospital are summarized in Figures 5-34 and 5-35. Status asthmaticus (poor response to emergency department treatment protocol) is treated with IV corticosteroids, oxygen, and a nebulized beta-agonist on a regular, frequent (every 1 to 2 hours), or even continuous basis. Patients are weaned from it as they improve. If the patient has been on chronic maintenance theophylline therapy as an outpatient, then parenteral theophylline therapy also should be instituted. Most pediatric patients improve on this therapeutic regimen and are discharged within 3 days, but adults frequently respond less rapidly and require longer periods of hospitalization. In general, beta-adrenergic dosing intervals of less than 2 hours require observation and monitoring in an intensive care facility. A patient with status asthmaticus must be monitored closely during the first 6 to 12 hours of hospitalization for impending respiratory failure so that therapy to prevent progression to respiratory failure can be instituted.

Therapy for impending respiratory failure consists of the correction of acid-base imbalances in the setting of an intensive care unit, where cardiac and respiratory function can be closely monitored. If respiratory failure supervenes despite intense medical management, artificial mechanical ventilation is indicated.

### Management of Asthma During Pregnancy

It is essential that sufficient lung function and blood oxygenation be maintained during pregnancy so that an adequate oxygen supply to the fetus is provided. Increased perinatal mortality, increased prematurity, and low birth weight can all result from poorly controlled asthma. For most drugs used to treat asthma, there is little evidence to suggest an increased risk to the fetus.

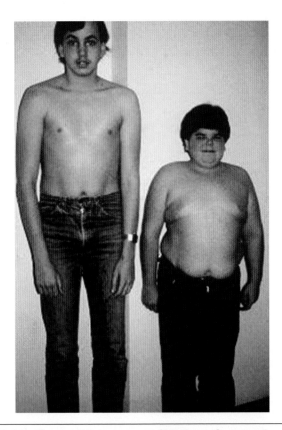

**Figure 5-33.** Short stature, a complication of systemic corticosteroid therapy for chronic asthma, is illustrated by the 16-year-old steroid-dependent asthmatic shown next to a nonasthmatic 16-year-old of normal size. (With permission from Skoner D, Stillwagon P, Friedman R, Fireman P: Pediatric Allergy and Immunology. In Davis H, Zitelli B (eds.): Atlas of Pediatric Physical Diagnosis. London, Gower Press, 1987.)

---

**BOX 5-4**
**Risk Factors for Death from Asthma**

**History of Severe Exacerbations**
- History of sudden severe exacerbations
- Prior intubation for asthma
- Prior admission for asthma to an intensive care unit

**Asthma Hospitalizations and Emergency Visits**
- Two or more hospitalizations in the past year
- Three or more emergency care visits in the past year
- Hospitalization or emergency visit in past month

**Beta-2 Agonist and Oral Steroid Usage**
- Use of more than two canisters per month of short-acting inhaled beta-2 agonist
- Current use of oral steroids or recent withdrawal from oral steroids

**Complicating Health Problems**
- Comorbidity (e.g., cardiovascular diseases or COPD)
- Serious psychiatric disease, including depression, or psychosocial problems
- Illicit drug use

**Other Factors**
- Poor perception of airflow obstruction or its severity
- Sensitivity to *Alternaria* (an outdoor mold)
- Low socioeconomic status and urban residence

COPD, chronic obstructive pulmonary disease.

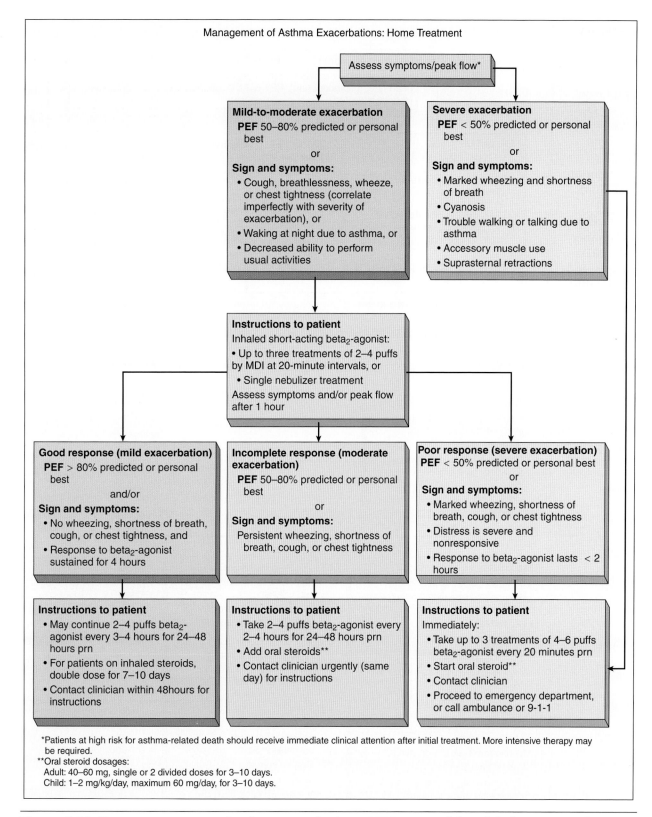

**Figure 5-34.** Home management of asthma exacerbations. MDI, metered dose inhaler; PEF, peak expiratory flow. (From National Asthma Education and Prevention Program: Practical Guide for the diagnosis and management of asthma. Bethesda, MD, NIH Publication Number 97-4053, October 1997, page 27; National Heart, Lung, and Blood Institute; National Institutes of Health, 1997.)

**Figure 5-35.** Emergency department– and hospital-based management of asthma exacerbations. FEV$_1$, forced expiratory volume in 1 second; O$_2$, oxygen; PEF, peak expiratory flow. (From National Asthma Education and Prevention Program: Practical Guide for the diagnosis and management of asthma. NIH Publication Number 97-4053. Bethesda, MD, National Heart, Lung, and Blood Institute of Health, 1997.)

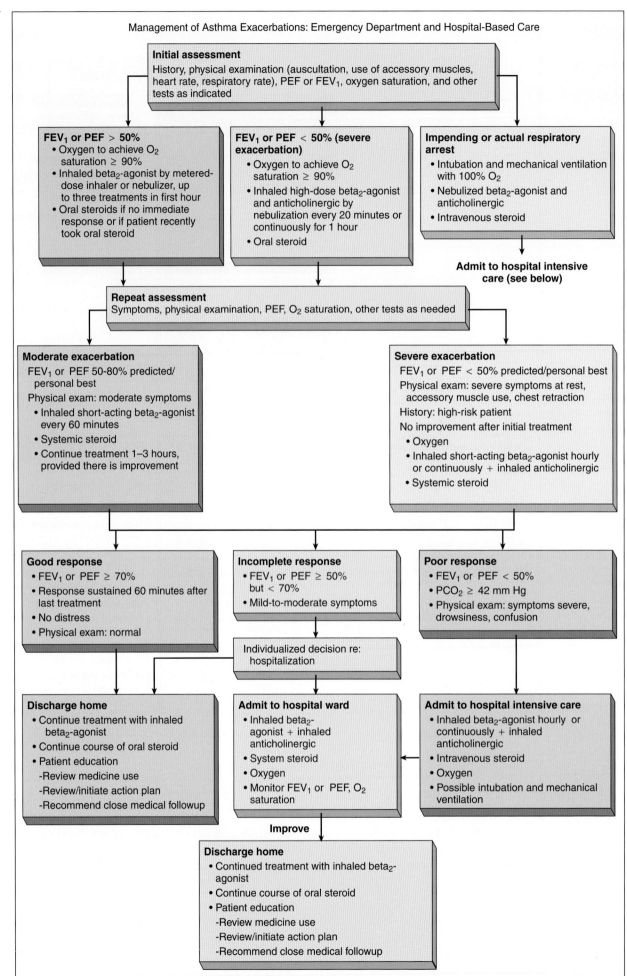

Management of Asthma Exacerbations: Emergency Department and Hospital-Based Care

**Initial assessment**
History, physical examination (auscultation, use of accessory muscles, heart rate, respiratory rate), PEF or FEV$_1$, oxygen saturation, and other tests as indicated

**FEV$_1$ or PEF > 50%**
- Oxygen to achieve O$_2$ saturation ≥ 90%
- Inhaled beta$_2$-agonist by metered-dose inhaler or nebulizer, up to three treatments in first hour
- Oral steroids if no immediate response or if patient recently took oral steroid

**FEV$_1$ or PEF < 50% (severe exacerbation)**
- Oxygen to achieve O$_2$ saturation ≥ 90%
- Inhaled high-dose beta$_2$-agonist and anticholinergic by nebulization every 20 minutes or continuously for 1 hour
- Oral steroid

**Impending or actual respiratory arrest**
- Intubation and mechanical ventilation with 100% O$_2$
- Nebulized beta$_2$-agonist and anticholinergic
- Intravenous steroid

**Admit to hospital intensive care (see below)**

**Repeat assessment**
Symptoms, physical examination, PEF, O$_2$ saturation, other tests as needed

**Moderate exacerbation**
FEV$_1$ or PEF 50-80% predicted/personal best
Physical exam: moderate symptoms
- Inhaled short-acting beta$_2$-agonist every 60 minutes
- Systemic steroid
- Continue treatment 1–3 hours, provided there is improvement

**Severe exacerbation**
FEV$_1$ or PEF < 50% predicted/personal best
Physical exam: severe symptoms at rest, accessory muscle use, chest retraction
History: high-risk patient
No improvement after initial treatment
- Oxygen
- Inhaled short-acting beta$_2$-agonist hourly or continuously + inhaled anticholinergic
- Systemic steroid

**Good response**
- FEV$_1$ or PEF ≥ 70%
- Response sustained 60 minutes after last treatment
- No distress
- Physical exam: normal

**Incomplete response**
- FEV$_1$ or PEF ≥ 50% but < 70%
- Mild-to-moderate symptoms

**Poor response**
- FEV$_1$ or PEF < 50%
- PCO$_2$ ≥ 42 mm Hg
- Physical exam: symptoms severe, drowsiness, confusion

Individualized decision re: hospitalization

**Discharge home**
- Continue treatment with inhaled beta$_2$-agonist
- Continue course of oral steroid
- Patient education
  -Review medicine use
  -Review/initiate action plan
  -Recommend close medical followup

**Admit to hospital ward**
- Inhaled beta$_2$-agonist + inhaled anticholinergic
- System steroid
- Oxygen
- Monitor FEV$_1$ or PEF, O$_2$ saturation

**Admit to hospital intensive care**
- Inhaled beta$_2$-agonist hourly or continuously + inhaled anticholinergic
- Intravenous steroid
- Oxygen
- Possible intubation and mechanical ventilation

**Improve**

**Discharge home**
- Continued treatment with inhaled beta$_2$-agonist
- Continue course of oral steroid
- Patient education
  -Review medicine use
  -Review/initiate action plan
  -Recommend close medical followup

Exceptions include corticosteroids and epinephrine. Therapy with the lowest possible doses of the fewest possible medications should be the goal of treatment of asthma during pregnancy.

## Identification of Patients at Risk for Asthma-Related Death

Care of asthmatic patients should include the identification of patients at risk for asthma-related death (Box 5-4). Clues include the presence of previous life-threatening exacerbations of asthma, the lack of adequate and ongoing medical care that provides appropriate follow-up and prophylactic therapy, and significant depression or psychosocial behavioral problems.

## Asthma as a Component of a Whole-Airway Disease

There is a strong relationship between events in the upper and lower airways, which are linked epidemiologically and patho-physiologically. The evolving concept is "one airway, one disease." This has led to the development of a set of guidelines termed *ARIA*, for Allergic Rhinitis and its Impact on Asthma.[17] These guidelines strongly recommend that persistent asthmatics be evaluated for nasal disease (allergic rhinitis) and vice versa (see Chapter 9). Moreover, a combined approach to therapy, considering both safety and efficacy, is recommended.

# REFERENCES

1. Executive Summary of the NAEPP Expert Panel Report: Guidelines for the diagnosis and management of asthma—Update on selected topics 2002. National Institutes of Health; National Heart, Lung, and Blood Institute. Bethesda, MD, Publication No. 02-5075, June 2002.
2. National Asthma Education and Prevention Program. Practical Guide for the diagnosis and management of asthma. Bethesda, MD, National Heart, Lung, and Blood Institute; National Institutes of Health, 1997.
3. National Heart, Lung, and Blood Institute: National Asthma Education Program: Guidelines for the Diagnosis and Management of Asthma. National Institutes of Health, Bethesda, MD, No. 91-3042, August, 1991.
4. Global Initiative for Asthma. Global strategy for asthma management and prevention. NIH Publ 02.3659. Bethesda, MD, National Heart, Lung, and Blood Institute. National Institutes of Health, 1998.
5. British Thoracic Society: The British guidelines on asthma management. Thorax 1997;52:51–521.
6. Szefler SJ: Asthma: The new advances. Adv Pediatr 2000;47:273–308.
7. Busse WW, Lemanske RF: Asthma. Advances in immunology. N Engl J Med 2001;344:350–362.
8. Von Mutius E, Martinez FD: Epidemiology of childhood asthma. In Murphy S, Kelly HW (eds): Pediatric Asthma. Series: Lung Biology in Health and Disease, Vol. 126. New York, Marcel Dekker, 1999, pp 1–39.
9. Martinez FD, Wright AL, Taussig LM, et al: Asthma and wheezing in the first six years of life. N Engl J Med 1995;332:133–138.
10. Lange P, Parner J, Vestbo J, et al: A 15-year follow-up study of ventilatory function in adults with asthma. N Engl J Med 1998;339:1194–1200.
11. Burrows B, Martinez FD, Halonen M, et al: Association of asthma with serum IgE levels and skin-test reactivity to allergens. N Engl J Med 1989;320:271–277.
12. Skoner DP, Caliguiri L: The wheezing infant. In Fireman P (ed): Pediatric Allergic Disease, Philadelphia, W.B. Saunders, 1988.
13. Djukanovic R, Roche WR, Wilson JW, et al: Mucosal inflammation in asthma. Am Rev Respir Dis 1990;142:434–457.
14. Kay AB: Allergy and allergic diseases: Advances in Immunology. N Engl J Med 2001;344:10–37.
15. Skoner DP: Growth effects of asthma and asthma therapy. Cur Opin Pulm Med 2002;8:45–49.
16. Castro-Rodriguez JA, Holberg CJ, Wright AL, Martinez FD: A clinical index to define risk of asthma in young children with recurrent wheezing. Am J Respir Crit Care Med 2000;162:1403–1406.
17. Bousquet J, Van Cauwenberge P, Khaltaev N: Allergic rhinitis and its impact on asthma. J Allergy Clin Immunol 2001;108:S147–S334.
18. Malstrom K, Rodriguez-Gomez G, Guerra J, et al: Oral montelukast, inhaled beclomethasone, and placebo for chronic asthma. Ann Intern Med 1999;130:487–495.
19. Szefler S, Weiss S, Tonascia A, et al: Long-term effects of budesonide or nedocromil in children with asthma. N Engl J Med 2000;343:1054–1063.
20. Suissa S, Ernst P, Benayoun S, et al: Low-dose inhaled corticosteroids and the prevention of death from asthma. N Engl J Med 2000;343:332–336.
21. Pauwels RA, Pedersen S, Busse WW, et al: Early intervention with budesonide in mild persistent asthma: A randomized, double-blind trial. Lancet 2003;361:1071–1076.
22. Lipworth BJ: Systemic adverse effects of inhaled corticosteroid therapy: A systematic review and meta-analysis. Arch Intern Med 1999;159:941–955.
23. Agertoft L, Pedersen S: Effect of long-term treatment with inhaled budesonide on adult height in children with asthma. N Engl J Med 2000;343:1064–1069.
24. Knorr B, Matz J, Bernstein JA, et al: Montelukast for chronic asthma in 6- to 14-year-old children: A randomized, double-blind trial. Pediatric Montelukast Study Group. JAMA 1998;279:1181–1186.
25. Milgrom H, Berger W, Nayak A, et al: Treatment of childhood asthma with anti-immunoglobulin E antibody (omalizumab). Pediatrics 2001;108:E36.
26. Busse W, Corren J, Lanier BQ, et al: Omalizumab, anti-IgE recombinant humanized monoclonal antibody, for the treatment of severe allergic asthma. J Allergy Clin Immunol 2001;108:184–190.

*Emil J. Bardana, Jr.*

# *6* Occupational Asthma and Allergies

The Occupational Safety and Health Administration (OSHA) has estimated that there are some 575,000 potentially hazardous chemicals in the workplace. More than 250 of these chemicals and organic dusts have been implicated in the causation of new-onset occupational rhinitis and asthma as well as other hypersensitivity disorders. In addition to the chemicals and industrial dusts, there are a variety of common environmental factors such as ambient pollution with cigarette smoke and other agents that also may contribute to the development of respiratory ill health in the workplace. This review focuses on the classification, pathogenesis, and evaluation of occupational asthma and associated respiratory disorders.

---

**BOX 6-1**

**Classification of Occupational Reactions with Selected Examples of the Types of Exposures Causing Them**

**Annoyance Reactions**
Perfumes
Exhaust fumes
Cleaning agents
Tobacco smoke on clothing

**Irritational Reactions**
Tobacco smoke
Pollution
Field/slash burning
Paint fumes

**Immunologic Reactions (IgE)**
Animal proteins
Papain
Latex
Platinum salts
Acid anhydrides

**Corrosive Reactions**
Chlorine
Anhydrous ammonia
Vinyl chloride
Hydrochloric acid

---

IgE, immunoglobulin E.

After the skin, the lungs are the organ most frequently affected by allergens and irritants in the workplace. The lungs are the point of initial impact for a wide array of industrial dusts, gases, fumes, and vapors. Exposures may induce dose-related symptoms in the exposed worker. At one end of a continuum of symptoms, low concentrations of mild irritants or disagreeable fragrances can provoke annoyance reactions. Modest concentrations of soluble irritants may induce transient inflammatory reactions of the upper airways. At the extreme end of the spectrum, numerous potent toxicants can cause dermatologic burns, conjunctivitis, and acute inflammatory changes of the upper airways because of their inherent corrosive properties. Finally, there are industrial agents that have the capacity to provoke an immunologic response; i.e., sensitization (Box 6-1).

The health sequelae following any given exposure to an airborne toxicant depend on the physiochemical properties of the agent; i.e., dust, gas, fume, or vapor (Fig. 6-1), as well as a myriad of host factors.[1] Some irritating gases or vapors have the capacity to evoke direct tissue injury, and the site and degree of injury are largely dependent on the inhalant's water solubility. Highly soluble gases such as ammonia and formaldehyde precipitate nasopharyngeal irritation and possibly laryngeal irritation. The skin and ocular tissues also are affected, with inflammatory injury; i.e., conjunctivitis and skin burns. Because highly soluble gases are significantly absorbed in the upper airways, lower airway health sequelae are usually milder with these agents (see Fig. 6-1). On the other hand, insoluble gases such as phosgene, ozone, and oxides of nitrogen cause little or no upper airway injury and significant distal small airway inflammation, in the form of conditions such as bronchiolitis, alveolitis, and even pulmonary edema. It may take weeks for some of the latter processes to fully declare themselves.

The hallmark of occupational asthma is variable airway obstruction associated with bronchial hyperresponsiveness. It is precipitated by bronchial inflammation secondary to inhalation of ambient dusts, gases, fumes, or vapors that are produced or incidentally present in the workplace.[2,3] Other preexistent pulmonary disease may be present (e.g., emphysema).

## EPIDEMIOLOGY

There are few long-term prospective longitudinal studies related to the prevalence of occupational asthma. Many of the epidemiologic

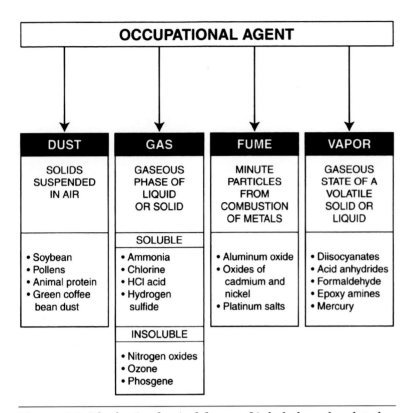

**OCCUPATIONAL AGENT**

| DUST | GAS | FUME | VAPOR |
|---|---|---|---|
| SOLIDS SUSPENDED IN AIR | GASEOUS PHASE OF LIQUID OR SOLID | MINUTE PARTICLES FROM COMBUSTION OF METALS | GASEOUS STATE OF A VOLATILE SOLID OR LIQUID |

SOLUBLE

| DUST | GAS | FUME | VAPOR |
|---|---|---|---|
| • Soybean<br>• Pollens<br>• Animal protein<br>• Green coffee bean dust | • Ammonia<br>• Chlorine<br>• HCl acid<br>• Hydrogen sulfide | • Aluminum oxide<br>• Oxides of cadmium and nickel<br>• Platinum salts | • Diisocyanates<br>• Acid anhydrides<br>• Formaldehyde<br>• Epoxy amines<br>• Mercury |

INSOLUBLE

• Nitrogen oxides
• Ozone
• Phosgene

**Figure 6-1.** The basic physical forms of inhaled work-related substances that determine which part of the lungs will likely be affected and the nature of that physiologic response. HCl, hydrochloric. (Adapted with permission from Bardana EJ: Occupational asthma and allergies. J Allergy Clin Immunol 2003;111:S530.)

studies in this area have relied on subjective data in identifying bronchial asthma. Hence, one cannot exclude the possibility of pre-existent minimally symptomatic but undiagnosed nonoccupational asthma being attributed to a certain work exposure. It is also not possible to exclude the presence of asymptomatic bronchial hyperreactivity that contributes to the development of asthma in association with a viral respiratory infection, an environmental irritant, or exposure to a non–work-related antigen. Recent observations have demonstrated that asymptomatic bronchial hyperreactivity persists through adolescent and young adult life and is not modified by inhaled corticosteroid therapy. It is simply not known whether the presence of bronchial hyperreactivity predisposes to the subsequent development of occupational asthma.[1]

Given these inadequacies in the information base, the prevalence of occupational asthma is said to account for between 2% and 6% of the asthmatic population. A recent large population-based study of occupational asthma estimated that between 5% and 10% of cases of asthma among European adults were secondary to occupational exposures.[4]

## PREDISPOSING FACTORS

A number of predisposing factors may influence or facilitate the development of occupational asthma (Table 6-2). These include industrial, climatic, and genetic factors.[5-7] In addition, personal habits such as tobacco and recreational drug use may have an adverse effect on lung health. Other medical issues such as respiratory viral infections, the presence of subclinical bronchial

---

**BOX 6-2**
**Predisposing Factors for Occupational Asthma**

**Industrial Factors**
Characteristics of the job.
Implementation of safety practices.
Availability of MSDS information.
Nature and concentration of chemical exposures.

**Meterological Conditions**
Presence of diesel exhaust particles.
High concentrations of oxidizing pollutants.
Wind conditions.
Temperature inversions.
Presence of seasonal allergens and incidental industrial irritants.

**Genetic Influences**
Atopic individuals more likely to develop occupational asthma when exposed to high-molecular-weight allergens.
Sensitization may be facilitated by HLA polymorphisms.

**Cigarette Smoking**
Tobacco abuse implicated as a potential predisposing and aggravating factor in development of occupational asthma.
Smoking facilitates morbidity associated with respiratory tract infections.

**Recreational Drug Use**
There is evidence that cannabis and tobacco abuse have an additive effect.

**Respiratory Infection**
Viral infections have been increasingly recognized as an important trigger of asthma exacerbations.
Sinusitis is also associated with deterioration of underlying asthma.

**Bronchial Hyperreactivity**
Bronchial hyperractivity is felt to represent the common physiological pathway of several mechanisms leading to a lowered threshold of airway narrowing to bronchoconstrictor stimuli.

**Miscellaneous Factors**
Aspirin sensitivity syndrome
Gastroesophageal reflux
Incidental drug therapy, eg., beta-adrenergic blockers

HLA, histocompatibility leukocyte antigen; MSDS, material safety data sheet.

hyperreactivity, and miscellaneous pharmacotherapy also may impact the lungs adversely.[8,9] These factors are outlined in Box 6-2.

# PATHOGENESIS

Occupational asthma can be classified in several ways. From a clinical and pathogenetic perspective, new-onset occupational asthma can be divided into immunologic and nonimmunologic variants.[1,9] The immunologic variant can be further divided into immunoglobulin (Ig) E–mediated or polyimmunologic types. The nonimmunologic variant can be divided into reactive airways dysfunction syndrome (RADS), pharmacologic bronchoconstriction, and reflex bronchoconstriction (Fig. 6-2).

# ALLERGIC OCCUPATIONAL ASTHMA

Allergic work-related asthma can be triggered by a large number of high-molecular-weight allergens. These are generally proteins derived from animals, plants, foods, and enzymes (Box 6-3). In the majority of cases, occupational asthma involves a specific T-helper type 2 lymphocyte response with production of specific IgE antibody. Usually, a latent period of sensitization must occur, which can vary from a few weeks to as long as several years. Only a selected number of exposed workers are generally affected. However, sensitivity to the causative allergen generally increases with time; the longer the worker is exposed, the more likely a severe reaction will occur.[1,9]

There are a number of low-molecular-weight allergens, including the isocyanates, the acid anhydrides, and plicatic acid, that are also capable of inducing occupational asthma. Although IgE and IgG antibodies are occasionally generated, the pathogenesis

remains only partly elucidated. Studies of bronchial tissue show significant numbers of activated T-lymphocytes in a peribronchial location, suggesting that they play an active role in eliciting immunologic inflammation.[10] The majority of these cells are of the CD8 phenotype capable of producing interferon gamma and interleukin 5, but little interleukin 4; i.e., the mechanism is polyimmunologic.

The clinical presentation of a worker with allergic occupational asthma would parallel the symptoms of most patients with classic allergic disorders. In many instances, there are preceding or concomitant ocular and upper airway symptoms of allergic rhinoconjunctivitis. Subsequently, symptoms of work-related airflow obstruction characterized by chest tightness, cough, and dyspnea that generally intensify over the course of the workweek may develop. Symptoms with work exposure may be immediate, delayed, or biphasic in nature (dual), consistent with the early- and late-phase allergic response (Fig. 6-3).

# NONALLERGIC OCCUPATIONAL ASTHMA

Nonallergic industrial asthma may be divided into several clinical variants depending on pathogenesis. The most common and best-understood variant was originally described by Gandevia in 1970 and referred to as "acute inflammatory bronchoconstriction."[11] The onset was related to the acute accidental exposure to high concentrations of a corrosive irritant; e.g., chlorine, hydrogen sulfide, and phosgene. Airflow obstruction manifested itself within hours of the exposure, secondary to a chemically induced bronchitis or bronchopneumonia.[12] Many afflicted workers continued to manifest chronic asthma or asymptomatic bronchial hyperreactivity, depending on the corrosive properties of the precipitating exposure.

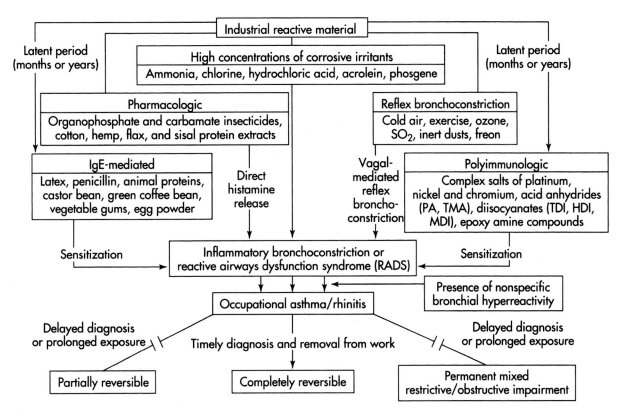

**Figure 6-2.** Several pathogenetic mechanisms of occupationally induced airway obstruction. FEV$_1$, forced expiratory volume in 1 second, HDI, hexamethylene diisocyanate; Ig, immunoglobulin; MDI, diphenylmethane diisocyanote; PA, phthalic anhydride; SO$_2$, sulfur dioxide; TDI, toluene diisocyanate; TMA, trimellitic anhydride. (Adapted with permission from Bardana EJ: Occupational asthma and allergies. J Allergy Clin Immunol 2003;111:S530).

**BOX 6-3**
**Classification of Selected Asthma-Producing Agents by Molecular Weight**

**High Molecular Weight**
Animal protein
Papain
Avian proteins
Fish-derived allergens
Wheat flour
Trypsin
Soybean dust
Psyllium
Natural rubber latex
Seeds (linseed, flaxseed)

**Low Molecular Weight**
Platinum salts
Nickel
Vanadium
Phthalic anhydride
Trimellitic anhydride
Colophony
Diisocyanates
Plicatic acid
Penicillins
Sulfonamides

In 1981, Brooks and Lockey coined the term *RADS* to describe a condition seen in 13 workers acutely exposed to an industrial irritant (see Fig. 6-2). Agents that have been incriminated in the induction of RADS are outlined in Box 6-4. In the ensuing years, RADS has replaced "inflammatory bronchoconstriction" as the label.[13] Although there has been significant controversy related to this diagnosis, it has gradually gained acceptance in the general medical community. Major and minor diagnostic criteria have been proposed for RADS (Box 6-5).[14,15] The mechanism of damage in RADS has been hypothesized to result from extensive denudation of the bronchial epithelium resulting in sustained airway inflammation. Over time, desquamation of epithelium with an influx of lymphocytes occurs, which can persist for months.[13]

Nonallergic occupational asthma also can be induced by substances that act by a direct pharmacologic action on the respiratory mucosa, such as organophosphate and carbamate insecticides. In sufficient doses, these agents can inhibit acetylcholinesterase, which in turn potentiates the effect of acetylcholine released from vagal fibers that innervate bronchial smooth muscle (see Fig. 6-2).[1,9]

The final mechanism operative in the induction of occupational asthma is called reflex bronchoconstriction. It is different from RADS by virtue of the intensity of the exposure. Reflex bronchoconstriction generally involves mild to moderate irritational reactions by agents described in Table 6-1. It is not likely to be a cause of de novo occupational asthma. However, workers who have preexisting asthma or bronchitis may respond in a nonspecific fashion to irritants. This reflex bronchoconstriction results from the direct effect of such substances on irritant receptors in the bronchial wall (see Fig. 6-2).[9]

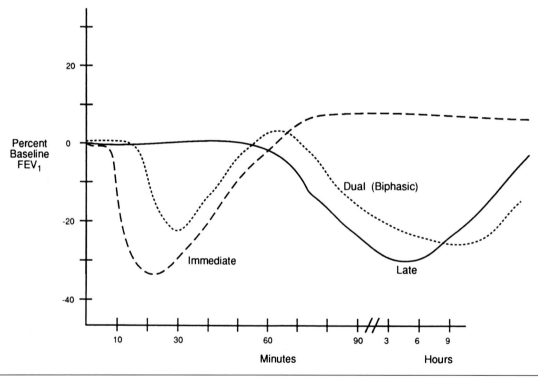

**Figure 6-3.** Allergic occupational asthma, where antigen activation of the mast cell is followed by the early- and late-phase responses. The immediate response is essentially bronchospastic with some mild, transient bronchial hyperreactivity. The late-phase response is characterized by an influx of inflammatory cells. (Adapted with permission from Bardana EJ: Occupational asthma and related respiratory disorders. Disease-a-Month 1995;61:141–2000.)

# DIAGNOSIS

## *MEDICAL HISTORY AND EXAMINATION*

In the evaluation of workers with suspected occupational asthma, it is critical to define the parameters of establishing a diagnosis that will distinguish it from a variety of closely allied conditions (Box 6-6). However, the initial hurdle is to be absolutely certain that the patient has asthma by virtue of the presence of reversible obstruction. Once the diagnosis of asthma is established, one must demonstrate that the asthma is due to an industrial agent. A detailed history must be taken of the worker's occupational environment. The clinician must elucidate not only the materials with which the patient works directly but also other agents that are incidentally encountered in the workplace. It is helpful to know if any co-workers are similarly afflicted. The temporality of symptoms to a work agent can be very helpful (e.g., if regression of symptoms occurs over weekends or holidays). Because a complete history is so critical, a detailed review of all prior medical records should be carried out. It is important to establish whether the worker has an atopic predisposition.[1,9]

The medical history should reflect all prior employers, prior work-related claims, and the industrial hygiene aspects of the workplace. The information acquired should provide a detailed understanding of the protective equipment used by the worker, including face mask, earplugs, goggles, gloves, and uniform (Fig. 6-4). The examiner must inquire about the details of any respiratory protection: Was the worker trained in its utilization? Was it fit-tested? What was the frequency of cartridge change? Were prefilters used? (Fig. 6-5). The presence or absence of facial hair is critical whenever a mask is worn.

## *SITE VISIT*

A site visit to the work area is of great value to establish the precise cause of the occupational allergy. The worker may have only partial knowledge of the industrial processes involved and the potential chemical substances that are generated (Fig. 6-6). Visiting the worksite enables the physician to see the worker in action and to obtain a much more accurate picture of the types of exposure and the industrial hygiene measures in place (Fig. 6-7). The 1986 OSHA "right to know" act makes it mandatory for the employer to provide Material Safety Data Sheets, which provide detailed information about the substances to which the worker may be exposed, the required protection that is recommended, and the potential adverse health effects of each (Fig. 6-8).

---

**BOX 6-4**
**Selected Agents That Have Been Cited in the Causation of RADS**

Anhydrous ammonia
Chlorine
Diethylene diamine
Glacial acetic acid
Hydrochloric acid
Hydrogen sulfate
Phosgene
Phosphoric acid
Sulfuric acid
Toluene diisocyanate

RADS, reactive airways dysfunction syndrome.

---

**BOX 6-5**
**Criteria for the Diagnosis of RADS (American College of Chest Physicians)**

**Major**
Absence of prior pulmonary disease or complaints
A single exposure precipitates onset of symptoms
Presence of high concentration of a corrosive chemical agent
Symptoms appear within 24 hr of the exposure and last 3 mo or more
Continuation of asthma-like symptoms
Spirometry with airflow obstruction and/or presence of nonspecific bronchial hyperreactivity
Alternative respiratory conditions excluded

**Minor**
There is no evidence of an allergic state
Pulmonary and peripheral eosinophilia are absent
The worker has not smoked for 10 years
Methacholine challenge positive at a $PC_{20}$ at or below 8 mg/mL
Histopathology and/or bronchoalveolar lavage demonstrating mild lymphocytic inflammation

RADS, reactive airways dysfunction syndrome.

---

**BOX 6-6**
**Diagnostic Criteria for New-Onset Allergic Occupational Asthma**

No preexisting diagnosis of asthma
Typical temporally related symptoms to a known occupational allergen
Demonstrated persistent variable airway obstruction
Demonstration of IgE-specific antibodies by standard skin testing or in vitro methodology
Physiologic demonstration of reversible airway obstruction with subirritant concentrations of the suspected agent
Improvement or cessation of symptoms with timely diagnosis and removal from incriminated allergen

IgE, immunoglobulin E.

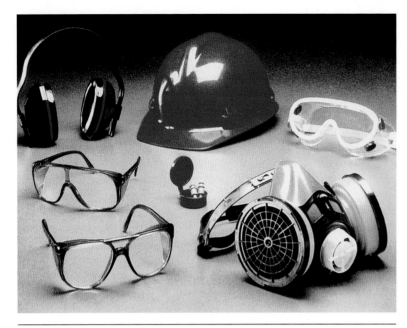

**Figure 6-4.** A variety of protective equipment used by workers. (Reproduced with permission from Bardana EJ: Occupational asthma. In Lieberman PI, Blaiss MS (eds): Atlas of Allergic Diseases. Philadelphia, Current Medicine, 2002, pp 191–201.)

## PHYSICAL EXAMINATION

The examination should address all major organ systems. The examiner should have a focus on the signs supporting underlying atopy; i.e., atopic dermatitis, dermatographism, evidence of allergic rhinoconjunctivitis, and, most importantly, evidence of bronchospasm. Signs of paranasal sinusitis with or without polyposis may be associated with asthma and may suggest the presence of aspirin idiosyncracy syndrome or immunodeficiency. Attention should be given to signs of current tobacco abuse, including nicotine stains of the teeth and fingers and the odor of smoke on the breath or clothes.

## LABORATORY STUDIES

The diagnostic value of skin testing and in vitro laboratory assays is limited to cases in which sensitivity involves either a high-molecular-weight allergen or selected low-molecular-weight agents where in vitro assays may be available. In the latter case, standardized assays are available and may have limited utility.

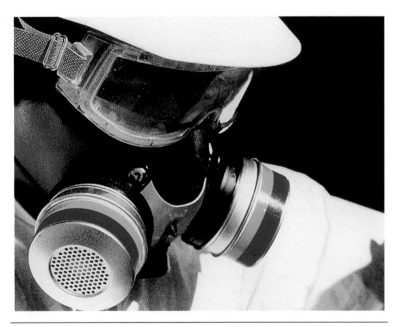

**Figure 6-5.** Partial face respirator. The evaluator must document a detailed understanding of the protective equipment used by the worker. Important data include the brand of mask worn, how it was test fitted, frequency of cartridge change, and types of prefilters used. (Reproduced with permission from Bardana EJ: Occupational asthma. In Lieberman PI, Blaiss MS (eds): Atlas of Allergic Diseases. Philadelphia, Current Medicine, 2002, pp 191–201.)

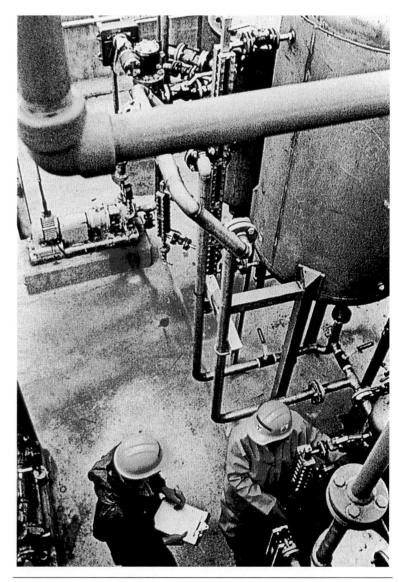

**Figure 6-6.** Visitation to an isocyanate foam plant with evidence of white spill.

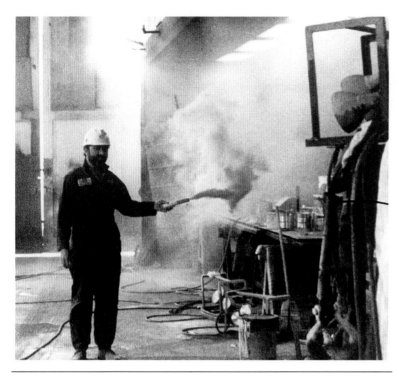

**Figure 6-7.** Visitation to a shipyard paint bench. Safety personnel are testing the suction exhaust with a smoke bomb. (Reproduced with permission from Bardana EJ: Occupational asthma. In Lieberman PI, Blaiss MS (eds): Atlas of Allergic Diseases. Philadelphia, Current Medicine, 2002, pp 191–201.)

| MATERIAL SAFETY DATA SHEET | | |
|---|---|---|
| **I PRODUCT IDENTIFICATION** | | |
| MANUFACTURER'S NAME | REGULAR TELEPHONE NO EMERGENCY TELEPHONE NO | |
| ADDRESS | | |
| **TRADE NAME** | | |
| **SYNONYMS** | | |
| **II HAZARDOUS INGREDIENTS** | | |
| MATERIAL OR COMPONENT | | HAZARD DATA |
| | | |
| | | |
| | | |
| | | |
| | | |
| | | |
| | | |
| **III PHYSICAL DATA** | | |
| BOILING POINT 760 MM HG | | MELTING POINT |
| SPECIFIC GRAVITY (H$_2$0•1) | | VAPOR PRESSURE |
| VAPOR DENSITY (AIR•1) | | SOLUBILITY IN H$_2$0 % BY WT |
| % VOLATILES BY VOL | | EVAPORATION RATE IBUTYL ACETATE II |
| APPEARANCE AND ODOR | | |

**Figure 6-8.** Format of a material safety data sheet. (Adapted with permission from Bardana EJ: Occupational asthma and allergies. J Allergy Clin Immunol 2003;111:S530.)

As in all laboratory testing, the weight that is placed on the data has to be judged in the context of the entire clinical picture. Cutaneous or serologic sensitization is not sufficient in itself to conclude that the putative allergen is responsible for the patient's occupational asthma. The presence of antibody cannot be interpreted as more than evidence of prior exposure to that allergen. It does not necessarily equate to a symptomatic state. By the same token, a negative test, especially with in vitro assays involving low-molecular-weight antigens, does not necessarily exclude sensitization.

## IMAGING STUDIES

The role of chest radiographs and other available sophisticated imaging studies lies principally in the exclusion of unrelated disorders such as pulmonary fibrosis, bronchiectasis, emphysema, and neoplasm. In adults with work-related asthma, x-ray findings are almost always normal.

## PULMONARY FUNCTION STUDIES

Pulmonary function studies are critical to the diagnosis and assessment of impairment in occupational asthma. The diagnosis demands an unequivocal finding of reversible airflow obstruction that has been defined as a minimum of 12% increase in forced expiratory volume in 1 second with a bronchodilator. It is important to be mindful that when evaluating spirometric data from primary care providers, less than 20% of spirometric tests performed in primary care settings meet American Thoracic Society criteria. A methacholine provocation test can be utilized to demonstrate the presence of underlying bronchial hyperreactivity. Although a positive test is not specific for asthma, a negative test, providing the worker is not taking any antiasthmatic drugs, would argue strongly against the presence of asthma.

A provisional cause-and-effect relationship to a workplace agent can be reached by serial determination of peak expiratory flow rates during a prescribed period of work abstinence followed by a return to work (Fig. 6-9). However, the results of such testing should be interpreted with caution, as the procedure is effort dependent, and recent studies have demonstrated that as many as 50% of submitted values are fabricated or inadequately recorded.[16]

A more dependable diagnostic approach would assess the degree of bronchial hyperreactivity before and after return to work after a period of 2 to 3 weeks off work. A change in bronchial hyperreactivity greater than two doubling concentrations is considered highly significant.[17]

A third approach might rely on cross-shift spirometric measurements. Performing spirometry to compare forced expiratory volume in 1 second before and after the work shift daily for at least a week has been used to verify work-specific degradation of lung function.[17]

## BRONCHIAL PROVOCATION STUDIES

Bronchial provocation tests are considered the gold standard in the diagnosis of bronchial asthma. The initial pragmatic approach was designed to recreate the workplace and suspected allergen;

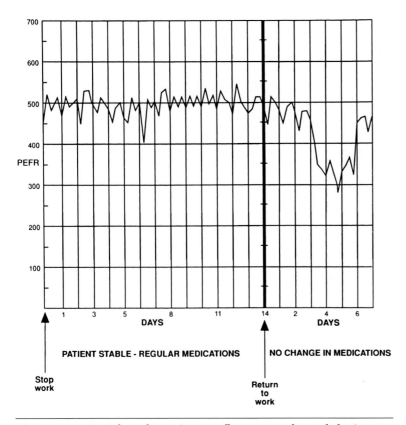

**Figure 6-9.** Serial peak expiratory flow rates charted during a period of work abstinence and after a return to work. PEFR, peak expiratory flow rate. (Reproduced with permission from Bardana EJ: Occupational asthma and allergies. J Allergy Clin Immunol 2003;111:S530.)

i.e., "simulated work provocation." These tests were carried out with chemical dusts, wood dust, flour, paint vapors, and other substances. Controls were devised to appear similar to the provocative agent. Despite the imprecision of provocative concentrations, work simulation was reasonably achieved and usable results obtained.

Direct bronchial challenge is used only rarely and generally in a specialized hospital center. There are several reasons to perform such a test. Most important is to study a previously unrecognized agent as a possible asthmogenic agent. Another reason is to segregate offending antigens from the frequently complex work environment. Finally, such a test may be employed to accurately confirm the diagnosis and identify the culprit agent (Fig. 6-10). The procedure is time consuming and potentially dangerous and requires carefully designed protocols and patient consent.[1,9,17]

## DIFFERENTIAL DIAGNOSIS

The clinician determining whether a worker's asthma is linked to his or her work environment must always eliminate the possibility that the asthma is secondary to triggers of a nonoccupational nature. The atopic worker who may have had preexisting subclinical asthma is always a diagnostic challenge. Recent studies have shown that patients who were thought to have "outgrown" their childhood asthma have shown the continued presence of asymptomatic pulmonary function abnormalities, as well as bronchial hyperreactivity. The transient expression of preexisting subclinical asthma by irritant triggers at the workplace is a commonplace occurrence. As well, other variants of asthma, such as allergic bronchopulmonary aspergillosis, aspirin-sensitivity

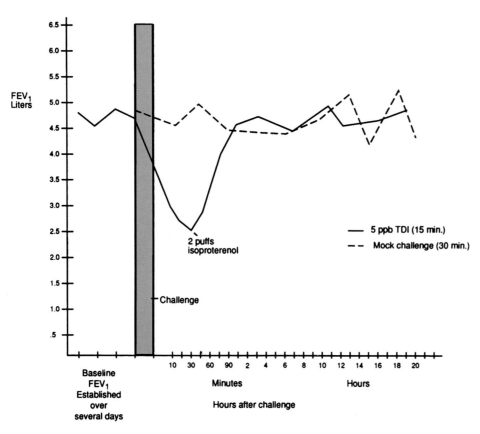

**Figure 6-10.** Controlled provocation study. Spirometric results of a controlled bronchial provocation study to toluene diisocyanate (TDI), indicating a positive immediate response. $FEV_1$, forced expiratory volume in 1 second. (Adapted from Bardana EJ: Occupational asthma. In Lieberman PI, Blaiss MS (eds): Atlas of Allergic Diseases. Philadelphia, Current Medicine, 2002, pp 191–201.)

syndrome, and Churg–Strauss allergic granulomatosis, must be excluded. Unrelated disorders masquerading as asthma also must be ruled out (Box 6-7).

# PREVENTION AND MANAGEMENT

Clearly, the most desirable method of reducing instances of occupational asthma is to insulate at-risk workers from potentially hazardous agents. Employers should implement and enforce use of state-of-the-art worker protection to substantially reduce or eliminate known irritants or immunogens. Furthermore, many industries conduct regular surveillance of production processes; i.e., measuring ambient levels of hazardous chemicals and mandatory monitoring of worker respiratory health.

The management of occupational asthma is identical to the management of non–work-related asthma (see Chapter 5). However, the most important issue with work-related asthma is removal of the worker from any further exposure to the causative agent.

# PROGNOSIS

The key factors operative in determining the prognostic outcome of the worker with occupational asthma include the duration of exposure to the putative allergen, severity of asthma at the time of diagnosis, and pathogenic mechanisms involved in the ongoing airway inflammation. A variety of other comorbid factors also play a role (Box 6-8).[18]

---

**BOX 6-7**

**Differential Diagnostic Considerations in the Setting of Occupational Asthma**

Allergic bronchopulmonary aspergillosis
Aspirin sensitivity syndrome
Churg–Strauss granulomatosis
Vocal cord dysfunction syndrome
Industrial bronchitis
Congestive heart failure
Hypersensitivity pneumonitis
Acute tracheobronchitis
Gastrointestinal reflux disease
Organic toxic dust syndrome

---

**BOX 6-8**

**Factors Affecting the Prognosis of Occupational Asthma**

Total duration of exposure to the offending work allergen
Severity of occupational asthma at the time of diagnosis
Degree of bronchial hyperreactivity at the time of diagnosis
Pathogenetic mechanisms that underlie the airway inflammation
History of prior (or concomitant) cigarette smoking
Presence of chronic sinusitis
Presence of gastroesophageal reflux

---

# REFERENCES

1. Bardana EJ, Montanaro A: Occupational asthma and related disorders. In Rich RR, Fleisher TA, Shearer WT, et al (eds): Clinical Immunology, Principles and Practice, 2nd ed. London, C.V. Mosby, 2001, pp 1–14.
2. Alberts WM, Brooks SM: Advances in occupational asthma. Clin Chest Med 1992;13:281–302.
3. Chan-Yeung M, Malo JL: Occupational asthma. N Engl J Med 1995; 333:107–112.
4. Kogevinas M, Anto JM, Sunyer J, et al: Occupational asthma in Europe and other industrialized areas: A population based study. Lancet 1999; 353:1750–1754.
5. Sunyer J, Anto JM, Sabria J, et al: Risk factors of soybean epidemic asthma: The role of smoking and atopy. Am Rev Respir Dis 1992;145:1098–1102.
6. Newman Taylor AJ: Role of human leukocyte antigen phenotype and exposure in development of occupational asthma. Cur Opin Allergy Clin Immunol 2001; 1:157–161.
7. Bignon JS, Aron Y, Ju LY, et al: HLA Class II alleles in isocyanate-induced asthma. Am J Respir Crit Care Med 1994;149:71–75.
8. Woolcock AJ: What is bronchial hyperresponsiveness from the clinical standpoint? In Page CP, Gardiner PJ (eds): Airway Hyperresponsiveness: Is It Really Important for Asthma? Oxford, Blackwell Scientific, 1993.
9. Bardana EJ: Occupational asthma and allergies. J Allergy Clin Immunol 2003; 111:S530–S539.
10. Frew A, Chang JH, Chan H, et al: T-lymphocyte responses to plicatic acid-human serum albumin conjugate in occupational asthma caused by western red cedar. J Allergy Clin Immunol 1998;101:841–847.
11. Gandevia B: Occupational Asthma (Part 1). Med J Aust 1970;2:332–333.
12. Smith DD: Acute inhalational injury: How to assess, how to treat. J Respir Dis 1999;20:405.
13. Brooks SM, Weiss MA, Bernstein IL: Reactive airways dysfunction syndrome (RADS): Persistent airways hyperreactivity after high-level irritant exposure. Chest 1985;88:376–384.
14. Alberts WM, doPico G: Reactive airways dysfunction syndrome. Chest 1996; 104:1618–1626.
15. Bardana EJ: Reactive airways dysfunction syndrome (RADS): Guidelines for diagnosis and treatment and insight into likely prognosis. Ann Allergy Asthma Immunol 1999;83:583–586.
16. Malo J-L, Trudeau C, Ghezzo H, et al: Do subjects investigated for occupational asthma through serial peak expiratory flow measurements falsify their results. J Allergy Clin Immunol 1995;601–607.
17. Tan RA, Spector SL: Diagnostic testing in occupational asthma. Ann Allergy Asthma Immunol 1999;83:587–592.
18. Montanaro A: Prognosis of occupational asthma. Ann Allergy Asthma Immunol 1999;83:593–596.

*Sergei N. Belenky and Carl R. Fuhrman*

# 7 Hypersensitivity Pneumonitis

The ready access to potent antigens and the presence of large numbers of immunocompetent cells, including sensitized lymphocytes, macrophages, neutrophils, eosinophils, plasma cells, and mediator substances, contribute to make the lung an important immunologic shock organ (Table 7-1). In addition to these categories, some immunologic diseases, such as hypersensitivity pneumonitis (HP), may represent a combination of immunologic responses.

Whereas the present era of interest in hypersensitivity lung disease began more than 50 years ago with the first description of farmer's lung, a great deal of study and an increased awareness of HP has been prompted recently by the availability of new immunologic techniques. These have aided in both the diagnosis and the better definition of the pathogenesis.

Synonyms for HP include *pulmonary hypersensitivity syndrome* and *extrinsic allergic alveolitis*. The latter term is perhaps the best and most descriptive. "Extrinsic" refers to an exogenous antigen or allergen. "Allergic" indicates that the disease has a hypersensitivity basis. "Alveolitis" refers to that part of the lung that is most affected by this disease process. Whichever term is used, we are referring to the same underlying pathogenic entity—namely, a condition caused by sensitivity to organic dust inhalation.

## EPIDEMIOLOGY

There are no definitive studies that delineate the prevalence of HP because the illness represents a group of syndromes rather than a single disease with etiology. The prevalence of one HP syndrome, farmer's lung disease, varies between and within countries and ranges from 1.6% to 7%.[1]

Several factors determine the nature of an individual's response to inhalation of organic dust (Box 7-1). First is the basic immunologic reactivity of the host. An atopic or allergic individual typically responds to organic dust inhalation with the production of an immunoglobulin (Ig) E skin-sensitizing antibody. A nonallergic or nonatopic individual tends to respond to organic dust inhalation with the production of an IgG precipitating antibody.

A second factor influencing the response is the nature and source of the antigen. Perhaps the most important is the particle size of the dust. The optimal size for penetration of the smaller airways is less than 5 μm. Particles larger than 10 μm are trapped in the upper airway and unable to reach the alveoli in amounts sufficient to cause injury.

A third factor determining the response to organic dust is the nature and circumstance of the exposure. An intense but intermittent exposure results in a clinical picture different from that of a less intense exposure of longer duration. A good example of this is the response to avian antigens. Intermittent, heavy exposure of short duration, such as experienced by a pigeon fancier who cleans out the coops twice a week, produces an acute form of HP that is usually reversible. However, a part-time employee in a pet store may have more continuous exposure of relatively shorter duration, which results in a subacute, insidious form that is also usually reversible. Long-term exposure, such as experienced by an elderly housebound person with two parakeets, may result in chronic, irreversible disease (Table 7-2).

| Gell and Coombs Classification | Immunologic Characteristic | Pulmonary Manifestation |
|---|---|---|
| Type I | IgE-mediated | Allergic bronchial asthma |
| Type II | Autoimmune, cytotoxic | Goodpasture's syndrome |
| Type III | Immune complex, precipitating antibody | Polyarteritis |
| Type IV | Lymphocyte, cell-mediated | Tuberculosis |

**TABLE 7-1**
The Lung as an Immunologic Shock Organ

IgE, immunoglobulin E.

A variety of antigens may result in HP.[2] As our awareness of the disease process increases and other forms of environmental exposure develop, the list continues to expand. Table 7-3 shows the general categories of antigens with selected examples of each.

# CLINICAL PRESENTATION

The clinical manifestations of HP are essentially the same regardless of the offending antigen but may vary depending on the intensity and frequency of exposure. Table 7-4 contrasts the features of the three forms of HP defined in Table 7-2.[3]

In the acute form associated with intermittent, intense antigen exposure, the main symptoms are fever, chills, cough, dyspnea, headache, body aches, and malaise, appearing 4 to 6 hours after organic dust inhalation. Remission of symptoms follows 12 to 18 hours later in the absence of further exposure.

Intermittent but longer-term exposure results in the subacute form of HP marked by progressively increasing fatigue, dyspnea, weight loss, and productive cough. Rales become more widespread.

In the chronic form caused by prolonged organic dust exposure, the symptoms seen in the subacute form progress, resulting in pulmonary fibrosis and respiratory failure.[4]

## *RADIOGRAPHIC FINDINGS*

Chest imaging findings in HP are conveniently classified by the three clinically recognized presentations of the disease: acute, subacute, and chronic. Radiographic documentation of progression between these stages is uncommon, and prior imaging studies in most patients with the chronic form have not confirmed the acute or subacute stage of the disease. Chest imaging, including high-resolution computed tomography (HRCT), is particularly useful in suggesting the correct diagnosis in patients with appropriate clinical symptoms and a history of antigen exposure. Improvement in the chest radiographs after removal from the antigen, and recurrence of radiographic abnormalities after reexposure to the antigen are important in confirming a clinically suspected diagnosis of HP.

The acute form of the disease usually occurs after a short, intense antigen exposure (4 to 8 hours). The chest x-ray may be entirely normal, even when a subsequent biopsy confirms interstitial disease. The typical radiographic appearance of acute HP consists of areas of extensive airspace consolidation, which usually involves the mid- and lower lung zones and usually spares the lung apices (Fig. 7-1A). There may be small micronodular opacities (Fig. 7-1B), but these nodules are usually not seen on routine chest radiographs. (However, they may be apparent on HRCT.) The chest radiographic findings are often mistaken for

---

**BOX 7-1**

**Factors Determining Response to Organic Dust Inhalation**

1. **Immunologic reactivity of host**
   Atopic, nonatopic

2. **Nature and source of antigen**
   Particle size, growth in airway

3. **Nature and circumstances of exposure**
   Intense and intermittent versus low grade; chronic

---

**TABLE 7-2**

**Nature of Disease Related to Exposure**

| Exposure | Example | Disease |
|---|---|---|
| Intermittent, short term | Pigeon breeder | Acute—reversible |
| Intermittent, long term | Pet store employee | Subacute—usually reversible |
| Long term | Parakeet owner | Chronic—irreversible |

---

**TABLE 7-3**
**Antigens Causing Hypersensitivity Pneumonitis**

| Category of Antigen | Disease | Category of Antigen | Disease |
|---|---|---|---|
| **Thermophilic organisms** | | **Animal** | |
| *Micropolyspora faeni* | Farmer's lung | Bird protein | Pigeon breeder's lung |
| *Thermoactinomyces sacchari* | Bagassosis | Gerbil protein | Gerbil keeper's lung |
| | | Amoeba (*Naegleria gruberi*) | Humidifier lung |
| **Mold** | | | |
| *Aspergillus clavatus* | Malt worker's lung | **Chemicals** | |
| *Penicillium roqueforti* | Cheese worker's lung | Toluene diisocyanate (TDI) | Paint finisher's lung |
| | | Phthalic anhydride | Epoxy resin lung |

acute bacterial or viral pneumonia. These patients are often admitted to the hospital, and the rapid clinical and radiographic improvement is then attributed to antibiotic therapy (rather than removal from the antigen). Radiographic resolution is usually complete by 7 to 10 days. Repeated hospital admissions for "bilateral pneumonia" that improves rapidly may be the first clue that the correct diagnosis is acute HP.

The subacute form of HP produces abnormal chest radiographs or CT scans in approximately 90% of patients. The most common finding is the presence of small bilateral pulmonary nodules (2 to 4 mm in diameter) involving all portions of both lungs, with greatest involvement in the mid- and lower zones (Fig. 7-2). The borders of the nodules may be either sharply or poorly defined. The nodules may be diffuse and produce a ground-glass pattern where individual nodules are not easily recognized. This form of the disease often causes a characteristic HRCT pattern suggestive of HP and will show the interstitial changes (including the centrilobular nodules) much better than routine chest radiographs,

**TABLE 7-4**
**Clinical Presentation of Hypersensitivity Pneumonitis**

| Features | Acute | Subacute | Chronic |
|---|---|---|---|
| Chills and fever | + | | |
| Dyspnea | + | + | + |
| Cough | Nonproductive | Productive | Productive |
| Malaise and myalagia | + | + | + |
| Weight loss | | + | + |
| Rales | Bibasilar | Widespread | Widespread |
| Chest radiograph | Nodular infiltrates | Nodular infiltrates | Pulmonary fibrosis |
| Precipitins | + | + | + |
| Pulmonary function | Restrictive | Restrictive and obstructive | Restrictive and obstructive |
| Reversible | Yes | Yes | No |

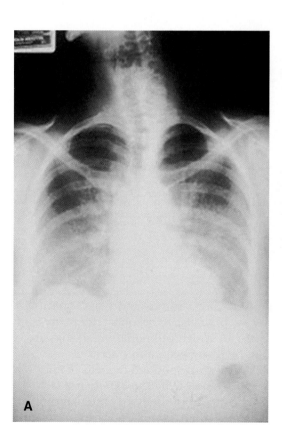

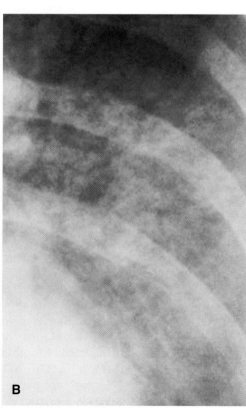

**Figure 7-1.** *A,* Chest radiograph showing diffuse, bilateral, finely granular infiltrates characteristic of alveolar or interstitial pneumonitis. Note the sparing of upper lung fields. *B,* Magnified view of chest radiograph demonstrating patchy micronodular densities. (Courtesy of Dr. Raymond Slavin, St. Louis University School of Medicine, St. Louis, MO)

A

B

which are often nonspecific. The HRCT findings include ground-glass opacities (Fig. 7-3), centrilobular nodules, subpleural nodules (Fig. 7-4), thickening of bronchovascular bundles, and focal areas of air trapping on CT images obtained during expiration (consistent with small airways disease and bronchiolitis). The subacute form of HP may show overlap with the acute form (areas of airspace consolidation) and the chronic form (fibrosis) (Fig. 7-5). The radiographic findings in subacute HP may resolve 10 days to 3 months after removal from the antigen. Any areas of scarring usually show no improvement. Subacute HP is often first suggested by characteristic HRCT findings in patients referred for CT scanning because of abnormal chest radiographs and pulmonary function tests suggesting interstitial lung disease.

In the chronic form of the disease, the interstitial changes reflect parenchymal fibrosis and consist of small irregular linear opacities, architectural distortion and traction bronchiectasis, honeycombing, and areas of emphysema adjacent to fibrosis. The fibrosis often involves the upper and mid-lung zones and can occur after several acute episodes. The fibrosis more commonly develops slowly related to chronic low-dose antigen exposure with no acute episodes. Often, there is overlap with the subacute phase of the disease, and the presence of micronodules and ground-glass opacities (in a mid- and lower-zone distribution) with fibrosis (in a mid- and upper-zone distribution) is an important radiographic finding that helps to distinguish the chronic form of HP from idiopathic pulmonary fibrosis and other chronic fibrotic interstitial lung diseases. The fibrosis may be so extensive that the chest x-ray resembles that of a patient with end-stage sarcoid or complicated pneumoconiosis with progressive massive fibrosis. The fibrosis is irreversible, but the associated features of subacute HP may improve following removal from the antigen.

## PULMONARY FUNCTION STUDIES

Pulmonary function studies in acute HP reveal a restrictive type of ventilatory impairment associated with low vital capacity and low arterial oxygen saturation that falls further with exercise. In the subacute and chronic forms, obstructive defects are observed also.

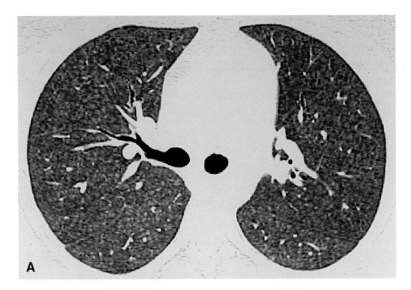

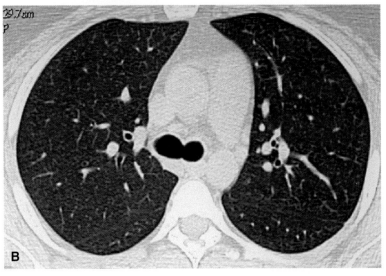

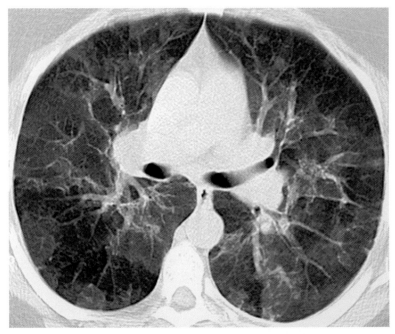

**Figure 7-2.** *A,* Note the innumerable tiny centrilobular nodules measuring 1 to 2 mm in diameter in this CT scan. These nodules are in the center of the pulmonary lobule corresponding to the location of the terminal bronchioles. This 30-year woman began to have respiratory symptoms shortly after moving to a new apartment where her roommate had a pet bird. *B,* Almost complete clearing of the nodules approximately 3 months later. (Courtesy of Dr. Carl Fuhrman.)

**Figure 7-3.** There are diffuse areas of "ground-glass" opacity in both lungs in this CT scan. *Ground-glass opacities* refer to areas of parenchymal opacification in which pulmonary markings are still visible. In addition, there are geographic areas of increased lung blackness that corresponded to areas of air trapping. This 45-year-old woman began to experience increasing severe respiratory symptoms shortly after starting a job as a cashier at a pet store. (Courtesy of Dr. Carl Fuhrman.)

## BRONCHOPROVOCATION TESTS

Bronchoprovocation tests may be helpful when the specific diagnosis is in doubt because of the relevance of the particular exposure. Under carefully controlled conditions, an aqueous extract of the antigen in question is delivered to the bronchi. A positive result is identified by temperature elevation, chills, cough, dyspnea, leukocytosis, and changes in pulmonary function after 4 to 6 hours (Fig. 7-6). Provocative bronchial challenges should not be performed on a routine basis and must be used with great caution because of their possible severe systemic effects, including cough, fever, and dyspnea.[5]

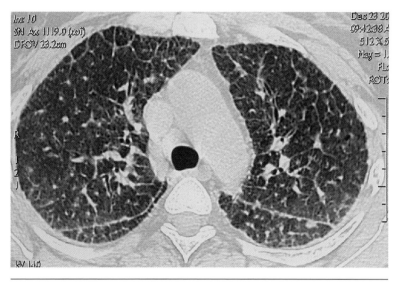

**Figure 7-5.** This CT scan was obtained 6 months after the start of pulmonary symptoms. In addition to interstitial thickening and subpleural nodularity, there is early fibrosis with architectural distortion of the bronchovascular bundles and pulmonary lobules. (Courtesy of Dr. Carl Fuhrman.)

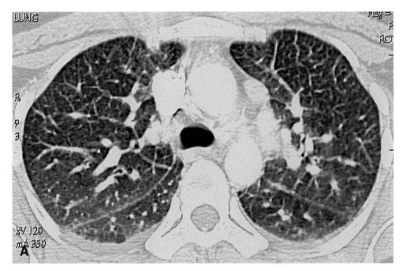

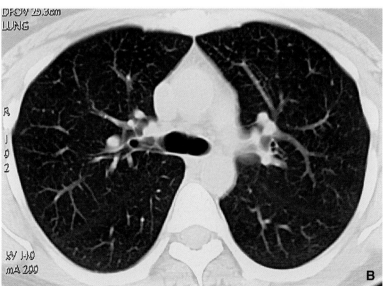

**Figure 7-4.** *A,* There is nodularity and "beading" along the fissures corresponding to granuloma formation in the subpleural lymphatics. In addition, there is thickening of the bronchovascular bundles and interstitial thickening with septal lines. This 39-year-old woman became symptomatic shortly after starting a new job at a pet store. The initial computed tomographic scan was obtained 6 weeks after 6 weeks of symptoms that did not respond to antibiotic therapy. *B,* Complete resolution 2 months later. (Courtesy of Dr. Carl Fuhrman.)

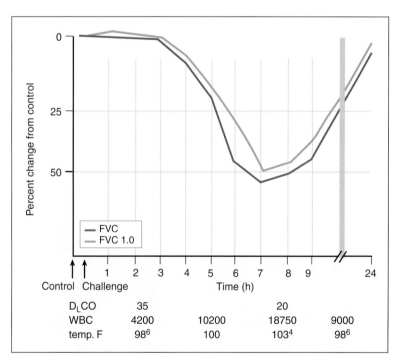

**Figure 7-6.** Bronchial challenge results from aqueous extract inhalation in a case of hypersensitivity pneumonitis. $D_LCO$, diffusion lung capacity to carbon monoxide; FVC, forced vital capacity; WBC, white blood cells. (Reproduced with permission Fink JN, Zacharisen MC: Hypersensitivity pneumonitis. In Adkinson NF, Yunginger JW, Busse WW, et al. (eds.): Middleton's Allergy Principles and Practices 6th ed. Philadelphia, Mosby, 2003, pp 1373–1390.)

# PATHOLOGIC PICTURE

The findings of HP on performance of a lung biopsy vary, depending on the stage of the disease.[6] Initially, there is patchy interstitial and peribronchial inflammation with a predominance of lymphocytes and plasma cells (Figs. 7-7 and 7-8). Frequently, macrophages with foamy cytoplasm and giant cells are seen (Fig. 7-9). In the subacute stage, noncaseating granulomas, which progress in the chronic stage to interstitial fibrosis, appear (Fig. 7-10).

## *PATHOGENESIS*

Serum-precipitating antibody directed against the offending antigen was previously considered an immunologic hallmark of HP

(Fig. 7-11). It was believed for some time that the type III immune response marked by the presence of immune complexes played a major role in the pathogenesis of HP. A good deal of evidence, as presented in (Box 7-2), disputes this. Precipitating antibody is generally seen in HP but is certainly not pathognomonic of the disease, because as many as 50% of exposed but asymptomatic individuals have titers as high as those in symptomatic individuals. Experimental models of HP have been created in the guinea pig, rabbit, mouse, and monkey. After immunization, which results in production of serum-precipitating antibody alone, transfer of serum to unaffected animals followed by an appropriate inhalation challenge does not result in disease production. When HP patients are challenged with antigen inhalation, serum complement does not decrease, and, finally, vasculitis is not ordinarily seen on lung biopsy of HP.

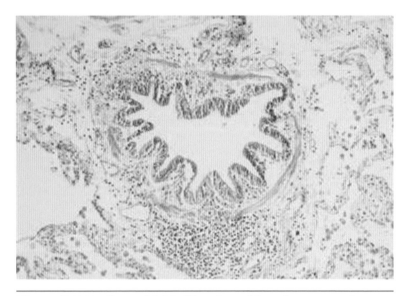

**Figure 7-7.** Peribronchial infiltration of lymphocytes and plasma cells. (Courtesy of Dr. Carlos Bedrossian, St. Louis University School of Medicine, St. Louis.)

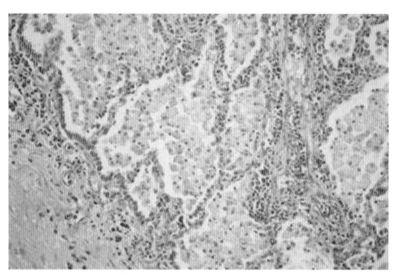

**Figure 7-9.** Lymphocytic and plasma cell infiltration of alveolar walls. The alveoli are filled with foamy macrophages. (Courtesy of Dr. Carlos Bedrossian, St. Louis University School of Medicine, St. Louis.)

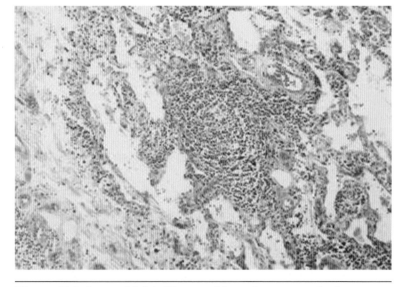

**Figure 7-8.** Interstitial infiltrate of lymphocytes and plasma cells around distal air spaces. (Courtesy of Dr. Carlos Bedrossian, St. Louis University School of Medicine, St. Louis.)

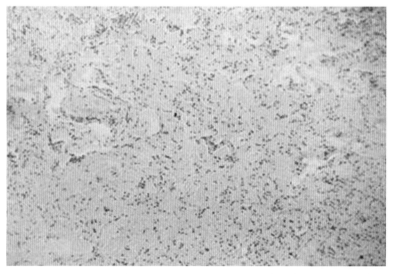

**Figure 7-10.** End stage of hypersensitivity pneumonitis, showing dense fibrosis.

It now appears that cellular immune responses constitute the primary mechanism for lung injury seen in HP. Box 7-3 summarizes the evidence for the vital contribution of type IV immune response. In a rabbit model of HP, acute disease is better correlated with immunization procedures favoring cell-mediated hypersensitivity than with the presence of serum-precipitating antibody. Pigeon breeders with symptomatic disease demonstrate in vitro proliferation of lymphocytes and production of macrophage-migration inhibition factor in response to pigeon antigen, in contrast to asymptomatic breeders with precipitins, who show no

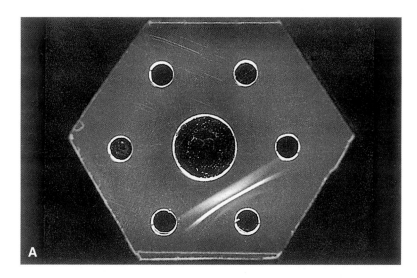

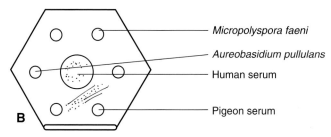

Micropolyspora faeni

Aureobasidium pullulans

Human serum

Pigeon serum

**Figure 7-11.** Double-gel diffusion plate showing positive precipitin bands between patient serum (center well) and pigeon serum. Two other hypersensitivity pneumonitis antigens are negative.

such reactivity. As previously noted, the lung biopsies of patients with HP show large numbers of lymphocytes and noncaseating granulomas, both of which are compatible with a cell-mediated immune response. Finally, bronchoalveolar lavage fluid from patients with chronic HP contains large numbers of lymphocytes, the majority of which are T-lymphocytes.[7] Further analysis reveals that the predominant T-cell subset is the CD8-positive or T-suppressor cell. Lavage fluid also contains significantly increased levels of total protein, IgG, and IgM. C4 and C6 complement levels in lavage fluid are similar to those in controls, indicating that there is no direct evidence of local, complement-mediated reactions.

One recent study has shown a marked increase, on the order of 1000-fold, in numbers of mast cells in lavage fluid of HP. The investigators suggest that mast cell degranulation is important in regulating the number of immune and inflammatory cells in the lung and that a late-phase reaction initiated by antigen-induced mast cell degranulation may be important in the pathogenesis of HP.

Figure 7-12 depicts the suggested pathogenesis of HP. It combines a nonimmunologic pathway (macrophage activation resulting in a release of enzymes, oxygen metabolites, fibronectin, and fibroblast growth factor) with an immunologic pathway (interleukins resulting in T-cell proliferation and lymphokine release).

## DIAGNOSIS

The diagnostic criteria of HP is summarized in Box 7-4. The diagnostic index of suspicion should be kept high and the disease strongly suspected in any case of recurrent pneumonia, interstitial pneumonitis, or pulmonary fibrosis. A careful history should elicit the signs and symptoms of the disease in association with exposure and remission on avoidance. A chest radiograph taken at the acute stage shows diffuse, finely granular infiltrates confined to the lower lung field. (See "Radiographic Findings.") A restrictive pattern is seen on pulmonary function testing, as are serum precipitins against the offending antigen. The history, chest radiograph, pulmonary function testing, and serum precipitin should

---

**BOX 7-2**

**Evidence Against Type III as the Most Important Immune Response in Hypersensitivity Pneumonitis**

1. Precipitating antibody is present in 50% of exposed but asymptomatic individuals

2. Serum alone cannot transfer disease from affected to unaffected experimental animals

3. Serum complement does not decrease when hypersensitivity pneumonitis patients are given inhalation challenge with antigen

4. Vasculitis is not seen on lung biopsy

---

**BOX 7-3**

**Evidence for Type IV as the Most Important Immune Response in Hypersensitivity Pneumonitis**

1. In experimental animals, development of hypersensitivity pneumonitis has better correlation with cell-mediated immunity

2. In vitro lymphocyte proliferation to antigen

3. In vitro production of macrophage-migration inhibitor factor

4. Large numbers of lymphocytes and noncaseating granulomas seen on lung biopsy

5. Bronchoalveolar lavage fluid shows large numbers of lymphocytes, with activated T-suppressor cells being predominant

offer presumptive evidence of HP. Only in unusual circumstances does one have to resort to bronchial challenge, bronchoalveolar lavage, or lung biopsy.[8]

In 1989 the subcommittee on HP of the American Academy of Allergy, Asthma and Immunology proposed guidelines for the clinical evaluation of HP.[9] In 1992, Schuyler and Cormier advanced these guidelines and proposed HP diagnosis confirmed if four of the major criteria and at least two of the minor criteria are fulfilled.[10] These guidelines also entail the ruling out of all other clinical conditions that have similar clinical signs and symptoms.

## DIFFERENTIAL DIAGNOSIS

A number of pulmonary illnesses must be ruled out when considering the diagnosis of HP (Box 7-5). A disease that is often confused in the clinician's mind with HP is allergic bronchopulmonary aspergillosis. Box 7-5 summarizes the rather clear distinction between these two entities. Sarcoidosis is an interstitial lung disease that also may be confused with HP. One distinguishing characteristic is seen on bronchoalveolar lavage. The lavage fluid of HP patients shows a preponderance of CD8-positive

**Figure 7-12.** Suggested pathogenesis of hypersensitivity pneumonitis. (Reproduced with permission from Stankus RP, DeShazo RD: Hypersensitivity pneumonitis. In Schwartz MI, King TE Jr (eds): Interstitial Lung Disease. Toronto, B.C. Decker, 1988, pp 111–121.)

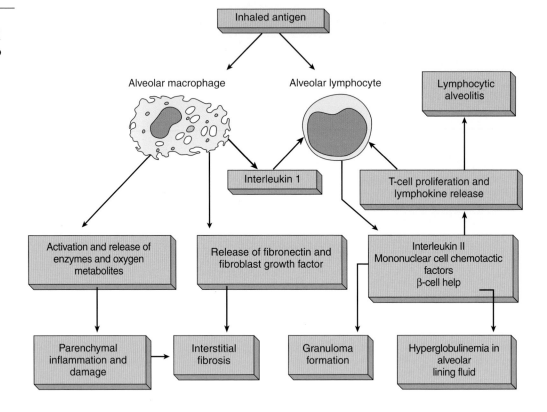

---

**BOX 7-4**
**Diagnostic Criteria for Hypersensitivity Pneumonitis**

**Major Criteria**

1. History of symptoms compatible with hypersensitivity pneumonitis that appear or worsen within hours after antigen exposure

2. Confirmation of exposure to the offending agent by history, investigation of the environment, serum precipitin test, and/or bronchoalveolar lavage fluid antibody

3. Compatible changes on chest radiography or high-resolution computed tomography of the chest

4. Bronchoalveolar lavage fluid lymphocytosis, if bronchoalveolar lavage performed

5. Compatible histologic changes, if lung biopsy performed

6. Positive "natural challenge" (reproduction of symptoms and laboratory abnormalities after exposure to the suspected environment) or by controlled inhalation challenge

**Minor Criteria**

1. Basilar crackles

2. Decreased diffusion capacity

3. Arterial hypoxemia, either at rest or with exercise

Adapted from Patel AM, Ryu JH, Reed CE: Hypersensitivity pneumonitis: Current concepts and future questions. J Allergy Clin Immunol 2001;108:661–670.

suppressor lymphocytes, whereas a predominance of CD4-positive T-lymphocytes is usually seen in bronchoalveolar lavage of sarcoidosis patients.

# PREVENTION AND TREATMENT

Clearly, the most important aspect in the management of HP is recognition and avoidance of the causative antigen. Once the disease is suspected, a careful environmental survey of the patient's occupational, home, and vocational life must be carried out to search for the presence of offending antigens.[11] When the disease is diagnosed and the antigens recognized, the definitive therapy is early avoidance. HP may cause an untimely death due to progressive respiratory insufficiency. A general approach to the prevention of HP is given in Box 7-6. A number of interventions decrease the formation of antigens in conducive environments. For example, the growth of thermophilic actinomycete spores in compost can be suppressed by treatment with a 1% solution of propionic acid. Water that remains for long periods of time in older air-conditioning or humidification units may become a fertile source for the growth of thermophilic organisms. Therefore, the water needs to be changed and the unit cleaned on a regular basis. Contaminated ventilation systems have to be thoroughly cleaned and replaced. Blowing cool air through stored hay helps to prevent the growth of mold. Harvesting crops when the moisture content is low also results in less exposure to organic dusts.

In occupational situations where organic dust generation is inevitable, every effort should be made to reduce the worker's exposure. In enclosed spaces, extremely dusty materials should be handled mechanically. Materials such as sugar cane should be stored outside, and cattle should be fed outside as much as possible so that the associated organic dusts can be diluted by the ambient air.

In terms of removal of dusts from the air, improved ventilation may aid considerably. Electrostatic air purifiers may be of help in instances where the concentration of dust is not too great. The use of personal dust respirators or masks is limited because of their inconvenience. A type IIB filter is quite effective in filtering small particles but causes so much resistance to the flow of air that people hard at work are unable to wear it. An airstream helmet in which an electrical pump blows air through a filter and into the breathing zone is heavy and uncomfortable to wear. Even the best device only has a maximum filtering capacity of 99% for fine particles. The remaining 1% can produce new attacks in highly sensitive individuals. When the disease is not yet manifest, even a filter with 95% filtering capacity is adequate. Good results have been reported with a 3M disposable mask, model 8719 (Fig. 7-13).

When these environmental control measures cannot be carried out or are inadequate, the patient should be removed from that work area. This may entail a change in the workplace or type of work or, in extreme cases, a change in occupation. It is not known what length or level of exposure is required to produce irreversible pulmonary changes. If the diffusing capacity has not returned to normal within 3 months, the individual should be advised to leave that particular workplace.

The treatment of HP is summarized in Box 7-7. In many cases, no treatment is necessary other than avoidance of the causative antigen. However, corticosteroid therapy can greatly accelerate the

---

**BOX 7-5**
**Differential Diagnosis of Hypersensitivity Pneumonitis**

**Acute Stage**
Acute tracheobronchitis, bronchiolitis, or pneumonia
Acute endotoxin exposure
Organic dust toxic syndrome
Allergic bronchopulmonary aspergillosis
Reactive airways dysfunction syndrome (RADS)
Pulmonary embolism/infarction
Aspiration pneumonitis
Bronchiolitis obliterans organizing pneumonia
Diffuse alveolar damage

**Subacute Stage**
Recurrent pneumonia
Allergic bronchopulmonary aspergillosis
Granulomatous lung disease
Infection (mycobacteria, fungi)
Berylliosis
Silicosis
Talcosis
Langerhans' cell histiocytosis
Churg–Strauss syndrome
Wegener's granulomatosis
Sarcoidosis

**Chronic Stage**
Idiopathic pulmonary fibrosis
Chronic obstructive pulmonary disease with pulmonary fibrosis
Bronchiectasis/bronchiolectasis
*Mycobacterium avium* complex pulmonary disease

Adapted from Patel AM, Ryu JH, Reed CE: Hypersensitivity pneumonitis: Current concepts and future questions. J Allergy Clin Immunol 2001;108:661–670.

---

**BOX 7-6**
**Prevention of Hypersensitivity Pneumonitis**

1. **Decrease formation of microbial antigens**
   Add chemicals to prevent growth of microbes
   Change water frequently in humidification or air-conditioning units
   Use storage dryers on hay and straw
   Harvest crops when moisture content is low

2. **Decrease exposure to organic dusts and chemicals**
   Mechanically handle dusty materials within closed spaces
   Remove dusts from ambient air
   Wear personal respirators or masks

3. **Remove worker from disease-producing environment**

Reproduced with permission from Terho EO; Extrinsic allergic alveolitis: Management of established cases. Eur J Respir Dis 1982;123:101.

clinical improvement and should be considered for very ill patients with gross radiographic or physiologic abnormalities, such as hypoxemia.[12] Oral prednisone in an initial daily dose of 40 to 60 mg is usually adequate and should be continued until there is significant improvement in clinical, radiographic, and pulmonary function tests. Prednisone may then be slowly tapered until the resolution of clinical and radiologic signs is complete. The total duration of therapy is generally no more than 4 to 6 weeks, providing exposure to the antigen is prevented. It must be emphasized and reemphasized to the patient that corticosteroids are not a substitute for antigen identification and avoidance.

In cases of severe hypoxemia in the acute stage, oxygen should be administered in amounts sufficient to keep the partial pressure of oxygen between 60 and 100 mm Hg. Other supportive measures include antitussives and antipyretics. On occasion, despite the physician's best efforts, the patient may elect to return to the same workplace or occupation. In these instances, long-term continuous administration of corticosteroids may be called for. One should strive for an alternate-day program utilizing the lowest dose that still controls the patient's symptoms. The chronic form of HP develops insidiously and occurs either after repeated acute episodes or as a result of long-term, low-grade exposure. A therapeutic trial of steroids can be given but should be continued only if the radiographic findings and the physiologic testing indicate a beneficial response.

## PROGNOSIS

The overall prognosis of HP is very good provided that diagnosis is made at an early stage of the disease and exposure to an offending agent is extinguished in a timely way.[13] Clinical improvement is then usually seen within 1 to 6 months. In acute HP, the restrictive defect in pulmonary function and decreased diffusion lung capacity to carbon monoxide reverse to normal levels in several weeks. In subacute HP, granuloma and bronchiolitis tend to resolve slower, even with steroid treatment. The long-term prognosis for the farmer's lung form of HP is poor; however, physiologic consequences of farmer's lung seem to progress even after removal of offending factors.[14] In Cormier and Belanger's study, 24 of 61 farmers with acute HP who did not farm for 3 to 5 years still demonstrated continuous decline in diffusion lung capacity to carbon monoxide and total lung capacity.[15] Several investigators found an increased risk of emphysema in the farmer's lung form of HP as well.[7] The chronic stage of HP—fibrosis—is a slowly progressive and irreversible form of the disease that leads to potentially fatal complications, including chronic respiratory insufficiency and cor pulmonale. Prognosis in children with HP who are diagnosed early and treated properly is excellent.[16] In one study of 67 cases of pediatric HP with reported outcomes, 65 children improved and became completely asymptomatic, 1 developed progressive disease, and 1 died after several years of exposure to budgerigars and other birds, despite combination therapy with corticosteroids and D-penicillamine.[17]

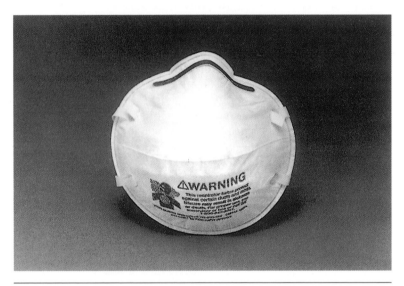

**Figure 7-13.** A 3M disposable mask, model 8710, found to be useful in prevention of hypersensitivity pneumonitis. (Courtesy of 3M Center, St. Paul, MN.)

**BOX 7-7**
**Treatment of Hypersensitivity Pneumonitis**

**Acute form**
Remove patient from exposure—may entail hospitalization
Administer oxygen if hypoxic or dyspneic
Prescribe oral prednisone 40–60 mg/day with slow taper
Use supportive measures—rest, antitussives, antipyretics

**Repeated acute or subacute form**
Decrease exposure as much as possible
Administer long-term corticosteroids emphasizing alternate-day therapy

**Chronic form**
Trial with corticosteroids but continue only if radiographic findings and physiologic testing indicate a response

## REFERENCES

1. Lopez M, Salvaggio JE: Epidemiology of hypersensitivity pneumonitis/allergic alveolitis. Monogr Allergy 1987;21:70–86.
2. Fink JN, Zacharisen MC: Hypersensitivity pneumonitis. In Adkinson NF, Yuninger JW, Busse WW, et al., (eds): Middleton's Allergy Principles and Practice 6th ed., Philadelphia, Mosby 2003;1373–1390.
3. Greech V, Vella C, Lenicker H: Pigeon breeder's lung in childhood, varied clinical picture at presentation. Pediatr Pulmonol 2000;30:145–148.
4. Lynch DA, Newell JD, Logan PM, et al: Can CT distinguish hypersensitivity pneumonitis from idiopathic pulmonary fibrosis. Am J Roentgenol 1995;165:807–813.
5. O'Grady NP, Preas HL, Pugin J, et al: Local inflammatory responses following bronchial endotoxin instillation in humans. Am J Respir Crit Care Med 2001;163:1591–1598.
6. Kawanami O, Basset F, Barrios R, et al: Hypersensitivity pneumonitis in man. Light- and electron-microscopic studies of 18 lung biopsies. Am J Pathol 1983;110:275–289.
7. Yamasaki H, Ando M, Brazer W, et al: Polarized type 1 cytokine profile in bronchoalveolar lavage T cells of patients with hypersensitivity pneumonitis. J Immunol 1999;163:3516–3523.
8. Krasnick J, Meuwissen HJ, Nakao MA, et al: Hypersensitivity pneumonitis: problems in diagnosis. J Allergy Clin Immunol 1996;97:1027–1030.
9. Richerson HB, Bernstein IL, Fink JN, et al: Guidelines for the clinical

evaluation of hypersensitivity pneumonitis. Report of the Subcommittee on Hypersensitivity Pneumonitis. J Allergy Clin Immunol 1989;84:839–844.

10. Schuyler M, Cormier Y: The diagnosis of hypersensitivity pneumonitis. Chest 1997;111:534–536.

11. Weltermann BM, Hodgson M, Storey E, et al: Hypersensitivity pneumonitis: a sentinel event investigation in a wet building. Am J Ind Med 1998;34:499–505.

12. Kokkarinen JI, Tukiainen HO, Terho EO: Effect of corticosteroid treatment on the recovery of pulmonary function in farmer's lung. Am Rev Respir Dis 1992;145:3–5.

13. Patel AM, Ryu JH, Reed CE: Hypersensitivity pneumonitis: Current concepts and future questions. J Allergy Clin Immunol 2001;108:661–670.

14. Braun SR, doPico GA, Tsiatis A, et al: Farmer's lung disease: Long-term clinical and physiologic outcome. Am Rev Respir Dis 1979;119:185–191.

15. Cormier Y, Belanger J: Long-term physiologic outcome after acute farmer's lung. Chest 1985;87:796–800.

16. Fan L: Hypersensitivity pneumonitis in children. Curr Opin Pediatr 2002; 14:323–326.

17. Vergesslich KA, Gotz M, Kraft D: Bird breeder's lung with conversion to fatal fibrosing alveolitis [German]. Dtsch Med Wochenschr 1983;108:1238–1242.

*Paul A. Greenberger*

# *8* Allergic Bronchopulmonary Aspergillosis

Allergic brochopulmonary aspergillosis (ABPA) typically occurs in patients with asthma or cystic fibrosis and results in pulmonary infiltrates seen on chest roentgenograms or chest tomography.[1] The infiltrates often affect the upper lobes or middle lobe and can cause relatively few symptoms compared with the same appearance from a bacterial pneumonia, which would cause chills, rigors, temperature elevation, productive cough, and even chest pain. In ABPA, the infiltrates may result in a mild cough or a cough productive of tenacious sputum plugs, with modest amounts of dyspnea. ABPA infiltrates may be asymptomatic or result in marked dyspnea if extensive bronchiectasis is already present. ABPA may be identified in some patients with allergic fungal sinusitis, but most ABPA patients do not have this form of sinusitis. ABPA has been detected in some patients with the hyper–immunoglobulin (Ig) E syndrome and chronic granulomatous disease.

Some examples of diseases caused by *Aspergillus* species are presented in Box 8-1. Patients with ABPA have asthma and are very reactive to inhalation of spores of *Aspergillus*. Indeed, dual (early and late) bronchial reactions have occurred, as seen in Figure 8-1, which demonstrates 50% and 75% declines in the forced expiratory volume in 1 second ($FEV_1$) during the early (20 minute) and late (8 hour) responses. Some patients also reported myalgias and malaise with temperature elevations. Peripheral blood eosinophilia was present within 15 minutes and during the late response. These intense responses may occur in patients with ABPA who are exposed to high concentrations of *Aspergillus*, such as in moldy mulches or wood chips, compost piles, and indoors if roof leaks causing water damage to walls have occurred.

## DEFENSES AGAINST *ASPERGILLUS*

In ABPA, the spores of *Aspergillus fumigatus* are inhaled and then grow saprophytically in the bronchial mucus. Other *Aspergillus* species or fungi may cause bronchopulmonary syndromes as well. Some of the host defenses against invasive aspergillosis include: (1) killing by polymorphonuclear neutrophils and alveolar macrophages; (2) an intact, seemingly nondamaged, pulmonary epithelium as a barrier; (3) the alternative pathway of complement, and perhaps (4) platelets. In patients who have received chemotherapy, the pulmonary epithelia cells may have become damaged, which could support entry of *Aspergillus* into the interstitium and vasculature of the lung. Fortunately, patients with ABPA are not neutropenic, so invasive aspergillosis is not seen. In allergic *Aspergillus* sinusitis, there may be mucoid impactions of the sinuses

---

**BOX 8-1**
**Conditions in Humans Caused by *Aspergillus* Species**

Allergic asthma
Allergic rhinitis
Allergic fungal sinusitis
Allergic bronchopulmonary aspergillosis
Hypersensitivity pneumonitis (malt workers' lung)
Chronic necrotizing pneumonia
Invasive aspergillosis
Pulmonary mycetoma (aspergilloma)
Ulcerative tracheitis

---

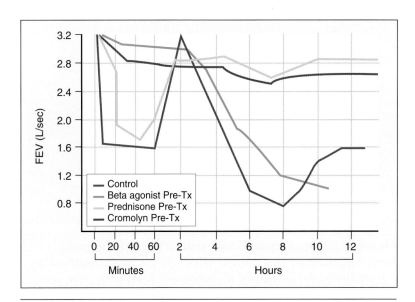

**Figure 8-1.** The dual-phase respiratory response after *Aspergillus* bronchial challenge. FEV, forced expiratory volume; Tx, treatment.

with thinning of bones or outright septal deviation if adequate surgical intervention has not been instituted.[2]

# PATHOGENESIS

Spores of *A. fumigatus* are inhaled and able to grow in bronchial mucus (Fig. 8-2). The growth is saprophytic as hyphae (2 to 3.5 μm) and seemingly converts the mucus into a tenacious substance. Specific survival or virulence factors are not yet known. Nevertheless, in experiments with some of the 22 recombinant *A. fumigatus* allergens, some insights have been observed, such as the enzymatic activity of these allergens. *Asp f 1* contains a ribonuclease that is cytotoxic, as it inhibits protein synthesis. *Asp f 2* damages epithelial cells, and *Asp f 5* is a metalloprotease. *Asp f 6* functions as a manganese superoxide dismutase, and *Asp f 13* and *Asp f 18* are serine proteases. Some of these allergens can serve as ribotoxins, which disrupt protein synthesis, and it has been shown that some *A. fumigatus* strains can be induced to produce a collagenase. *A. fumigatus* can stimulate B and T cells to produce isotypic antibodies IgE, IgG, and IgA, as well as total IgE. *A. fumigatus*, when incubated with eosinophils and its growth factors interleukin-3, interleukin-5, and granulocyte-macrophage colony-stimulating factor supports additional survival of eosinophils. T-cell clones generated from ABPA patients are of the Th2 phenotype and in some patients are major histocompatibility complex class II restricted.[6] The role of these individual actions in producing bronchial wall widening and pulmonary cavities or fibrosis is not clear but is certainly suggestive. One could speculate that host genetics—immunologic responses being initially inadequate and then hyperresponsive—perhaps impaired defenses against *A. fumigatus* hyphae, and *A. fumigatus* virulence factors all participate in allowing exposures to this ubiquitous fungus to produce ABPA in 1% to 2% of patients with persistent asthma and in 1% to 13% of patients with cystic fibrosis.[7]

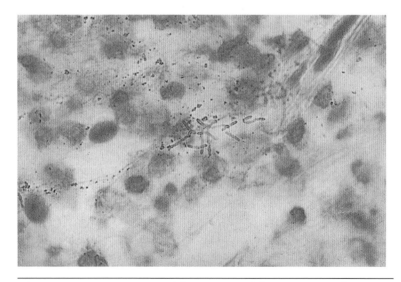

**Figure 8-2.** Immunoperoxidase stain with anti–*Aspergillus fumigatus* antibody in a patient with allergic brochopulmonary aspergillosis. Fragments of dichotomous septate hyphae are seen in the lung parenchyma. (Reproduced with permission from Slavin RG, Bedrossian CW, Hutcheson PS, et al: A pathologic study of allergic bronchopulmonary aspergillosis. J Allergy Clin Immunol 1988;81:718–725.)

*Aspergillus fumigatus* hyphae are present in the sputum plugs but are not present after treatment with oral corticosteroids or remission of ABPA. They then return when there is an exacerbation of ABPA (doubling of the total serum IgE concentration and new radiologic infiltrates, as in Figures 8-4 and 8-5). The hyphae shed enzymes, proteins, and allergens and induce the intense immunologic responses locally in the bronchi. Mast cell activation occurs along with the activation of T- and B-lymphocytes, eosinophils, and macrophages. *A. fumigatus* antigens range from 10 to 100 kD in weight, and some 40 components have been recognized to bind with IgE antibodies.

# CLINICAL CRITERIA FOR ALLERGIC BRONCHOPULMONARY ASPERGILLOSIS

## *DIAGNOSTIC CRITERIA*

The diagnostic criteria for both asthma and cystic fibrosis are presented in Box 8-2 and Box 8-3.[1] Nearly every patient with ABPA has a history of asthma; however, occasionally, there seem to be no recognized symptoms and the patient presents with an abnormal chest roentgenogram and has lobar collapse. The

---

**BOX 8-2**
**Diagnostic Criteria for Allergic Bronchopulmonary Aspergillosis**

**In Patients with Asthma**

***Minimal Essential Criteria***
Asthma
Central bronchiectasis (inner 2/3 of chest CT field)
Total serum IgE concentration >417 KU/L (1000 ng/mL)
Immediate skin reactivity to *A. fumigatus* or Aspergillus species
Elevated serum IgE–*A. fumigatus* antibody and/or IgG–*A. fumigatus* antibody*

***Other Criteria (Not Essential for Diagnosis)***
Chest or CT infiltrates
Serum precipitating antibodies to *A. fumigatus*

**In Patients with Asthma Without Bronchiectasis (ABPA-Seropositive)**
Asthma
Total serum IgE concentration >417 KU/L (1000 ng/mL)
Immediate skin reactivity to *A. fumigatus* or *Aspergillus* species
Elevated serum IgE–*A. fumigatus* antibody and/or IgG–*A. fumigatus* antibody*

---

*Sera are compared with sera from patients with asthma and immediate skin reactivity to *Aspergillus* but without sufficient criteria for ABPA.
ABPA, allergic bronchopulmonary aspergillosis; CT, computed tomography; Ig, immunoglobulin.

recognition of peripheral blood eosinophilia leads to the diagnosis of ABPA with the possibility of the patient not having either intermittent or persistent asthma. While this condition may occur, it is the exception to the rule! Some patients only admit to mild exercise-induced asthma prior to the onset of pulmonary infiltrates and therefore would have been categorized as having intermittent asthma had it been recognized. Conversely, asthma may range from mild to severe, including prednisone-dependent asthma.

## SYMPTOMS AND SIGNS

Allergic brochopulmonary aspergillosis should be suspected in highly atopic patients, and those with allergic rhinitis, allergic asthma, food or medication allergies, or asthma that has worsened for unexplained reasons. Conversely, in some patients with asthma, the presence of a cough will lead the physician to order a chest roentgenogram, which reveals a mass that is suspected of being a lymphoma, thus leading to the diagnosis of ABPA. In some patients, it is not clear that excessive exposures to fungi have occurred.

The physical examination ranges from a normal chest examination to detecting crackles localized to the areas of pulmonary infiltrates. In patients with bronchiectasis, there will be crackles that do not clear after coughing, and the crackles may be present in the apices of the lung. This location may mimic pulmonary tuberculosis. Clubbing of digits and cyanosis may be present if there is extensive bronchiectasis with or without cystic fibrosis. Patients with ABPA may have acute or chronic (more than 12 weeks of symptoms) sinusitis and should be examined for nasal polyps or enlarged nasal turbinates. Rarely, a patient with ABPA presents when in status asthmaticus; in that case, there are widespread rhonchi on auscultation but no clear evidence of egophony or crackles. The admitting chest roentgenogram demonstrates one or more infiltrates that raise the possibility of ABPA.

## SKIN TESTING

All patients have immediate skin reactivity to *Aspergillus* species (mixes) or to *Aspergillus fumigatus*. An example of a positive re-

action to *A. fumigatus* on prick (percutaneous) testing is presented in Figure 8-3. It remains critical to use reactive extracts. If the prick test is nonreactive, an intradermal injection is used. Some extracts of mixes of *Aspergillus* species for intradermal injection do not contain *A. fumigatus*; thus, it is important to use an extract containing *A. fumigatus*. About 25 percent of patients with asthma will have positive immediate reactions to skin tests with *A. fumigatus*. Properly performed skin testing with prick and intradermal injections, if negative, essentially excludes ABPA. However, if there are pulmonary infiltrates on chest roentgenogram with peripheral blood eosinophilia and a bronchopulmonary syndrome is suspected, another species of *Aspergillus* or another fungus genus, such as *Curvularia* or *Pseudoallescheria*, could be the etiology of the ABPA.

## LABORATORY TESTING

The total serum IgE concentration is elevated in ABPA, especially when there are new pulmonary infiltrates. The total serum IgE concentration should be more than 417 KU/L (1000 ng/mL) and often is much higher. Some patients have nonexacerbation total IgE concentrations of 2000 to 7000 KU/L with doubling or tripling at the time of radiologic infiltrates. Conversely, in patients with ABPA who have prednisone-dependent persistent asthma and no current infiltrates, the total IgE may be less than 417 KU/L. Nearly all of the total IgE is not reactive with epitopes of *A. fumigatus*. This has led to the notion that *A. fumigatus* produces "nonspecific" IgE antibodies. Conversely, the sera of patients with ABPA contain large quantities of anti–*A. fumigatus* IgG and IgA antibodies as well

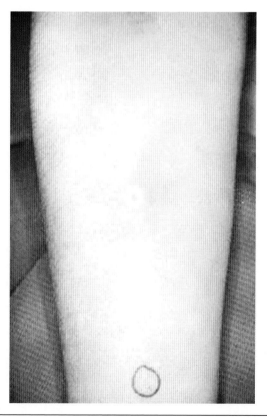

**Figure 8-3.** A positive prick test with *Aspergillus fumigatus* in a patient with allergic brochpulmonary aspergillosis. The wheal and erythema reaction at 15 minutes after performing the skin test.

---

BOX 8-3
**Diagnostic Criteria for Allergic Bronchopulmonary Aspergillosis in Patients with Cystic Fibrosis**

Clinical deterioration consisting of increased cough, exercise intolerance, reductions in pulmonary function parameters, increased sputum production
Total serum IgE concentration >417 KU/L or (1000 ng/ml)
Immediate skin reactivity to *A. fumigatus* or serum IgE–*A. fumigatus* antibody
Abnormal chest roentgengram (change from previous films, infiltrates, or mucous plugging)

Ig, immunoglobulin.

as IgE antibodies, compared with sera from patients with asthma who do not have ABPA. Sera from patients with ABPA and allergic asthma both have far greater quantities of anti–*A. fumigatus* IgE than does sera from nonatopic controls.

Serum IgG antibodies to *A. fumigatus* precipitate in gel diffusion in as many as 97% of ABPA patients. Sera should be concentrated up to fivefold, and reactive *A. fumigatus* extracts are necessary. Precipitating antibodies have been questioned as to their diagnostic utility, as essentially 100% of patients with aspergilloma, 9% of hospitalized patients, and 10% of outpatients with asthma can have precipitating antibodies to *A. fumigatus*. An example of a precipitin-in-gel reaction to *A. fumigatus* is presented in Figure 8-4. The precipitin-in-gel reaction is representative of large quantities of anti–*A. fumigatus* IgG antibodies. The anti–*A. fumigatus* IgG antibodies detected by enzyme-linked immunosorbent assay (ELISA) discussed earlier help differentiate ABPA serum from asthma serum and are different in the sense that the serum is diluted 1:1000 and 1:5000. A patient's serum may have very high amounts of these anti–*A. fumigatus* IgG antibodies by ELISA compared with sera from patients with asthma and nonatopics but have no precipitating antibodies in gel. Because of differences in these determinations (one concentrated sera, one very dilute sera), it is possible to have a patient with ABPA who has no precipitating antibodies but has very high anti–*A. fumigatus* IgG by ELISA.

Peripheral blood eosinophilia (more than 1000/μL) can be expected at the time of radiologic infiltrates, especially if the patient has not been treated with oral corticosteroids. For example, most patients have an eosinophil level between 1000 and 3000/μL, whereas a small number have eosinophil counts of more than

3000/μL. Sputum eosinophilia can be expected in all the patients who produce sputum. The total white blood cell count may be normal or elevated, with most patients at less than 15,000/μL. If obtained, the erythrocyte sedimentation rate is more than 20 mm/hr.

## PULMONARY FUNCTION TESTS

When there are pulmonary infiltrates, the lung function tests can appear to be restrictive in nature, with reductions in forced vital capacity, $FEV_1$, total lung capacity, diffusing capacity, and functional residual capacity. The diffusing capacity should be normal or even elevated in most patients who have asthma without ABPA. However, with pulmonary fibrosis and bronchiectasis in ABPA, the diffusing capacity will be reduced. After treatment and resolution of the infiltrates, the pulmonary function tests may manifest some degree of obstruction as occurs with asthma. If there is end-stage, fibrocavitary ABPA, then there may be severe airway obstruction, with reductions in $FEV_1$ less than 0.8 L and forced vital capacity (FVC) with $FEV_1/FVC$ less than 50%. There may be more than 12% improvement with albuterol in these patients, but there is very little additional improvement in spirometric values or respiratory status.

As shown in Figure 8-1, when bronchoprovocation challenges were performed with an extract of *A. fumigatus*, severe reductions in $FEV_1$ occurred during the early and late responses, even resulting in status asthmaticus in some patients. Thus, it is not appropriate to perform these tests, as they may cause severe obstructive responses. Cromolyn is known to inhibit some of the early and late responses as it does with other allergens. Albuterol can inhibit the early response, and inhaled corticosteroids can inhibit the late response. Oral or inhaled corticosteroids, if administered for a week or more during other allergen challenges in patients with asthma but not ABPA, also can inhibit some of the early responses. Such data do not exist for ABPA.

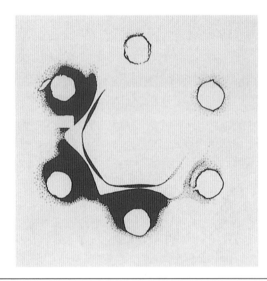

**Figure 8-4.** *Aspergillus fumigatus* 10 mg/mL is placed in the center well. Normal serum is in the top well. Sera from a patient with allergic brochopulmonary aspergillosis are placed in the other wells with dates indicating when the sera were drawn. With time and clinical improvement, the precipitin band diminishes. The large, indistinct precipitin band appearing close to and curving around the well in which the test serum is placed represents a reaction between serum C-reactive protein and a somatic polysaccharide substance in certain *Aspergillus* extracts. It is of no immunologic significance. (Reproduced with permission from Slavin RG, Laird TS, Cherry JD: Allergic bronchopulmonary aspergillosis in a child. J Pediatr 1970;76:416.)

## RADIOGRAPHIC FINDINGS

Chest roentgenography and high-resolution chest tomography (HRCT) are useful modalities in ABPA. HRCT utilizes thin (1–2-mm) sections rather than conventional 10-mm sections.[3] Slices may be obtained every 10 mm. Proximal or central bronchiectasis refers to dilated bronchi compared with the adjacent bronchial artery in the inner two thirds of the field of view. Bronchiectasis may be cyclindrical if the bronchus does not taper and is at least 1.5 times the diameter of the comparison bronchial artery. Bronchiectasis can be cystic or varicoid as well. On the chest roentgenogram, bronchiectasis may be detected when dilated bronchi show up as ring shadows 1 to 2 cm in diameter. These bronchi are visualized in the en face perspective; when the bronchus is identified in a coronal plane, the bronchiectatic area is referred to as a parallel-line shadow.

In ABPA, the presentation chest roentgenogram may reveal large areas of homogeneous infiltrates, typically in upper lobes or the middle lobe. The infiltrates can be widespread (Figs. 8-5 and 8-6) and transient (Figs. 8-7 and 8-8). These infiltrates may resemble a lymphoma but are from mucoid impactions, which result in lobar or even whole lung collapse. Repeated infiltrates, especially if not treated with oral corticosteroids, may cause additional bronchiectasis, pulmonary fibrosis, bulla, or cavities with air fluid levels. The infiltrates can be attributable to mucous plugs causing distal obstruction or from parenchymal conditions such as eosinophilic pneumonia or bronchocentric granulomatosis.

Recent studies with HRCT have shown some dilated bronchi consistent with bronchiectasis, even in patients with persistent asthma who do not have ABPA. In one study, 29% of patients did have a few dilated, cylindrical bronchi. In comparison, in ABPA, there are multiple dilated bronchi in different lobes with cylindrical, varicose, and cystic bronchiectasis (Figs. 8-9 and 8-10). Some patients will have varicose and cystic bronchiectasis, mucous accumulation, and inflammatory scarring that will show little improvement with oral corticosteroids (Fig. 8-11). The bronchiectasis can be extensive and result in restrictive findings on pulmonary

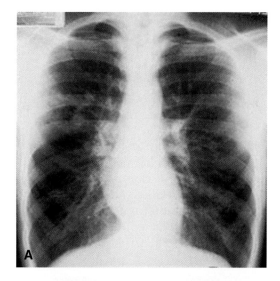

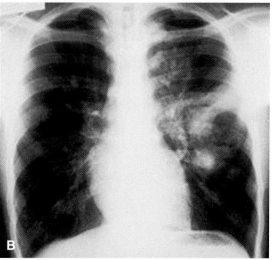

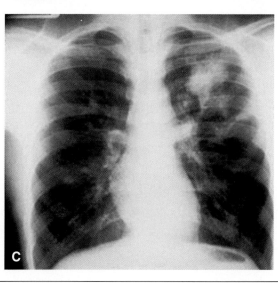

**Figure 8-7.** Chest radiographs demonstrating fleeting infiltrates in the case of allergic brochopulmonary aspergillosis. *A,* Soft nodular infiltrates in the right upper lobe suggest tuberculosis. *B,* Fourteen days later, there is some clearing on the right with a new infiltrate present in the left mid-lung field. *C,* Ten days later, the left mid-lung has cleared, but a new infiltrate is present in the upper lobe. (Reproduced with permission from Slavin RG: Allergic bronchopulmonary aspergillosis. Clin Rev Allergy 1985;3:167.).

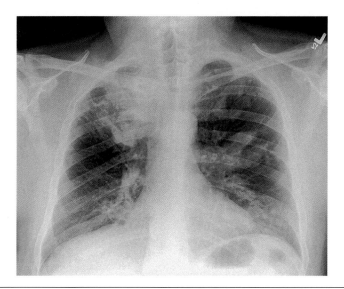

**Figure 8-5.** Posterior–anterior chest roentgenogram in a 60-year-old man with an exacerbation of allergic brochopulmonary aspergillosis. The total serum immunoglobulin E concentration increased from 7160 KU/L to 15,160 KU/L over a 2-month period. He was dyspneic and coughing up sputum plugs. There are bilateral infiltrates.

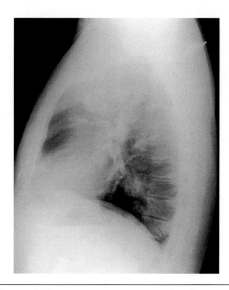

**Figure 8-6.** Lateral chest roentgenogram in the same patient as in Figure 8-5 showing upper and lower lobe infiltrates.

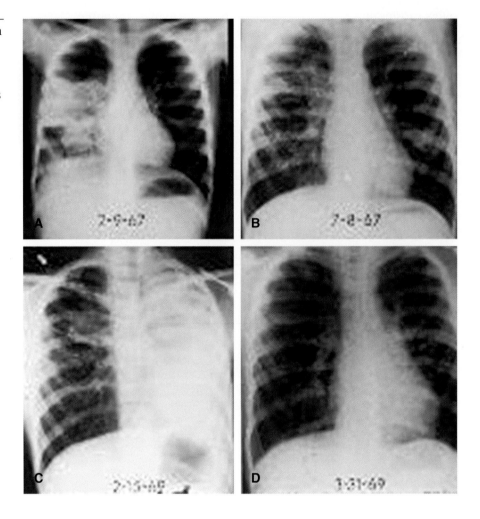

**Figure 8-8.** Chest radiographs of a 9-year-old girl with allergic brochopulmonary aspergillosis. *A,* Right middle and right lower lobe consolidations are seen. *B,* General involvement of all lobes on the right with left upper lobe and left lingular involvement 5 months later. *C,* After an interval of 1 to 1.5 years, there is a right upper lobe infiltrate with atelectasis and total collapse of the left lung with herniation across the middle. *D,* Six weeks after institution of therapy, infiltrates have cleared, but dilated bronchi are seen. (Reproduced with permission from Slavin RG, Laird TS, Cherry JD: Allergic bronchopulmonary aspergillosis in a child. J Pediatr 1970;76:416.).

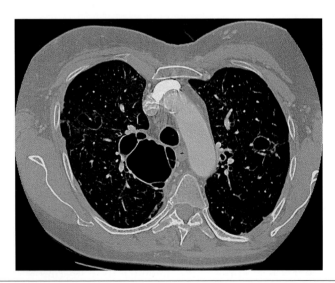

**Figure 8-9.** High-resolution computed tomograph of the lung in a 59-year-old woman with longstanding allergic brochopulmonary aspergillosis. There are large cystic areas on the upper lobe, especially on the right. This case was managed with prednisone 20 mg on alternate days, and the patient had no major respiratory symptoms, despite the abnormalities.

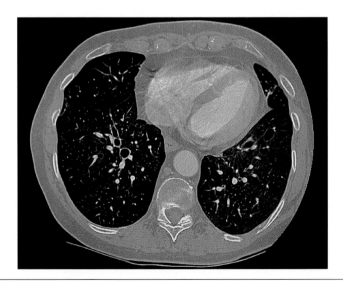

**Figure 8-10.** The same patient as in Figure 8–11, but the computed tomograph is at a lower level. There is cystic and varicose bronchiectasis of the lower lobes.

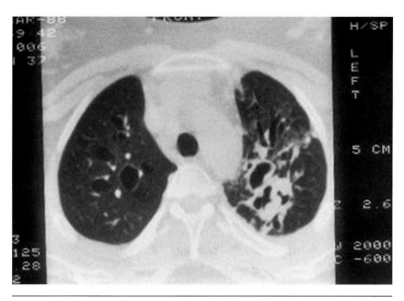

**Figure 8-11.** Computed tomographic scan of the chest in a patient with allergic brochopulmonary aspergillosis. Dilated bronchi are seen bilaterally, with a marked inflammatory response in the left posterior lung field.

function tests because of loss of lung volume. Formerly, bronchography was used to demonstrate dilated, irregular bronchi. As illustrated in Figure 8-12, there is radiographic contrast material in multiple proximal bronchi, none of which would be present in a patient without bronchiectasis.

## SPUTUM

Sputum may be expectorated as tenacious, golden brown plugs that contain eosinophils and septate hyphae of *A. fumigatus* (see Fig. 8-13).[4] In other patients, such mucus may be obtained during bronchoscopy. However, ABPA may be suspected by the physician after examining a patient with pulmonary infiltrates whose bronchi are obstructed by thick "nonextractable" mucus. A limited number of patients with ABPA will have allergic fungal sinusitis and produce thick nasal secretions that contain eosinophiles. *A. fumigatus* from sputum or sinus secretions is not diagnostic of ABPA, as *A. fumigatus* is detectable in patients with asthma or other lung conditions and with chronic sinusitis.

## LUNG BIOPSY

There is infrequent need for lung biopsies in patients with ABPA. However, when they are obtained, there is evidence of bronchiectasis with mucous plugging and a variety of histologic diagnoses. For example, there may be areas of eosinophilic pneumonia (Fig. 8-14), granulomatous bronchiolitis, bronchocentric granulomatosis, bronchiolitis obliterans, exudative bronchiolitis, lipid pneumonia, or combinations of these findings.[5] It is unclear why certain patients have these various histologic patterns.

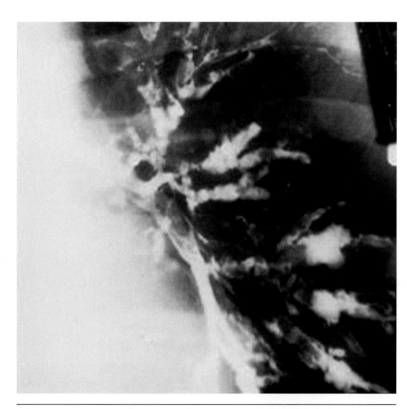

**Figure 8-12.** Bronchogram of a patient with allergic brochopulmonary aspergillosis, showing saccular proximal involvement with peripheral sparing. (Reproduced with permission from Slavin RG: Allergic bronchopulmonary aspergillosis. In Fireman P, Slavin RG (eds): Atlas of Allergies, 2nd ed. London, Mosby-Wolfe, 1996, p 134.)

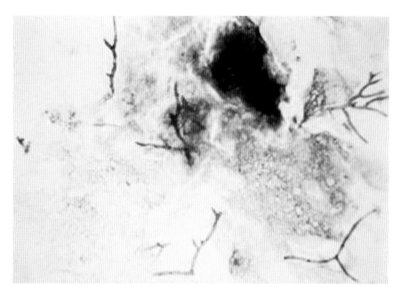

**Figure 8-13.** Sputum smear of patient with allergic brochopulmonary aspergillosis showing eosinophila with good preservation of cytoplasm. Gomorimethenamine silver-Giemsa counterstain. (Reproduced with permission from Slavin RG, Laird TS, Cherry JD: Allergic bronchopulmonary aspergillosis in a child. J Pediatr 1970;76:416.)

# DIFFERENTIAL DIAGNOSIS OF ABPA

Classic cases of ABPA have all the criteria listed in Table 8-1 or Box 8-2 and may have sputum plugs and peripheral blood eosinophilia. Some conditions that may be in the differential diagnosis are presented in Box 8-4. In patients with asthma who have pulmonary infiltrates and eosinophilia but do not have ABPA, an allergic bronchopulmonary mycosis may be present. Culture of sputum for fungi or identification of a particular fungus on immediate skin testing or by testing for precipitins may help lead to the etiology.

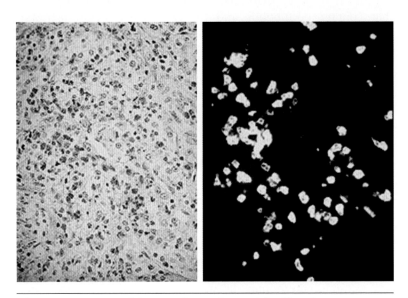

**Figure 8-14.** Lung biopsy of a patient with allergic brochopulmonary aspergillosis. Hematoxylin and eosin stain is on the *left*. On the *right*, the same section is stained with flourescein-labeled, anti–major basic protein antibody. Positive staining corresponds to eosinophils (×400). (Reproduced with permission from Slavin RG, Bedrossian CW, Hutcheson PS, et al: A pathologic study of allergic bronchopulmonary aspergillosis. J Allergy Clin Immunol 1988;81:718–725.)

# TREATMENT

After the diagnosis is made, it is helpful to determine the stage of ABPA (Table 8-1). Avoidance measures are indicated for fungi, animals, and dust mites, as for any patient with asthma. Water leaks in the house from roofs, basements, and plumbing should be remedied. The patient should be informed about the need, at least initially, for oral corticosteroids for management of the pulmonary infiltrates. An empiric approach is presented in Box 8-5 beginning with 2 weeks of daily prednisone. Then, alternate-day prednisone can be employed, which avoids the major adverse effects of corticosteroids, such as cushingoid obesity, diabetes mellitus, hypertension, and serious infections. After 2 to 3 months, the prednisone can be tapered and discontinued. In treatment of ABPA patients, inhaled corticosteroids are recommended for asthma. However, even high doses of potent inhaled cortiocosteroids have not been successful at treatment or prevention of new radiologic infiltrates. Prednisone treatment will result in resolution of the acute infiltrates, as shown in Figures 8-5 and 8-6, clearing or reduction of the sputum plugs if they were expectorated, improvement in overall respiratory status and pulmonary function parameters, and a decline of at least 33% in the total serum IgE concentration. Prednisone can be discontinued after a taper. Some patients will in fact have developed prednisone-dependent asthma after the onset of ABPA. Many patients will not need continued prednisone, however. Subsequent total serum IgE concentrations can be determined every 2 to 3 months the first year to establish the baseline from which 100% elevations are often associated with new radiologic infiltrates.

---

**TABLE 8-1**
**Stages of Allergic Bronchopulmonary Aspergillosis**

| Stage | Signs/Comments |
|---|---|
| 1. Acute | Infiltrates clear with prednisone; total IgE declines by 33% in 6 wk |
| 2. Remission | No infiltrates and no prednisone for 6 mo; total IgE can be normal or elevated |
| 3. Exacerbation | New infiltrates resolve with prednisone; total IgE is double baseline or remission concentrations and declines with prednisone, as in the acute stage |
| 4. Corticosteroid-dependent asthma | Asthma requires prednisone and inhaled corticosteroids; infiltrates may still occur; scarring may be present on chest roentgenograms; total IgE concentration can be low to elevated |
| 5. End-stage fibrotic | Fixed obstructive or restrictive disease; fibrocavitary lesions on chest roentgenograms; new infiltrates may be from *Pseudomonas aeruginosa*; if the $FEV_1$ is <0.8 L, the prognosis is poor |

$FEV_1$, forced expiratory volume in 1 sec; IgE, immunoglobulin E.

The evidence for concomitant treatment with antifungal therapy with itraconazole for pulmonary infiltrates is almost nonexistent. This author has seen multiple failures, so many successes would be needed to achieve any clinical or statistical significance. One controlled trial actually concluded that the patients who benefited the most were those without bronchiectasis.[8] Furthermore, itraconazole, a fungistatic drug, may have anti-inflammatory, antieosinophilic effects for treatment of asthma in patients with ABPA.[9] Perhaps a fungicidal drug, voriconazole, may be of true clinical benefit, likely as adjunctive to oral corticosteroids.

Allergen vaccine immunotherapy with *A. fumigatus* has not been studied in ABPA and has been avoided for fear of inducing either local or systemic allergic reactions or worsening pulmonary disease. ABPA patients are highly atopic and often have allergic rhinitis along with allergic asthma. Thus, allergen vaccine immunotherapy without *Aspergillus* species can be administered if indicated.

The prognosis of ABPA is good if the condition is diagnosed early before there is much bronchiectasis. Alternatively, if there is extensive bronchiectasis (see Figs. 8-9 and 8-10), the patient's respiratory status will be impaired and purulent sputum might be from *Staphylococcus*, *Pseudomonas*, or atypical mycobacteria. In end-stage patients, supportive care, DNAase, pulmonary toilet procedures, and oxygen may be necessary. Fortunately, with earlier diagnosis and treatment of ABPA, there are few patients who evolve to this stage. Alternatively, one should not overtreat the ABPA patient with prednisone who has no radiologic infiltrates but whose total IgE concentration is 3000 KU/L. That concentration may be the patient's baseline values, although elevated, from which future 100% increases will be seen.

# REFERENCES

1. Greenberger PA: Allergic bronchopulmonary aspergillosis. J Allergy Clin Immunol 2002;110:685–692.
2. DeShazo RD, Chapin K, Swain RE: Fungal sinusitis. N Engl J Med 1997;337:254–259.
3. Ward S, Heyneman L, Lee MJ, et al: Accuracy of CT in the diagnosis of allergic bronchopulmonary aspergillosis in asthmatic patients. Am J Roentgenol 1999;173:937–942.
4. Slavin RG, Laird TS, Cherry JD: Allergic bronchopulmonary aspergillosis in a child. J Pediatr 1970;76:416–421.
5. Bosken CH, Myers JL, Greenberger PA, et al: Pathologic findings of allergic bronchopulmonary aspergillosis. Am J Surg Pathol 1988;12:216–222.
6. Chauhan B, Santiago L, Hutcheson PS, et al: Evidence for the involvement of two different MHC class II regions in susceptibility or protection in allergic bronchopulmonary aspergillosis. J Allergy Clin Immunol 2000;106:723–729.
7. Marchand E, Verellen-Dumoulin C, Mairesse M, et al: Frequency of cystic fibrosis transmembrane conductance regulator gene mutations and 5T allele in patients with allergic bronchopulmonary aspergillosis. Chest 2001;119:762–767.
8. Stevens DA, Schwartz HJ, Lee JY, et al: A randomized trial of itraconazole in allergic bronchopulmonary aspergillosis. N Engl J Med 2000;342:756–762.
9. Wark PA, Hensley MJ, Saltos N, et al: Anti-inflammatory effect of itraconazole in stable allergic bronchopulmonary aspergillosis: A randomized controlled trial. J Allergy Clin Immunol 2003;111:952–957.

*Philip Fireman*

# *9* Allergic Rhinitis

Allergic rhinitis is the most common allergic disease, chronically affecting more than 40 million people in the United States and many more worldwide.[1] Although not life threatening, this frequent illness causes considerable morbidity and results in the expenditure of billions of dollars in direct and indirect health care and the loss of millions of work and school days.[2]

Allergic rhinitis is provoked by exposure to antigenic environmental factors referred to as allergens, with resultant sneezing, nasal pruritus, rhinorrhea, nasal mucosal edema, and subsequent nasal obstruction induced by an immunoglobulin (Ig) E–mediated response. Symptoms can be episodic or perennial; because symptoms recur annually during certain months, the syndrome is sometimes called *seasonal* allergic rhinitis (Table 9-1). The predominate allergens causing seasonal allergic rhinitis are outdoor pollens, such as tree, grass, or ragweed pollen. Typically, seasonal allergic rhinitis does not develop until after the patient has been sensitized by two or more seasons. Seasonal allergic rhinitis is frequently referred to as *hay fever* or *summer cold*, but these descriptive terms are misleading and should be discarded because fever is not a symptom of allergic rhinitis, and the common cold virus is not the etiology. Perennial allergic rhinitis can be constant or recurrent and occurs year-round. It can also be associated with seasonal exacerbations.

Recent guidelines for the management of allergic rhinitis have redefined the illness as intermittent or persistent rather than seasonal and perennial (see Box 9-1).[3] A major impetus for this reclassification is that sensitization to multiple pollens is common with individuals sensitized to several pollen allergens, such as trees, grasses, and weeds. These multiple allergies can be associated with long-lasting disease that can extend for many months in various temperate climates of the world. In subtropical and tropical climates, prolonged pollen exposure may also provoke disease year-round. Thus, typical seasonal allergens in one climate may provoke perennial disease in another climate. Conversely, sensitization to typical perennial allergens such as animal allergens may provoke intermittent or transient symptoms in those sensitized who do not have daily exposure to pet animals.

Intermittent rhinitis is defined on the basis of symptoms that are present for less than 4 days per week and for less than 4 weeks (see Table 9-1). If symptoms are present for more than 4 days per week or have lasted for more than 4 weeks regardless of the number of days per week, the illness is classified as *persistent* allergic rhinitis. In addition, the severity of symptoms should be designated as mild or moderate to severe (Box 9-1). A large body of published literature on the pharmacotherapy of allergic rhinitis was developed during the past 25 years examining patients categorized as having either seasonal or perennial disease. This new classification of allergic rhinitis as intermittent and persistent may cause confusion when reviewing this literature.

## EPIDEMIOLOGY

Allergic rhinitis was relatively uncommon prior to the Industrial Revolution at the turn of the 20th century, whereas it is much more common now. Data from many sources and countries support these observations. In addition, diagnostic recognition of the illness has improved remarkably in the past 100 years. Swedish army recruits showed a prevalence of seasonal allergic rhinitis of 4.4% in 1971, increasing to 8.4% in 1981.[4] Broder and colleagues,[5] in a 1970 questionnaire study of a well-defined population in Tecumseh, Michigan, found that the incidence of allergic rhinitis increased during childhood from less than 1% during

---

**BOX 9-1**
**Clinical Classification of Allergic Rhinitis**

1. Duration
   a. Intermittent (seasonal): Symptoms present
      - Less than 4 days/wk or
      - Less than 4–6 wk/yr
   b. Persistent (perennial): Symptoms present
      - More than 4 days/wk and
      - More than 6 wk

2. Severity
   a. Mild: Symptoms do not affect lifestyle
   b. Moderate–severe: Symptoms affect lifestyle
      - Sleep disturbance
      - Impair leisure or sport activities
      - Impair school or work

From Bousquet J, van Cauwenberge P, Khaltaev N: Allergic rhinitis and its impact on asthma. ARIA Workshop report. J Allergy Clin Immunol 2001;108:S147–S374.

infancy to 4% to 5% from ages 5 to 9 years to 9% during adolescence to 15% to 16% after adolescence. Even though seasonal allergic rhinitis is infrequent in very young children, persistent allergic rhinitis has been recognized in infancy and even in neonates. In a more recent prospective study of children followed from birth in a Tucson, Arizona, HMO, physicians diagnosed allergic rhinitis in 40% of children by 6 years of age and confirmed it by allergy skin testing in 40% of those children whose families agreed to the procedure.[6] Whereas seasonal (intermittent) allergic rhinitis in the Tecumseh study was shown to be almost twice as common as perennial (persistent) allergic rhinitis, the more recent Tucson study showed the reverse. In Britain, a community-based questionnaire survey of adolescents and adults showed a prevalence of 16% for allergic rhinitis, with 8% having only perennial (persistent), 6% having a combination of both seasonal (intermittent) and perennial (persistent), and 2% having only seasonal (intermittent).[7] The incidence of allergic rhinitis remains constant in young adults but gradually declines during middle age and in the elderly (Fig. 9-1).

For reasons that are not clear, more male than female children, in a ratio of 2 to 1, are affected with allergic rhinitis before adolescence, whereas females are slightly more often affected with nasal allergy after adolescence. The prevalence of allergic rhinitis may vary both within and between countries. For example, allergic rhinitis is more frequently diagnosed in metropolitan areas than in rural areas. In addition, allergic rhinitis is more common in industrialized developed countries in contrast to underdeveloped nations.

Allergic rhinitis is a familial, genetically influenced illness. However, migration studies suggest environmental factors may be just as important. Children born to immigrants in a new country resemble native children in both prevalence and natural history of their rhinitis. In the United States, no differences were found in self-reported allergic rhinitis among white and nonwhite adults.

The basis for the increase in prevalence of allergy in recent years has not been established, but some studies suggest that the modern lifestyle, fewer infections, or the environment is important. Studies of Swiss children have shown that symptoms of allergic rhinitis as well as allergen-specific IgE antibodies were lower in offspring of farmers than in other children in the same rural areas.[8] Another concept, the so-called "hygiene hypothesis," proposes that the decline of childhood infections or lack of exposure to infectious agents or their products (i.e., endotoxin) during the first few months or years of life is responsible for the increase in allergic disease. Children born into families with several older siblings have reduced risk for allergic sensitization at school age than school-age children with no siblings.[9] Studies of preadolescent children who attended day care during infancy have less allergic disease than children who did not attend day care. These observations may well be compatible with the immunopathogenetic aspects of allergic disease discussed later in this chapter.

# ETIOLOGY

The development of allergic rhinitis requires two conditions: the atopic familial predisposition to develop allergy and the environmental exposure of the sensitized patient to the allergen. Patients are not born with allergies but have the capacity to develop symptoms spontaneously through repeated exposure to allergens in their environment. Therefore, an understanding of the environmental factors—allergens—that provoke allergy are essential for diagnosing and treating allergic diseases (see Chapter 2). Inhalants are the principal allergens responsible for allergic rhinitis and may be present outdoors and indoors. These microscopic airborne particles include the pollens from weeds, grasses, and trees; fungi (mold) spores; animal products; and environmental dusts, either household or occupational. Intermittent (seasonal) allergic rhinitis is primarily induced by pollens from the germination of "nonflowering" vegetation. In temperate climates, the most important are tree pollens in the spring, grass pollens in the late spring and early summer, and weeds—especially ragweed in the United States—in the late summer and early fall. Because there is variation from one geographic area to another, it is necessary for each clinician to become familiar with the pollination patterns in their region. "Flowering" vegetation, such as roses and fruit blossoms, rarely causes allergic rhinitis because its pollens are too heavy to be airborne and its germination is facilitated by the action of bees and other insects. However, these flower pollens cannot be ignored as potential allergens in florists, gardeners, and flower fanciers or hobbyists.

In warm subtropical or tropical climates, mold spores may be airborne year-round. In those climates in which snow and freezing occur in the winter months, airborne mold spores are present intermittently during the spring, summer, and fall and decrease after a significant frost. In patients with persistent (perennial) allergic rhinitis, mold spores may be a significant inhalant allergen indoors, along with house dust. The principal allergen in household dust can vary, but the major portion is due to the house dust mite *Dermatophagoides*. Several species of house dust mite have been identified with different geographic distribution. The specific house mite allergens have been identified in its cuticle and feces.

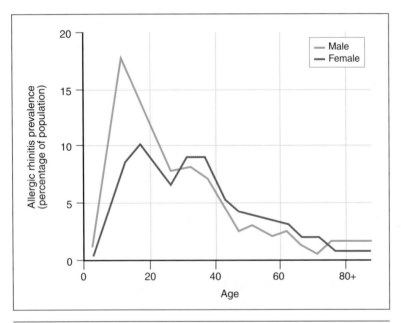

**Figure 9-1.** Prevalence of allergic rhinitis. Peak incidence occurs in the postadolescent patient. Because immunoglobulin E antibodies do not traverse the placenta, infants are not born with allergic rhinitis but acquire the syndrome after exposure to allergens during the first several years of life. The prevalence stabilizes during the adult years and gradually decreases during middle and advanced age. (Bousquet J: Allergic rhinitis and its impact on asthma. J Allergy Clin Immunol 2001;108:S147–S336.)

Animal epidermal danders, as well as salivary proteins, urinary proteins, feces, and feathers, especially from pets such as cats, dogs, and birds, are potential inhalant allergens. Most allergens, including the pollens, have been only partially chemically characterized, and each consists of multiple antigenic determinants.

Food allergens cannot be ignored, especially in young children, but are of lesser importance in the etiology of allergic rhinitis than inhalants. Foods are especially important allergens in infancy, probably because of immaturity of the digestive and immune process of the gut that increases the sensitization to ingested substances. Food allergy can appear at any age but most commonly occurs in early life. Gastrointestinal complaints are the most common symptoms, but food allergy can produce upper respiratory complaints of allergic rhinitis, as well as asthma, urticaria, angioedema, eczema, and even anaphylaxis. Sensitivity to food frequently decreases as the child becomes older but can be lifelong, especially allergic reactions to nuts, fish, and shellfish.

Patients may be sensitive to one or multiple allergens. Although it is a well-established fact that exposure to an allergen is necessary for the development of sensitivity and symptoms, it is not known why allergic individuals, sometimes even twins with similar exposures, become sensitive to certain allergens but not to others. The threshold of reactivity to each allergen varies greatly from one patient to another; certain individuals react to small allergenic challenges, whereas others tolerate a large allergen dose before developing symptoms. In addition to allergens, other nonallergenic factors can provoke nasal symptoms that resemble nasal allergy, except that there are no specific IgE antibodies to these nonallergenic substances. These factors include cigarette smoke; aerosolized cosmetics; industrial fumes; and changes in temperature, humidity, and barometric pressure. Psychological and social stresses and anxiety can also contribute to or exacerbate nasal symptoms. The importance of these additional contributory factors varies greatly from patient to patient and should not be neglected in patient management.

Even though it is not possible to predict with certainty the potentially atopic patient, the familial autosomal nature of allergic rhinitis has been recognized for years, and a positive family history of atopy has been noted in 50% to 75% of allergic rhinitis patients. Elevated serum levels of IgE are frequently associated with allergic diseases, and a recessive genetic influence has been suggested. Most investigators feel that several genetic loci are involved in the expression of allergic disease, and inheritance is multifactorial. A variety of population-based studies using positional cloning techniques and genetic mapping have identified candidate genes or loci that may be involved in allergic rhinitis. One candidate loci for allergy is on chromosome 5q, near the site of the gene cluster encoding interleukin (IL)-3, IL-4, IL-5, IL-9, IL-13, and the IL-4 receptor.[10] Another candidate locus is on chromosome 11q13, which is the location of the gene encoding the high-affinity IgE receptor.[11] Animal studies have shown that synthesis of specific antibodies to well-characterized antigens is controlled in part by immune response (Ir) genes, which are linked to the major tissue histocompatibility locus (HLA). The studies by Levine and co-workers have suggested that ragweed allergic rhinitis and immune responses to purified ragweed antigen E were linked to a particular histocompatibility locus haplotype in successive generations of allergic families.[12] Marsh and colleagues reported a significant correlation between haplotype histocompatibility locus 7 and increased IgE antibodies to a low-molecular-weight purified ragweed antigen (Ra5) in a group of allergic rhinitis patients

sensitive to this small portion of the ragweed allergen.[13] Similar studies of other purified allergens are indicated in allergic rhinitis patients because the responses to the more complex allergens, such as those used in clinical practice, may or may not be controlled by similar or different genetic influences.

# IMMUNOPATHOLOGY

Allergic rhinitis, allergic asthma, and allergic urticaria are described immunologically as immediate hypersensitivity syndromes and are mediated in large part by IgE antibodies. Allergic (atopic) individuals produce high levels of IgE antibodies in response to particular allergens, whereas nonallergic individuals generally synthesize other Ig isotypes, such as IgM and IgG antibodies and minimal IgE antibodies to the specific allergen. Regulation of the IgE synthesis depends on the propensity of an individual to mount a response of specific T-helper ($Th_2$) lymphocytes to an allergen. This propensity is influenced by a variety of factors, including familial genes, the nature of the allergen, and the history of prior allergen exposure. Thus, the allergic patient inherits the risk, but environmental factors, including exposure, determine the nature and extent of the allergic rhinitis.

On the first exposure to an antigen, an individual with a genetic predisposition to mounting an allergic response becomes sensitized to that antigen. During this exposure, those cells responsible for initiating the inflammatory response are recruited to the site of exposure. At subsequent exposures to the same antigen, these cells are considered to be "primed" and can rapidly respond to antigen through immediate release of factors that cause inflammatory changes. In the case of allergic rhinitis, there can be a dual temporal reaction with an immediate or early-phase response clinically manifested by nasal itching, sneezing, rhinorrhea, and congestion. In addition, 50% of patients with allergic rhinitis have a late-phase response characterized mainly by congestion. On a cellular level, this represents the long-term consequences of cellular upregulation that began in the early phase.

The cellular interactions of allergic rhinitis begin with antigen uptake and processing via the antigen-presenting cell. Antigen-presenting cells are identified as macrophages and dendritic cells in the nasal mucosa and submucosa, and they display processed peptides in the form of major histocompatibility complex class II–associated peptides. Naïve T-lymphocytes, also called $T_h0$ cells, migrate toward antigen-presenting cells and processed antigen and are stimulated by recognition of the peptide–major histocompatibility complex on the antigen-presenting cell. On antigen recognition, the $T_h0$ cell becomes activated and will clonally expand. The progeny of antigen-stimulated $T_h0$ cells differentiate into effector cells that produce different sets of cytokines and perform different functions. These subsets include two populations, T-helper 1 ($T_h1$) and $T_h2$ cells.[15] The $T_h1$ cells are involved in the production of interferon gamma and tumor necrosis factor beta, and the $T_h2$ cells have the capacity to produce IL-4, IL-5, IL-6, IL-9, IL-10, IL-13, and granulocyte-macrophage colony-stimulating factor. IgE production is facilitated by IL-4, IL-6, and IL-13; eosinophil production, by IL-4 and IL-5; and mast cells and basophils, by IL-4, IL-9, and IL-10. As the allergic response continues, mast cells, B cells, natural killer cells, eosinophils, and epithelial cells may also release $Th_2$ cytokines. Thus, the $Th_2$ cell and its cytokines are critical and responsible for creating and sustaining the allergic response (Fig. 9-2).

On subsequent allergen challenge, the allergen combines with its specific IgE antibody at the cell membrane of the sensitized tissue mast cell and blood basophil. When allergen cross-links the bound IgE, this triggers mast cell degranulation.[16] The degranulation begins a cascade that is characterized by two phases: an immediate or early reaction that occurs within 60 minutes and a late-phase reaction that peaks in 3 to 6 hours but may be present for 8 to 24 hours (Fig. 9-3).

The combination of allergen and IgE antibody results in a sequence of calcium- and energy-dependent enzyme reactions, with alteration of the mast cell or basophil membrane, which initiates a process of mediator release, synthesis, and transcription. Those factors that are released immediately include the preformed mast cell inflammatory mediators, such as histamine and tryptase. Newly generated lipid mediators, such as leukotriene C4 and prostaglandin D2, are synthesized from the phospholipid constit-

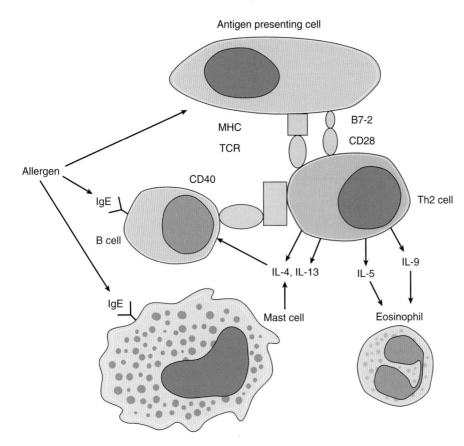

**Figure 9-2.** The T-helper (Th₂) cell recognizes allergen bound to the antigen-presenting cell and will produce various cytokines as diagrammed. Interleukin (IL)-4 and IL-13 promote B-cell switching to produce immunoglobulin E (IgE). IL-5 promotes eosinophil production and survival. IL-9 acts on the eosinophil to increase IL-5 expression. Mast cells, basophils, and eosinophils also produce Th₂-type cytokines that will amplify the allergic inflammatory response. Once IgE is cross-linked on basophils and mast cells, histamine is released, eosinophils are degranulated, and lipid mediators are produced, thus increasing allergic inflammation. MHC, major histocompatibility complex; TCR, T-cell receptor. (Adapted from Robinson DS: Th-2 cytokines in allergic disease. Brit Med Bull 2000;56:956–968.)

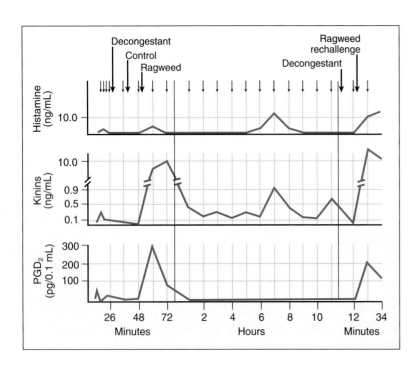

**Figure 9-3.** Profile of selected mediators present in nasal secretions collected by nasal wash from allergic rhinitis patients during early, late, and rechallenge responses to ragweed allergen. The time of each nasal wash is indicated by an *arrow.* Pretreatment with decongestants is necessary, as there are some mediators present in the nasal washes after the initial challenges. Histamine, kinins, tryptase, and prostaglandin D₂ (PGD₂) are present within minutes (early phase) of challenge with the ragweed allergen. In these experiments, without additional allergen, histamine and kinins reappear in nasal washes 2 to 8 hours after the initial exposure (late phase). Note that PGD₂ is not present in secretions during the late-phase reaction. On subsequent reexposure to the allergen during rechallenge, there are prompt increases in these mediators in nasal washes. These data help explain the almost continual (daily) symptoms that many allergic rhinitis patients experience.

uents of the mast cell membrane via arachidonic acid metabolism. In addition, cytokines, including IL-4 and IL-13, are transcribed.[16] The interaction of antigen (allergen) and antibody (IgE) at the mast cell membrane also promotes the synthesis of additional mediators, including platelet activating factor (PAF), bradykinin, and the interleukins IL-4 and IL-5, as well as tumor necrosis factor and granulocyte-macrophage colony-stimulating factor. The expression of the early- and late-phase allergic reactions is diagrammed in Figure 9-3. The mediators shown in Figure 9-3 cause the increased vascular permeability, increased local edema, and increased eosinophil-laden secretions seen in allergic rhinitis. The early phase of the allergic reaction occurs within minutes after exposure to the allergens. In contrast, patients who manifest the late-phase IgE allergic reaction show prolonged tissue inflammation. The total allergic inflammation can resolve within hours but may persist for days, weeks, or months, depending on the extent and duration of allergen exposure.

Histamine promptly released from mast cells, as well as from basophils, appears to be a major chemical mediator in nasal allergy. The mechanism by which histamine produces tissue edema is based on its ability to produce vasodilation and to increase capillary permeability. Histamine stimulates both $H_1$ and $H_2$ receptors in the nose, although the $H_2$ effect in the nose is probably minimal. The increased vascular permeability generated by histamine indirectly leads to the production of kinins, including bradykinin, which require kallikrein for their formation. Leukotrienes (LTs), $LTC_4$, $LTD_4$, and $LTE_4$, are found in nasal secretions after both allergen and cold air challenges. All have been found to increase vascular permeability and mucous secretion. $LTB_4$ has also been found to increase leukocyte adhesion molecule expression and to act as a neutrophil and eosinophil chemoattractant. Prostaglandin $D_2$ is the only currently studied mediator found to be elevated during the immediate nasal reaction but not during the late phase.[17] Since this prostaglandin is produced by mast cells and not basophils, it has been suggested that mast cells are involved primarily in the early allergic reaction, whereas basophils contribute to the late reaction. These mediators can directly affect the vascular bed of the nose, and the edema and congestion of the nasal tissues can disturb the balance of autonomic nervous control of nasal function. Because patients with allergic disease overreact to cholinergic stimuli, it may be that vascular dilation and hypersecretion are aggravated by the disturbance and resultant imbalance of autonomic control. The participation of neurohumors and vasoactive peptides, including factors such as substance P and vasoactive intestinal peptide, has been suggested, but their role needs definition.

The immunologic effectors of the immediate hypersensitivity allergic reaction have been shown to be IgE antibodies in most situations. However, it should be emphasized that it is the mediators, such as histamine, leukotrienes, prostaglandins, and eosinophil chemotactic factor of anaphylaxis, that are responsible for the pathophysiology of the immediate hypersensitivity reaction.

The hallmark of allergic pathology is the eosinophil.[18] Histologic examination of nasal mucosa after allergen challenge demonstrates that tissues are infiltrated with eosinophils and T-lymphocytes with a paucity of neutrophils. There are distended goblet cells in the presence of enlarged, congested mucous glands, as well as impaired ciliary beating and some epithelial exfoliation. The intracellular spaces are enlarged, and the basement membrane is thickened. Mast cells are present in both the nasal epithelium and the lamina propria and represent more than 80% of the metachromatic cells (mast cells and basophils) seen in nasal biopsies, with degranulated mast cells significantly increased 20 minutes after a provocative allergen challenge. Heterogeneity of mast cells has been proposed, with mucosal mast cells in the epithelium and connective tissue mast cells in the lamina propria. Basophils are the predominant metachromatic cell type found in nasal secretion and may be increased during the late-phase reactions.

# PATHOPHYSIOLOGY

Allergic rhinitis adversely affects normal nasal function which, besides its role as an airway (Fig. 9-4*A* and *B*) includes filtration of particulate matter from inspired air, humidification of air, olfaction, and phonation. The patient with allergic rhinitis has compromise not only of nasal function but also of other portions of the contiguous respiratory tract, including the eustachian tube, sinuses, and bronchi, which can be affected (Fig. 9-5). Allergen-provoked eustachian tube obstruction has been detected not only after intranasal provocation but also during seasonal, natural pollen exposure[19] (see Chapter 11). Allergen, methacholine, or histamine bronchial challenge provokes lower airway obstruction (i.e., asthma) in 30% or patients with allergic rhinitis (see Chapter 5). That allergic rhinitis contributes to the pathogenesis of sinusitis has also been suggested (see Chapter 10).

# CLINICAL PRESENTATION

Seasonal (intermittent) allergic rhinitis begins with frequent sneezing, nasal pruritus, and clear rhinorrhea and then progresses to nasal obstruction (Table 9-1). Perennial (persistent) allergic rhinitis tends to manifest more stuffiness. Patients emphasize early morning and late evening symptoms, and nasal obstruction may interrupt sleep. They also complain of itching of the eyes, throat, ears, and nose (Fig. 9-6). To relieve the nasal itch, some children may press the palm or arm upward against the nose in an "allergic salute" (Fig. 9-7). Constant rubbing of the itchy nose may produce a transverse nasal crease, a horizontal groove across the lower third of the nose (Fig. 9-8). With nasal obstruction, the patient becomes a mouth breather, so snoring is a nighttime symptom (Fig. 9-9). Mouth breathing may contribute to orofacial dental abnormalities that require orthodontic procedures, but this has not been established definitely.

Seasonal (intermittent) allergic rhinitis is frequently accompanied by allergic conjunctivitis (see Chapter 12). When symptoms of nasal obstructin are severe, adjacent sinuses may be involved, causing facial discomfort or headaches. Patients with eustachian tube dysfunction complain of fullness or popping sounds in the ears. Hearing loss in a child with perennial (persistent) allergic rhinitis suggests a conductive hearing deficit associated with otitis media with effusion (see Chapter 11). Loss of sense of smell and taste is also described. A few patients may complain of generalized malaise, irritability, and fatigue, which may be related to interrupted sleep.

Patients with seasonal (intermittent) pollinosis describe increased symptoms as the season progresses, especially on dry, windy days; symptoms may continue well beyond the season. Repeated exposure to allergens increases nasal reactivity and

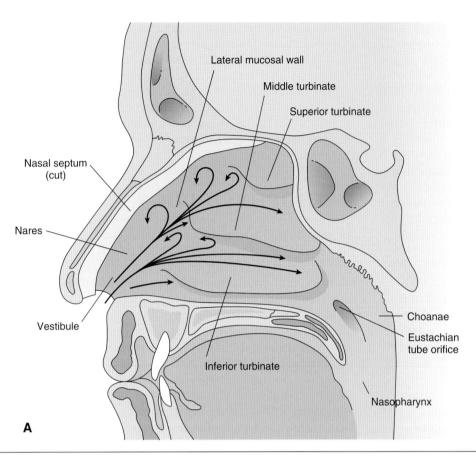

**NASAL FUNCTION: IMPORTANT ASPECTS**

1. Passage of air
2. Humidification
3. Warming of air
4. Filtering of air
5. Mucociliary action
6. Olfaction
7. Phonation

**Figure 9-4.** *A,* The inside of the nose, illustrating how the inspired air, after entering the nose, circulates over, under, and around the inferior, middle, and superior nasal turbinates. This pattern of circulation enables the nasal mucosa to more effectively filter, humidify, and warm the air. *B,* Major aspects of the nasal function.

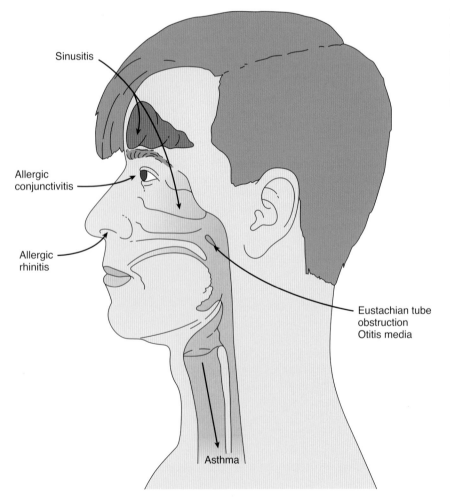

**Figure 9-5.** The clinical conditions that can be associated with allergic rhinitis due to their continuous anatomic relationships within the respiratory tract. When evaluating a possible cause of allergic rhinitis, the clinician should thoroughly examine all respiratory organs and related anatomic structures.

**TABLE 9-1**
Allergic Rhinitis: Symptoms, Pathophysiology, and Effector Mediators

| Symptoms | Pathophysiology | Effector Mediators |
|---|---|---|
| Tickling, itchiness, nose rubbing, allergic "salute" | Pruritus | Histamine, prostaglandins |
| Sneezing | Sneezing | Histamine, leukotrienes |
| Nasal congestion, stuffy nose, mouth breathing, snoring | Mucosal edema, increased vascular permeability | Histamine, leukotrienes, bradykinin, PAF |
| Runny nose, postnasal drip, throat clearing | Rhinorrhea, mucous secretion | Histamine leukotrienes |

PAF, platelet-activating factor.

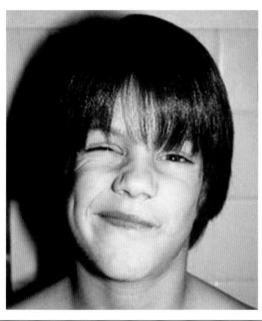

**Figure 9-6.** Nasal itching in patients with allergic rhinitis frequently causes facial grimacing and twitching. These symptoms are recognized by family and friends and also may be quite obvious during the physical examination. (Reproduced with permission from Skoner DP, Stillwagon PK, Friedman R, Fireman P: Pediatric allergy and immunology in Zitelli BJ and Davis HW (eds): Atlas of Pediatric Diagnosis, 3rd ed. New York, Gower, 1987.

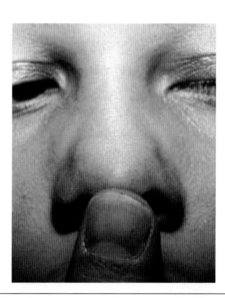

**Figure 9-8.** The chronic rubbing of the nose often results in a nasal crease in patients with allergic rhinitis. (Reproduced with permission from Skoner DP, Stillwagon PK, Friedman R, Fireman P: Pediatric allergy and immunology in Zitelli BJ and Davis HW (eds): Atlas of Pediatric Diagnosis, 3rd ed. New York, Gower, 1987.)

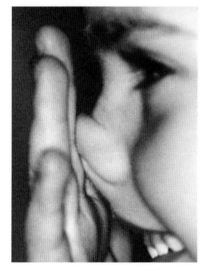

**Figure 9-7.** Children with allergic rhinitis are especially prone to forcibly rubbing the nose in an upward direction, using the fingers and palm of the hand. This "allergic" salute may become a habit and is frequently noted by parents. (Reproduced with permission from Skoner DP, Stillwagon PK, Friedman R, Fireman P: Pediatric allergy and immunology in Zitelli BJ and Davis HW (eds): Atlas of Pediatric Diagnosis, 3rd ed. New York, Gower, 1987.)

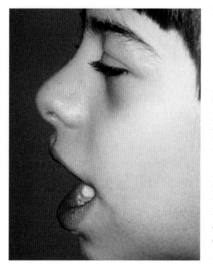

**Figure 9-9.** Open-mouthed breathing is typical in patients with longstanding allergic rhinitis. This behavior is also seen in patients with adenoidal hypertrophy causing posterior pharyngeal nasal obstruction. (Reproduced with permission from Skoner DP, Stillwagon PK, Friedman R, Fireman P: Pediatric allergy and immunology in Zitelli BJ and Davis HW (eds): Atlas of Pediatric Diagnosis, 3rd ed. New York, Gower, 1987.)

"primes" nasal mucosa, so that ordinarily innocuous concentrations of allergens and other environmental factors provoke symptoms. The pattern of symptoms helps distinguish seasonal (intermittent) from perennial (persistent) allergic rhinitis. In subtropical climates, a seasonal aeroallergen exposure pattern may not be obvious, as pollen seasons extend for many months and fungi can be airborne year-round. In much of the United States, as well as other temperate climates, trees pollinate in spring, grasses in late spring and summer, and weeds during late summer and early fall (see Chapter 2). The arid southwestern United States was traditionally pollen free, but the advent of irrigation and increased vegetation has changed the ecology. Increased pollen concentrations—and thus, frequent complaints of more symptoms—are noted in areas of high plant density. Yet, windblown, airborne pollens can spread for miles and cause symptoms. If they have direct contact with considerable amounts of pollen, patients can have angioedema, especially of the eyes and throat.

Patients with perennial (persistent) symptoms are more of a diagnostic challenge. Continuous exposure to home or occupational factors induces persistent symptoms, because congestion of the mucosal tissues does not return to normal during the few hours free of allergen exposure. In these patients, nonallergenic aerosolized irritants, such as cigarette smoke, fumes, industrial pollutants, and cosmetics, provoke increased symptoms. Additional nonallergenic factors include changes in barometric pressure, temperature, and humidity.

Examination of nasal mucosa requires the use of a nasal speculum with an appropriate light source (Fig. 9-10). Although fiberoptic rhinoscopy is not needed for most cases, it can be a valuable adjunct in a more thorough inspection of the nose and nasopharynx (Fig. 9-11A and B). With development of nasal allergy, clear nasal secretions are evident. The mucosa appear pale, boggy, blue-gray, and edematous without much erythema (Fig. 9-12A and B). The turbinates become swollen and obstruct the nasal airway. When this occurs, it may be necessary to shrink the mucosa and to use a vasoconstrictor to document nasal polyps, which occur in 10% to 15% of adult patients (Fig. 9-13). Conjunctival edema and hyperemia, along with Dennie's lines (Fig. 9-14), are frequent findings. Allergic rhinitis patients with considerable nasal obstruction and venous congestion, particularly children, demonstrate edema and darkening of the tissues beneath the eyes (Fig. 9-15). These so-called "allergic shiners" are not pathognomonic for allergic rhinitis; they can also be seen in patients with recurrent nasal and sinus congestion of any cause.

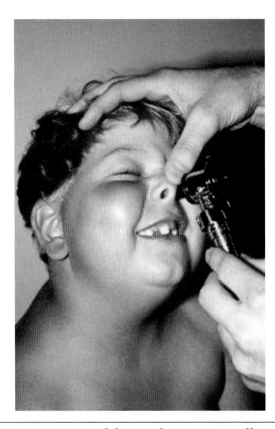

**Figure 9-10.** Inspection of the nasal mucosa. An illuminated nasal speculum is inserted into the nares for magnified visualization of the anterior nasal structures. This allows the clinician to view the anterior nares and to inspect the middle turbinate. The speculum must be directed to allow visualization of the inferior or superior turbinate. This mode of examination does not allow visualization of the anterior or posterior nasopharynx. (Reproduced with permission from Skoner DP, Stillwagon PK, Friedman R, Fireman P: Pediatric allergy and immunology in Zitelli BJ and Davis HW (eds): Atlas of Pediatric Diagnosis, 3rd ed. New York, Gower, 1987.)

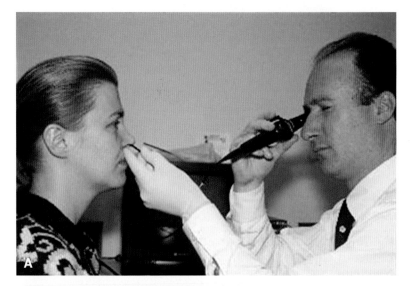

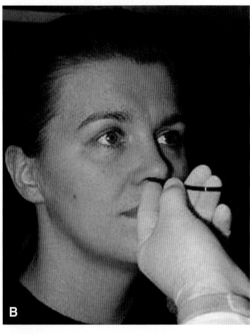

**Figure 9-11.** Lateral (*A*) and frontal (*B*) view of the fiberoptic rhinoscopic procedure that can be used for a more thorough examination of the nares, especially the anterior and posterior nasopharynx, which cannot be seen with a speculum. This examination also provides magnification of the nasal structures.

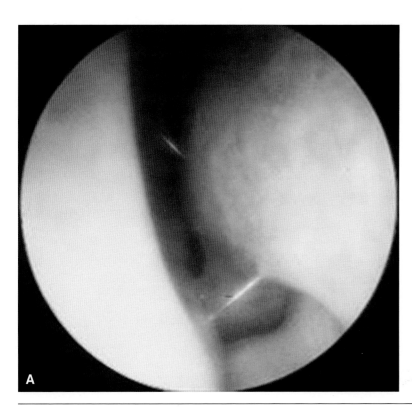

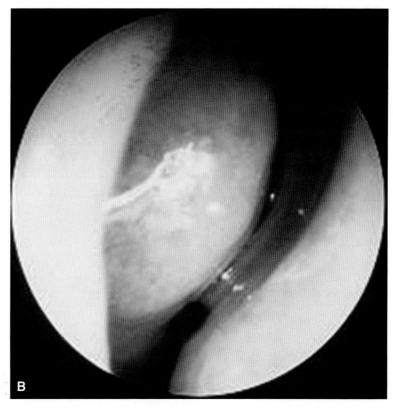

**Figure 9-12.** *A,* The inferior nasal turbinate of a patient with allergic rhinitis as seen through a fiberoptic rhinoscope. The mucosa are swollen, pale, and edematous, with increased nasal secretions, which may be watery to mucoid. *B,* Nasal obstruction due to the engorged and swollen nasal mucosa. Note the clear, watery secretions of allergic rhinitis.

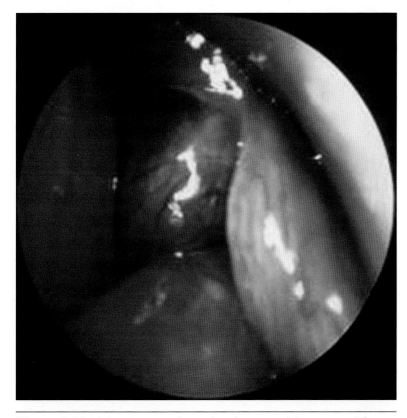

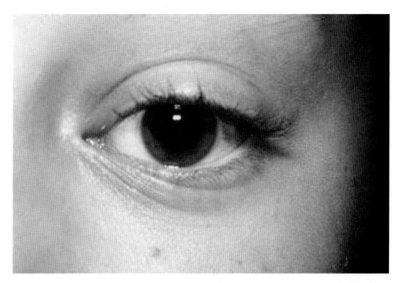

**Figure 9-14.** Dennie's lines on lower eyelid of a patient with allergic rhinoconjunctivitis. These lines originate at the inner canthus and traverse one half to one third of the length of the lower lid in an arc nearly parallel with its margin. (Reproduced with permission from Skoner DP, Stillwagon PK, Friedman R, Fireman P: Pediatric allergy and immunology in Zitelli BJ and Davis HW (eds): Atlas of Pediatric Diagnosis, 3rd ed. New York, Gower, 1987.)

**Figure 9-13.** Appearance of nasal polyps on rhinoscopy. They are pale, bluish gray, and almost gelatinous. These polyps, which obstruct the nasal airway, are best seen after application of a vasoconstrictor to shrink the nasal mucosa. (Photo courtesy of Dr. Sylvan Stool, Department of Otolaryngology, University of Pittsburgh School of Medicine, Pittsburgh, PA.)

# DIAGNOSIS

Analysis of cytology of expelled nasal secretions or scraping of nasal mucosa obtained with a flexible plastic nasal probe can help in the differential diagnosis of selected patients with recurrent rhinitis. Expelled nasal secretions during exacerbation of allergic rhinitis contain increased eosinophils of more than 3% on stained smears (Fig. 9-16). Nasal eosinophilia may not be evident during a superimposed infection or during steroid therapy. Increased nasal mucosal basophils (Fig. 9-17), mast cells, and eosinophils are found in nasal scraping, not only from allergic rhinitis but also from nonallergic eosinophilic rhinitis and primary nasal mastocytosis. The cytology of bacterial or viral infections shows a predominance of polymorphonuclear leukocytes (Fig. 9-18).

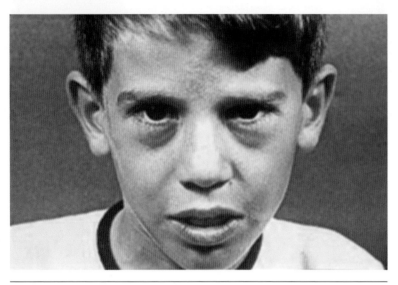

**Figure 9-15.** Suborbital venous congestion, edema, and darkening of the tissues under the eyes. This condition is frequently seen in patients with chronic allergic rhinitis and is referred to as an "allergic shiner." This patient's allergic rhinitis obstructed nasal breathing, resulting in open-mouthed breathing. (Photo courtesy of Dr. Meyer B. Marks, Division of Pediatric Allergy and Immunology, University of Miami School of Medicine, Miami, FL.)

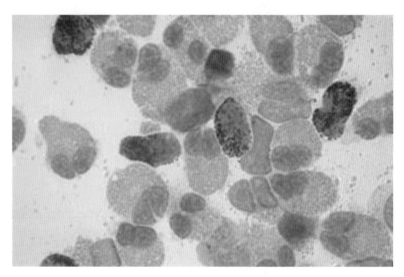

**Figure 9-17.** Nasal scrapings from a patient with allergic rhinitis. Obtained by using a flexible plastic probe, this material was spread on a microscope slide and stained with Wright's stain. This high-power photomicrograph shows several basophilic leukocytes, with their dark-blue cytoplastic granules, among a cluster of eosinophilic leukocytes, with reddish cytoplasmic granules. (Courtesy of Drs. A. Jalowaryski and E. Meltzer, Division of Allergy and Immunology, University of California, San Diego, San Diego, CA.)

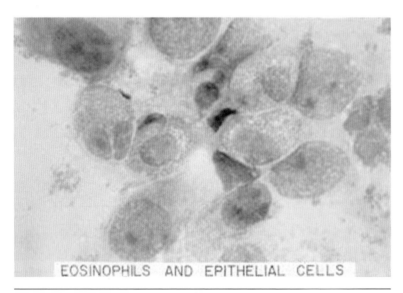

**Figure 9-16.** Nasal secretions from a patient with allergic rhinitis, stained with Wright's stain. This high-power photomicrograph shows typical eosinophils, with red-staining granules, among the blue-staining nasal epithelial cells. (Courtesy of Drs. A. Jalowaryski and E. Meltzer, Division of Allergy and Immunology, University of California, San Diego, San Diego, CA.)

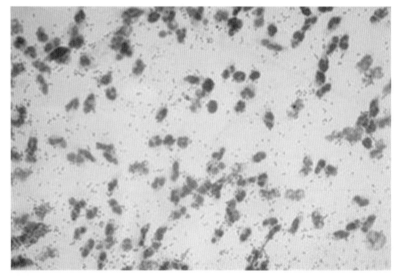

**Figure 9-18.** Nasal secretions photographed at low power from a patient with nasal infection. Typically, one sees many polymorphonuclear leukocytes, as well as bacteria, without any eosinophils. Viral rhinitis can also involve many polymorphonuclear leukocytes. (Courtesy of Drs. A. Jalowaryski and E. Meltzer, Division of Allergy and Immunology, University of California, San Diego, San Diego, CA.)

Laboratory confirmation of the presence of IgE antibodies to specific allergens is often helpful in confirming the clinical diagnosis of allergic rhinitis and in reinforcing patient compliance (see Chapter 3). Testing should be performed when a seasonal pattern is not evident. Skin testing with the suspected allergens is mandatory in all patients prior to immunotherapy (hyposensitization) with allergen extracts, because the intensity of the skin reaction helps determine the initial treatment dose. End-point titration has been suggested as a guide for the initial dosage. However, this author does not recommend it because it is expensive and lacks sufficient controlled data to document its validity. Clinicians should be selective; only common allergens of clinical relevance should be chosen on the basis of prevalence in the patient's environment (see Chapter 2). The most useful allergens in the study of allergic rhinitis are the inhalants, especially the pollens, the molds (fungi), house dust, and animal products (Box 9-2). Food testing is infrequently indicated.[20]

The in vitro serum immunoassay tests (the radioallergosorbent test [RAST], fluorescent allergosorbent test [FAST], and enzyme-linked immunosorbent assay [ELISA]) for assessing the presence of serum IgE antibodies to various allergens are 10% to 20% less sensitive than skin tests, and their increased cost is another disadvantage. Only rarely are IgE antibodies present in nasal secretions but not detected in serum or evident by skin testing. The in vitro cytotoxic serum leukocyte test with foods and other allergens is unproven and not recommended.

A nasal provocation test performed by introducing the allergen into the nostril of the allergic patient elicits local pruritus, sneezing, rhinorrhea, and edema. The sublingual challenge with allergen is not a useful diagnostic test for allergic rhinitis. The provoked nasal obstruction can be measured by rhinomanometry. There are two approaches, anterior and posterior, to the measurement of air pressure and flow relationships in the nose (Fig. 9-19A and B). Anterior rhinomanometry requires minimum patient cooperation but is compromised by the normal nasal cycling phenomenon in which airflow is predominant in one nostril for 2 to 3 hours and then alternates to the other side (Fig. 9-20A and B). This requires measurement of the resistance of both nostrils or of total nasal airway resistance. Alternatively, posterior rhinomanometry measures posterior pharyngeal pressure via an oral tube as nasal airflow is being monitored using a tightly fitting facial mask over the nose. However, 10% of adults cannot perform this test. Posterior rhinomonometry requires a storage oscilloscope because it is necessary to establish that an artifact-free pressure-flow curve has been achieved before nasal resistance measurements can be made. The development of computer-assisted

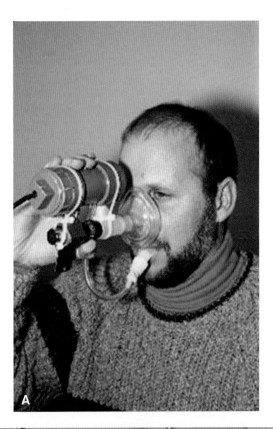

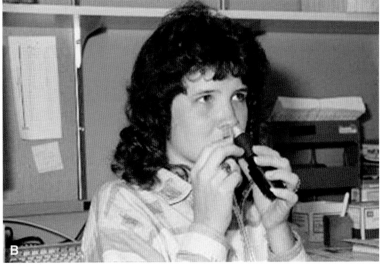

**Figure 9-19.** *A,* Posterior rhinomanometry utilizes a facemask, which fits securely around the nose. Nasal airflow is measured via a transducer attached to the nasal facemask. Nasopharyngeal pressure is measured via a plastic mouthpiece held securely between the teeth, with the lips closed. Nasal resistance is calculated from the airflow and pressure measurements that can be monitored and calculated with computer assistance. *B,* Anterior rhinomanometry utilizes a system whereby nasal airflow is measured in one naris, while nasal pressure is measured in the other.

---

**BOX 9-2**
**Selected Inhalant Allergens Useful in Evaluation and Testing for Allergic Rhinitis**

**Pollens (vary with geographic area)**
Weeds (ragweed, plantain, etc.)
Grasses (timothy, rye, etc.)
Trees (oak, maple, etc.)

**Fungi (molds)**
Seasonal (*Alternaria*, etc.)
Storage (*Aspergillus*, etc.)

**Animal products**
House dust mites (cuticle, feces)
Dogs, casts (dander, saliva)
Birds (feathers, droppings)

rhinomanometry has now made this a fast, accurate system. Whereas it seems likely that rhinomanometry will be utilized more widely in the future, it has not yet been standardized for routine clinical practice.

# DIFFERENTIAL DIAGNOSIS

Patients who present to the clinician with complaints of rhinorrhea and nasal obstruction may have symptoms due not only to allergy but also to a variety of other conditions, including infections, structural changes, drug reactions, neoplasms, or foreign bodies (Box 9-3). At its onset, an upper respiratory viral infection, with its clear, watery rhinorrhea and sneezing, resembles allergic rhinitis (Fig. 9-21). Redness of the nasal mucosa is characteristic, and, after several days, the purulent nasal discharge indicates infection. Demonstration of the predominance of neutrophils on a smear of nasal secretions (see Fig. 9-18) confirms this impression, but remember that nasal infections can be superimposed on allergic rhinitis.

## *OBSTRUCTIONS*

Nasal obstruction and purulent rhinorrhea can also occur with foreign objects in the nares (Fig. 9-22), but the unilateral symptoms differentiate this condition from allergic or infectious rhinitis. Beside nasal polyps (see Fig. 9-13), causes of unilateral nasal obstruction include deviation of the nasal septum (Fig. 9-23) and neoplasm; both are detectable on visual examination. Drugs such as reserpine can simulate allergic rhinitis, and withdrawal establishes this diagnosis. The most common drug rhinopathy

---

**BOX 9-3**
**Differential Diagnosis of Chronic Rhinitis and Nasal Obstruction**

**Rhinitis**
Allergic rhinitis: Seasonal or perennial
Infectious rhinitis: Chronic or acute (frequent recurrences)
Obstructive foreign body
Rhinitis secondary to topical decongestants, rhinitis medicamentosa
Nonallergic rhinitis with eosinophilia (NARES)
Nonallergic vasomotor rhinitis (cholinergic)
Hormonal rhinitis: Pregnancy or hypothroidism
Atrophic rhinitis

**Other Causes of Nasal Obstruction**
Rhinosinusitis
Anatomical abnormality (e.g., deviated septum, enlarged adenoids)
Nasal polyps
Tumor (e.g., angiofibroma)
Cerebrospinal fluid leakage secondary to perforation of the cribriform plate by fracture or tumor
Granulomatous disorders (e.g., Wegener's granulomatosis, sarcoidosis)

---

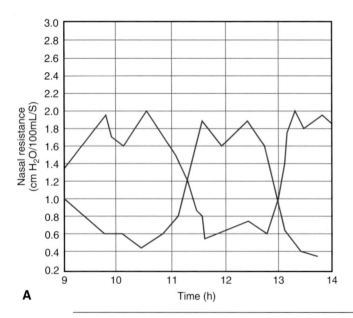

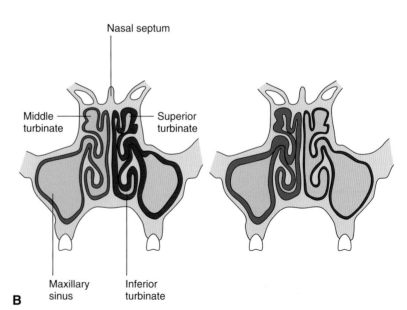

**Figure 9-20.** *A,* The normal nasal cycle during which the individual breathes predominantly through one and the other nostril. For several hours, breathing occurs through one nostril, as indicated by the lower nasal resistance. The nasal resistance then increases in that nostril but decreases in the other, as the breathing cycles to the second nostril. *B,* The alternating change in nasal airflow is accompanied by a functionally decreased nasal airway in one naris and an increased airway in the other.

is rhinitis medicamentosa following administration of topical vaso-constrictors for more than 3 to 5 days. The mucosa become red and irritated or pale and edematous. Other causes of nasal congestion include pregnancy, hypothyroidism, and nonallergic perennial rhinitis.

## ALLERGIC AND NONALLERGIC PERENNIAL (PERSISTENT) RHINITIS

The differential diagnosis between allergic and nonallergic persistent rhinitis often can be difficult. Nonallergic perennial rhinitis is more common in adults, and no immunologic etiology can be implicated. Allergy testing does not reveal a specific cause for the symptoms. In nonallergic rhinitis, the edematous mucous membranes are often pale with watery secretions but contain no eosinophils. When eosinophilia is present, the syndrome is diagnosed as nonallergic rhinitis with eosinophilia (NARES). Vasomotor rhinitis is a vague category of chronic nonallergic nasal disease typically seen in adult women. These patients seem to have unusual awareness of their symptoms and complain of over-responsiveness of the nose to minimal changes of temperature, humidity, and odors. Immunotherapy (hyposensitization) is not to be used in these diseases, and drug therapy with antihistamine decongestants controls the symptoms inconsistently. Intranasal ipratropium or steroids may benefit some of these patients. A comparison of these different types of rhinitis is made in Table 9-2.

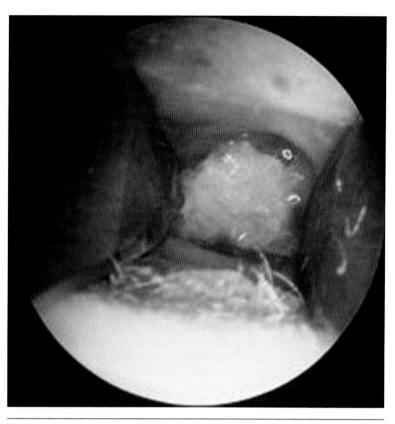

**Figure 9-22.** Yellow plastic foam lodged in a child's naris. This foreign body, which caused unilateral nasal obstruction and a mucopurulent discharge, could not be seen until a speculum was introduced into the nares to inspect the mucosa. (Photo courtesy of Dr. Sylvan Stool, Department of Otolaryngology, University of Pittsburgh School of Medicine, Pittsburgh, PA.)

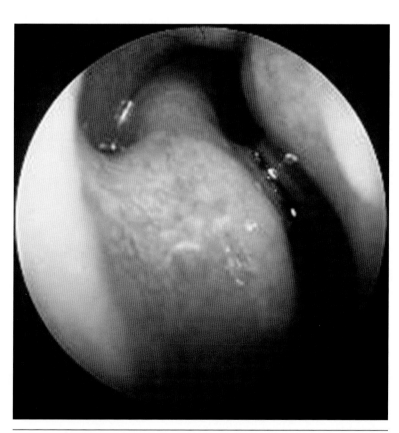

**Figure 9-21.** Clear, watery nasal secretions with swollen, reddish turbinates seen via fiberoptic rhinoscopy in a patient during the first few days of viral rhinitis. Often the secretions become mucopurulent after several days.

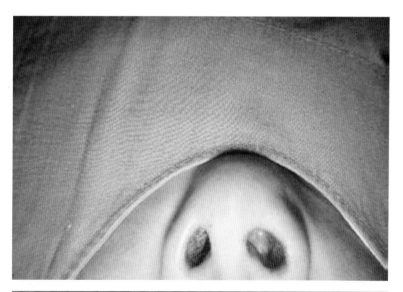

**Figure 9-23.** Deviation of the nasal septum. This condition can be seen on visual inspection of the nose. It frequently causes unilateral nasal obstruction. If severe, it can be corrected surgically. (Photo courtesy of Dr. Sylvan Stool, Department of Otolaryngology, University of Pittsburgh School of Medicine, Pittsburgh, PA.)

# THERAPY

## GENERAL CONSIDERATIONS

Successful therapy for allergic rhinitis involves three primary considerations: environmental control by identification and avoidance of the specific allergens and other contributory factors,[1] pharmacologic management,[2] and immunotherapy (desensitization) to alter the patient's immune response to the allergen[3,20] (Box 9-4). An algorithm for the therapy of allergic rhinitis is outlined in Table 9-7. Successful management includes identifying the specific precipitants and initiation of appropriate environmental control measures (see later). At the same time, the patient's history should be evaluated and based on symptoms. Cases should be categorized as intermittent (seasonal) or persistent (perennial) and should be further defined as mild, moderate, or severe, based on symptomatology and response to pharmacotherapy. Mild symptoms can be controlled with over-the-counter medication, whereas moderate rhinitis will require daily treatment with prescription therapy to control the patient's symptoms. Severe intermittent or persistent symptoms are those that severely affect everyday activities, especially adverse effects on school and work performance, difficulty with sleep, or failure of previous medications to control symptoms. Patients with moderate-to-severe symptoms not kept in check with environmental control and prescription medications require in-depth evaluation through referral to an allergy specialist. Additional therapy may include consideration of allergen injection immunotherapy. Although rhinomanometric measurements of nasal airflow have been used in clinical and laboratory research, they have not been clinically validated to help the physician in better defining these categories of mild, moderate, and severe rhinitis.

## ENVIRONMENTAL CONTROL

Complete avoidance of the allergens is the best therapy for allergic disease: Without exposure the allergic reaction will not take place.[21] Once the specific allergens responsible for the symptoms are identified, the patient should make an effort to reduce the exposure to these allergens. Elimination of exposure to an animal dander by disposal of a feather pillow or removal of a pet from the house or elimination of a food allergen from the diet may provide complete or partial relief of symptoms. Avoidance of more ubiquitous allergens such as pollens, dusts, and molds may be more difficult. Patients sensitive to grass pollens should avoid increased exposure through gardening and grass-cutting during the grass pollen season. Camping trips and picnics in the countryside should be avoided by ragweed-sensitive patients during the ragweed pollen seasons. Pollen rubbed into the nose and eyes can produce severe local edema, a point particularly important to remember

**TABLE 9-2**

Comparison of Allergic and Nonallergic Rhinitis

| | Allergic | Nonallergic | |
| --- | --- | --- | --- |
| | | NARES | Vasomotor |
| **History** | | | |
| Occurrence | Seasonal, perennial | Perennial | Perennial |
| Age | Children, adults | Mostly adults | Mostly adults |
| Sex | Male, female | Male, female | Mostly female |
| **Physical examination** | | | |
| Edema | Moderate, marked | Moderate | Moderate |
| Secretions | Watery | Watery | Mucoid, watery |
| **Laboratory tests** | | | |
| Nasal eosinophils | Common | Common | Coincidental |
| Allergen tests | Positive | Coincidental | Coincidental |
| **Therapy** | | | |
| Antihistamines | Beneficial | Rarely help | Rarely help |
| Decongestants | Helpful | Sometimes help | Sometimes help |
| Steroids | Beneficial | Helpful | Rarely help |
| Cromolyn | Beneficial | Not helpful | Not helpful |
| Ipratropium | Not helpful | Not studied | Helpful |
| Immunotherapy | Beneficial | Not indicated | Not indicated |

NARES, nonallergic rhinitis with eosinophilia.

in dealing with children, who often play outdoors in close contact with pollinating plants. Patients should avoid direct contact with pollinating plants. House dust mite control measures, especially in the bedroom, can be effective for patients allergic to these mites. Such steps include providing rubberized or plastic airtight enclosures for pillows, mattresses, and box springs; the use of synthetic bedding fabrics; and the removal from the bedroom of stuffed toys, stuffed furniture, heavy drapery, and dust catchers, such as bookshelves.

Environmental control measures should also include removal of hair carpet underpads and, if feasible, sealing of the forced-air heating ducts and vents in the bedroom. Thorough weekly cleaning and vacuuming of the bedding and rugs in the bedroom effectively reduces the house dust mite allergen concentration. Washing bedding in hot water (130°F or hotter) will kill the house dust mite. High-efficiency particulate air (HEPA) filters placed in central forced-air heating or cooling systems are the most effective means of removing allergens from room air. Single-room air filter units are less efficient. Electrostatic precipitrons can be installed in central forced-air heating and cooling systems, and these can substantially reduce house dust, pollens, and other airborne particles. Single-room air conditioners, which recirculate the air, can also effectively reduce pollen in the bedroom. Because single-room electrostatic precipitron units are less effective and may generate irritating ozone, they are not recommended. Mold-sensitive patients should be advised against raking leaves, since the outdoor molds, especially *Alternaria* and *Cladosporium*, thrive on dead leaves and cut vegetation. Damp basements and wallpaper, as well as glass-enclosed shower stalls, are often sources of molds in the home, and removal of the source of moisture will eliminate mold proliferation. If the moisture cannot be eliminated, mold retardants can be incorporated into the house paints or used in washing the walls. Molds in damp basements can be reduced by aerosolized paraformaldehyde or other antifungal agents. It is unfortunate that many patients do not have sufficient motivation to carry out adequate avoidance procedures to control their symptoms.

## PHARMACOLOGIC MANAGEMENT

If the patient cannot or does not want to avoid the allergens responsible for his or her symptoms, the allergic symptoms can be relieved in many instances with medications. However, for several reasons, not all patients improve or respond to the same medicines. Medications shown to be clinically useful in the therapy of allergic rhinitis differ in their mechanisms. These differences translate into differences in patients' symptom improvement. Table 9-3 lists the various categories of medications used in the therapy of nasal allergy and compares their benefit in relieving the various symptoms of allergic rhinitis. Whereas one patient may respond to one family of medications, another may respond in part or not at all. For example, oral antihistamines are effective for the relief of sneezing, pruritus, and rhinorrhea but not for nasal congestion. If the allergic rhinitis patient has nasal congestion in addition to the nasal itch and sneezing, the antihistamine will provide only partial relief because it is not a decongestant. It would be appropriate to use combination therapy of an antihistamine

---

**BOX 9-4**
**Therapy of Allergic Rhinitis: General Considerations**

**Avoidance**
Specific allergens
Nonspecific factors

**Pharmacologic management**
Reverse symptoms
Present symptoms

**Immunotherapy (hyposensitization)**
Prevent symptoms

---

**TABLE 9-3**
**Comparison of Medications in Relieving Allergic and Nonallergic Rhinitis Symptoms**

|  | Oral Antihistamine | Intranasal Antihistamine | Oral or Nasal Decongestant | Nasal Steroid | LT Receptor Antagonist | Intranasal Anticholinergic | Intranasal Cromolyn | Allergen Immunotherapy |
|---|---|---|---|---|---|---|---|---|
| Sneezing | + | + | – | + | + | – | – | + |
| Itching | + | + | – | + | – | – | + | + |
| Rhinorrhea | + | + | + | + | + | + | + | + |
| Congestion | – | – | + | + | + | – | – | + |
| Conjunctivitis | + | – | – | – | + | – | – | + |
| Vasomotor rhinitis | – | – | + | + | – | + | – | – |
| Infectious rhinitis | – | – | + | – | – | + | – | – |

LT, leukotriene.

with a decongestant or use an intranasal corticosteroid. Allergic eye symptoms should not be ignored and often require combinations of therapy. Intranasal medications usually have modest benefit on relieving ocular allergy. Systemic (oral) antihistamine therapy and topical eye drops are needed for management of allergic conjunctivitis (see Chapter 12).

As outlined in the algorithm (see Table 9-4), mild intermittent symptoms can be controlled with antihistamines on an as-needed basis or over-the-counter intranasal cromolyn, along with environmental control. If symptoms are moderate to severe and persistent, the use of intranasal steroids along with a second-generation antihistamine is recommended. Patients with inadequate responses to environment control and pharmacotherapy should be referred to a specialist for allergy testing and considered for allergen immunotherapy. Cases of severe persistent allergic rhinitis frequently are controlled with the combination of intranasal steroids and a second-generation antihistamine with decongestant. Recent studies suggest that montelukast, an LT receptor antagonist, is also beneficial in the management of allergic rhinitis.[21] Occasionally, treatment with a short burst of oral corticosteroids may be required to gain control of symptoms. Most clinicians do not recommend intranasal injection of corticosteroids or intramuscular steroid depot injection. Each category of medication is discussed in greater detail.

## ANTIHISTAMINES

Antihistamines block the $H_1$ receptor and function by competing with histamine for $H_1$ receptors on cells. They are often used as the first-line medication for treating mild allergic rhinitis and are currently the most prescribed treatment for allergic rhinitis.[22] Most clinicians categorize them as first- and second-generation products (Table 9-5). The older first-generation antihistamines are lipophilic, cross the blood–brain barrier, and cause sedation. They have a shorter duration of action and have anticholinergic effects but are as effective as the newer second-generation antihistamines. These agents are available in oral formulations, and lower doses are available without a prescription. Representatives of first-generation antihistamines include diphenhydramine (Benedryl), azatidine (Optimine), clemastine (Tavist), chlorpheniramine (Chlor-Trimeton), brompheniramine (Dimetane), and hydroxyzine (Atarax, Vistaril). Many of these medications are available in combination with a decongestant or an analgesic. Antihistamines taken early in the morning and at bedtime may provide good symptomatic control of pruritus, sneezing, and rhinorrhea but do not relieve congestion or stuffiness. Additional doses may be taken at 4- to 6-hour intervals. Side effects, which include drowsiness and anticholinergic effects, frequently interfere with the effectiveness of the classic antihistamines. Patients should be warned against driving an automobile or operating machinery after taking first-generation antihistamines.

Second-generation antihistamines are preferred by most allergists because they are generally less sedating and do not interfere with school or work performance when compared with the first-generation antihistamines. They are lipophobic, have a larger molecular size, possess an electrostatic charge, and do not readily enter the central nervous system. They have longer duration of action, lack the anticholinergic side effect profile of first-generation drugs, and are well tolerated in the elderly. Products currently approved by the Food and Drug Administration include loratadine (Claritin); desloratadine (Clarinex), the metabolite of

---

**TABLE 9-4**
**Stepwise Algorithm for Management of Allergic Rhinitis**

| Intermittent (Seasonal) | | Persistent (Perennial) | |
|---|---|---|---|
| **Mild** | **Moderate–Severe** | **Mild** | **Moderate–Severe** |
| Environmental control | Environmental control | Environmental control | Environmental control |
| *plus* | *plus* | *plus* | *plus* |
| Antihistamine (PRN) | Antihistamine | Antihistamine | Antihistamine |
| ± decongestant | ± decongestant | ± decongestant | ± decongestant |
| *or* | *plus* | *or* | *plus* |
| Nasal corticosteroid | Nasal corticosteroid | Nasal corticosteroid | Nasal corticosteroid |
| *or* | *or* | *or* | *or* |
| Nasal cromolyn | LT receptor antagonist | LT receptor antagonist | LT receptor antagonist |
| *or* | *plus* | *consider* | *plus* |
| LT receptor antagonist | Specialist referral | Specialist referral | Specialist referral |
| | *consider* | | *consider* |
| | Allergen immunotherapy | | Allergen immunotherapy |

LT, leukotrine; PRN, as needed.

loratadine; cetirizine (Zyrtec), the metabolite of hydroxyzine; and fexofenadine (Allegra), the metabolite of terfenadine. Sedation is similar to placebo (5%) in studies of loratadine, desloratadine, and fexofenadine. Cetirizine's sedation effects are greater and affect approximately 10% to 15% of patients. Each of these second-generation antihistamines is efficacious when compared with placebo in double-blind placebo-controlled studies. Data also have shown similar benefit from intranasal spray formulations of antihistamines, Azelatin (Astelin), and levocabastine (Livostin).[23] However, 10% to 15% of patients complained of sedation with use of these intranasal antihistamines. Astemizole (Hismanal) and terfanadine (Seldane) were the first second-generation antihistamines introduced and have been removed by the Food and Drug Administration from the U.S. market because of drug-to-drug interactions and their association with torsades de pointes.

Antihistamine effectiveness is enhanced if the drugs are taken prophylactically or at the onset of symptoms. Contrary to popular belief, tachyphylaxis does not develop, and insufficient benefit is usually related to noncompliance. There are currently no double-blind placebo-controlled head-to-head trials that compare the clinical efficacy of the four available second-generation oral antihistamines. Several have compared two of the second-generation antihistamines with placebo, and slight differences

have been described. Each of these products and their dosages are outlined in Table 9-5.

## INTRANASAL CORTICOSTEROIDS

Intranasal (topical) corticosteroids are highly effective in the treatment of allergic rhinitis.[24] It has been shown that each of the intranasal steroids is effective in reducing the nasal symptoms of itching, sneezing, rhinorrhea, and obstruction compared with placebo. Intranasal corticosteroids can affect both the early-phase and late-phase allergic responses after experimental challenge with allergen. Prolonged treatment may inhibit allergen-induced late responses that are associated with the recruitment and activation of T-lymphocytes, $Th_2$ cytokine secretion, and eosinophilia.[25] Intranasal steroids have been shown to reduce the number of eosinophils and basophils in nasal lavages and decrease the number of activated lymphocytes and chemical mediators. Use of the intranasal corticosteroids as first-line therapy has been hampered by the misconception that they are unsafe or that they take a long time to take effect. Newer agents have higher lipid solubility, increased potency, a better safety profile, better efficacy, and a quicker onset of action. Examples of newer agents with

---

**TABLE 9-5**
**Formulations and Dosages of Selected $H_1$ Antagonists**

| $H_1$-Receptor Antagonist | Formulation | Recommended Dose |
|---|---|---|
| **First Generation (Selected)** | | |
| Chlorpheniramine (Chlor-Trimeton) | Tablets: 4 mg, 8 mg, 12 mg<br>Syrup: 10 mg/5 mL<br>Parenteral solution: 10 mg/mL | Adult: 8–12 mg 2×/day<br>Child: 0–0.35 mg/kg/24 hr |
| Hydroxyzine Atarax | Capsules: 25 mg, 50 mg<br>Syrup: 10 mg/5 mL | Adult: 25–50 mg 2×/day<br>Child: 2 mg/kg/24 hr |
| Diphenhydramine (Benadryl) | Capsules: 25 mg, 50 mg<br>Elixir: 12.5 mg/5 mL<br>Syrup: 6.25 mg/5 mL<br>Parenteral solution: 50 mg/mL | Adult: 25–50 mg 3×/day<br>Child: 5 mg/kg/24 hr |
| **Second Generation** | | |
| Cetirizine (Zyrtec) | Tablet: 10 mg<br>Syrup: 5 mg/5 mL | Adult: 10 mg/day<br>Child 2–6 yr old: 2.5–5 mg/day<br>>6 yr old: 5–10 mg/day |
| Fexofenadine (Allegra) | Tablets: 30 mg, 60 mg, 180 mg* | Adult: 60 mg 2 ×/day or 180 mg/day<br>Child 6–11 yr old: 30 mg 2 ×/day<br>>12 yr old: 60 mg 2 ×/day or 180 mg/day |
| Loratadine (Claritin) | Tablets: 10 mg<br>SL Tablets: 10 mg<br>Syrup: 1 mg/1 mL | Adult: 10 mg/day<br>Child >3 yr old, >30 kg: 5 mg/day<br>>3 yr old, >30 kg: 10 mg/day |
| Desloratadine (Clarinex) | Tablets: 5 mg | Adult: 5 mg/day<br>Child: ≥12 yr old: 5 mg/day |

*Timed-release formulation.
$H_1$, histamine receptor type 1; SL, sublingual.

these features include budesonide (Rhinocort), flunisolide (Nasalide, Nasarel), fluticasone propionate (Flonase), mometasone furoate (Nasonex), and trimacinolone (Nasacort). Table 9-6 lists these intranasal steroids and their dosages. Studies comparing intranasal steroids versus placebo showed decreased histamine levels in nasal lavages of those treated with the steroids, which was associated with significant improvements in nasal symptom scores, use of rescue medications, and number of symptom-free days. These agents have been shown to be effective in adults, adolescents, and children. A 3- to 5-day course of a topical decongestant such as oxymetazalone may be used when starting intranasal corticosteroid therapy in patients with severe allergic rhinitis to optimize intranasal corticosteroid delivery to the nasal mucosa.

Concerns about steroid systemic side effects in children have led to numerous growth studies using intranasal steroids. In a year-long study of prepubertal children 6 to 9 years old with perennial allergic rhinitis treated with beclomethasone dipropionate 168 μg twice daily, overall growth rate was significantly slower, by 1 cm, than in the placebo-treated group.[26] The difference in growth rate was evident as early as 1 month into treatment. No significant between-group difference was found in the hypothalamic-pituitary-adrenal axis assessment. In a similar 1-year study, prepubertal patients between 3 and 9 years of age with perennial allergic rhinitis were treated with mometasone furoate agueous nasal spray 100 μg once a day. After 1 year, no suppression of growth was seen in subjects treated with mometasone furoate agueous nasal spray, and mean standing heights were actually higher in the mometasone furoate agueous nasal spray group than in the placebo group at all time points.[27]

Local adverse events associated with intranasal corticosteroid include rare nasal-septal perforation, usually related to improper administration directed toward the septum instead of to the lateral area of the nasal cavity. More commonly, there is dissatisfaction with smell, taste, and a drip sensation.

## DECONGESTANTS

Decongestants contain sympathomimetic agents that activate alpha-adrenergic receptors and cause vasoconstriction, thus reducing nasal congestion (see Table 9-8). Available oral formulations include pseudophedrine and phenylephrine. Based on a recent report regarding the risk of hemorrhage stroke in patients receiving phenylpropanolamine, the U.S. Food and Drug Administration has removed it from the market. The effective dose for pseudophedrine is 1 mg/kg four times a day in children younger than 6 years; 30 mg four times a day in children 6 to 12 years old; and 60 mg four times a day or 120 mg extended release twice a day in patients older than 12 years. Unfortunately, some patients experience side effects with pseudophedrine, including nervousness, irritability, tachycardia, palpitations, headache, and insomnia. These drugs should be used with caution, as they may cause urinary retention and increased blood pressure in older individuals and prostate hypertrophy in men. Prolonged use of oral decongestants may lead to withdrawal symptoms of headache and fatigue when the drug is discontinued. They have limited action on the other symptoms of rhinitis, including rhinorrhea, sneezing, and itching. Combinations of antihistamines and decongestants

**TABLE 9-6**
Formulations and Dosages of Intranasal Corticosteroids

| Generic Name | Brand Name | Formulation | Pediatric Dose | Adult Dose |
|---|---|---|---|---|
| Beclomethasone | Beconase AQ | Spray 42 μg | 6–12 yr old 1 spray bid | >12 yr old 1–2 sprays bid |
| Dipropionate, monohydrate | Vancenase AQ | 84 μg | >6 yr old 1–2 sprays qd | 1–2 sprays qd |
| Beclomethasone Dipropionate | Beconase | Inhalation Aerosol 42 μg | 6–12 yr old 1 spray bid | >12 yr old 1 spray bid–qid |
| Budesonide | Rhinocort AQ | Spray 32 μg | >6 yr old 1 spray qd | 1 spray qd |
| Flunisolide | Nasarel | Solution 0.025% | 6–14 yr old 2 sprays bid | >14 yr old 2 sprays bid |
| Fluticasone Propionate | Flonase | Spray 50 μg | >4 yr old 1 spray qd | 1–2 sprays qd |
| Mometasone Furoate, monohydrate | Nasonex | Spray 50 μg | 3–11 yr old 1 spray qd | >12 yr old 2 sprays qd |
| Triamcinolone | Nasacort | Spray 55 μg | 6–12 yr old 1 spray qd | >12 yr old 2 sprays qd |
| Acetonide | Tri-Nasal | 50 μg | >12 yr old 2 sprays qd | 2 sprays qd |

↑ AU: Make sure rows all aligned correctly

provide patient convenience and additional relief of symptoms of allergic rhinitis. Pseudophedrine combined with fexofenadine (Allegra D), ceterizine (Zyrtec D), and lortradine (Claritin D) are examples, of these products.

## MAST CELL STABILIZERS

Intranasal cromolyn sodium is a nonsteroid mast cell stabilizer agent that is available without a prescription. Although the mechanism of action remains uncertain, it has anti-inflammatory properties and clearly blocks the early- and late-phase responses in a laboratory setting. It has been shown clinically to relieve sneezing, rhinorrhea, nasal congestion, and pruritis. Yet in head-to-head clinical trials, intranasal corticosteroids are more effective than cromolyn. Cromolyn has an excellent safety profile, may be used immediately prior to an anticipated exposure to prevent symptoms, and is recommended to be administered four times a day. Intranasal cromolyn is considered first-line treatment for the pregnant patient with allergic rhinitis.

## LEUKOTRIENE RECEPTOR ANTAGONISTS

Several studies have identified clear increments in leukotriene levels in nasal lavage fluid in association with the immediate nasal response to allergen.[29] Nasal insufflations provocation studies show that both $LTC_4$ and $LTD_4$ induce an increase in nasal airway resistance, as measured by rhinometry. The leukotriene receptor antagonist montelukast is currently approved in the United States for the therapy of allergic rhinitis. Montelukast selectively blocks the receptor that mediates the function of the various leukotrienes. Several clinical trials have documented the efficacy of montelukast in the management of allergic rhinitis versus placebo, and its efficacy is comparable to that of the antihistamines.[30]

## ORAL CORTICOSTEROIDS

A short burst (3 to 5 days) of oral steroids may be appropriate for some patients with very severe symptoms or to gain control of symptoms during acute exacerbations. Generally, the Prednisone dosage is 1 mg/kg/day for pediatric patients to a maximum of 60 mg/day. Adults may be treated with 40 to 60 mg/day in divided doses for 3 to 5 days. Long-term daily treatment with oral steroids is contraindicated, and instead, maintenance control of symptoms with intranasal steroids is recommended to gain control of symptoms. The intranasal steroids should be started at the same time as the short oral steroid burst.

# IMMUNOTHERAPY

When symptomatic drug therapy and avoidance cannot control symptoms, immunotherapy (hyposensitization) should be considered (see Chapter 22 for a more detailed discussion of immune therapy). Several double-blind controlled studies have shown immunotherapy to be 80% effective in reducing the symptoms of seasonal (Table 9-6) as well as perennial allergic rhinitis. The patient's symptoms should closely correlate with the presence of specific IgE antibodies. Positive allergy tests that do not confirm

the clinical presentation are false-positive reactions and contribute to unnecessary and unsuccessful immunotherapy.

After the decision is made to initiate immunotherapy, the magnitude of the local skin reaction should be a guide to determining the initiating dose of allergen. This author does not agree with suggestions that immunotherapy can be initiated based on the results of in vitro serum IgE antibody. Not only does this hypothesis lack adequate documentation and clinical confirmation, but it also promotes provision of clinical care by non-physician health providers who do not see or examine the patient. Endpoint titration skin testing also has been recommended as a guide for initiation of immunotherapy, but this adds significantly to the cost of skin testing and requires more controlled documentation prior to acceptance.

The clinician begins with relatively weak subcutaneous injections of aqueous or alum-precipitated solutions of allergens. These are gradually increased in volume and concentration to the maximally tolerated dose, as indicated by a moderate local reaction. A typical treatment protocol is outlined in Table 9-7. It is imperative that the treatment does not induce systemic symptoms or provoke exacerbation of allergic rhinitis. After reaching the maximally tolerated dose, the time interval between injections is gradually increased from weekly to biweekly to monthly. Treatment is given perennially for several years. Box 9-5 outlines several potential mechanisms behind immunotherapy, though it is not known precisely how immunotherapy promotes clinical improvement in allergic rhinitis.

**TABLE 9-7**
**Perennial Immunotherapy Dosage Schedule**

| Interval (Date) | Allergen Concentration | Volume Dosage (mL) |
|---|---|---|
| Weekly | 1:10,000* | 0.05 |
| " | | 0.10 |
| " | | 0.20 |
| " | | 0.40 |
| " | | 0.50 |
| " | 1:1000 | 0.05 |
| " | | 0.10 |
| " | | 0.20 |
| " | | 0.40 |
| " | | 0.50 |

Progress from

1:100

↓

1:10 in similar sequence†

*Very sensitive patients should begin at 1:100,000; this situation is rare.
†When maximum tolerated allergen dose is achieved, begin q 2 wk then gradually advance q 3 wk and ultimately q 4 wk.

Immunotherapy may be expected to provide significant clinical improvement in more than 80% of patients with pollen-induced allergic rhinitis. If improvement is not obtained after a 2-year trial, the patient should be reevaluated and discontinuation of immunotherapy should be considered. The duration of immunotherapy injections in patients who achieve clinical benefits is dependent on the patient's overall clinical response. In response to clinical improvements, the patient should be given the opportunity to stop treatment after approximately 3 to 5 years of injections. Many children with allergic rhinitis tend to improve with age and time. They are not "growing out" of the allergy, because improvement is related not to physical growth but to an as-yet-undefined age-related phenomenon.

There is no place for immunotherapy with allergens that can be easily removed or avoided. This is especially true for food allergens. The use of animal danders for immunotherapy should be limited to those individuals, such as veterinarians, who cannot avoid exposure to animal allergens.

It has been claimed that immunotherapy in children for seasonal allergic rhinitis may reduce their chances of developing pollen-induced asthma, but this hypothesis is open to many questions and needs to be substantiated. In general, patients with seasonal allergic rhinitis are more responsive to immunotherapy than those with perennial allergic rhinitis. The factors responsible for clinical improvement are multiple. Certain patients have exacerbations of symptoms after a spontaneous or induced remission for several seasons, and immunotherapy can be reinstituted without complication. In general, the prognosis for allergic rhinitis is better than that for nonallergic rhinitis.

---

**BOX 9-5**
**Immunologic Responses Associated with Allergen Immunotherapy**

Allergen-specific blocking (IgG) antibodies increase
Rise and then decrease in IgE-specific antibodies
Decreased basophil histamine release in response to allergen
Increased allergen-specific suppressor T cells
Decreased lymphocyte-cytokine response to allergen

---

Ig, immunoglobulin.

# REFERENCES

1. Dykewicz MS, Fineman S, Skoner DP, et al: Diagnosis and management of rhinitis: Complete guidelines of the joint task force on practice parameters in allergy, asthma and immunology. Ann Allergy Clin Immunol 1998;81:478–518.
2. Malone DC, Lawson KA, Smith DH, et al: A cost of illness study of allergic rhinitis in the United States. J Allergy Clin Immunol 1997;99:22–27.
3. Bousquet J, van Cauwenberge P, Khaltaev N: Allergic rhinitis and its impact on asthma. From allergic rhinitis and its impact on asthma: ARIA workshop report. J Allergy Clin Immunol 2001;108:S147–S374.
4. Burney PG, Luczynska C, Chinn S, Jarvis D: The European Community Respiratory Health Survey. 1994;7:954–960.
5. Broder I, Higgins MW, Matthews KP, Keller JB: Epidemiology of asthma and allergic rhinitis in a total community, Tecumseh, Michigan: IV. Natural history. J Allergy Clin Immunol 1974;54:100–110.
6. Wright AL, Holberg CJ, Martinez FD, et al: Epidemiology of physician-diagnosed allergic rhinitis in childhood. Pediatrics 1994;94(6 Pt 1):895–901.
7. Sibbald B, Strachan D: Epidemiology of rhinitis. In Busse W, Holgate S (eds): Asthma and Rhinitis. London, Blackwell Scientific, 1995, pp 32–43.
8. Braun-Fahrlander, CH, Gassner M, Grize L, et al: Prevalence of hay fever and allergic sensitization in farmers' children and their peers living in the same rural community. Clin Exp Allergy 1999;29:28–34.
9. Strachan DP: Epidemiology of hay fever: Towards a community diagnosis. Clin Exp Allergy 1995;25:296–303.
10. Marsh DG, Nelly JD, Breazeale DR: Linkage analysis of IL-4 and other chromosome 5q31.1 markers and total serum immunoglobulin E concentrations. Science 1994;264:1152–1156.
11. Cookson WO, Sharp PA, Faux JA, Hopkin JM: Linkage between immunoglobulin E responses underlying asthma and rhinitis and chromosome 11q. Lancet 1989;1:1292–1295.
12. Levine BB, Stember RH, Fotino M: Ragweed hay fever, genetic control and linkage to HLA haplotypes. Science 1972;178:1201.
13. Marsh DG, Bias WB, Hsu SH: Association of the HLA7 crossreacting group with a specific reaginic antibody response in allergic man. Science 1973;179:691.
14. Pearlman DS: Pathophysiology of the inflammatory response. J Allergy Clin Immunol 1999;104:S132–S137.
15. Abbas AK, Lichtman AH, Pober JS: Cellular and Molecular Immunology, 4th ed. Philadelphia, W.B. Saunders, 2000.
16. Broide DH: Molecular and cellular mechanisms of allergic disease. J Allergy Clin Immunol 2001;108:S65–S71.
17. Naclerio RM, Proud D, Togias AG: Inflammatory mediators in late antigen-induced rhinitis. N Engl J Med 1985;313:65–70.
18. Frigas E, Gleich GJ: The eosinophil and the pathophysiology of allergy. J Allergy Clin Immunol 1986;77:527.
19. Fireman P: Eustachian tube obstruction and allergy: A role in otitis media with effusion. J Allergy Clin Immunol 1985;76:137–140.
20. Frigas E, Gleich GJ: The eosinophil and the pathophysiology of allergy. J Allergy Clin Immunol 1986;77:527–537.
21. Philip G, Malmstrom K, Hampel FC: Montelukast for treating seasonal allergic rhinitis, a randomized double-blind, placebo controlled trial performed in the spring. Clin Exp Allergy 2002;32:1020–1028.
22. Simon EF: Antihistamine in Middleton's Allergy Principals and Practice, 6th ed. Philadelphia, C.V. Mosby, 2003, pp 834–869.
23. LaForce C, Dockhorn RJ, Prenner BM, et al: Safety and efficacy of azelastine nasal spray (Astelin NS) for seasonal allergic rhinitis: A 4-week comparative multicenter trial. Ann Allergy Asthma Immunol 1996;76:181–188.
24. Spahn JD, Covan R, Szefler SJ: Glucocorticoids. Clinical Science in Middleton's Allergy Principles and Practice, 6th ed. Philadelphia, C.V. Mosby, 2003, pp 887–914.
25. Fokkens WJ, Godthelp T, Holm AF, et al: Allergic rhinitis and inflammation: The effect of nasal corticosteroid therapy. Allergy 1997;52:S29–S32.
26. Skoner DP, Rachelefsky GS, Meltzer EO, et al: Detection of growth suppression in children during treatment with intranasal beclomethasone dipropionate. Pediatrics 2000;105:E23.
27. Schenkel EJ, Skoner DP, Bronsky EA, et al: Absence of growth retardation in children with perennial allergic rhinitis after one year of treatment with mometasone furoate aqueous nasal spray. Pediatrics 2000;105:E22.
28. Welsh PW, Stricker WE, Chu CP, et al: Efficacy of beclomethasone nasal solution, flunisolide, and cromolyn in relieving symptoms of ragweed allergy. May Clin Proc 1987;62:125–134.
29. Creticos PS, Peters SP, Adkinson NF, Jr, et al: Peptide leukotriene release after antigen challenge in patients sensitive to ragweed. N Engl J Med 1984;310:1626–1630.
30. Meltzer EO, Malmstrom K, Lu S, et al: Concomitant montelukast and loratadine as treatment for seasonal allergic rhinitis: A randomized, placebo-controlled clinical trial. J Allergy Clin Immunol 2000;105:917–925.

*Ellen R. Wald*

# *10* Sinusitis

Infection of the paranasal sinuses is an extremely common medical condition in both children and adults. In this chapter, we discuss the structure and function of the paranasal sinuses, how they protect themselves from infection, and how general and local conditions may predispose an individual to sinusitis. The clinical presentation of sinusitis may be quite subtle; therefore, the clinician must have a high diagnostic index of suspicion. In this chapter, clinical symptoms, physical findings, and diagnostic aids—particularly imaging—are placed in perspective. Appropriate medical therapy is generally effective in treating acute sinusitis, recurrent acute sinusitis, and acute exacerbations of chronic sinusitis. On occasion, surgical intervention is required. Finally, a complication of sinusitis (namely, bronchial asthma) is discussed.

## STRUCTURE AND FUNCTION

There are four paired paranasal sinuses: ethmoid, maxillary, frontal, and sphenoid. The paranasal sinuses form as invaginations of the mucous membrane of the nasal cavity, so the mucous lining of the sinuses contains the same ciliated pseudostratified columnar epithelium, with goblet cells, as the nose. The relationship of the nose and paranasal sinuses is shown in Figure 10-1. The nose is divided in the midline by the nasal septum. From the lateral wall of the nose come three shelf-like structures designated as the inferior, middle, and—seen best on the sagittal section—superior turbinates. Beneath the middle and superior turbinates is a meatus that drains two or more of the paranasal sinuses. The maxillary,

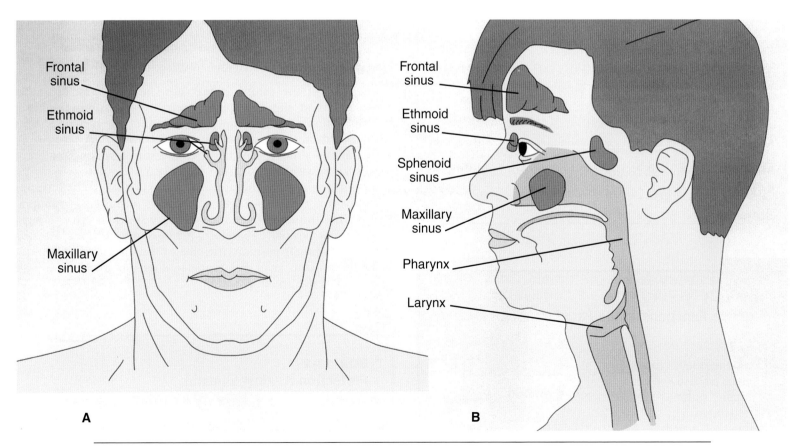

**Figure 10-1.** Frontal (*A*) and lateral (*B*) views of the head showing the anatomy of the four paired paranasal sinuses.

frontal, and anterior ethmoids drain to the middle meatus; the posterior ethmoids and sphenoid drain to the superior meatus; and only the lacrimal duct drains to the inferior meatus. It is important to note the outflow tract of the maxillary sinus high on the medial wall of that sinus. This awkward positioning of the outflow tract predisposes to maxillary sinusitis as a complication of a viral upper respiratory tract infection. The numerous ethmoid sinuses each drain by a tiny independent ostium into the middle meatus. The very narrow caliber of these draining ostia sets the stage for obstruction to occur easily and often during a viral upper respiratory tract infection.

Figure 10-2 shows the anatomy of the turbinates. *Part A* shows the inferior and middle turbinates in the coronal plane. The ethmoid bulla is the most inferior of the ethmoid air cells. If enlarged, it can impinge on the outflow tract of the maxillary sinus. The osteomeatal complex is the area between the inferior and middle turbinates; it represents the confluence of the drainage from the frontal, ethmoid, and maxillary sinuses. Within the osteomeatal complex, there are several areas in which mucosa abuts mucosa. When this occurs, ciliary function may be impaired even without actual physical obstruction. In *part B*, we see a sagittal view of the nose and paranasal sinuses, depicting the relationship of the inferior, middle, and superior turbinates, which originate from the lateral wall of the nose. Beneath the middle and superior turbinates, there is a meatus that drains two or more of the paranasal sinuses.

Table 10-1 shows the development of the paranasal sinuses. At birth, the maxillary sinus is a slitlike cavity running in an anteroposterior direction parallel to the middle third of the nose.

Gradually, the maxillary sinus increases in width and height until in the adult it holds a volume of 15 mL. The frontal sinuses develop embryologically from an anterior ethmoid and move from an infraorbital to supraorbital position sometime between 6 and 10 years of age. The frontal sinuses evaginate the frontal bone and may not be completely formed until late adolescence.

The precise functions of the paranasal sinuses are not clear (Box 10-1). Some suggestions have included a role in olfaction, voice resonance, production of protective mucus, dampening of sudden pressure changes in the nose during respiration, lessening of skull weight, and conditioning of the inhaled air by supplying warmth and humidification.

# PROTECTION AGAINST INFECTION

While secretory immunoglobulins and lysosomes play some role in the protection of the sinuses against infection, the major defense mechanism is an active mucociliary apparatus (Box 10-2). Micro-organisms and foreign particles that escape the filtering mechanism in the nose are trapped in the mucus of the sinuses. The underlying cilia then propel the mucous blanket or layer out of the sinus cavity through the ostium. Bacterial infection occurs when this self-cleansing mechanism becomes impaired. Mucus accumulates, stagnates, and becomes infected by bacteria that are normally present in the nose and nasopharynx. Retention of secretions in the paranasal sinuses may be due to several different factors:

- Swelling of the mucous membrane of the nose, leading to reduced patency of ostia
- A quantitative reduction of cilia, retardation of ciliary movement, and insufficient coordination of cilia, followed by reduced transport capacity
- Overproduction or a change in viscosity of secretions

Patency of the ostium is the most important factor in the development of sinusitis. Obstruction of the ostium results in a prolongation of sinus emptying time and gas exchange, thus leading to decreased oxygen tension and a negative pressure in the paranasal sinuses. This negative pressure favors aspiration of mucus laden with bacteria from the nose and nasopharynx.

Returning now to the previous discussion of paranasal sinus anatomy, it is easy to see why maxillary sinusitis is so common. The ostium, through which the maxillary sinus drains, is located in a superior position. Therefore, for discharge to occur into the nose in an upright position, the cilia of the maxillary sinus must move the mucous layer in a cephalad direction, against the force of gravity, to the draining ostium.

---

**TABLE 10-1**
**Development of the Paranasal Sinuses**

|  | Anatomic Appearance | Radiographic Appearance |
|---|---|---|
| Maxillary | 3rd–5th prenatal mo | Infancy |
| Ethmoid | 3rd–5th prenatal mo | Infancy |
| Frontal | 6th–12th postnatal mo | 6th–10th yr of life |
| Sphenoid | 3rd yr of life | 9th yr of life |

---

**BOX 10-1**
**Possible Functions of the Paranasal Sinuses**

Olfaction
Provide resonance to voice
Produce protective mucus
Dampen sudden pressure changes in nose during respiration
Lessen skull weight
Condition inhaled air with warmth and humidification

---

**BOX 10-2**
**Protection Against Sinusitis**

Mucus of the proper viscosity
Adequate number of actively beating cilia
Patent ostia

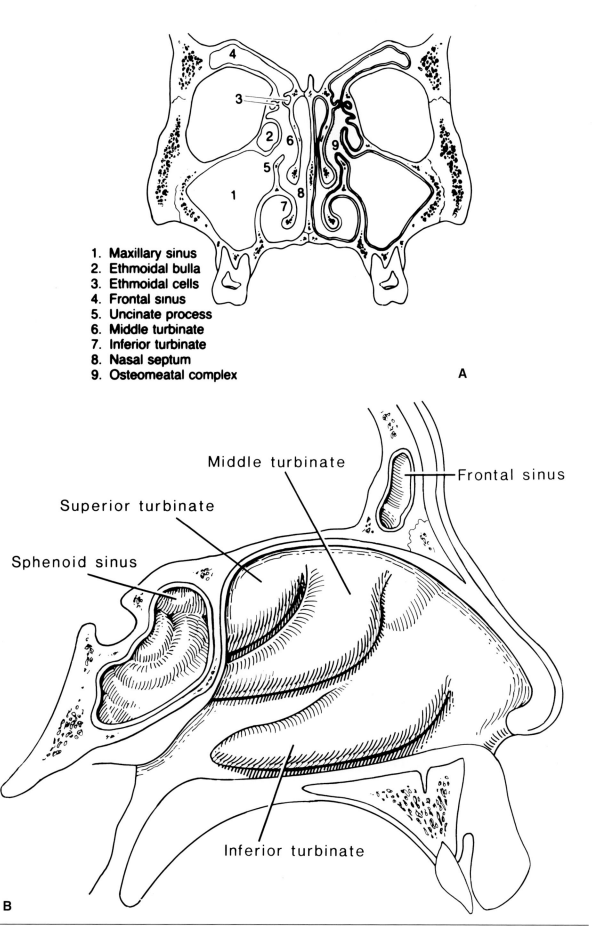

1. **Maxillary sinus**
2. **Ethmoidal bulla**
3. **Ethmoidal cells**
4. **Frontal sinus**
5. **Uncinate process**
6. **Middle turbinate**
7. **Inferior turbinate**
8. **Nasal septum**
9. **Osteomeatal complex**

**A**

**B**

**Figure 10-2.** Anatomy of the nasal turbinates. *A,* Coronal diagram of relation of nasal turbinates and sinus anatomy. *B,* Sagittal diagram of relation of nasal turbinates and sinus anatomy. (From Wald ER: Sinusitis. In Brook I (ed): Atlas of Infectious Disease, vol IV: Upper Respiratory and Head and Neck Infections.)

Given the mechanism that protects the sinuses against infection, it is now appropriate to look at Table 10-2 for a list of those conditions that may predispose an individual to sinusitis. Heading the list of local conditions are upper respiratory infection and allergic rhinitis. Both of these conditions result in edema of the nasal mucosa and obstruction of the ostium, with a decrease in action of the mucociliary apparatus in the sinuses. Negative pressure in the sinuses set the stage for secondary bacterial infection and the conversion of mucus into mucopus. Mucopus further impairs ciliary function and increases the swelling around the ostium when it discharges into the nose, thus perpetuating a vicious cycle. There are also other systemic factors that serve to predispose an individual to sinusitis, such as cystic fibrosis, immune disorders, and immotile cilia. Additional factors predisposing to sinusitis by sinus ostial obstruction include deviated nasal septum, nasal polyps, tumor, foreign body, and enlarged adenoids.

## MICROBIOLOGY OF SINUSITIS

Knowledge of the microbiology of sinusitis (Table 10-3) has come from maxillary sinus aspirates obtained by direct antral puncture or direct sampling during surgery.[1] Nasal smears and cultures are not helpful in predicting the microbiology of sinus infection.

Part one of Table 10-3 shows the microbiology of acute sinusitis in adults. *Streptococcus pneumoniae* and *Haemophilus influenzae* account for about one half of all cases in adults as well as in children. Less-frequent causes include *Staphylococcus aureus, Streptococcus pyogenes*, rhinovirus, influenza virus, and anaerobic bacteria.

Part two of Table 10-3 shows the microbiology of acute sinusitis in children. The data are derived from maxillary sinus aspirations performed on 50 symptomatic patients. *S. pneumoniae* is the most common cause of acute sinusitis in all age groups, both children and adults, with *H. influenzae* (nontypeable) being the next most common cause in both groups. *Moraxella catarrhalis* (previously known as *Neisseria catarrhalis* or *Branhamella catarrhalis*) is also a frequent maxillary sinus isolate in children.

Currently, nearly 100% of *M. catarrhalis* are β-lactamase positive. Staphylococci and anaerobes are less frequently recovered from patients with acute sinusitis. Viral agents, recovered from maxillary sinus aspirates in approximately 20% of patients, include adenovirus, parainfluenza, and influenza virus.

## HISTORY AND PHYSICAL EXAMINATION

Figure 10-3 shows the three clinical presentations of acute sinusitis that must be differentiated from that of a simple uncomplicated viral upper respiratory tract infection.[2] In the patient with a viral upper respiratory tract infection, fever, if present, occurs early in the illness, usually in concert with other constitutional symptoms such as myalgia and headache. The fever resolves in a day or two, and then the respiratory symptoms become prominent. Respiratory symptoms such as nasal discharge (of any quality—serous, mucoid, or purulent), nasal congestion, and cough peak in 5 to 7 days. Although the patient may not be symptom free at 10 days, the symptoms usually have diminished and improvement is

---

**TABLE 10-2**
**Factors Predisposing to Sinusitis via Sinus Ostial Obstruction**

| Mucosal Swelling | Mechanical Obstruction |
| --- | --- |
| Systemic disorder | Choanal atresia |
|   Viral URI | Deviated septum |
|   Allergic inflammation | Nasal polyp |
|   Cystic fibrosis | Foreign body |
|   Immune disorders | Tumor |
|   Immotile cilia | Hypertrophied adenoids |
| Local insult | |
|   Facial trauma | |
|   Swimming or diving | |
|   Rhinitis medicamentosa | |

URI, upper respiratory tract infection.

---

**TABLE 10-3**
**Microbiology of Acute Maxillary Sinusitis in Adults**

| Bacterial Species | Percentage |
| --- | --- |
| *Streptococcus pneumoniae* | 31 |
| *Haemophilus influenzae* (unencapsulated) | 21 |
| Gram-negative bacteria | 9 |
| Anaerobic bacteria | 6 |
| Combined *S. pneumoniae* and *H. influenzae* | 5 |
| *Moraxella catarrhalis* | 2 |
| **Virus Species** | |
| Rhinovirus | 15 |
| Influenza virus | 5 |

**Microbiology of Acute Maxillary Sinusitis in Children**

| Bacterial Species | Percentage |
| --- | --- |
| *S. pneumoniae* | 30 |
| *H. influenzae* (50% of isolates β-lactamase positive) | 20 |
| *M. catarrhalis* (100% of isolates β-lactamase positive) | 20 |
| Other | 6 |
| Sterile | 30 |
| **Virus Species** | 10 |

apparent. In patients with "severe" acute sinusitis, the fever persists and the nasal discharge is purulent (thick, colored, and opaque). In patients with "persistent acute sinusitis," fever is low grade or absent, but respiratory symptoms (nasal discharge of any quality, daytime cough, or both) persist beyond 10 days without evidence of improvement. In "worsening" sinusitis, a patient who was beginning to recover suddenly becomes worse, as manifest by fever and an increase in respiratory symptoms (cough and nasal

discharge). Box 10-3 shows the ways in which the diagnosis of sinusitis may be suspected and confirmed.

If treatment is not initiated or is only partially effective, then acute sinusitis may enter a subacute or chronic phase. A patient's lack of pain or systemic symptoms makes the diagnosis of chronic sinusitis difficult for the physician to make on history alone. The patient with chronic sinusitis generally presents with nasal stuffiness, hyposmia, purulent nasal and postnasal secretions, sore throat, fetid breath, malaise, and on occasion, cough. On physical examination, an edematous and hyperemic nasal mucosa is generally bathed in mucopus (Box 10-4).

## DIAGNOSTIC TECHNIQUES

### NASAL SECRETIONS

Nasal secretions in acute sinusitis may be of any quality—thick, thin, serous, mucoid, or purulent. The technique of fiberoptic nasopharyngoscopy (Figs. 10-4 to 10-6) affords an excellent opportunity for better visualization of the draining ostia of infected sinuses and for obtaining specimens for culture. However, there are only a few studies correlating the results of sinus aspirate and cultures obtained from the middle meatus.

---

**BOX 10-3**
**Diagnosis of Sinusitis**

History
Physical examination
Fiberoptic rhinopharyngoscopy
Images
    Plain radiographs
    Computed tomography (CT) scan
    Ultrasound
Sinus aspiration

---

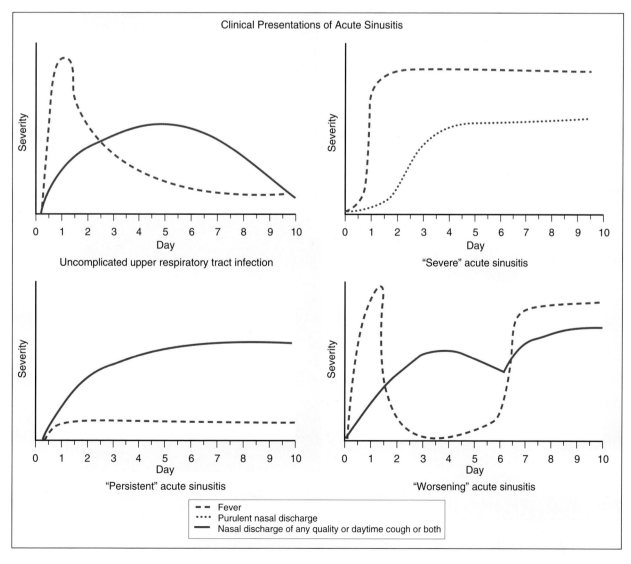

**Figure 10-3.** Three clinical presentations of acute sinusitis (*B, C, D*) that must be differentiated from that of a simple uncomplicated viral upper respiratory tract infection (*A*).

## RADIOGRAPHS

A commonly used adjunct in the diagnosis of sinusitis is radiography. The occipitomental, or Waters, view—with the head slightly tilted back—affords the best image of the maxillary sinuses. The occiptofrontal, or Caldwell, view demonstrates both the ethmoid and frontal sinuses. The sphenoid sinus is seen on the lateral view. A normal Waters view is shown in Figure 10-7, demonstrating the total radiolucency of the maxillary sinuses with a thin mucoperiostium. Studies correlating radiographic findings with direct antral puncture have shown positive aspirates (bacteria in high density) with mucosal thickening of more than 4 mm in children and 5 to 8 mm in adults (Fig. 10-8), air-fluid levels (Fig. 10-9), and diffuse opacification (Fig. 10-10).

Special mention should be made of sinus radiographs in children. Contrary to an earlier belief, crying is not a cause of abnormal maxillary sinus radiographs in children older than 1 year of age; in children older than 1 year, abnormal sinus radiographs are generally related to inflammation of the sinuses secondary to viral or bacterial infection.

### BOX 10-4
### Presenting Findings in Chronic Sinusitis

Nasal obstruction
Purulent nasal and/or paranasal drainage
Co-existent otitis media (in children)
Hyposmia
Fetid breath
Sore throat
Malaise
Cough
Wheeze

## COMPUTED TOMOGRAPHY

It is accepted that computed tomography (CT) scans can delineate sinus pathology more clearly than plain radiography, revealing the extent of disease and bony destruction and distinguishing opacification from membrane thickening (Fig. 10-11). CT scans of patients with normal sinus radiographs may show areas of anterior ethmoidal disease (Fig. 10-12). A four-slice coronal CT scan of the sinuses has been shown to provide excellent views of the paranasal sinuses. The cost has been reduced so dramatically that in the future it will undoubtedly replace plain radiography in the diagnosis of sinusitis. Indications for sinus CT scans are listed in Box 10-5.

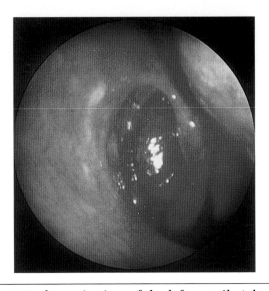

**Figure 10-5.** Endoscopic view of the left nostril. A large polyp arising from the hiatus semilunaris fills the anterior portion of the left middle meatus. (Courtesy of Dr. David W. Kennedy, University of Pennsylvania, Philadelphia, PA.)

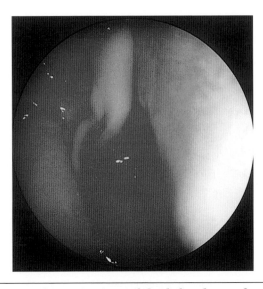

**Figure 10-6.** Endoscopic view of the left sphenoethmoidal recess. Pus is seen draining from the area of the sphenoid sinus ostium. (Courtesy of Dr. David W. Kennedy, University of Pennsylvania, Philadelphia, PA.)

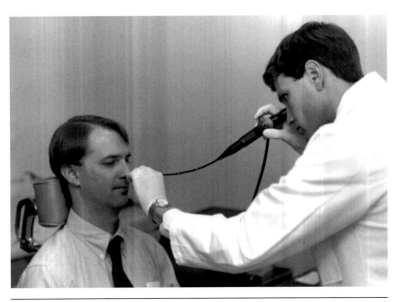

**Figure 10-4.** Insertion of a fiberoptic nasopharyngoscope.

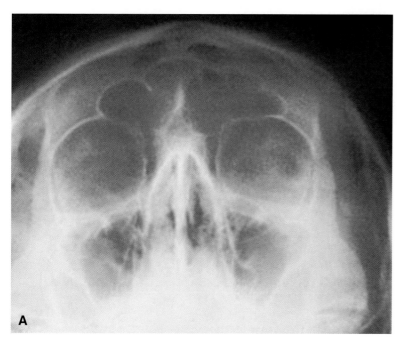

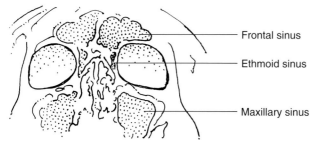

- Frontal sinus
- Ethmoid sinus
- Maxillary sinus

**Figure 10-7.** *A,* Radiographic Waters view of normal paranasal sinuses. The frontal, ethmoid, and maxillary sinuses are radiolucent, and the mucoperiostium is thin. *B,* Diagram of radiograph (*A*) with frontal, ethmoid, and maxillary sinuses identified.

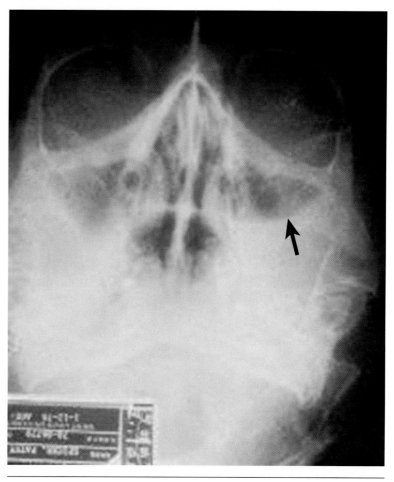

**Figure 10-9.** Waters view of the sinuses. An air-fluid level (*arrow*) is seen in the left maxillary sinus.

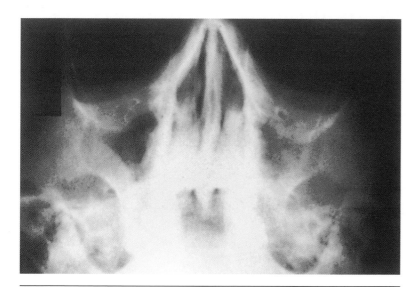

**Figure 10-8.** Waters view of the sinuses. There is marked mucoperiostial thickening of both maxillary sinuses.

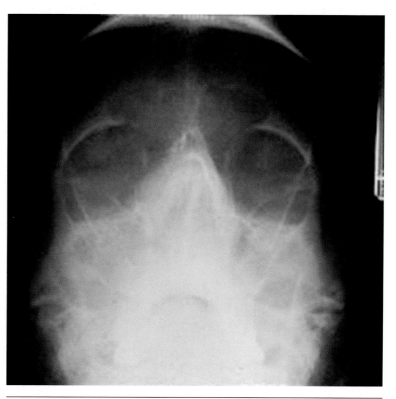

**Figure 10-10.** Waters view of the sinuses. Both maxillary sinuses are opacified.

It is essential to remember that images of any kind (plain x-rays, CT, or magnetic resonance imaging) cannot stand alone as evidence of sinus disease. These studies can only be confirmatory in patients with signs and symptoms suggesting the diagnosis. There are numerous examples of studies in which significant abnormalities have been observed when CT of the sinuses has been done on patients with an active upper respiratory infection or recently recovered from an upper respiratory infection. The images disclose abnormalities of the mucosa but do not inform regarding the etiology of the mucositis, that is, whether it was caused by virus, bacteria, allergy, or chemical inflammation.

## SINUS ASPIRATION

Sinus aspiration is the gold standard for diagnosis of acute sinusitis (Fig. 10-13). The trocar is passed beneath the inferior turbinate and across the lateral nasal wall. Secretions are aspirated into the syringe and sent to the laboratory for Gram's stain and culture. The area beneath the inferior turbinate must be sterilized so that the culture is not contaminated by normal nasal flora. An infection is defined as the recovery of bacteria in very high colony counts of at least $10^4$ colony-forming units per mL. However, aspiration is only performed on selected patients who are either seriously

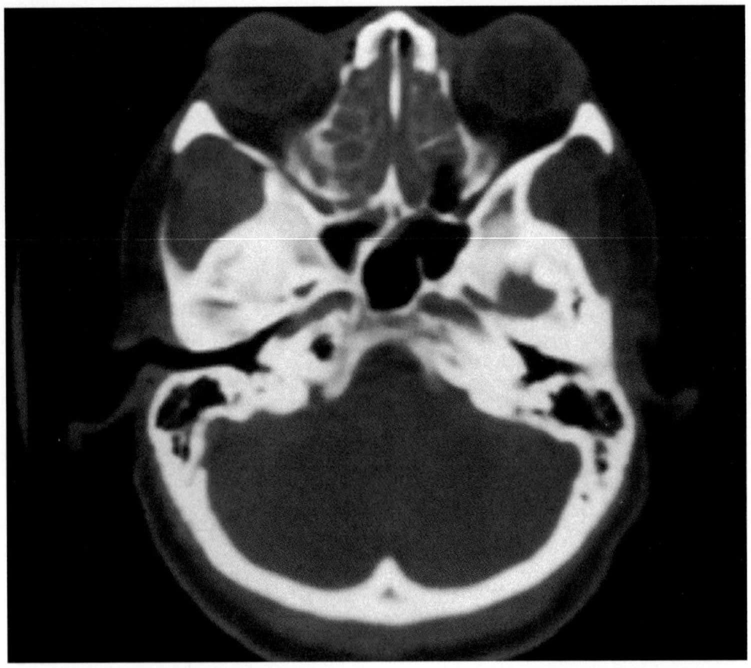

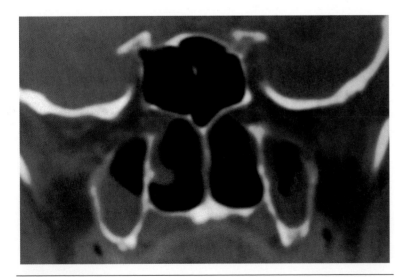

**Figure 10-11.** Transaxial computed tomography scan. Both ethmoid sinuses are opacified.

> **BOX 10-5**
> **Indications for Sinus Computed Tomography**
>
> Failure to respond to therapy
> To demonstrate anatomic abnormalities
> To localize disease for possible surgery
> To evaluate for infectious complications

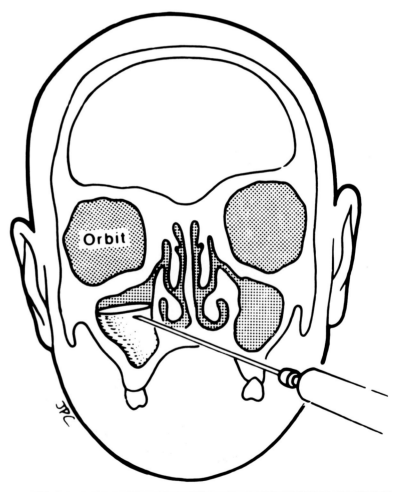

**Figure 10-12.** Coronal computed tomography scan showing air-fluid level in right maxillary sinus and marked mucoperiosteal thickening in the left maxillary sinus.

**Figure 10-13.** Sinus aspiration. (From Wald ER: Sinusitis. In Brook I (ed): Atlas of Infectious Disease, vol IV: Upper Respiratory and Head and Neck Infections.)

ill or likely to harbor unusual microbiologic agents in their sinus cavities. Aspiration is indicated in patients who fail to respond to antimicrobial therapy, those who present with serious intracranial complications, or immunosuppressed persons in whom a broad range of pathogens may be causative (Box 10-6).

## ANCILLARY LABORATORY TESTS

For resistant chronic sinusitis, other diagnostic tests must be considered. Humoral immune deficiency can be diagnosed by quantitation of serum immunoglobulins, specific serum antibody responses, and immunoglobulin (Ig) G subclasses. Underlying allergy can be determined by appropriate allergy skin testing. Information on the causative pathogens of chronic sinusitis can only be gained by sinus aspirates, not by nasopharyngeal culture (Box 10-7).

# MEDICAL TREATMENT

Medical therapy of sinusitis includes analgesics and antibiotics for the control of infection (Box 10-8). Adjunctive therapies may include topical or oral decongestants in selected cases. Topical decongestants may help greatly in promoting sinus drainage but may cause the so-called rebound phenomenon if used chronically. In this situation, the medication causes immediate vasoconstriction. After this subsides, the resultant vasodilation and consequent nasal congestion may exceed that which was present initially.

Longer-acting preparations used in the prescribed fashion at 12-hour intervals do not cause the vasodilating rebound phenomenon over several days' usage. In some cases of hyperplastic rhinosinusitis, topical or systemic corticosteroids over a short period may be indicated. Non-specific aids include humidification and local irrigation or nasal saline wash.

The antibiotic of first choice for treatment of uncomplicated acute sinusitis is amoxicillin because it is effective most of the time, safe, inexpensive, and narrow spectrum.[3] In many instances, bacteria responsible for sinusitis have become resistant to penicillin and cephalosporins by producing β-lactamase enzymes that destroy the β-lactam nucleus of these antibiotics or by alteration of penicillin-binding proteins. Clavulanic acid, an inhibitor of the β-lactamase enzyme, has been introduced in combination with amoxicillin. Other antibiotics useful in infections due to β-lactamase–producing organisms are cefuroxime, cefprozil, and cefdinir. Clarithromycin and azithromycin can be used in patients with type 1 hypersensitivity to β-lactams. The duration of treatment has received little systematic study. Antibiotics should be prescribed for at least 10 days or until the patient is symptom free plus 7 days, whichever is longer.

# SURGICAL TREATMENT

Persistent or recurrent episodes of sinusitis, despite appropriate medical therapy, necessitate consideration of surgical intervention. The tasks of the otolaryngologist are to relieve the obstruction of the ostia, resect inflamed or infected tissues, and provide an airway with drainage for all nasal and sinus compartments.[4] A

---

**BOX 10-6**
**Indications for Sinus Aspiration**

Suppurative complications of acute sinusitis
  Orbital
  Central nervous system
Failure to improve on appropriate antimicrobial therapy
Severe symptoms or toxicity
Immunocompromised host

---

**BOX 10-7**
**Ancillary Laboratory Tests for Chronic Sinusitis**

**Immunologic studies**
Quantitative immunoglobulins
Specific antibody responses: diphtheria, tetanus, *Streptococcus pneumoniae*
IgG subclasses

**Allergy skin tests**

**Bacteriologic studies: Antral puncture**

IgG, immunoglobulin G.

---

**BOX 10-8**
**Medical Treatment of Sinusitis**

**Analgesics**
Nonspecific—fluids, rest, steam inhalation, hot washcloths to nasal area

**Antibiotics**
Amoxicillin
Amoxicillin/K Clavulanate
Cefdinir
Cefuroxime
Cefpodoxime
Clarithromycin
Azithromycin

**Consider decongestants**
Topical—oxymetazoline, phenylephrine
Oral—pseudoephedrine, phenylephrine

**Consider corticosteroids in patients with underlying allergic disease**
Topical—beclomethasone, flunisolide, budesonide, fluticasone for patients with underlying allergic disease
Oral—prednisone for patients with underlying allergic disease

variety of surgical procedures have been used for the treatment of sinusitis, but functional endoscopic surgery has emerged as the technique of choice in most instances. The usefulness of the technique is predicated on the evidence that the middle meatus–anterior ethmoid complex (osteomeatal unit) is heavily involved in the pathogenesis of sinusitis. The availability of endoscopes with a variety of angles of view has greatly expanded the usefulness of this technique. Its advantage is that minimal trauma to the normal nasal sinus structures occurs with the conservative removal of diseased tissue, resulting in a quicker and more complete return to the natural physiology and mucociliary clearance and function of the sinuses.

An overall approach to the management of sinusitis is given in the flow diagram (Fig. 10-14).

# SINUSITIS AND ASTHMA

The relationship of nasal and paranasal sinus disease to bronchial asthma has been recognized for many years. Numerous observations have been made of the increased incidence of radiographically demonstrated sinusitis in both childhood and adult asthmatics. This, however, does not necessarily mean that there is a cause-and-effect relationship. A large number of studies performed both in experimental animals and humans have demon-strated that reflex bronchoconstriction can result from stimulation of receptors in the nose and nasopharynx. This could account for the clinical association of sinusitis and asthma.

This association has been examined both in children and adults. Rachelefsky and colleagues,[6] in a study of 48 children with

**Figure 10-14.** Management of sinusitis. CT, computed tomography.

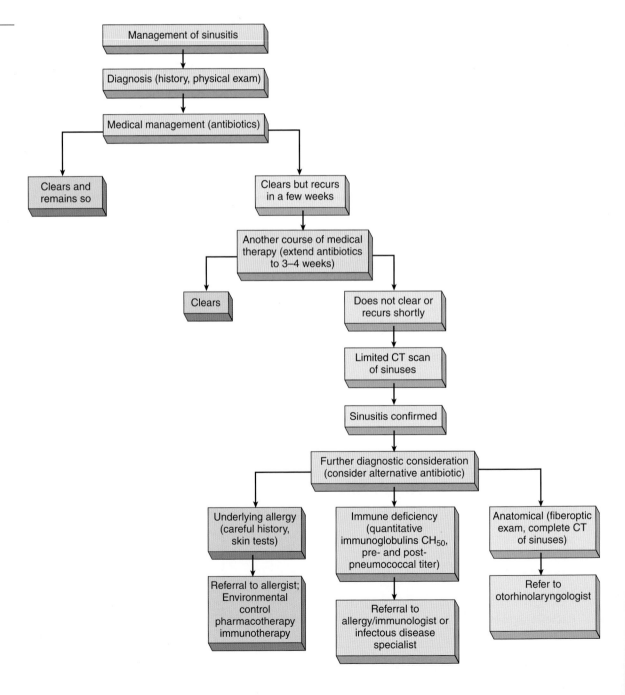

**TABLE 10-4**

Disease Characterization Before and After Treatment for Sinusitis in 48 Children with Asthma

| Characteristic | Before (%) | After (%) |
|---|---|---|
| Cough | 100 | 29 |
| Wheeze | 100 | 15 |
| Normal PFT | 0 | 67 |
| Bronchodilator use | 100 | 21 |

Adapted with permission from Rachelefsky GS, Katz RM, Siegel SC: Chronic sinus disease with associated reactive airway disease in children. Pediatrics 1984;73:526. PFT, pulmonary function tests.

**BOX 10-9**

## Characteristics of Adult Patients with Sinusitis and Asthma

Sinusitis preceded asthma in more than 90%.
Two thirds were nonatopic, based on history and skin tests.
More than half were aspirin sensitive.
More than half were receiving corticosteroids.
Two thirds noted improvement in their asthmatic state after medical and/or surgical treatment of sinusitis.

sinusitis and asthma, showed that 70% were able to discontinue taking bronchodilators after resolution of their sinusitis through antimicrobial therapy (Table 10-4). Characteristics of adult patients with sinus disease and asthma are seen in Box 10-9.[7] In the great majority of cases, asthma historically followed the occurrence of sinusitis. Most of the patients were nonatopic and more than half were sensitive to aspirin. A clinical clue to the association of sinusitis and asthma is steroid dependency, and this should prompt the clinician to consider underlying sinusitis.

In summary, there is suggestive evidence, both in children and adults, that medical or surgical therapy of sinusitis results in significant improvement in the asthmatic state. In any instance of corticosteroid-dependent asthma, consideration should be given to underlying sinusitis.

## REFERENCES

1. Wald ER: Microbiology of acute and chronic sinusitis in children and adults. Am J Med Sci 1998;316:13–20.
2. Nash DR, Wald ER: Pediatric sinusitis. Pediatr Rev 2001;22:111–116.
3. American Academy of Pediatrics. Subcommittee on Management of Sinusitis and Committee on Quality Improvement: Clinical practice guideline: Management of sinusitis. Pediatrics 2001;108:798–808.
4. Sinus and Allergy Health Partnership: Antimicrobial treatment guidelines for acute bacterial rhinosinusitis. Supplement to Otolaryngol Head Neck Surg 2004;130:1–45.
5. Orlandi RR, Kennedy DW: Surgical management of rhinosinusitis. Am J Med Sci 1998;316:29–38.
6. Rachelefsky GS, Katz RM, Siegel SC: Chronic sinus disease with associated reactive airway disease in children. Pediatrics 1984;73:526.
7. Slavin RG: Complications of allergic rhinitis: Implications for sinusitis and asthma. J Allergy Clin Immunol 1998;101:S357–S360.

*Ellen Mandel, Margaretha Casselbrant, and Philip Fireman*

# *11* Otitis Media

Otitis media (OM) is a very common disease characterized by acute or chronic inflammation of the middle-ear mucosa.[1] The term *OM* includes acute otitis media (AOM) and OM with effusion (OME). The diagnosis of AOM is usually based on the finding of at least one symptom and one otoscopic sign of middle-ear inflammation. Symptoms include fever, earache (or recent onset of ear tugging), and irritability. Otoscopic signs include erythema and/or white opacification (other than from scarring) of the tympanic membrane, fullness or bulging of the tympanic membrane, a white fluid level, and otorrhea from a perforation of a previously intact tympanic membrane. OME is defined as asymptomatic middle-ear effusion (MEE; i.e., without the symptoms of inflammation found in AOM) and may be diagnosed on routine examination as an occult condition, perhaps following a subclinical or protracted inflammation of the middle ear. OME may be a recurrent or chronic condition and is frequently recognized as a sequela of AOM. Many synonyms have been used during the past 50 years to designate OME, including *serous OM, secretory OM, mucoid otitis, "glue ear," nonsuppurative OM, catarrhal otitis, tubotympanic catarrh,* and *allergic OM.* These descriptive terms have created much confusion. It is difficult to determine by history and visual inspection of the tympanic membrane alone the specific characteristics of the middle-ear effusion. Without a diagnostic aspiration, the clinician cannot be certain whether the fluid is serous, mucoid, or purulent, and without a culture of the aspirate, the microbial characteristics of an effusion cannot be identified. Therefore, these descriptive terms should be discarded, and the generic term, *OME,* is recommended.

The possibility that allergy contributes to OM is not a new concept; its role has been suggested for years.[2] Therefore, this disease is of considerable interest to allergists. If a causal relationship between allergy and middle-ear disease were to be established, then one would expect that antiallergic therapy would reduce the morbidity associated with OM. Such therapy might be able to prevent or resolve the disease and thereby reduce the time with hearing loss and prevent possible speech and language delays that may result in infants and children from the presence of fluid in the middle-ear cavity. This chapter reviews the history, physical findings, and laboratory studies associated with OM and develops the concept that OM is a multifactorial disease. As illustrated in Figure 11-1, not only infection and eustachian tube dysfunction but also allergy and host-defense defects must be considered in understanding the basis of OM.

## STRUCTURE AND FUNCTION OF THE MIDDLE-EAR SYSTEM

Otitis media appears to be related to abnormal functioning of the eustachian tube.[3] Understanding and diagnosing this disease requires familiarity with the anatomy and physiology of the upper airway, which is made up of the nasal cavity, nasopharynx, eustachian tube, middle ear, and mastoid air cells (Fig. 11-2). The eustachian tube provides an anatomic communication between the nasopharynx and the middle ear and is in a unique position to effect changes in the middle ear secondary to reactions in the nose. In relation to the middle ear and the nasopharynx, the eustachian tube may be considered to be analogous in part to the bronchial tree in relation to the lung and nasopharynx. Like mucosa elsewhere in the respiratory tract, the mucosa lining the eustachian tube contains mucus-producing cells, ciliated cells, plasma cells, and mast cells. Unlike the bronchial tree, the eustachian tube is usually collapsed and thus closed to the nasopharynx and its contents (see Fig. 11-2B). Active opening of the eustachian tube

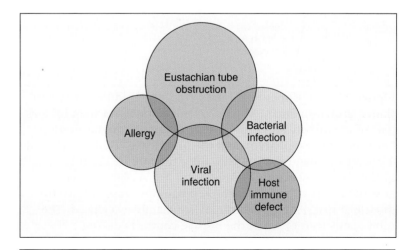

**Figure 11-1.** Pathogenesis of otitis media with illustration of the proposed interactions among eustachian tube obstruction, viral infection, bacterial infection, host immune defect, and allergy.

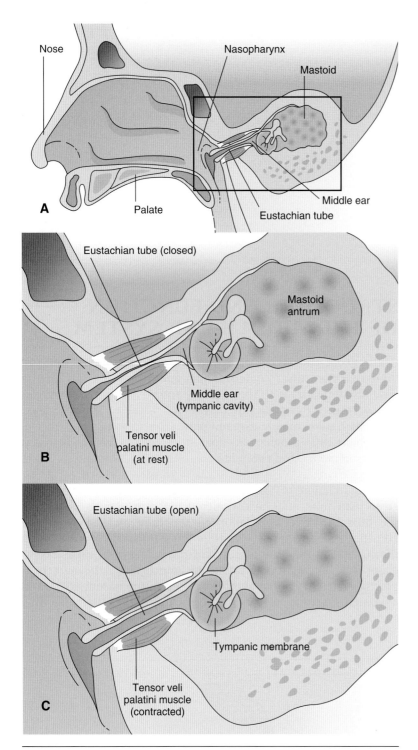

**Figure 11-2.** *A,* Upper respiratory tract and middle-ear system (latter shown in *insert*). The *insert* shows the eustachian tube as part of the airway and provides an anatomic communication between the nasopharynx and the middle ear. *B* and *C,* The role of the eustachian tube in ventilating the middle ear is shown in the enlargements of the *insert* from *part A.* Tubal function is governed in part by the tensor veli palatini muscle. With this muscle at rest *(part B),* the tube is almost always closed. The tube opens *(part C)* when the muscle contracts during swallowing, yawning, crying, or sneezing. Obstruction of the tube plays a central role in the pathogenesis of otitis media. (Adapted with permission from Fireman P: New concepts in the pathogenesis of otitis media with effusion. Immunol Allergy Clin Noth Am 1987;7:133–150.)

is accomplished by contraction of the tensor veli palatini muscle during swallowing, yawning, or crying (see Fig. 11-2C). In this regard, the eustachian tube, like the bronchial airway, serves several physiologic functions—protection, drainage, and ventilation: protection from nasopharyngeal secretions, drainage into the nasopharynx of secretions produced within the middle ear, and ventilation of the middle ear to equilibrate air pressure with atmospheric pressure (Fig. 11-3).

# EPIDEMIOLOGY

Otitis media is a worldwide health problem; in the United States, it is the most common diagnosis in physician office practices in children younger than 15 years. While not as common as in young children, OM does occur in older children and adults. Approximately 3% to 15% of OM patients referred to otolaryngology clinics are adults. Various studies have shown that from 20% to 62% of children have had at least one episode of AOM by the age of 1 year; by 3 years of age, 50% to 84% have had at least one episode.[4] Recurrent episodes of AOM are common. By 1 year of age, three or more episodes of AOM have been reported in 10% to 19% of children. By ages 3, 5, and 7 years, three or more episodes of AOM have been found in 50%, 65%, and 75% of children, respectively. The incidence of OME, which is by definition "asymptomatic," is more difficult to ascertain but has been estimated in various populations using tympanometry alone or tympanometry and otoscopy. In a study of 4-year-old Danish children, 32% of ears were diagnosed with OME at least once on five screenings during a 1-year period.[5] In the United States, MEE was found at least once in 22% of 111 school-age children (5 to 12 years of age) on monthly examinations consisting of otoscopy and tympanometry.[6]

Various risk factors are considered important in the occurrence and persistence of middle-ear disease. These factors can be viewed as *host related* (age, sex, race, craniofacial abnormalities, genetic predisposition, allergy, and immunocompetence) or *environmental* (upper respiratory infection, seasonality, daycare, siblings, tobacco smoke exposure, breastfeeding, pacifier use, and socioeconomic status) (Box 11-1). The highest incidence of AOM occurs between 6 and 11 months of age. Children whose first episode of AOM occurs before 6 months of age are more likely to have recurrent AOM. Male children have been found in some studies to have a higher incidence of AOM and more recurrent episodes than female children, but this has not been consistent in all studies. Some populations, such as Native Americans and Native Alaskans, have higher rates of middle-ear disease. African-American children have been thought to have lower rates of OM than white American children, but when studies have examined children of both races who came from the same socioeconomic background, there was little or no difference in their experience with OM.[7] Children with craniofacial abnormalities, such as cleft palate and Down syndrome, have high rates of middle-ear disease. A genetic component to OM has been found using twin studies, which found a higher concordance of disease histories in monozygotic twins compared with dizygotic twins.[8] Other evidence for a genetic component includes familial clustering of OM and the finding of certain histocompatibility locus antigens (HLAs) more frequently in children with recurrent AOM or chronic OME than in children without those problems.

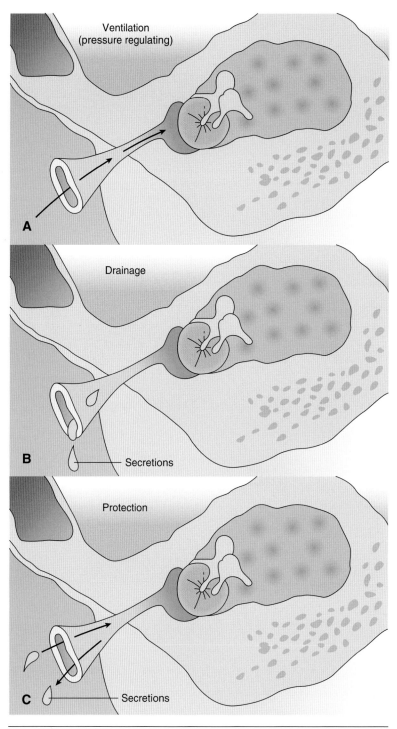

**Figure 11-3.** Physiologic functions of the eustachian tube as related to the middle ear. *A,* Opening of the eustachian tube provides for ventilation of the middle ear and equilibrates middle-ear pressure with atmospheric pressure. *B,* Opening of the tube allows for drainage and clearance of middle-ear secretions. *C,* In the closed state, the eustachian tube protects the middle ear from nasopharyngeal secretions. These functions are analogous to those of the bronchial tree. Like other respiratory tract mucosa, the lining of the eustachian tube contains mast cells, lymphocytes, macrophages, and plasma cells. (Adapted with permission from Bluestone CD, Doyle WJ: Anatomy and physiology of eustachian tube and middle ear related to otitis media. J Allergy Clin Immunol 1988;81:997–1006.)

Environmental factors figure prominently in the occurrence of middle-ear disease. AOM and OME have long been known to occur most frequently in the fall and winter months, paralleling the occurrence of viral upper respiratory tract infection (URI).[9] Viral URI has been shown to be a risk factor for eustachian tube dysfunction and the development of OM. URI associated with respiratory syncytial virus, influenza virus, or adenovirus often precedes episodes of AOM. Children attending daycare have been shown to be at higher risk for the development of OM than children cared for at home and also are more likely to undergo tympanostomy tube insertion.[10] Furthermore, birth order has been shown to be associated with risk for OM and, like daycare, is probably a matter of exposure. Firstborn children have lower rates of OM and shorter duration of MEE than do children with older siblings. The relationship of passive cigarette smoke exposure to the development of OM is not clear, but higher rates of middle-ear disease have been found with higher levels of cotinine (a metabolite of nicotine and a marker for smoke exposure), rather than with exposure measured by questionnaire given to parents. Pacifier use also has been linked to higher rates of OM. Breastfeeding has been found in most studies to be protective for OM, but the duration of breastfeeding necessary for this protective effect is not known. The effect of socioeconomic status, another factor frequently mentioned in connection with the development of OM, is unclear.

# PATHOGENESIS

As illustrated in Figure 11-1, eustachian tube dysfunction and infection, both bacterial and viral, are the best understood etiologies.[11] In addition, allergies and host-defense defects may participate either directly or indirectly in the development of OM.[12,13]

---

**BOX 11-1**
**Risk Factors for Otitis Media in Children**

**Host Related**
Age
Sex
Race
Craniofacial abnormalities
Genetic predisposition
Allergy
Immunocompetence

**Environmental**
Upper respiratory infection
Seasonality
Day care
Siblings
Tobacco smoke exposure
Breast feeding
Pacifier use
Socioeconomic status

## EUSTACHIAN TUBE DYSFUNCTION

In normal tubal function, intermittent opening of the tube maintains near-ambient pressure in the middle-ear cavity. When active opening of the tube is inadequate to overcome tubal resistance, the tube remains collapsed, resulting in progressively negative middle-ear pressure. If negative middle-ear pressure persists and effective ventilation does not occur, transudation of sterile middle-ear effusion into the tympanum can result, as a consequence of the constant absorption of nitrogen by the middle-ear epithelium. Since tubal opening is possible in a middle ear with effusion, aspiration of nasopharyngeal secretions might occur, thus creating the clinical condition in which persistent effusion and recurrent AOM occur together. Moderate-to-high negative middle-ear pressures have also been identified by tympanometry in many children who have no MEE, probably as a result of tubal opening that occurs but is infrequent. Persistently high negative middle-ear pressure with severe retraction or collapse of the tympanic membrane has been termed *atelectasis of the tympanic membrane;* effusion may or may not be present. Thus, abnormal eustachian tube function may predispose the middle ear to atelectasis, infection, or effusion.

## EUSTACHIAN TUBE OBSTRUCTION

Two types of eustachian tube obstruction could result in acute or chronic OM—mechanical or functional obstruction.[14] Figure 11-4 shows a classification of common conditions associated with eustachian tube obstruction. Intrinsic mechanical obstruction may result from the inflammation of infection or allergy, whereas extrinsic obstruction may result from enlarged adenoids or tumors. Experimentally, allergic rhinitis provoked in patients with a history of allergy has been associated with the development of eustachian tube obstruction.[15] This obstruction, related to edema and inflammation of the posterior nasopharynx, could be both extrinsic and intrinsic. A persistent collapse of the eustachian tube during swallowing may result in functional obstruction, which appears to be related to increased tubal compliance, an inefficient active opening mechanism by the tensor veli palatini muscle, or both. Functional eustachian tube obstruction is common in infants and younger children, as the amount and stiffness of the cartilage support of the eustachian tube are less than in older children and adults. Also, there appear to be marked age differences in the angulation of the craniofacial base, which renders the tensor veli palatini muscle less efficient before puberty. The pathogenesis of MEE in infants and children with cleft palate is related to a functional obstruction of the eustachian tube.

## INFECTION

Bacteria have been cultured from 70% to 80% of MEEs in children with AOM and have been shown to be similar to those found in the nasopharynx (Fig. 11-5A).[16] *Streptococcus pneumoniae* has been cultured from approximately 35% and is clearly the most common infectious agent in all age groups; approximately 30% to 50% are resistant to penicillin, but this figure varies with the population studied. *Haemophilus influenzae*, nontypable, has been found in approximately 23% of acute middle-ear effusions, of which about 30% to 45% are β-lactamase–producing. In the past,

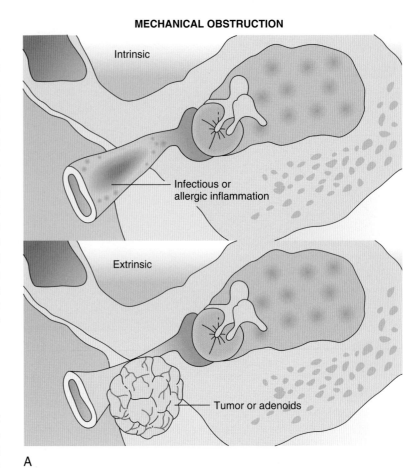

**MECHANICAL OBSTRUCTION**

Intrinsic

Infectious or allergic inflammation

Extrinsic

Tumor or adenoids

A

**FUNCTIONAL OBSTRUCTION**

"Floppy tube"

Poor TVP function

B

**Figure 11-4.** Pathophysiology of eustachian tube dysfunction, showing that the tube may be abnormally patent or obstructed. This illustrates several types of eustachian tube problems that contribute to MEE. *A,* Mechanical obstruction may be either intrinsic, due to inflammation produced by infection or allergy, or extrinsic, produced by peritubular conditions such as enlarged adenoids or tumors. *B,* Functional obstruction, common in infants, leads to failure of the eustachian tube to open during swallowing. This can be due to persistent collapse of the tubal cartilage due to lack of stiffness of the cartilage ("too floppy") or to poor tensor veli palatini muscle function. (Adapted with permission from Bluestone CD, Doyle WJ: Anatomy and physiology of eustachian tube and middle ear related to otitis media. J Allergy Clin Immunol 1988;81:997–1006.)

the incidence of *Moraxella catarrhalis* has been about 5%, but it is now about 14%, with more than 90% of strains producing β-lactamase. The frequency of group A β-hemolytic *Streptococcus* was 3%. The emergence of antibiotic-resistant organisms has had an important impact on the choice of antibiotics for therapy.

Anaerobic bacteria and viruses have been cultured infrequently from middle-ear aspirates of children with AOM, but viral antigens have been identified using immune assay in 10% to 20% of MEE in patients with AOM and in about 50% using reverse transcriptase polymerase chain reaction (PCR).[17] Why viruses have been difficult to culture from MEE is not known. That bacterial OM is secondary to a preceding viral URI that resulted in eustachian tube obstruction has been suggested by the observations that children have more severe obstruction of the eustachian tube during a viral URI than before the URI. Rhinovirus- or influenza A–provoked experimental viral URI in susceptible normal young adult volunteers produced eustachian tube obstruction and negative middle-ear pressures in 70% to 80%.[18,19] Less than 5% of volunteers infected with rhinovirus developed MEE, whereas 20% of susceptible volunteers infected with influenza A virus developed MEE. One subject developed AOM; the middle-ear aspirate contained genomic DNA sequences of influenza A virus and *S. pneumoniae* bacteria (as detected by polymerase chain reaction) even though this aspirate grew no bacterial or viral pathogens in culture. In addition, many children have symptoms of URI prior to their symptoms of AOM.

Previously, it had been assumed incorrectly that chronic middle-ear effusions were sterile, especially after apparently adequate antimicrobial therapy. In several studies, bacteria were found in about 50% of the chronic, persistent middle-ear effusions. The microbiology was similar to that found in AOM, except that *H. influenzae* was recovered more often than *S. pneumoniae* (see Fig. 11-5B).

An inadequate host defense system can contribute to recurrent respiratory infections as well as to OM. The most common of these unusual problems is immunoglobulin (Ig) A deficiency, but other Ig or cellular immunodeficiencies, as well as the immotile cilia syndrome, cannot be overlooked (see Chapter 20).

## ALLERGY

That IgE-mediated allergic reactions participate in the pathogenesis of OM has been suggested by clinical observations reporting a higher prevalence of OM in allergic patients, but these studies were retrospective and lacked appropriate controls and experimental

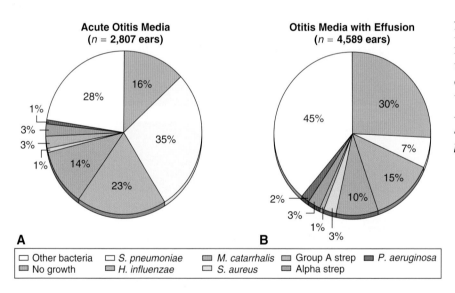

**A**, Acute Otitis Media (*n* = 2,807 ears)

**B**, Otitis Media with Effusion (*n* = 4,589 ears)

☐ Other bacteria  ☐ S. pneumoniae  ▨ M. catarrhalis  ▨ Group A strep  ▪ P. aeruginosa
▨ No growth  ▨ H. influenzae  ☐ S. aureus  ☐ Alpha strep

**Figure 11-5.** *A,* Percentage of bacteria cultured from middle ears of children with acute otitis media at the time of tympanocentesis. *B,* Percentage of bacteria cultured from middle ears of children with otitis media with effusion at the time of tympanocentesis. *H, Haemophilus; M., Moraxella; P., Pseudomonas; S. aureus, Staphylococcus aureus; S. pneumoniae, Streptococcus pneumoniae;* strep, *Streptococcus.*

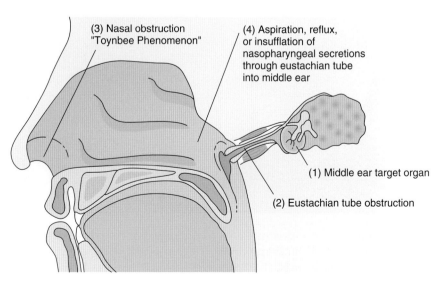

(3) Nasal obstruction "Toynbee Phenomenon"

(4) Aspiration, reflux, or insufflation of nasopharyngeal secretions through eustachian tube into middle ear

(1) Middle ear target organ

(2) Eustachian tube obstruction

**Figure 11-6.** The four possible mechanisms involving allergy in the pathogenesis of otitis media.

design. The role of allergy in OM may involve one or more of the following mechanisms (Fig. 11-6):

- Middle-ear mucosa functioning as a target organ
- Inflammatory swelling of the eustachian tube with resultant obstruction
- Inflammatory obstruction of the nose and nasopharynx
- Reflux, insufflation, or aspiration of bacteria-laden allergic nasopharyngeal secretions into the middle-ear cavity

The last three mechanisms would be associated with abnormal function of the eustachian tube. Although histamine and other mediators of inflammation are present in middle-ear effusions, there is little evidence that the middle-ear mucosa functions as the allergic "shock organ" via IgE antibody and allergen reaction. However, there appears to be a relation between URIs and allergy and eustachian tube dysfunction. A prospective study of children with recurrent or chronic middle-ear disease and functional obstruction of the eustachian tube showed more severe obstruction (mechanical) of the tube when a URI developed.[20] A similar relationship has been reported between upper respiratory tract allergy and eustachian tube obstruction in a series of provocative, intranasal, allergen-inhalation challenge studies.[21]

Nasal obstruction also may be involved in the pathogenesis of OM. Swallowing when the nose is obstructed (inflammation or obstructive adenoids) creates a closed nasopharyngeal chamber. During swallowing, an initial positive nasopharyngeal air pressure is followed by a negative pressure phase within the closed system. There are two possible effects of these pressures on a pliant tube: With positive nasopharyngeal pressure, secretions might be insufflated into the middle ear, especially when the middle ear has high negative pressure, or with negative nasopharyngeal pressures, such a tube could be prevented from opening and become further functionally obstructed. This has been termed the *Toynbee phenomenon.*

The following sequence of events is postulated to occur in patients who have respiratory allergy and OM. Most likely, a basic eustachian tube dysfunction is present in certain infants and children whose tubal function becomes compromised in the presence of upper respiratory tract allergy, similar to eustachian tube obstruction caused by a URI. Upper respiratory tract allergy may cause some intrinsic as well as extrinsic mechanical obstruction in patients who have normal eustachian tube function, but their normal active opening mechanism (i.e., tensor veli palatini muscle pull) is able to overcome the obstruction. Therefore, patients who have functional obstruction due to poor muscular opening would be at highest risk for developing sufficient mechanical obstruction to give rise to middle-ear disease. Many children, as part of normal development, have difficulty actively opening their eustachian tubes; they are the population most at risk for manifesting OM.

## DIAGNOSIS OF OTITIS MEDIA

### HISTORY

The earliest signs of AOM are most frequently ear pain and discomfort, which may be difficult to discern in a child who is too young to speak. The child may be irritable and pull on the affected

ear. With MEE due either to AOM or OME, a conductive hearing loss can be present; increased clumsiness may or may not be present. With OME, there are usually no associated ear symptoms other than hearing loss or clumsiness.

Acute otitis media and OME often occur with an associated rhinitis, and it is important to decide whether the rhinitis is infectious or allergic (Fig. 11-7A and B). The differentiation between infection and perennial allergic rhinitis can be difficult. Symptoms

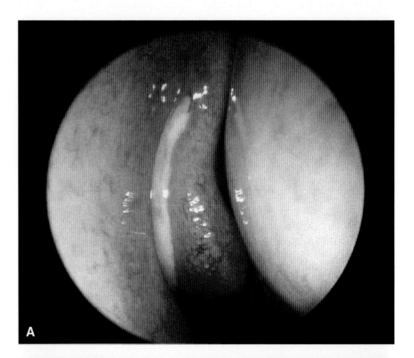

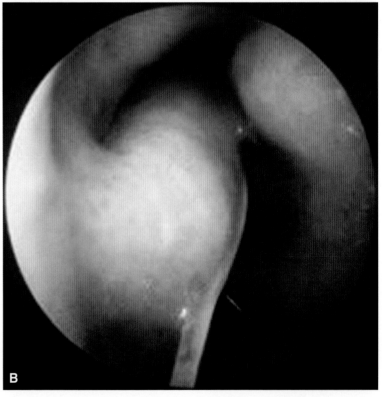

**Figure 11-7.** Otitis media is frequently associated with rhinitis. *A,* Photograph of nasal mucosa of a child with infectious rhinitis. *B,* Photograph of nasal mucosa from a child with allergic rhinitis.

of a URI, such as fever and malaise with profuse acute rhinorrhea, would suggest an infection. The presence of a similar acute illness in immediate family members or contacts would also indicate an infection. Of course, a purulent rhinorrhea or pharyngitis would suggest an infection. However, prolonged or recurrent seasonal rhinitis with itching and sneezing would suggest an allergic basis, as would bilateral red, itchy, swollen, nonpurulent inflammation of the eyes, all of which are manifestations of allergic rhino-conjunctivitis (see Chapter 9).

Even if eustachian tube obstruction is minimal, patients with allergic rhinitis may have mild symptoms of eustachian tube dysfunction, such as "popping" and "snapping" sounds in the ear.

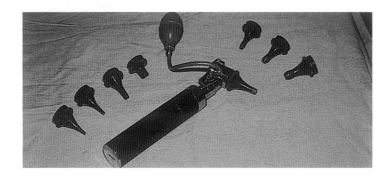

**Figure 11-8.** Pneumatic otoscope and various sizes of specula. Pneumatic otoscopy requires the proper equipment, including a pneumatic otoscope head with attached bulb and appropriately sized speculum to achieve a good air seal. When, despite proper speculum size, a seal is difficult to obtain, the head and tubing should be checked for air leaks. If none are found, application of a piece of rubber tubing to the end of the speculum (shown on speculum attached to the otoscope) or use of a softer speculum may solve the problem. (Reproduced with permission from Bluestone CD: Pediatric otolaryngology. In Zitelli BJ, Davis HW (eds): Atlas of Pediatric Diagnosis. St. Louis, Mosby, 1987, p 20.7.)

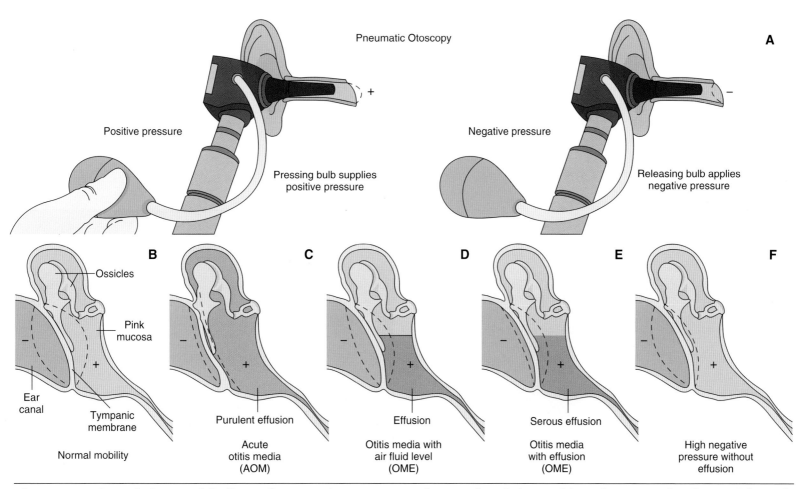

**Figure 11-9.** The technique and findings of pneumatic otoscopy. *A,* The speculum is inserted into the ear canal to form a tight seal. The bulb is then gently and slowly squeezed and released, while the mobility of the drum is assessed. Pressing on the bulb applies positive pressure; letting up applies negative pressure. *B,* With normal mobility, the drum moves inward and then back. *C,* In cases of acute otitis media in which the middle ear is filled with purulent material, the drum bulges toward the examiner and moves minimally. *D,* In cases of otitis media with an air-fluid level, mobility may be nearly normal. In some patients, however, the drum may be retracted, indicating increased negative pressure. Mobility may be reduced with applied positive pressure while mobility is nearly normal or only mildly decreased with applied negative pressure, as seen in otitis media with effusion *(part E). F,* In cases of high negative pressure with no effusion, application of positive pressure produces little or no movement. On negative pressure, the drum billows back toward the examiner. (Adapted with permission from Bluestone CD: Pediatric otolaryngology. In Zitelli BJ, Davis HW (eds): Atlas of Pediatric Diagnosis. St. Louis, Mosby, 1987, p 20.7.)

These symptoms may be aggravated during airplane travel. Many patients experience these symptoms and go on to have more problems, such as hearing loss, ear discomfort, tinnitus, and, sometimes, dizziness during the worst periods of their allergic rhinitis. These symptoms may not be manifest in the nonverbal child. A family history of allergy along with a seasonal runny nose or a constant "cold" should raise suspicions of an allergic diathesis. Other allergic conditions associated with allergic rhinitis include atopic dermatitis and allergic asthma. Seasonal allergic rhinitis occurs episodically, most typically in temperate North America during the grass and ragweed pollen seasons, whereas perennial allergic rhinitis evokes symptoms all year and can be due to non-seasonal allergens present in the home, especially the bedroom, or the workplace. These include house dust, dust mites, storage mold spores, animal products, or occupational allergens.

## DIAGNOSTIC TECHNIQUES

### Pneumatic Otoscopy

Recognition of MEE during the physical examination requires the use of the pneumatic otoscope with an attached air bulb (Fig. 11-8). The physician must choose the correct size speculum to fit each patient's ear canal. It is necessary to obtain a good, airtight seal during an otoscopic examination to ascertain mobility of the tympanic membrane with gentle application of air pressure via the handheld bulb. The technique and findings of pneumatic otoscopy are shown in Figure 11-9. Reduced or absent mobility of the eardrum during this procedure indicates loss of compliance of the eardrum due to either MEE behind the drum or increased stiffness because of scarring or thickening of the tympanic

membrane. Total absence of mobility of the tympanic membrane also may be caused by an opening in the eardrum due to a tube or perforation.

Otoscopic inspection requires visualization of the tympanic membrane and, frequently, cerumen may have to be removed from the external ear canal to permit an adequate examination. The equipment necessary to clean the ear canal is shown in Figure 11-10. The normal tympanic membrane is thin, translucent, neutrally positioned, and mobile. The ossicles, particularly the malleus, are generally visible through it. Adequate assessment

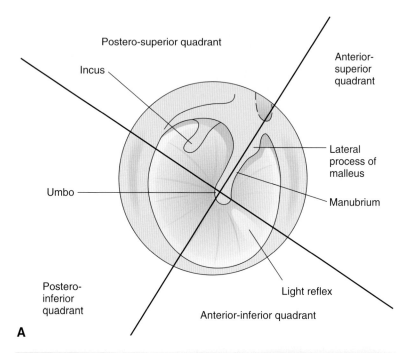

A

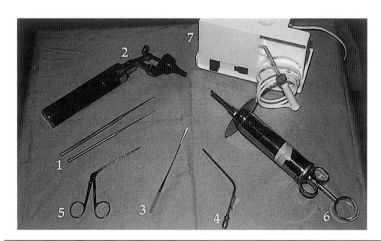

**Figure 11-10.** Equipment for cleaning the external auditory canal. The curette *(1)* is the implement most commonly used to remove cerumen. Use of a surgical otoscope head *(2)* makes the process considerably easier. Additional implements include cotton wicks *(3)* and a suction tip *(4)* for removal of discharge or moist wax, alligator forceps *(5)* for the removal of foreign bodies, an ear syringe *(6)*, and a motorized irrigation apparatus *(7)* for the removal of firm objects or impacted cerumen. Lavage is contraindicated when there is a possible perforation of the tympanic membrane. If the motorized apparatus is used for irrigation, it must be kept on the lowest power setting to avoid traumatizing the eardrum.

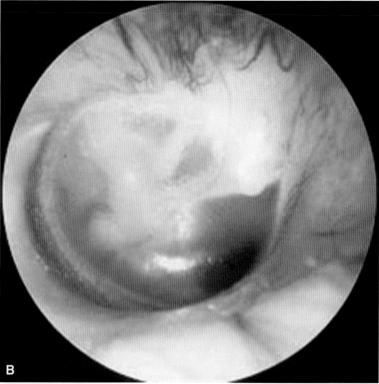

B

**Figure 11-11.** *A,* The normal landmarks of the tympanic membrane. *B,* Photograph of a normal tympanic membrane.

requires that the physician take note of the major characteristics of the tympanic membrane—its thickness, degree of translucence, position, and mobility to applied pressure. The normal tympanic membrane and landmarks are illustrated in Figure 11-11A and can be easily recognized in the normal eardrum shown in Figure 11-11B.

Fullness of the tympanic membrane is caused by increased air pressure or effusion or both and is initially seen in the postero-superior portion of the membrane, as this is the most highly compliant part of the tympanic membrane. The bulging drum in Figure 11-12 indicates the presence of middle-ear fluid filling the middle-ear–mastoid system. The presence of marked erythema and hyperemia with fullness or bulging, accompanied by symptoms of acute inflammation (fever, otalgia, or irritability) point to a clinical diagnosis of AOM. AOM may, by virtue of increasing middle-ear pressure, result in acute perforation of the tympanic membrane. On presentation, the canal may be filled with pus. Careful removal of the pus with a cotton wick usually reveals an inflamed drum with perforation. Air bubbles (Fig. 11-13) or fluid levels are obvious indicators of MEE. The presence of a retracted eardrum suggests negative pressure and possibly atelectasis within the middle ear. Figure 11-14 shows a severely retracted eardrum with effusion. Cholesteatoma, an accumulation of keratinized epithelium can be acquired or congenital. An acquired cholesteatoma is often the result of a severe retraction pocket in the posterior-superior quadrant or in the pars flaccida. A congenital cholesteatoma may be intratympanic (appearing as a "pearl" on top of an intact eardrum, as seen in Figure 11-15) or may appear as a white mass behind an intact eardrum (Fig. 11-16).

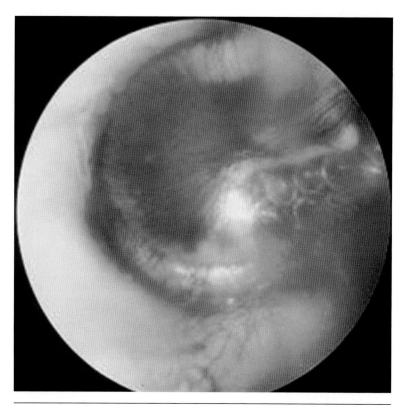

**Figure 11-13.** Obvious air bubbles seen on otoscopy lead to the diagnosis of otitis media with effusion. There is a loss of normal landmarks.

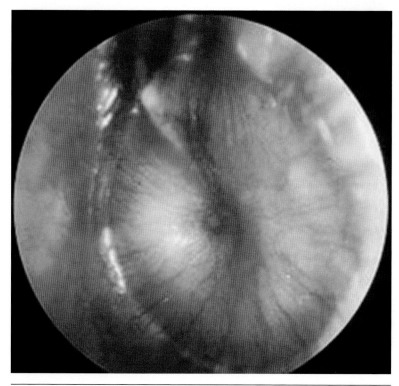

**Figure 11-12.** Acute otitis media. This is a typical erythematous, bulging tympanic membrane, as seen by otoscopy. Mobility and light reflex are reduced, and landmarks are partially obscured.

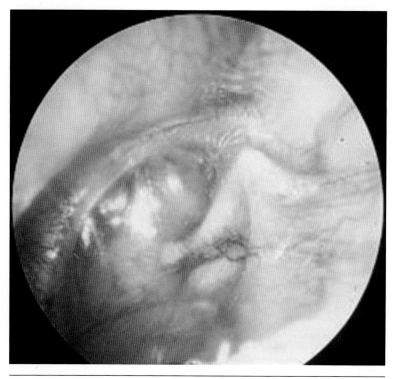

**Figure 11-14.** Severely retracted, opaque, right tympanic membrane with loss of typical landmarks, an example of otitis media with effusion.

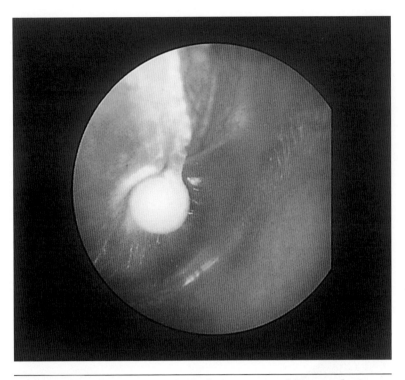

**Figure 11-15.** Intratympanic cholesteatoma. This mass lesion, which consists of an epithelial cyst, is growing within the tympanic membrane. (Reproduced with permission from Bluestone CD: Pediatric otolaryngology. In Zitelli BJ, Davis HW (eds): Atlas of Pediatric Diagnosis. St. Louis, Mosby, 1987, p 20.7.)

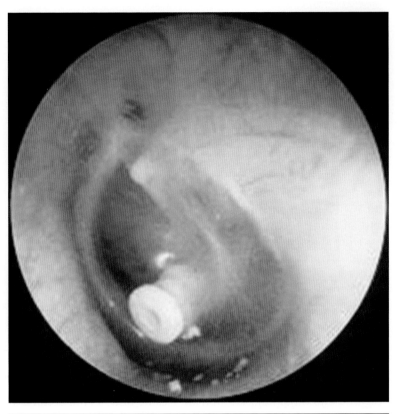

**Figure 11-17.** Tympanic membrane with tympanostomy tube in place. The tube serves to ventilate the middle ear, improve hearing, and reduce the frequency of infection.

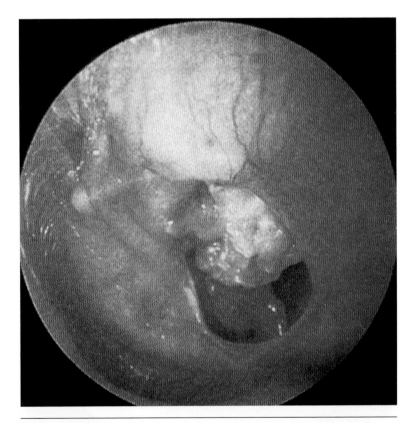

**Figure 11-16.** Middle-ear cholesteatoma visualized through perforation of the right tympanic membrane. (From Bluestone CD, Klein JO: Otitis Media in Infants and Children, 3rd ed. Philadelphia, W.B. Saunders, 2001; with permission.)

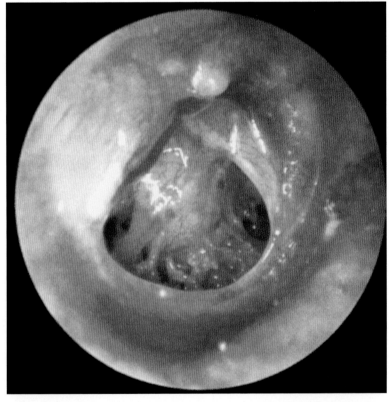

**Figure 11-18.** Large "dry" central perforation of the right tympanic membrane. (From Bluestone CD, Klein JO: Otitis Media in Infants and Children, 3rd ed. Philadelphia, W.B. Saunders, 2001, Fig. 7.15; with permission.)

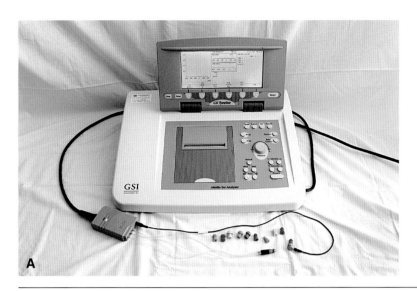
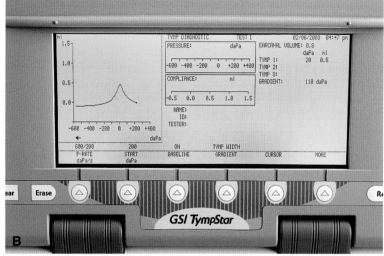

**Figure 11-19.** *A,* Example of one of the types of tympanometers (GSI Tympstar, Grason-Stadler, Inc., Milford, NH) and ear tips that are available. *B,* Example of tympanometer readout from a normal middle ear. Measures obtained on tympanometry include canal volume, middle-ear pressure, tympanic membrane compliance, and gradient (including tympanometric width), which are used to describe middle-ear status. The peak reflects the middle-ear pressure.

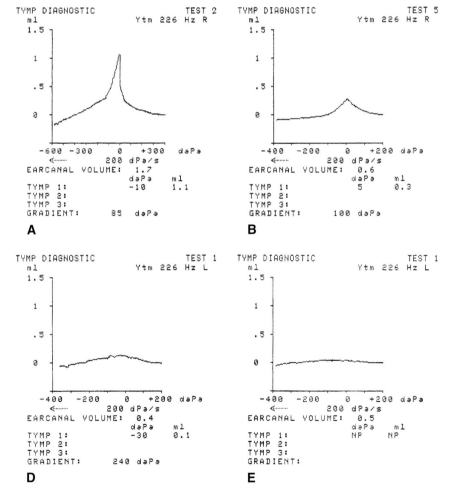

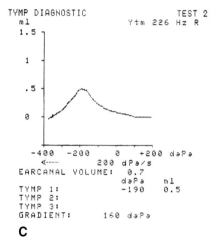

**Figure 11-20.** Admittance tympanogram. *A,* Normal-hearing adult ear. Ear-canal volume was estimated at +400 dPa, air pressure was swept positive-to-negative starting at +400 dPa, and a 226-Hz probe tone was used. (Tympanometric peak pressure = −10 dPa; peak admittance = 1.1 ms or mL; and gradient [measured as the tympanometric width] = 85 dPa.) *B,* Admittance tympanogram for a normal-hearing adult ear with low peak admittance (0.3 mL) but with tympanometric peak pressure and tympanometric width (gradient) within normal limits. *C,* Admittance tympanogram with peak admittance and tympanometric width (gradient) within normal limits but with high negative tympanometric peak pressure. *D,* Admittance tympanogram for a child's ear with OME. The tympanogram has a low, rounded shape, with peak admittance at 0.1 mL and tympanometric width (gradient) equal to 240 dPa. *E,* Admittance tympanogram for the ear of a 12-month-old infant with OME. The lack of a discernible peak causes the instrument to record "NP" (no peak) for the admittance values. (From Nozza RJ: The assessment of Hearing and Middle Ear Function in Children. In Bluestone CD, Casselbrandt ML, Stool SE, et al (eds.): Pediatric Otolaryngology. Philadelphia, PA, Saunders, 2003, p 197)

Persistence of MEE despite adequate therapy for more than 4 to 6 months or the occurrence of more than three episodes of AOM in 6 months or more than four episodes of AOM in 12 months is an indication for myringotomy and insertion of tympanostomy tubes (Fig. 11-17).[22] Perforation of the tympanic membrane may be the result of trauma, AOM, or chronic suppurative OM (with or without otorrhea, drainage from the ear) or may remain after a tympanostomy tube has extruded. A large central perforation is shown in Figure 11-18.

## Tympanometry

The use of the tympanometer in the assessment of potential ear disease has been recognized as a valuable adjunct in the management of OM. When otoscopic findings are unclear or otoscopy difficult to perform, tympanometry can be very useful in evaluating children older than 6 months. This instrument (Fig. 11-19A), which uses acoustic immittance, provides measures such as peak compensated (static) admittance, tympanometric peak pressure, acoustic reflex, and tympanometric width (a measure of gradient) (see Fig. 11-19B). A tympanogram is a plot of the immittance of the middle ear as a function of air pressure in the ear canal (Fig. 11-20). Tympanometry can be combined with otoscopy to assess the status of the middle ear, particularly to determine the presence or absence of middle-ear effusion and the presence or absence of a perforation of the tympanic membrane.

## Audiometry

A hearing test (audiogram) is also necessary for the management of recurrent and chronic MEE. The evaluation of a potential conductive hearing deficit as a result of MEE is an important aspect of patient management. Figure 11-21 illustrates audiograms of patients with, (A) conductive loss, (B) sensorineural loss, and (C) hearing mixed loss.

## Allergy

If allergy—specifically, allergic rhinitis—is suspected from the history and confirmed by physical examination as a risk factor for the development of OM, then an allergic evaluation is suggested to confirm this suspicion. Prick skin testing is preferred to serologic tests (e.g., radioallergosorbent test, fluoroallergosorbent test, enzyme-linked immunosorbent assay) for the detection of IgE antibodies to specific allergens because of its increased sensitivity and lower cost (see Chapter 3). Total serum IgE levels are usually not especially helpful for the evaluation of allergic rhinitis, because only a third of patients with allergic rhinitis have elevated total serum IgE. In addition, total serum IgE does not assist in defining specific allergen sensitivity.

## Immune Deficiency Syndrome

The possibility of an immune deficiency syndrome should be included in the differential diagnosis if the physician decides that the child has had undue susceptibility to infections. When a child with recurrent AOM has had recurrent sinusitis, pneumonia, or other infections in addition to the recurrent URIs, then immunologic assessment is indicated to evaluate potential immune deficiency syndromes. The initial laboratory test performed should include quantitation of serum IgG, IgA, and IgM, as well as a

complete blood count, including a leukocyte count and differential to ascertain the absolute lymphocyte count. A delayed skin test to candida can be applied to assess cell-mediated immunity. Additional laboratory tests to assess specific functional serum antibodies, serum IgG subclasses, T- and B-lymphocytes, as well as complement function, are discussed in detail in Chapter 20.

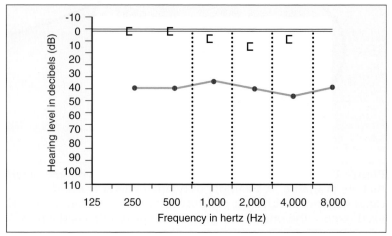

A

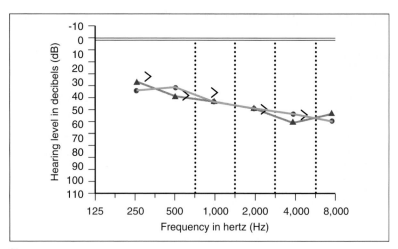

B

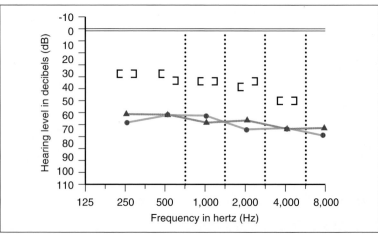

C

**Figure 11-21.** Sample audiograms showing three different types of hearing loss. *A,* Conductive hearing loss (right ear); *B,* sensorineural hearing loss (bilateral); *C,* mixed hearing loss (bilateral). Bone conduction ([ ]); Right ear air conduction (•); Left ear air conduction (▲).

# TREATMENT

## *ACUTE OTITIS MEDIA*

The approach to the treatment of AOM is shown in the algorithm in Figure 11-22.[23] Antimicrobial therapy is still the mainstay of treatment for AOM. In uncomplicated AOM, amoxicillin (45 mg/kg divided into two doses per day) is considered the drug of first choice. If the child has been treated for OM in the previous month or resides in an area known to have high rates of penicillin-resistant *S. pneumoniae*, a resistant organism may be suspected, and a "second-line" antibiotic should be used, such as amoxicillin-clavulanate, "high-dose" amoxicillin (90 mg/kg/day), or one of the cephalosporins.[24] For complicated AOM, the etiologic agent should be sought by obtaining middle-ear fluid for culture via tympanocentesis (needle aspiration of the middle-ear fluid). Treatment can be begun presumptively and changed, if necessary, when the culture results are known.

If a child has recurrent AOM, defined as more than three episodes in 6 months or more than four episodes in 12 months, risk factors such as daycare, secondary tobacco smoke exposure, allergy, immune deficiency, and enlarged adenoids should be considered. Immunizations for *S. pneumoniae* and influenza may be beneficial. For children who continue to have recurrent AOM, surgical treatment with tympanostomy tubes, with or without adenoidectomy, is an option. Prophylaxis with an antimicrobial agent, such as amoxicillin, has been shown to be efficacious in reducing the number of AOM episodes, but because of increasing antimicrobial resistance in bacterial pathogens, this method is reserved for only highly selected children who are not considered good surgical candidates.

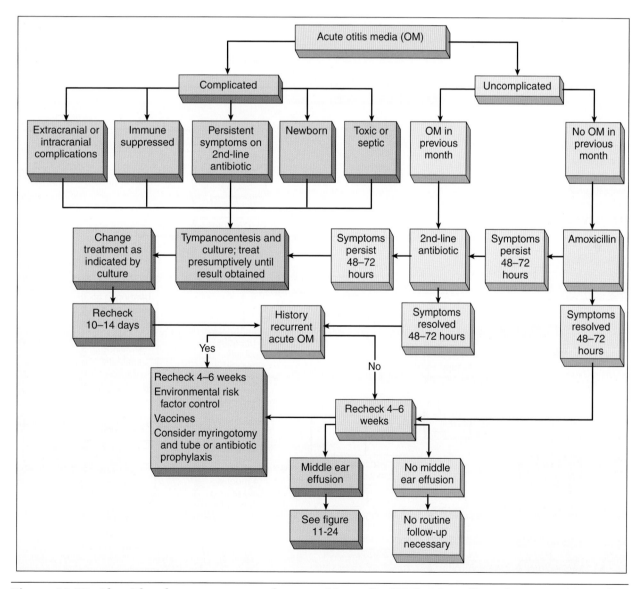

**Figure 11-22.** Algorithm for management of acute otitis media (OM). "Complicated" acute otitis media indicates that tympanocentesis (needle aspiration through the tympanic membrane of the middle-ear contents) is needed before starting medical therapy to establish with certainty the diagnosis of acute otitis media or the precise bacteriologic diagnosis. (Modified from Mandel EM, Casselbrant ML: Acute otitis media in decision making. In Alper CM, Myers EN, Eibling DE (eds): Decision Making in Ear, Nose, and Throat Disorders. Philadelphia, W.B. Saunders, 2001, p 32.)

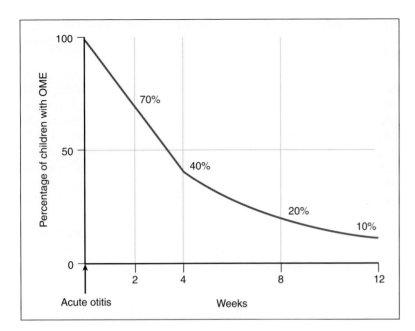

**Figure 11-23.** The persistence of middle-ear effusion after an initial episode of otitis media with effusion (OME) treated with amoxicillin for 10 days. Seventy percent of the children still had middle-ear effusion after 2 weeks; 40% had middle-ear effusion after 1 month; 20% had it after 2 months; and 10% had it after 3 months. (Modified with permission from Teele DW, Klein JO, Rosner BA: Epidemiology of otitis media in children. Ann Otol Rhinol Laryngol 1980; 89:5.)

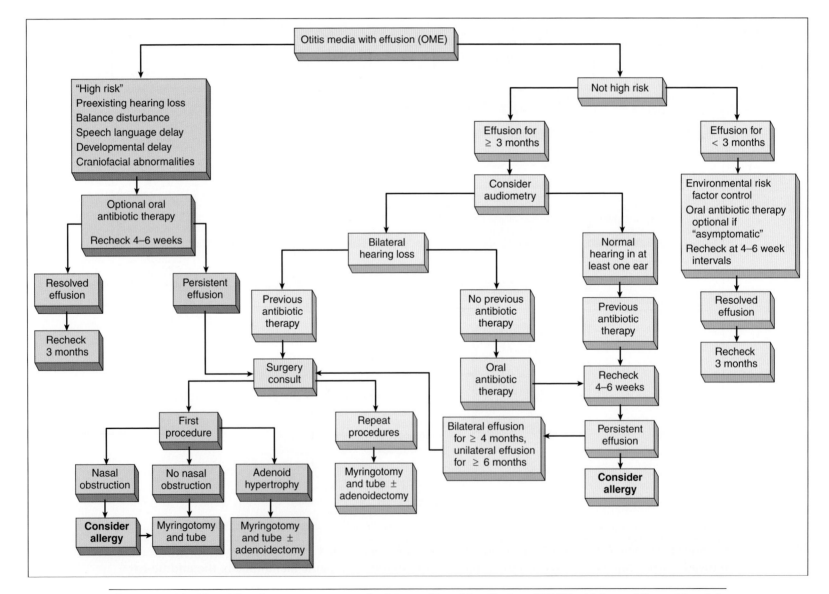

**Figure 11-24.** Algorithm for management of otitis media with effusion (OME). (Adapted from Mandel EM, Casselbrant ML: Acute otitis media. In Alper CM, Myers EN, Eibling DE (eds): Decision Making in Ear, Nose, and Throat Disorders. Philadelphia, W.B. Saunders, 2001, pp 32–33; with permission.)

## *OTITIS MEDIA WITH EFFUSION*

Otitis media with effusion, asymptomatic MEE, is a common finding in children and does not usually require immediate treatment. OME is a common finding following a treated episode of AOM, but only about 10% of children will continue to have effusion 3 months after the episode without any further treatment (Fig. 11-23). An approach to the management of OME is shown in Figure 11-24.[25] Due to the high rate of spontaneous resolution, children not at high risk can be observed. If bilateral MEE persists for 3 months or unilateral MEE persists for 6 months, a hearing test should be obtained and a course of antibiotic should be considered prior to surgical intervention if the child has not previously received antibiotics for this episode. If the child has not had previous surgery for OM, bilateral myringotomy and tube insertion (BM&T) is recommended; if the child has nasal obstruction, an adenoidectomy could also be considered. If the child has had previous tube insertion, adenoidectomy is recommended in addition to tube insertion, regardless of the presence or absence of nasal obstruction.

Allergy evaluation and management may also be warranted for OM accompanied by nasal symptoms. While decongestants may help alleviate nasal symptoms, they have not shown efficacy for resolution of OME in controlled clinical trials. Systemic and intranasal steroids are also effective in the treatment of allergic nasal symptoms and have been suggested for management of chronic OME. However, the efficacy of steroids has not been adequately confirmed in controlled trials, and therefore, steroids are not recommended for long-term management of OME.

# REFERENCES

1. Bernstein JM: Recent advances of immunologic reactivity in otitis media with effusion. J Allergy Clin Immunol 1982;81:1004.
2. Fireman P: Eustachian tube obstruction and allergy: A role in otitis media with effusion. J Allergy Clin Immunol 1985;75:137–139.
3. Bluestone CD, Klein JO: Otitis media and eustachian tube dysfunction. In Bluestone CD, Stool SE, Alper CM, et al (eds): Pediatric Otolaryngology, 4th ed. Philadelphia, W.B. Saunders, 2002, pp 474–685.
4. Casselbrant ML, Mandel EM: Epidemiology. In Rosenfeld RM, Bluestone CD (eds): Evidence-based otitis media, 2nd ed. Hamilton, Ontario, B.C. Decker, 2003, pp 147–162.
5. Tos M, Holm-Jensen S, Sorensen CH, Mogensen C: Spontaneous course and frequency of secretory otitis in four-year-old children. Arch Otolaryngol 1982;108:4–10.
6. Casselbrant ML, Brostoff LM, Cantekin EI, et al: Otitis media in children in the United States. Acute and secretory otitis media. In Proceedings of the International Conference on Acute and Secretory Otitis Media, Part I. Amsterdam, Kugler Publications, 1986, pp 161–164.
7. Casselbrant ML, Mandel EM, Kurs-Lasky M, et al: Otitis media in a population of black American and white American infants, 0–2 years of age. Int J Pediatr Otorhinolaryngol 1995;33:1–16.
8. Casselbrant ML, Mandel EM, Fall PA, et al: The heritability of otitis media: A twin and triplet study. JAMA 1999;282:2125–2130.
9. Tos M, Holm-Jensen S, Sorensen CH: Changes in prevalence of secretory otitis from summer to winter in four-year-old children. Am J Otol 1981;2(4):324–327.
10. Wald ER, Guerra N, Byers C: Upper respiratory tract infections in young children: Duration of and frequency of complications. Pediatrics 1988;87:129–133.
11. Henderson FW, Collier AM, Sanya MA, et al: A longitudinal study of respiratory viruses and bacteria in the etiology of acute otitis media with effusion. N Engl J Med 1982;306:1377–1382.
12. Tomonaga K, Kurono Y, Mogi G: The role of nasal allergy in otitis media with effusion: A clinical study. Acta Otolaryngol (Stockh) 1998;458(Suppl):41–47.
13. Stiehm ER, Ochs HD, Winkelstein JA: Immunodeficiency disorders: General considerations. In Stiehm ER, Ochs HD, Winkelstein JA (eds): Immunologic Disorders in Infants and Children. Philadelphia, Elsevier Saunders, 2004, pp 289–355.
14. Bluestone CD: Role of eustachian tube function: Physiology and role in otitis media. Ann Otol Rhinol Laryngol Suppl 1985;120:1–60.
15. Friedman RA, Doyle WJ, Casselbrant M, et al: Immunologic mediated eustachian tube obstruction: A double blind crossover study. J Allergy Clin Immunol 1983;71:4442–4477.
16. Giebink GS: The microbiology of otitis media. Pediatr Infect Dis J 1989;8:518–520.
17. Post JC, Preston RA, Aul JL, et al: Molecular analysis of bacterial pathogens in otitis media with effusion. JAMA 1995;273:1598–1604.
18. Buchman CA, Doyle WJ, Skoner DP, et al: Otologic manifestations of experimental rhinovirus infection. Laryngoscope 1994;104:1295–1299.
19. Doyle WJ, Skoner DP, Seroky JR, et al: Nasal and otologic effects of experimental influenza A virus infection. Ann Otol Rhinol Laryngol 1994;103:59–69.
20. Sanyal MA, Henderson FW, Stempel EC, Collier AM, Denny FW: Effect of upper respiratory tract infection on eustachian tube ventilatory function in the preschool child. J Pediatr 1980;1:11–15.
21. Skoner DP, Doyle WJ, Chamovitz AH, et al: Eustachian tube obstruction after intranasal challenge with house dust mite. Arch Otolaryngol 1986;112:840–842.
22. Bluestone CD, Klein JO: Otitis media and Eustachian tube dysfunction. In Bluestone CD, Stool SE, Alper CM, et al (eds): Pediatric Otolaryngology, 4th ed. Philadelphia, W.B. Saunders, 2002, p.640.
23. Mandel EM, Casselbrandt ML: Acute otitis media. In Alper CM, Myer EN, Eibling DF (eds): Decision Making in Ear, Nose and Throat Disorders. Philadelphia, W.B. Saunders, 2001, pp 32–33.
24. Dowel SF, Butler JC, Giebink GS: Acute otitis media: Management and surveillance in an era of pneumococcal resistance. Pediatr Infect Dis 1999;18:1–9.
25. Casselbrant ML, Mandel EM, Alper CM: Otitis media with effusion. In Alper CM, Myer EN, Eibling DF (eds): Decision Making in Ear, Nose and Throat Disorders. Philadelphia, W.B. Saunders, 2001, pp 36–37.

*Lee A. Wiley, Robert C. Arffa, and Philip Fireman*

# *12* Allergic Immunologic Ocular Diseases

Allergic and immunologic ocular diseases are influenced by the unique anatomy and physiology of the eye and ocular adnexa. For appropriate diagnosis and therapy, it is important for the clinician to be thoroughly familiar with the anatomy of the eye and its associated structures, as illustrated in Figures 12-1, 12-2, and 12-3. In this chapter, we describe how immunologic processes have been adapted to deal efficiently with the environmental antigens that continually impact on the eye and how these processes can contribute to allergic disease. These ocular diseases are then discussed in terms of their clinical presentations, pathologies, and treatments.

## NORMAL OCULAR ANATOMY

### *CONJUNCTIVA*

Conjunctiva, the mucosa of the ocular surface, is comparable to other epithelia, such as those lining the gut and bronchi. The ocular surface is subjected to a barrage of antigens and microorganisms. The conjunctiva and associated regional lymphoid tissues acquire and process antigens to produce sensitized T and B cells, thus providing a mechanism of immune response well adapted to the surveillance of an exposed surface.[1]

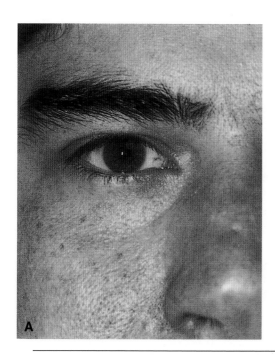

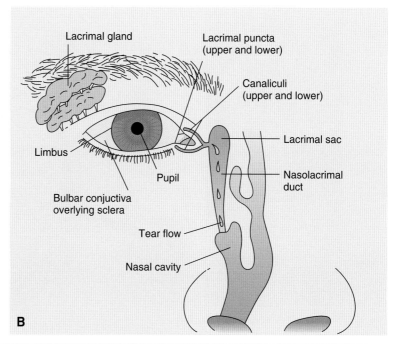

**Figure 12-1.** *A,* The external landmarks of a normal eye. *B,* Diagrammatic representation of the external landmarks of a normal eye and lacrimal system.

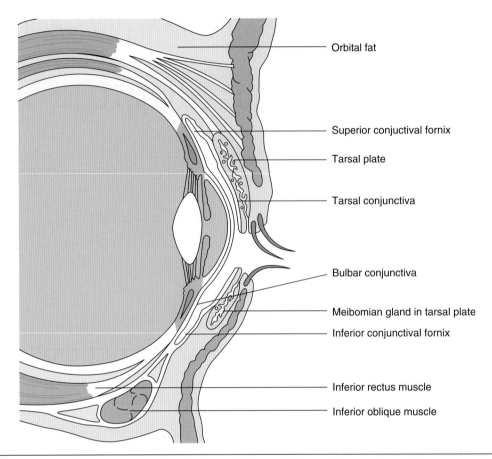

**Figure 12-2.** Sagittal view of the eyelids and the ocular orbit.

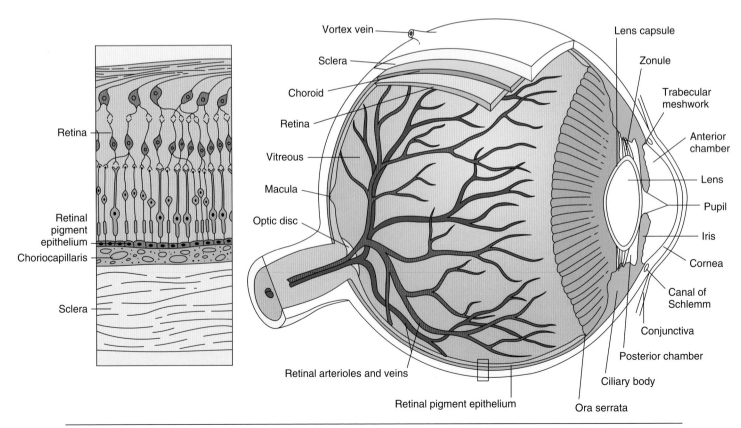

**Figure 12-3.** The internal structures of the eye.

Immunoreactive cell populations vary within the different layers and anatomic regions of conjunctiva (Fig. 12-4). The lymphocytes of the conjunctival epithelium are mainly CD8 cells, Langerhans' dendritic cells, which function in the afferent limb as antigen-presenting cells, are most plentiful in the epibulbar and forniceal conjunctiva. The substantia propria of the conjunctiva is populated by a nearly equal proportion of CD8 (cytotoxic/suppressor) and CD4 (helper/inducer) T cells. A smaller population of B cells arranged in lymphoid aggregates is present in the fornices (see Fig. 12-4). Mast cells are present in the substantia propria of the conjunctiva and tissues of the eyelid, as are dendritic cells. Plasma cells are adjacent to the accessory lacrimal tissue. Lymphatics of the conjunctiva and eyelid drain laterally to the preauricular and parotid nodes and medially to the submandibular nodes.

Sensitization to an allergen occurs when an antigen diffuses through the conjunctival mucosa and is then processed by antigen-presenting cells (Langerhans cells or macrophages). T-lymphocytes respond to the antigen-presenting cell–processed allergens by elaborating cytokines which, in turn, stimulate B-lymphocytes to produce antigen-specific immunoglobulin (Ig) E. The allergen-specific IgE molecules are then associated with the surface of mast cells, which are now primed for an allergic response.[2]

## THE LACRIMAL GLANDS

The lacrimal glands are located in the superotemporal orbits and are responsible for production of the aqueous component of tears (see Fig. 12-1; Fig. 12-5). The tears contain secretory IgA

antibodies and many other substances, such as lysozyme, that may be important to host defense.

Lymphoid aggregates composed of B cells, macrophages, dendritic cells, and CD4 (helper/inducer) T cells are active in local antigen processing, which leads to the development of IgA-producing plasma cells. The aggregates associated with the intralobular ducts of the lacrimal gland have a high proportion of plasma cells, the majority producing IgA (see Fig. 12-5). This IgA is taken up by the lacrimal gland acinar cells, which contribute the IgA secretory pieces that allow transport of the dimeric secretory IgA to the gland lumen. The components of the classic and alternative complement system are also present in tears. The lymphatic channels of the lacrimal gland drain to the preauricular and cervical nodes.

## THE CORNEA

The cornea is the transparent and avascular major optical component of the eye (see Fig. 12-3). It has no blood or lymphatic vessels, but in the noninflamed eye, Langerhans cells are found in the epithelium, with greatest density at the limbus and decreasing toward the central cornea. As in the conjunctiva, the Langerhans cells express MHC Class II antigen. Langerhans cells with antigen migrate to draining lymph nodes, where they participate in T cell activation. Complement components are found throughout the corneal stroma. Immune complex–mediated disease often initially affects the peripheral cornea, presumably as a result of its proximity to the limbal vasculature. Vascularization of the cornea

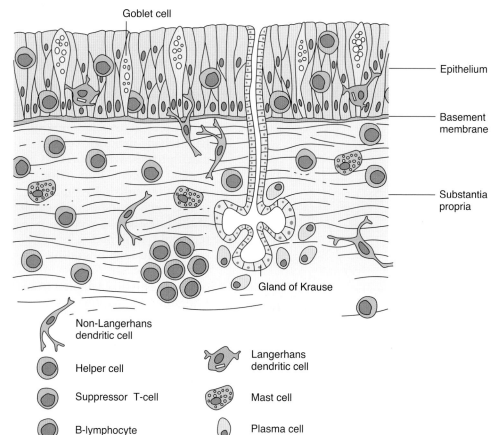

Goblet cell

Epithelium

Basement membrane

Substantia propria

Gland of Krause

Non-Langerhans dendritic cell

Helper cell

Suppressor T-cell

B-lymphocyte

Langerhans dendritic cell

Mast cell

Plasma cell

**Figure 12-4.** A diagram of the immunohistology of the conjunctiva. Only T-lymphocytes are present in the epithelium, with a preponderance of suppressor/cytotoxic T cells. Dendritic Langerhans cells are also present in the epithelium. The substantia propria contains an equal proportion of helper and suppressor T-lymphocytes. Non-Langerhans dendritic cells and mast cells reside in the substantia propria as well. Aggregates of lymphoid cells, including B-lymphocytes and plasma cells, are found in association with the accessory lacrimal glands, also known as glands of Krause. (Adapted from Sacks EH, Wieczorek R, Jakobiec FA, Knowles DM: Lymphocyte subpopulations in the normal human conjunctiva: A monoclonal antibody study. Ophthalmology 1986;93(10):1276–1283; with permission.)

is accompanied by the development of lymphatic channels, and both of these diminish the relative immune privilege of the cornea (see Figs. 12-16 and 12-17).

## THE LENS

The lens is a biconvex structure located in the posterior chamber behind the pupil. It aids in forming a focused image on the photoreceptor area, the retina (see Fig. 12-3). It has been proposed that because proteins of the lens are "sequestered" from the immune system, they might be recognized as foreign antigens. The tolerance to lens antigens may be overcome when a large amount of lens material is released in combination with trauma-induced inflammation and/or microbial contamination.

## CONJUNCTIVAL AND CORNEAL ALLERGIC DISEASES

The most commonly encountered allergic ocular disorders are allergic conjunctivitis (hay fever), vernal keratoconjunctivitis, atopic keratoconjunctivitis, and giant papillary conjunctivitis. These conditions can range in severity from the minimally symptomatic allergic conjunctivitis to the visually threatening atopic keratoconjunctivitis. Although the immunopathogenesis of these diseases varies, mast cells play a significant role, as many of them are present in the substantia propria of the conjunctiva and eyelid (see Fig. 12-4). Basophils are also involved in the cellular infiltrate of several allergic ocular disorders. The distinguishing clinical features of the conditions are shown in Table 12-1.

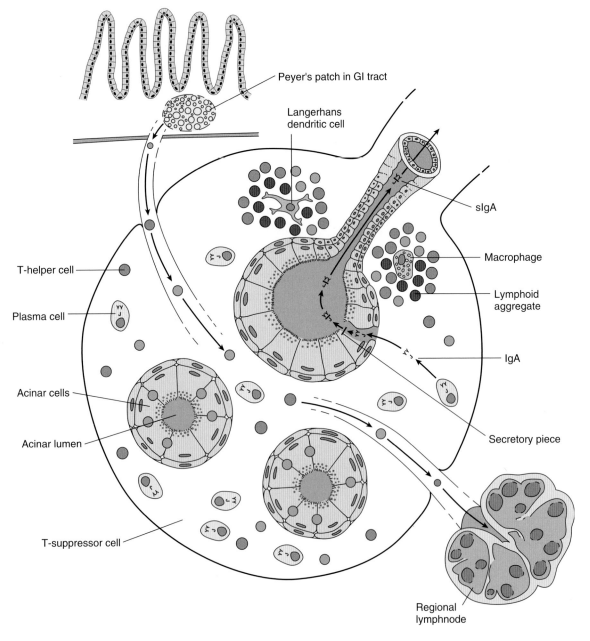

**Figure 12-5.** The immunologic structure of the lacrimal gland. Plasma cells are distributed throughout the lacrimal gland interstitium. They produce dimeric immunoglobulin A (IgA), which diffuses into the acinar cells. A secretory piece is added, allowing transport of the immunoglobulin into the acinar lumen (Sig A). Within the lacrimal gland epithelium, T-suppressor cells outnumber T-helper cells, and in the gland interstitium, T-suppressor cells remain more numerous. B-lymphocytes are found in periductular aggregates, sometimes in association with Langerhans dendritic cells or macrophages, which process and present antigens. Interaction with other mucosal lymphoid tissue, such as the Peyer's patch of the intestine, as well as regional lymph nodes, is possible through migrating lymphocytes. GI, gastrointestinal. (Adapted from Wieczorek R, Jakobiec FA, Sacks EH, Knowles DM: Immunoarchitecture of the normal human lacrimal gland: Relevancy for understanding pathologic conditions. Ophthalmology 1988;95(1):100–109; with permission.)

# ALLERGIC CONJUNCTIVITIS (HAY FEVER)

## Clinical Presentation

Patients with allergic conjunctivitis complain of itching, tightness, and swelling around their eyes. Affecting people of all ages, this very common condition is often associated with other atopic disorders, such as allergic rhinitis (see Chapter 9). It may be seasonal or perennial, depending on the provocative antigens, and often, there is a family history of allergy. Whereas there may be conjunctival edema, injection, and lid swelling, the symptoms often far exceed the objective findings (Fig. 12-6). Although eosinophils may be present in the conjunctival substantia propria, they are seldom found in the epithelium and are not routinely detected in a conjunctival scraping. In addition to the history, skin testing or in vitro IgE antibody determinations is the chief method of identifying the offending allergens (see Chapter 3).

## Pathogenesis

The pathogenesis of allergic conjunctivitis involves a type I hypersensitivity reaction initiated by the binding of an antigen to a specific IgE receptor molecule on the sensitized mast cell. The specific binding of the allergen results in the generation and release of mast cell inflammatory mediators, such as histamine, leukotrienes, prostaglandins, and neutrophil, and eosinophil chemotactic factors. The ocular tissues can manifest both early- (15 to 60 minutes) and late-phase (2 to 6 hours) IgE-mediated allergic reactions.

## Treatment

The treatment of allergic conjunctivitis can be greatly facilitated by identification and elimination of the offending allergen. Cool compresses applied to the orbital areas provides some symptomatic relief, and patients should be counseled that rubbing intensifies the symptoms. Topical antihistamine-vasoconstrictor combinations such as 0.05% antazoline phosphate/0.5% naphazoline hydrochloride (Vasocon-A) may be sufficient in mild cases. Levocarbastine 0.05% (Livostin) is a potent $H_1$ antihistamine with proven efficacy for relief of ocular itching. This antihistamine is often combined with a mast cell stabilizing agent such as lodoxamide 0.1% (Alomide) for those subject to chronic allergen exposure.[3] Combination mast cell stabilizer/antihistamine agents

**TABLE 12-1**
**Clinical Characteristics of Allergic, Vernal, and Atopic Conjunctivitis**

| | Allergic Conjunctivitis | Vernal Kerato Conjunctivitis | Atopic Kerato Conjunctivitis |
|---|---|---|---|
| Pathogenesis | Type 1 IgE-mediated hypersensitivity reaction to environmental antigen | Combination of type 1 IgE-mediated and type 4 cell-mediated hypersensitivity reaction | Chronic, type 1 IgE-mediated hypersensitivity Depressed cell-mediated immunity |
| Seasonal variation | Often seasonal; worsens with high pollen counts Associated with allergic rhinitis | Exacerbation in spring or summer More prevalent in warm climates | No seasonal variation |
| Ages affected | All ages | 3–25 yr; 80% of cases occur in patients younger than 14 yr | Begins in late teens; many cases remit at ages 40–50 yr |
| Conjunctival eye disease | Conjunctival injection and edema (chemosis) | Upper tarsal conjunctiva with giant papillae Limbal form shows gelatinous papillae at limbus | Papillary conjunctivitis of lower palpebral conjunctiva Conjunctival scarring and symblepharon may occur |
| Corneal complications | No corneal ulceration or scarring | Shallow vernal ulcer with vascularization | Deep corneal vascularization and corneal melting in severe cases |
| Conjunctival scraping | Eosinophils rarely seen | Often many eosinophils and free eosinophilic granules More than two eosinophils per high-power field is pathognomonic | Rare eosinophils and no free eosinophilic granules |
| Eyelids | Periorbital and eyelid edema | Swelling and ptosis of upper lids | Atopic dermatitis of lids Poor apposition of lids to globe resulting from scarring of eyelid skin |

Ig, immunoglobulin.

(Table 12-2) provide the convenience of twice-a-day dosing but tend to be more active for the relief of itching than redness. Loteprednol etabonate 0.2% (Alrex) is a modified corticosteroid designed to minimize steroid-induced side effects yet still provide control of superficial ocular inflammation. More potent topical corticosteroid preparations may precipitate steroid induced glaucoma and cataracts or may exacerbate microbial infections. Patients with allergic rhinoconjunctivitis may benefit from allergen hypersensitization.

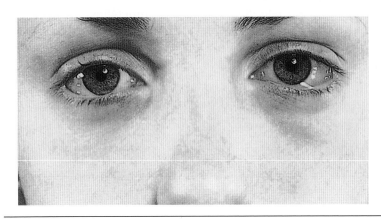

**Figure 12-6.** Allergic conjunctivitis with marked conjunctival edema and slight injection. This is often associated with allergic rhinitis (hay fever). (Reproduced from Spalton DJ, Hitchings RA, Hunter PA: Atlas of Clinical Ophthalmology. London, Gower, 1984, pp 5.2, 10.9; with permission.)

## VERNAL KERATOCONJUNCTIVITIS

### Clinical Presentation

Vernal keratoconjunctivitis is a bilateral, recurrent conjunctivitis that affects young people 3 to 25 years of age. The term *vernal* refers to the seasonal (spring and summer) exacerbation of symptoms. However, there may not be a direct association between symptoms and seasonal allergens. This disorder is more prevalent in warm climates and may remit in cooler ones. The symptoms of itching and photophobia may be severe, and it is fortunate that most patients become less symptomatic in their 20s. There are two forms of the disease: palpebral and limbal.

The palpebral form affects the upper tarsal conjunctiva, with the appearance of large flat-topped elevations, termed *giant papillae*. Generally more than 1 mm in diameter, these papillae can be seen easily (without magnification) on eversion of the upper lid (Fig. 12-7).

The limbal form exhibits a gelatinous papillary hypertrophy of the limbal conjunctiva (Fig. 12-8), often with chalk-white concretions of eosinophils, called Trantas' dots. The cornea may be affected, with a fine punctate epithelial cell loss or a vernal corneal ulcer (Fig. 12-9). Lens opacities develop in some patients. Conjunctival scraping typically reveals many eosinophils. Increased levels of serum IgE can be present, as well as specific IgE antibodies to environmental allergens. The majority of patients have a history of other atopic conditions and familial allergic disease.

**TABLE 12-2**
**Ophthalmic Allergy Medications**

| Drug Category | Medication | Dose Frequency |
|---|---|---|
| Antihistamine and vasoconstriction combination | Naphcon-A (naphazoline)<br>OcuHist (naphazoline with pheniramine)<br>Opcon-A (naphazoline HCl/pheniramine maleate)<br>Vasocon-A (naphazoline HCl/antazoline phosphate) | Up to 4/day |
| Topical NSAID | Acular (ketorolac tromethamine 0.5%) | 4/day |
| H₁: Receptor antagonists | Livostin (levocabastine HCl)<br>Emadine (emedastine difumerate) | Up to 4/day |
| Mast cell stabilizers | Crolom (cromolyn sodium)<br>Opticrom (cromolyn sodium 4%)<br>Alomide (lodoxamide tromethamine 0.1%) | 4/day |
| H₁: Receptor antagonist and mast cell stabilizer | Patanol (olopatandine hydrochloride) | 2/day |
| H₁: Receptor antagonists, mast cell stabilizer, and NSAID | Optivar (azelastine HCl 0.05%)<br>Alocril (nedocromil 2%)<br>Alamast (pemirolast potassium 0.1%)<br>Zaditor (ketotifen fumarate 0.025%) | 2/day |
| Modified corticosteroid | Alrex (loteprednol etabonate 0.2%) | 4/day |

HCl, hydrochloric acid; NSAID, nonsteroidal anti-inflammatory drug.

## Pathogenesis

Although the large number of eosinophils and degranulated mast cells in the tissue suggests an important role for type I hypersensitivity, this mechanism cannot explain all the findings. The giant papillae contain newly synthesized collagen and massive numbers of mast cells, eosinophils, basophils, and lymphocytes. It has been suggested that a T cell–mediated, delayed hypersensitivity contributes to the process. Inflammatory chemical medicators such as eosinophilic major basic protein are cytoxic to the corneal epithelium and may contribute to the formation of the vision-threatening vernal ulcer.

## Treatment

The sustained mast cell degranulation with subsequent recruitment of eosinophils suggests that mast cell stabilization is a key component of treatment. Agents such as lodoxamide 0.1% or disodium cromoglycate 2% are often combined with a short course of topical corticosteroids for an effective regimen. Combination antihistamine/mast cell stabilizers (see Table 12-2) may enhance compliance with their twice-a-day dosing, a particular advantage in this pediatric population. Other topical immunomodulations, such as cyclosporine, may offer other therapeutic options, particularly in those in whom topical corticosteroids cannot be tapered.

The vernal ulcer can become a vision-threatening problem, especially in children still susceptible to the development of amblyopia. Once the ocular inflammation is controlled, superficial keratectomy to remove the vernal plaque often promotes the growth of healthy epithelium. The second component of therapy requires the involvement of an allergist who can help identify and eliminate allergen in the environment.

## *ATOPIC KERATOCONJUNCTIVITIS*

### Clinical Presentation

Atopic keratoconjunctivitis is a chronic bilateral keratoconjunctivitis that occurs in patients with atopic dermatitis. The symptoms of itching and burning may be severe. Advanced cases often have a stringy, mucopurulent discharge. This allergic disorder is most common in men and teenage boys, tending to remit by the age of 50 years. The lids are thickened, indurated, and lichenified (Fig. 12-10A), sometimes with sufficient scarring to prevent apposition of the eyelid to the globe. There is often a chronic staphylococcal infection of the eyelid margins, with lid margin hyperemia and crusty deposits on the lashes. The inferior palpebral and forniceal conjunctiva are affected by a chronic papillary conjunctivitis (see Fig. 12-10B). The limbal conjunctiva may be thickened with gelatinous elevations. Corneal changes can be severe: Superficial scarring, vascularization, recurrent epithelial ulceration, and corneal perforation are vision-threatening complications (see Fig. 12-10C). Approximately 10% of patients with atopic dermatitis develop cataracts (Fig. 12-11).

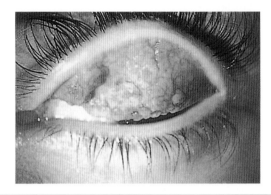

**Figure 12-7.** Vernal conjunctivitis, palpebral form. The giant papillary elevations are seen easily without magnification.

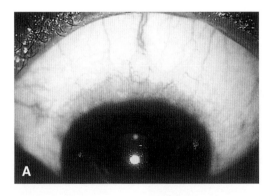

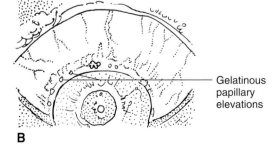

Gelatinous papillary elevations

**Figure 12-8.** Vernal conjunctivitis, limbal form. Note the gelatinous papillary elevations of the limbal tissue.

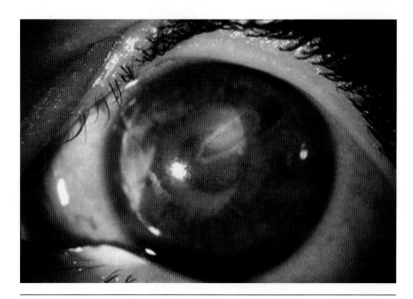

**Figure 12-9.** Vernal conjunctivitis with vernal corneal ulcer.

## Pathogenesis

The pathogenesis of atopic keratoconjunctivitis may be similar to that of atopic dermatitis (see Chapter 15). Serum IgE and allergen-specific IgE antibodies are elevated in the majority of patients, sometimes waxing and waning with the symptoms. Mast cell counts are increased in inflamed tissues. In atopic dermatitis, surface IgE has been detected not only on mast cells and basophils but also on macrophages and dendritic cells, suggesting another pathway by which IgE may trigger inflammation. The deficiency of suppressor T cells in the related condition of atopic dermatitis provides further evidence of abnormal cell-mediated immunity.

## Treatment

A regimen similar to that for the other allergic diseases, hinging on a mast cell stabilizer and antihistamines, may be employed. Topical cyclosporine (Restasis) can be added to the regimen in resistant cases. A special caution with topical corticosteroids must be exercised due to the propensity for corneal melting and infection. The predisposition of patients to acquire herpes simplex infections is a constant threat, with eczema herpeticum requiring therapy with oral acyclovir and topical triflurothymidine. Occasionally, systemic corticosteroid or cyclosporine are required.

## OTHER RELATED CONDITIONS

There are several other conjunctival and corneal diseases of note. Giant papillary conjunctivitis (Fig. 12-12) occurs when the upper lid meets a foreign body, such as a contact lens, prosthesis, or exposed suture. The papillae, composed of collagen, are heavily infiltrated with eosinophils, basophils, and mast cells. Scrupulous cleansing to remove contact lens protein deposits, a change to a different lens design, and the use of cromolyn or topical anti-inflammatory agents may allow a patient to continue wearing lenses.

Inflamed, scaly, periocular skin; lid margin hyperemia; and conjunctival injection are characteristic of contact dermato-conjunctivitis (Fig. 12-13). Scarring of the forniceal conjunctiva, punctal closure, and foreshortening of the lower eyelid skin, with poor apposition to the globe, may occur. This type IV hypersensitivity response may occur in reaction to topical application of many substances, including cosmetics and ophthalmic medications, such as neomycin, epinephrine, and atropine.

In phlyctenular keratoconjunctivitis (Fig. 12-14), an elevated, actively inflamed corneal lesion usually ulcerates and then

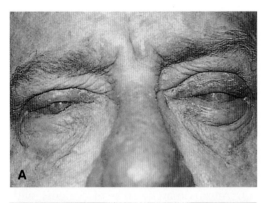

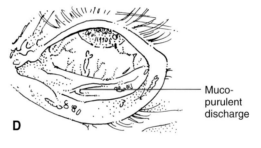

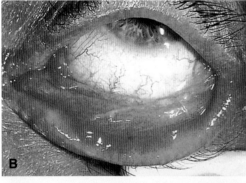

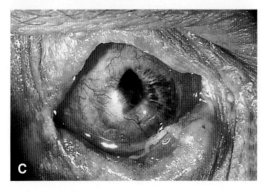

**Figure 12-10.** *A,* Atopic keratoconjunctivitis with thickened, indurated eyelids. Note the loss of lashes. The left eye has undergone application of tissue adhesive for a corneal perforation. *B,* Atopic keratoconjunctivitis with chronic papillary conjunctivitis. Note the stringy mucopurulent discharge often seen in this disorder. *C,* Atopic keratoconjunctivitis with corneal scarring and vascularization.

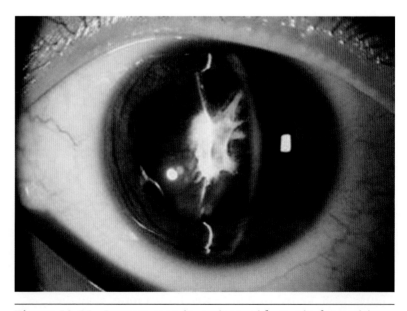

**Figure 12-11.** Cataract seen in patient with atopic dermatitis.

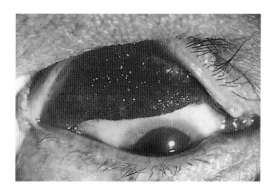

**Figure 12-12.** Characteristic lesions of giant papillary conjunctivitis. These hobnail-like elevations of the upper tarsal conjunctiva, evident on eversion of the upper eyelid, occur when the upper lid meets a foreign body, such as a contact lens, prosthesis, or exposed suture.

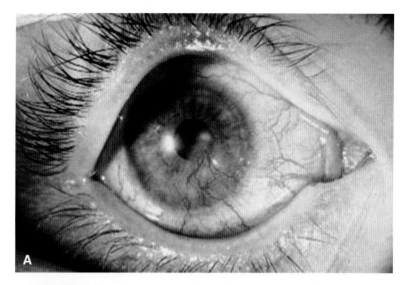

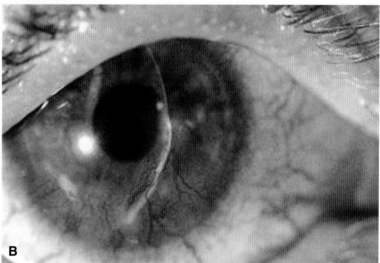

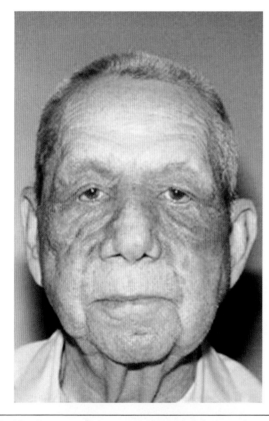

**Figure 12-13.** Contact dermatoconjunctivitis reaction to neomycin, with characteristic inflamed, scaly, periocular skin, lid margin hyperemia, and conjunctival injection. Scarring of the forniceal conjunctiva, punctal closure, and foreshortening of the lower eyelid skin with poor apposition to the globe may occur.

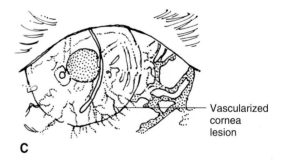

**Figure 12-14.** *A,* The characteristic triangular, vascularized corneal scar of phlyctenular keratoconjunctivitis. *B,* Closer view detailing the elevated, actively inflamed corneal lesion. This elevated area usually ulcerates and then spontaneously resolves within several weeks, leaving a visually disabling scar.

spontaneously resolves within several weeks, leaving a visible scar. This condition is believed to be a type IV hypersensitivity response to microbial antigens from *Staphylococcus* spp., *Candida* spp., or tuberculosis. Lid scrubs and topical antibiotics may decrease exposure to the inciting antigen, and topical corticosteroids may speed resolution of the inflammation, limiting the scarring of the visual axis.

Catarrhal marginal infiltrates begin in the anterior corneal stroma, parallel with the limbus, and show a lucid interval of clear cornea (Fig. 12-15). Often multiple, these lesions can spread circumferentially and ulcerate, mimicking an infectious corneal ulcer. This self-limited process may be due to immune complex deposition in the cornea provoked by antigens from infectious agents. The condition often responds to treatment of the associated blepharitis with lid scrubs, antibiotics, and judicious use of topical corticosteroids.

Peripheral ulcerative keratitis (Fig. 12-16) occurs in conjunction with collagen vascular diseases, such as rheumatoid arthritis, relapsing polychondritis, progressive systemic sclerosis, Wegener's granulomatosis, and polyarteritis nodosa. It manifests as inflammation, ulceration, and thinning of the cornea and adjacent sclera. Control of the systemic disease is the most effective therapeutic approach. In a series of patients with rheumatoid arthritis and necrotizing scleritis or peripheral ulcerative keratitis, reduced mortality was observed with the use of systemic immunosuppressive medications.

Mooren's ulcer (Fig. 12-17) is a rare, chronic, inflammatory disease of the peripheral cornea characterized by progressive thinning and loss of the anterior corneal stroma. Topical steroids, resection of the inflamed limbal conjunctiva adjacent to the ulcer, and systemic immunosuppression represent the stepwise approach most often used to treat this disease. Mooren's ulcer has recently been associated with chronic hepatitis C infections—these cases have responded to interferon α-2b therapy.

# SCLERAL DISEASES

The opaque wall of the globe is called the *sclera* (see Fig. 12-3). It is avascular, composed primarily of collagen and elastic tissue. The episclera is a fibrovascular membrane that encases the sclera, provides nutrition, allows smooth movement of the globe, and, together with the muscle sheaths to which it is fused, prevents excess movement. The eye and orbit can be thought of as a modified ball-and-socket joint, the episclera being analogous to a synovial membrane. Many of the collagen vascular diseases that cause inflammation of joints may also cause scleritis or episcleritis (Box 12-1).

Usually, inflammation of these deeper structures can be differentiated from conjunctival inflammation by history and clinical examination. Deep eye pain occurs with scleral inflammation but does not occur with conjunctivitis. Most important is examination of the sclera in daylight. Deep vascular inflammation appears violet, and with increased scleral thinning, the dark choroid may be better observed. Because scleritis is often bilateral and recurrent, scleral thinning may be apparent in the fellow eye or in uninflamed areas of the same eye. The involved tissue is tender: This does not occur in conjunctivitis. Blanching of the more superficial conjunctival vessels may be obtained with topical

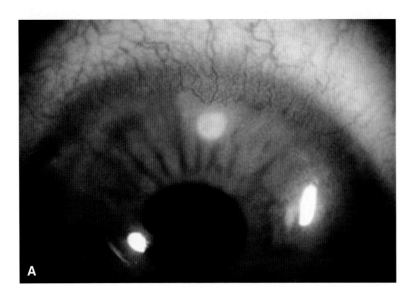

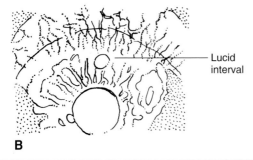

**Figure 12-15.** Catarrhal marginal infiltrates. These begin in the anterior corneal stroma, parallel with the limbus, and show a lucid interval of clear cornea. Often multiple, these lesions can spread circumferentially, and when ulcerated, they resemble infectious corneal ulcers.

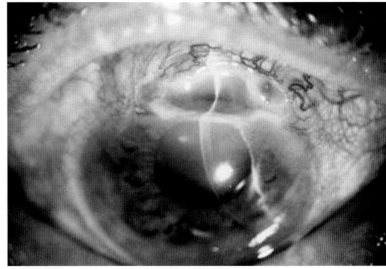

**Figure 12-16.** Inflammation, ulceration, and thinning of the cornea and adjacent sclera, characteristic of peripheral ulcerative keratitis. This condition occurs in conjunction with other collagen vascular diseases, including rheumatoid arthritis (as in this case), systemic lupus erythematosus, relapsing polychondritis, progressive systemic sclerosis, Wegener's granulomatosis, and polyarteritis nodosa.

phenylephrine 10% (Fig. 12-18), revealing persistent inflammation of the episcleral vessels.

## *EPISCLERITIS AND SCLERITIS*

### Clinical Presentation

Episcleritis is often asymptomatic but may be accompanied by a sensation of warmth or pricking in the eye. The onset is usually sudden. Episcleral vascular engorgement may occur in three patterns: sectoral, diffuse, or nodular (Fig. 12-19). No scleral edema or necrosis is observed. The eye is rarely tender to the touch, and vision is always normal.

In contrast, scleritis is usually gradual in onset, developing over several days. In most cases, the predominant symptom is a deep, penetrating pain that may be severe, radiating outward to adjacent structures. Lacrimation and photophobia may occur, and visual acuity may be reduced, particularly in posterior scleritis.

Clinically, scleritis can be divided into five different types[4]:

1. Nodular anterior scleritis has one or more localized areas of scleral inflammation without necrosis. In contrast to nodular episcleritis, these nodules are tender and immovable over underlying tissue.
2. Diffuse anterior scleritis is characterized by more widespread anterior scleral involvement (Fig. 12-20).
3. Necrotizing anterior scleritis with inflammation is associated with the greatest morbidity, owing to regions of vascular occlusion and loss of scleral substance (Fig. 12-21). Attacks can lead to total destruction of the sclera, with bulging of the ocular contents or even perforation and loss of the eye.
4. Scleromalacia perforans cause scleral loss without signs or symptoms of inflammation and occurs almost exclusively in chronic rheumatoid arthritis patients (Fig. 12-22).
5. Posterior scleritis is not associated with anterior inflammation, and the diagnosis is frequently missed. Retinal examination may indicate exudative detachments, choroiditis and choroidal folds, or vitritis (Fig. 12-23). A computed tomography scan of a patient with posterior scleritis is shown in Figure 12-24, demonstrating the increased radiodensity of the involved right sclera.

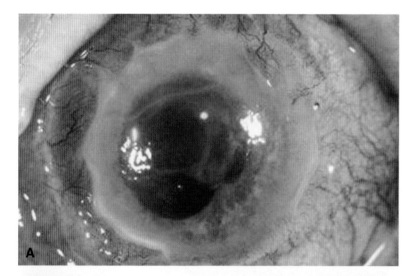

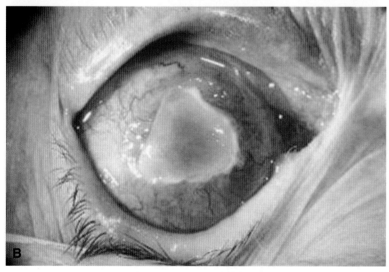

**Figure 12-17.** Mooren's ulcer is a rare, chronic inflammatory disease of the peripheral cornea, characterized by progressive thinning and loss of the anterior corneal stroma. Circumferential and central progression is illustrated by the appearance on presentation (*A*) and 3 months later (*B*). The cellular infiltrate in the conjunctiva adjacent to the ulcer and evidence of lymphocyte stimulation by corneal antigen suggest a local autoimmune phenomenon.

---

**BOX 12-1**
### Diseases Associated with Episcleritis and Scleritis

**Infectious Diseases**
Herpes simplex
Herpes zoster
Tuberculosis
Lyme disease
Syphilis

**Cutaneous Diseases**
Pyoderma gangrenosum
Porphyria
Acne rosacea

**Rheumatologic Diseases**
Rheumatoid arthritis
Wegener's granulomatosis
Inflammatory bowel disease
HLA-B27–associated rheumatologic diseases
Relapsing polychondritis
Polyarteritis nodosa
Giant cell arteritis
Behçet's disease
Sarcoidosis
Polymyositis
IgA nephropathy

HLA, histocompatibility locus antigen; Ig, immunoglobulin.

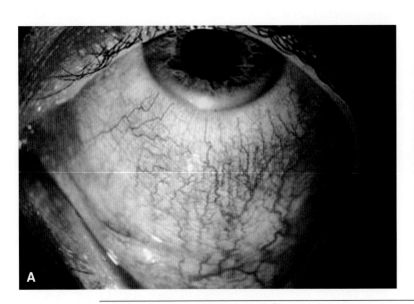 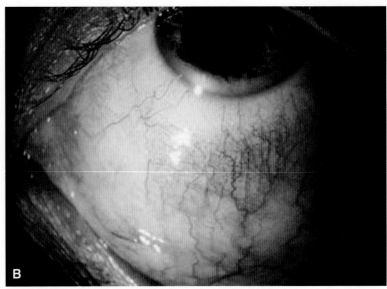

**Figure 12-18.** Diffuse episcleritis (*A*) and the same eye several minutes after application of topical phenylephrine 10% (*B*). Note that the topical vasoconstrictor blanches the conjunctival vessels, but the inflamed episcleral vessels persist.

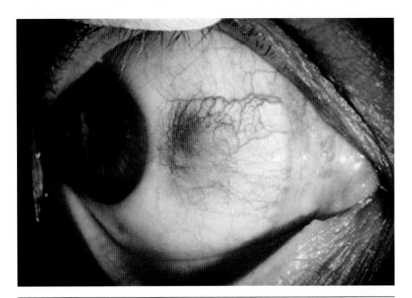

**Figure 12-19.** Nodular episcleritis.

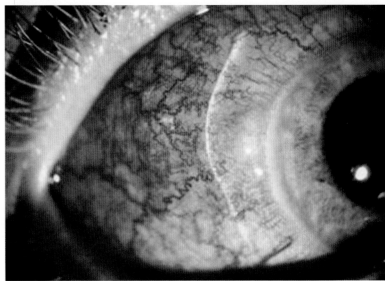

**Figure 12-20.** Diffuse anterior scleritis.

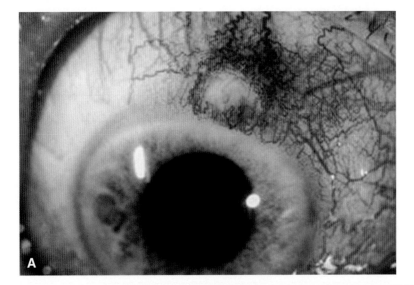 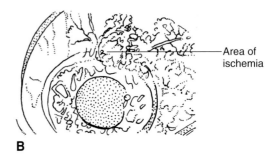

**Figure 12-21.** Necrotizing anterior scleritis with a nodular inflammation pattern. Note the ischemic area of the nodule.

## Pathogenesis

A number of diseases have been associated with scleritis and episcleritis (see Box 12-1). Rheumatoid arthritis is the most common, but no single etiology can be identified in more than 50% of patients. A lymphocytic infiltrate has been observed in episcleritis, but in scleritis, the inflammatory response is granulomatous, with fibrinoid necrosis surrounded by palisading fibroblasts, lymphocytes, plasma cells, polymorphonuclear cells, and occasional giant cells. Immune complex vasculitis is also seen and may play a role in the scleral inflammation associated with connective tissue diseases. Scleritis in rheumatoid arthritis patients with severe articular and extra-articular disease indicates a poor prognosis; if untreated, most of these patients die within 5 years.[5] Scleritis may indicate systemic activity in lupus erythematosus.

## Treatment

Episcleritis usually resolves without treatment in 2 to 3 weeks, although the nodular form may last up to 2 months. If the symptoms warrant, topical steroids speed its resolution. Attacks often recur but do not cause permanent damage or affect vision. Only very rarely does episcleritis progress to scleritis.

Topical steroids are seldom sufficient for treatment of scleritis. Systemic nonsteroidal anti-inflammatory agents are often effective in non-necrotizing disease and should be the first choice in primary episodes or mild recurrences; indomethacin, 70 to 100 mg/day, or tolmetin, 600 to 1800 mg/day, is often effective. If avascular areas are present or in severe or unrelenting disease, systemic prednisone 80 to 120 mg/day is required. Sufficient treatment is given to obtain quiescence of inflammation, allowing taper to nonsteroidal anti-inflammatory drugs or immunosuppressive agents, such as methotrexate or azathioprine. Scleritis may be an important warning of the need to treat a systemic autoimmune disease.

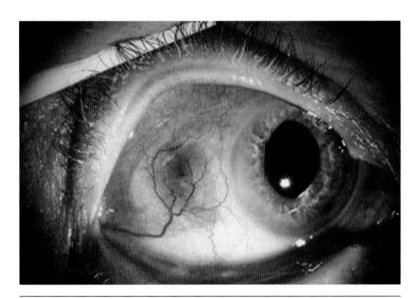

**Figure 12-22.** Scleromalacia perforans in a patient with rheumatoid arthritis.

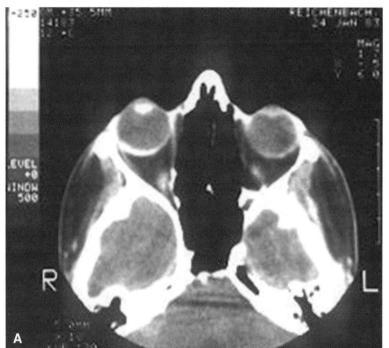

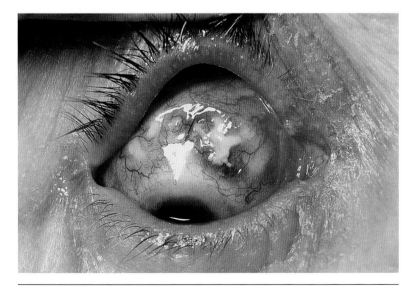

**Figure 12-23.** Retina of a patient with posterior scleritis. Note the areas of choroidal inflammation.

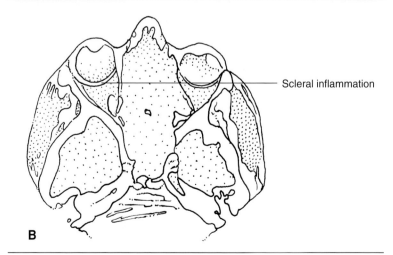

**Figure 12-24.** Computed tomographic scan of patient with posterior scleritis. Note the area of inflammation of the right sclera.

# UVEITIS

The uvea is composed of the iris, ciliary body, and choroid (see Fig. 12-3). They are densely pigmented, vascular structures whose main function is to supply nutrition to the eye. In addition, the muscles of the iris and ciliary body, respectively, control the pupillary aperture and the accommodative status of the lens. Uveitis is inflammation of any portion of the uvea or retina and can be caused by a wide variety of infectious agents and systemic diseases (Box 12-2). However, in many cases, no etiology can be found.[6]

Uveitis is often classified according to the primary focus of the inflammation. Iritis (anterior uveitis) frequently occurs in the histocompatibility locus antigen, (HLA)-B27–related diseases, including ankylosing spondylitis, Reiter's syndrome, and psoriatic arthritis. Iridocyclitis is characterized by inflammation of the iris

and ciliary body. The chronic iridocyclitis seen in pauciarticular juvenile rheumatoid arthritis (Fig. 12-25) exemplifies the damaging sequelae of this inflammation. Ocular inflammation is most frequent in seronegative, antinuclear antibody test–positive, pauciarticular disease, and it may cause severe damage despite apparently normal, noninflamed sclera and conjunctiva. Regular ophthalmic evaluation of patients with juvenile rheumatoid arthritis is important, as early diagnosis and prompt therapy with topical steroids and dilating agents appear to lessen the ocular complications (Table 12-3).

Intermediate uveitis manifests a more widespread inflammation of the vitreous, with many vitreous cells coalescing to form clumps and veils (Fig. 12-26). A fibrovascular membrane and a layer of cellular debris may begin to form on the peripheral retina, a condition known as pars planitis (see Fig. 12-26B).

In retinitis and choroiditis (posterior uveitis), the major sites of inflammation are the retina and the vascular choroid. Signs of inflammation may be present in the anterior chamber and vitreous. Behçet's disease commonly exhibits an occlusive retinal arteritis and periphlebitis (Fig. 12-27). Patients with Behçet's disease frequently show aphthous ulcers of the mouth and genitalia, erythema nodosum, polyarthritis, and central nervous system disorders, in addition to the retinal abnormality. There is a strong

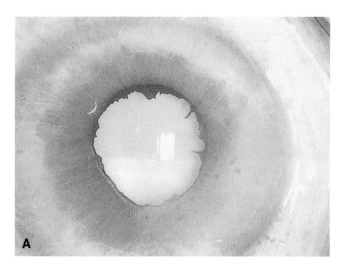
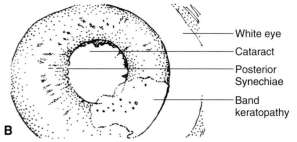

**Figure 12-25.** The chronic iridocyclitis of juvenile rheumatoid arthritis. This disease process can cause adhesions of the iris to the lens, cataract, calcium deposition in the cornea, and glaucoma. Severe damage may result despite apparently normal, noninflamed sclera and conjunctiva. Early diagnosis and prompt therapy with topical steroids and dilating agents are essential to prevent or limit ocular damage. (Reproduced from Spalton DJ, Hitchings RA, Hunter PA: Atlas of Clinical Ophthalmology. London, Gower, 1984, pp 5.2, 10.9; with permission.)

---

**BOX 12-2**
**Diseases Associated with Anterior and Posterior Uveitis**

**Anterior Uveitis (Iritis, Iridocyclitis)**

**Connective Tissue Diseases**
Ankylosing spondylitis
Reiter's syndrome
Psoriatic arthritis
Juvenile rheumatoid arthritis
HLA-B27–associated diseases

**Infectious Diseases**
Herpes zoster
Herpes simplex
Syphilis

**Other**
Sarcoidosis
Glaucomatocyclitis crisis
Heterochromic iridocyclitis

**Predominantly Posterior Uveitis (Affecting Choroid, Retina, Retinal Vessels, Optic Nerve, Vitreous)**

**Infectious diseases**
Toxoplasmic retinochoroiditis
Herpes zoster
Herpes simplex
Cytomegalovirus
Syphilis
Candida
Tuberculosis
Presumed ocular histoplasmosis
Nematode granuloma

**Other**
Pars planitis
Sarcoidosis
Bird-shot chorioretinitis
Behçet's disease
Vogt-Koyanagi-Harada syndrome
Sympathetic ophthalmia

association between this disease and HLA-B51. Short-term therapy with corticosteroids is helpful, but long-term systemic immunosuppression with azathioprine or cyclosporine seems more effective.

Vogt-Koyanagi-Harada syndrome (Fig. 12-28) and sympathetic ophthalmia (Fig. 12-29) primarily involve the choroid. The former, a diffuse granulomatous uveitis, involves the choroidal vessels and overlying pigmented epithelium, as well as the retina. Patients with this syndrome often show a loss of pigmentation of the eyelashes (poliosis) along with vitiligo and alopecia. The central nervous system manifestations of Vogt-Koyanagi-Harada include deafness, tinnitus, and seizures. Systemic corticosteroids, given topically and via periocular injection, are the proper modalities for this disease.

Sympathetic ophthalmia is characterized by the presence of Dalens-Fuchs nodules—collections of inflammatory cells beneath the retinal pigmented epithelium—which arise bilaterally, following the injury of one of the eyes. Through an unknown mechanism, the penetration of one eye provokes the formation of these nodules in the fellow (sympathizing) eye. The process can begin anywhere from 10 days to decades after surgical or traumatic ocular penetration. If, however, the injured eye is removed prior to the onset of inflammation in the fellow eye, sympathetic ophthalmia does not occur.

## CLINICAL MANIFESTATIONS

A patient with acute iritis usually experiences sudden onset of redness, photophobia, tearing, pain, and decreased vision. This can be difficult to differentiate from conjunctivitis without biomicroscopic (slit lamp) examination, but the pain and light sensitivity are more marked in iritis. The conjunctiva is injected, especially surrounding the cornea (Fig. 12-30). The pupil may be smaller in the inflamed eye. Inflammatory precipitates, called keratitic precipitates (Fig. 12-31), may form on the back of the cornea. Inflammatory nodules can develop on the iris or at the pupillary margin (Koeppe nodules) (Fig. 12-32), and adhesions may form between the iris and the cornea or the lens (see Fig. 12-25).

Inflammatory cells may be observed in the vitreous and may coalesce to form opacities visible to the patient as "floaters" (see Table 12-3). Vasculitis is characterized by exudation, sheathing of vessels, hemorrhage, and vascular closure (Fig. 12-33). The retina may become edematous from the leaking vessels, resulting in

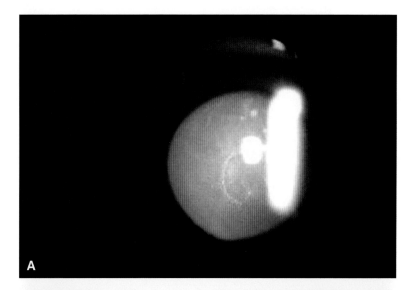
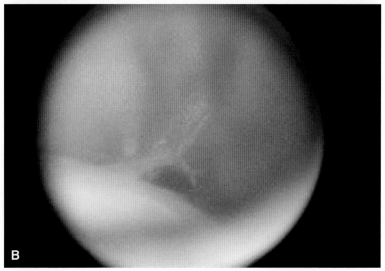

**Figure 12-26.** *A,* Opacities of intermediate uveitis. Vitreous inflammatory debris can coalesce to form vitreous opacities, visible to the patient as dark "floaters." These inflammatory vitreous opacities can be seen by the examiner via retroillumination as shiny particles against the retinal red reflex. *B,* By pressing on the inferior-anterior sclera near the limbus, the anterior retina (pars plana) of this patient can be brought into view. It is covered with a white inflammatory membrane extending into the vitreous. This condition may also be associated with optic nerve papillitis and macular edema.

---

**TABLE 12-3**
**Guidelines for the Frequency of Ophthalmologic Examinations in Children with JRA***

| JRA Subtype at Onset | Age of Onset | |
|---|---|---|
| | <7 yr[†] | ≥7 yr[‡] |
| **Pauciarticular** | | |
| +ANA | H[§] | M |
| −ANA | M | M |
| **Polyarticular** | | |
| +ANA | H[§] | M |
| −ANA | M | M |
| **Systemic** | L | L |

*High risk (H) indicates ophthalmologic examinations every 3–4 mo. Medium risk (M) indicates ophthalmologic examinations every 6 mo. Low risk (L) indicates ophthalmologic examinations every 12 mo.
[†]All patients are considered at low risk 7 yr after the onset of their arthritis and should have yearly ophthalmologic examinations indefinitely.
[‡]All patients are considered at low risk 4 yr after the onset of their arthritis and should have yearly ophthalmologic examinations indefinitely.
[§]All high-risk patients are considered at medium risk 4 yr after the onset of their arthritis.
ANA, antinuclear antibody test; JRA, juvenile rheumatoid arthritis.
From Guidelines for ophthalmologic examinations in children with juvenile rheumatoid arthritis. Sections on rheumatology and section on ophthalmology. Pediatr 1993;92:295.

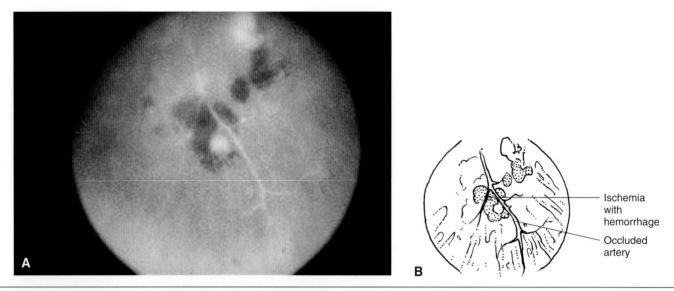

**Figure 12-27.** Occlusive retinal vasculitis in Behçet's disease. Note the occluded, whitened artery. Distal to the vascular occlusion is an area of retinal ischemia with hemorrhage.

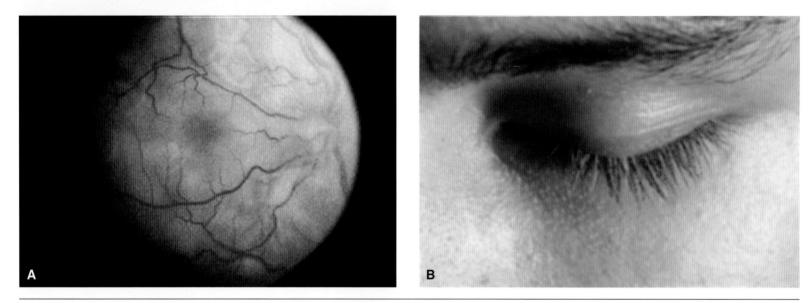

**Figure 12-28.** *A,* The diffuse exudative choroiditis of Vogt-Koyanagi-Harada syndrome. This chronic, diffuse, granulomatous uveitis involves the choroidal vessels, the overlying pigmented epithelium, and the retina. *B,* Loss of pigmentation of the eyelashes (poliosis) is often seen, along with vitiligo and alopecia.

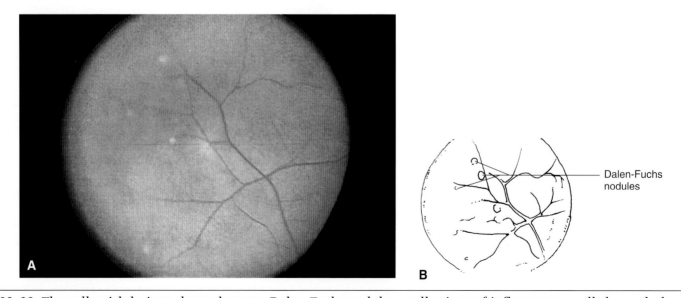

**Figure 12–29.** The yellowish lesions shown here are Dalen-Fuchs nodules—collections of inflammatory cells beneath the retinal pigmented epithelium. They are characteristic of sympathetic ophthalmia. This condition is a bilateral chronic panuveitis that follows penetrating injury of one eye. The mechanism by which penetration of one of the eyes provokes this response in the sympathetic eye is as yet unknown.

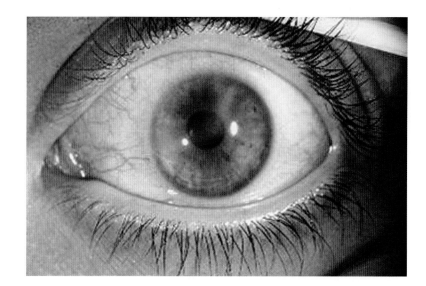

**Figure 12-30.** Iritis with circumlimbal flush. Note the ring of perilimbal injection so characteristic of iritis.

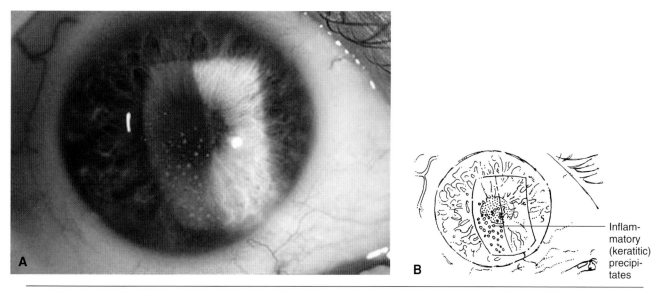

**Figure 12-31.** Inflammatory (keratitic) precipitates seen on the posterior surface of the cornea.

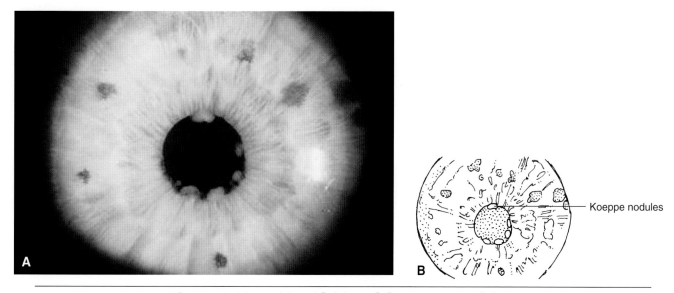

**Figure 12-32.** Uveitis with iris nodules (Koeppe nodules).

decreased vision. Inflammatory exudate in the retina and choroid appears white or yellow.

Leakage from inflamed choroidal vessels often results in the collection of fluid beneath the retina, causing a serous detachment. In eyes with hazy media, examination by an ophthalmologist skilled in the use of the indirect ophthalmoscope is necessary to assess the full extent of the diseases.

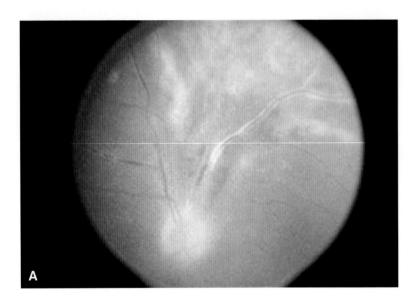

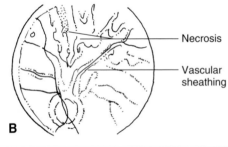

**Figure 12-33.** Vascular sheathing, edema, necrosis, and hemorrhage of the retina. These findings are characteristic of cytomegalovirus retinitis.

## TREATMENT

Therapy is best approached by the identification and treatment of any underlying systemic condition. Often, however, this is not possible, and nonspecific treatment of uveitis is usually initiated with a topical corticosteroid, such as prednisolone acetate 1% and pupillary dilatation/cycloplegia with atropine or scopolamine. More severe inflammation may require oral nonsteroidal anti-inflammatory agents (e.g., indomethacin) or corticosteroids. Periocular corticosteroid injections may control inflammation while minimizing the side effects. In recalcitrant cases or steroid-intolerant patients, methotrexate or cyclosporine may be successful.[7,8]

Topical therapy is not sufficient for inflammation of the posterior uvea, retina, and choroid. Systemic or periocular corticosteroid administration is required. If this is not successful, other immunosuppressive agents may be used.

## ACKNOWLEDGMENT

The authors acknowledge the excellent photographic assistance of Diane Curtin and Joseph Warnicki.

## REFERENCES

1. Smolen G, O'Connor GR (eds): Ocular Immunology, 2nd ed. Boston, Little, Brown & Co., 1986.
2. Abelson MB, Schaefer K: Conjunctivitis of allergic origin—immunologic mechanisms and current approaches to therapy. Surv Ophthalmol 1993; 38(suppl):115–132.
3. Allansmith MR, Ross RN: Ocular allergy and mast cell stabilizers. Surv Ophthalmol 1986;34(4):229–244.
4. Watson P: Diseases of the sclera and episclera. In Duane TD (ed): Clinical Ophthalmology, vol. 4. Philadelphia, Harper & Row, 1987, pp 1–43.
5. Foster, CS, Forstot SL, Wilson LA: Mortality rate in rheumatoid arthritis patients developing necrotizing scleritis or peripheral ulcerative keratitis: Effects of systemic immunosuppression. Ophthalmology 1984;9:1253–1263.
6. Nussenblatt RB, Palestine AG: Uveitis: Fundamental and Clinical Practice, Chicago, Year Book, 1989.
7. Dinning WJ: Therapy-selected topics. In Kraus-Mackiw E, O'Connor GR (eds): Uveitis: Pathophysiology and Therapy. New York, Thieme, 1986, pp 211–219.
8. Jabs DA, Rosenbaum JT, Foster CS, et al: Guidelines for the use of immunosuppressive drugs in patients with ocular inflammatory disorder: Recommendations of an expert panel. Am J Ophthalmol 2000;130(4):492–512.

*Amy M. Scurlock and A. Wesley Burks*

# *13* Food Hypersensitivity

Food hypersensitivity is a common clinical allergic problem. Adverse reactions to foods are classified as either food allergies or food intolerance.[1,2] The utilization of these terms has allowed better communication regarding various reactions to food components. *Adverse food reaction* is a general term that can be applied to a clinically abnormal response to an ingested food or food additive. Adverse food reactions may be secondary to *food hypersensitivity (allergy)* or *food intolerance*.

*Food hypersensitivity (allergy)* (Box 13-1) is an immunologic reaction resulting from the ingestion of a food or food additive. This reaction occurs only in some patients, may occur after only a small amount of the substance is ingested, and is unrelated to any physiologic effect of the food or food additive. To most physicians, the term is synonymous with reactions that involve the immunoglobulin E (IgE) mechanism, of which anaphylaxis is the classic example.

*Food intolerance* (Box 13-2) is a general term describing an abnormal physiologic response to an ingested food or food additive. This reaction has not been proven to be immunologic in nature and may be caused by many factors, including toxic contaminants (e.g., histamine in scromboid fish poisoning, toxins secreted by *Salmonella*, *Shigella*, and *Campylobacter* spp.), pharmacologic properties of the food (e.g., caffeine in coffee, tyramine in aged cheeses), characteristics of the host such as metabolic disorders (e.g., lactase deficiency), and idiosyncratic responses.

The term *food intolerance* has often been overused and, like the term *food allergy*, has been applied incorrectly to all adverse reactions to foods. IgE-mediated (type I) hypersensitivity accounts for the majority of well-characterized food allergic reactions, although non–IgE-mediated immune mechanisms are believed to be responsible for a variety of hypersensitivity disorders. In this chapter, we examine adverse food reactions that are IgE mediated, non–IgE mediated, or have characteristics of both.

## PREVALENCE

The true prevalence of adverse food reactions is still unknown. As many as 25% of people believe that they may be allergic to some food. However, the best available studies suggest that the actual prevalence of food allergy is 1.5% to 2% of the adult population.[3] The prevalence of adverse food reactions in young children is estimated at between 6% and 8%. Several well-controlled studies have revealed that the vast majority of food allergic reactions present in the 1st year of life.

---

**BOX 13-1**
**Food Hypersensitivity (Allergy): Immunologic Spectrum**

IgE mediated ⟶ Non–IgE mediated

Oral allergy syndrome
Anaphylaxis
Urticaria
    Eosinophilic esophagitis
    Eosinophilic gastritis
    Eosinophilic gastroenteritis
    Atopic dermatitis
        Protein-induced
          enterocolitis
        Protein-induced
          enteropathy
        Eosinophilic proctitis
        Dermatitis
          herpetiformis

---

**BOX 13-2**
**Food Intolerance: Non-Immunologic Adverse Reactions**

| Toxic/Pharmacologic | Nontoxic/Intolerance |
|---|---|
| Bacterial food poisoning | Lactase deficiency |
| Heavy metal poisoning | Galactosemia |
| Scromboid fish poisoning | Pancreatic insufficiency |
| Caffeine | Gallbladder/liver disease |
| Tyramine | Hiatal hernia |
| Histamine | Gustatory rhinitis |
| | Anorexia nervosa |

# PATHOPHYSIOLOGY

## *IMMUNOGLOBULIN E*

A variety of hypersensitivity responses to an ingested food antigen may result from the genetically predisposed patient's lack of development of oral tolerance or a breakdown of oral tolerance in his or her gastrointestinal tract. Either a failure to develop or a breakdown in oral tolerance results in excessive production of food-specific IgE antibodies (Fig. 13-1). These food-specific antibodies bind high-affinity FcɛI receptors on mast cells and basophils and low-affinity FcɛII receptors on macrophages, monocytes, lymphocytes, eosinophils, and platelets.[2] After the food allergen binds to the food-specific antibodies on mast cells or basophils, mediators such as histamine, prostaglandins, and leukotrienes are released. These mediators then promote vasodilatation, smooth muscle contraction, and mucus secretion, resulting in the symptoms

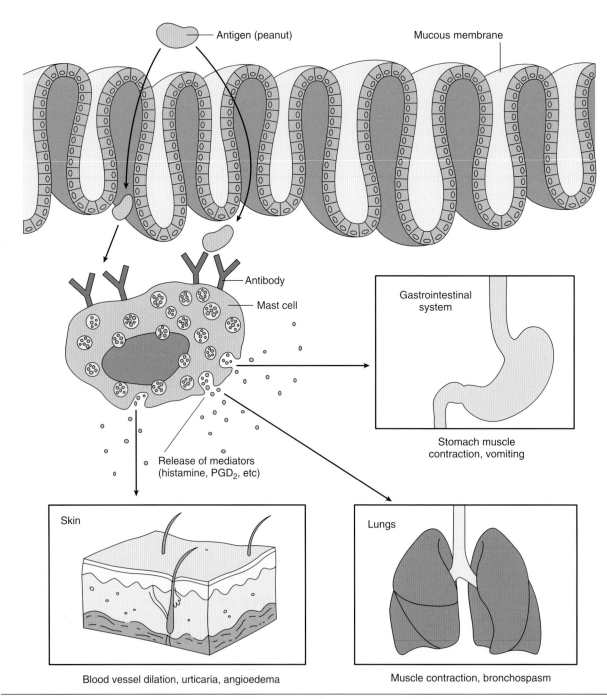

**Figure 13-1.** Schematic representation of the immunologic events underlying the clinically recognizable symptoms of food hypersensitivity. These processes are set in motion when a hypersensitive individual is exposed to an antigenic food such as peanuts. The antigenic component of the food, usually protein, binds to the immunoglobulin antibody on the surface of the mast cells. This triggers the degranulation and activation of the mast cells and the release and generation of a wide range of inflammatory mediators (histamine, $PGD_2$ [prostaglandin $D_2$], etc.). This results in the various end organ changes characteristic of food allergy.

of immediate hypersensitivity. The activated mast cells also may release various cytokines that play a part in the IgE-mediated late-phase response. With repeated ingestion of a specific food allergen, mononuclear cells are stimulated to secrete histamine-releasing factors. The "spontaneous" generation of histamine-releasing factors by the activated mononuclear cells in vitro has been associated with increased cutaneous irritability in children with atopic dermatitis. A rise in plasma histamine has been associated with the provocation of IgE-mediated allergic symptoms after blinded food challenges (Fig. 13-2). In IgE-mediated gastrointestinal reactions, endoscopic observation has revealed local vaso-dilatation, edema, mucus secretion, and petechial hemorrhaging. Increased stool and serum prostaglandin $E_2$ and $F_2$ have been seen after food challenges causing diarrhea.

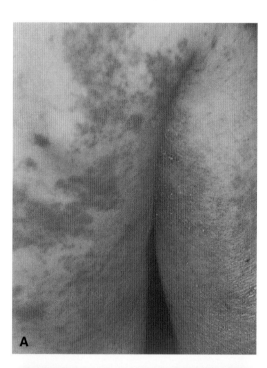

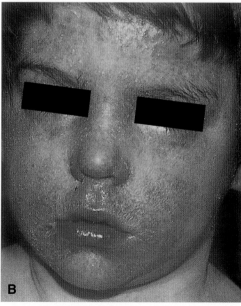

**Figure 13-2.** Exacerbation of atopic dermatitis of the arms (*A*) and the face (*B*) of a child following blinded food challenge. (Photos courtesy of Dr. Hugh A. Sampson, Johns Hopkins University School of Medicine, Baltimore, MD.)

## *NON–IMMUNOGLOBULIN E*

Although a variety of reports have discussed other immune mechanisms causing food-allergic reactions, the scientific evidence supporting these mechanisms is limited. Type III (antigen-antibody complex–mediated) hypersensitivity reactions have been examined in several studies. Whereas IgE–food antigen complexes are seen more commonly in patients with food hypersensitivity, there is little support for food antigen–immune complex–mediated disease. Type IV (cell-mediated) hypersensitivity has been discussed in several disorders where the clinical symptoms do not appear until several hours after the ingestion of the suspected food. This type of immune response may contribute to some adverse food reactions (i.e., enterocolitis), but significant supporting evidence of a specific cell-mediated hypersensitivity disorder is lacking.

# CLINICAL MANIFESTATIONS OF FOOD HYPERSENSITIVITY

## *IMMUNOGLOBULIN E–MEDIATED HYPERSENSITIVITY*

### Gastrointestinal Food Hypersensitivity Reactions

The signs and symptoms of food-induced IgE-mediated gastrointestinal allergy in humans may be secondary to a variety of syndromes, including the oral allergy syndrome, immediate gastrointestinal hypersensitivity, and a small subgroup of allergic eosinophilic gastroenteritis.[4]

The *oral allergy syndrome* (Box 13-3) is considered a form of contact urticaria that is confined almost exclusively to the oropharynx and rarely involves other target organs. The symptoms include rapid onset of pruritus and angioedema of the lips, tongue, palate, and throat. The symptoms generally resolve quite rapidly. This syndrome is most commonly associated with the ingestion of fresh fruits and vegetables, not processed foods. Interestingly, patients with allergic rhinitis secondary to certain airborne pollens (especially ragweed and birch pollens) are frequently afflicted with this syndrome. Patients with ragweed allergy may experience these symptoms following contact with certain melons (e.g., watermelon, cantaloupe, honeydew) and bananas. Those patients with birch sensitivity often have symptoms following the ingestion of raw potatoes, carrots, celery, apples, and hazelnuts. The diagnosis of this syndrome is made after a suggestive history and positive prick skin tests with the implicated fresh fruits or vegetables.[5] The caveat in this syndrome is that the commercially available allergen extracts for fruits and vegetables may be heat labile and often do not have the reliability of an allergen from the fresh food. It may be necessary to use the "prick-by-prick" method, where the device used for introducing the allergen into the skin may have to initially be "pricked" into the food.

*Immediate gastrointestinal hypersensitivity* (Box 13-4) is a form of IgE-mediated gastrointestinal hypersensitivity that may accompany allergic manifestations in other target organs.[6,7] The symptoms vary but may include nausea, abdominal pain or cramping, vomiting, and diarrhea. In studies of children with atopic dermatitis and food allergy, the frequent ingestion of a food allergen appears to induce partial desensitization of gastrointestinal mast cells, resulting in less pronounced symptoms.

The diagnosis of these symptoms is made by a suggestive clinical history, positive prick skin tests, complete elimination of the suspected food allergen for up to 2 weeks with resolution of symptoms, and oral food challenges. After avoidance of a particular food for 10 to 14 days, it is not unusual for symptoms of vomiting to occur during a challenge even when the patient had previously ingested that food without vomiting.

## Respiratory and Skin Food Hypersensitivity Reactions

*Respiratory* and *ocular* symptoms are common concurrent manifestations of IgE-mediated reactions to foods.[2,7] Symptoms may include periocular erythema, pruritus, and tearing; nasal congestion, pruritus, sneezing, and rhinorrhea; and coughing, voice changes, and wheezing. Isolated naso-ocular symptoms are an uncommon manifestation of food hypersensitivity reactions.

The *skin* is a frequent target organ in IgE-mediated food hypersensitivity reactions. The ingestion of food allergens can either lead to immediate cutaneous symptoms or aggravate more chronic symptoms. Acute *urticaria* and *angioedema* (see Chapter 18) are probably the most common cutaneous manifestation of food hypersensitivity reactions, generally appearing within minutes of ingestion of the food allergen (Fig. 13-3). The foods commonly causing these reactions in children include eggs, milk, peanuts, and tree nuts. In adults, this list includes fish, shellfish, tree nuts, and peanuts.

*Atopic dermatitis* (see Chapter 15) is a chronic skin disorder that generally begins in early infancy and is characterized by typical distribution, extreme pruritus, chronically relapsing course, and association with asthma and allergic rhinitis.[8] As many as one third of children with atopic dermatitis have at least one food allergic reaction. Foods to which they typically react include milk, egg, peanut, soy, wheat, fish, and tree nuts (Box 13-5). Food

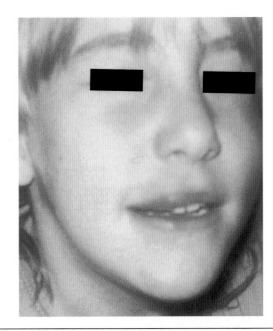

**Figure 13-3.** Angioedema of the lip. This reaction occurred in a child following ingestion of fish during an objective food challenge.

challenges may be needed to help with the diagnosis of food allergy in these children.

## MIXED IMMUNOGLOBULIN E MEDIATED AND NON–IMMUNOGLOBULIN E MEDIATED

*Allergic eosinophilic gastroenteropathy* (Box 13-6) is a disorder characterized by infiltration of the gastric or intestinal walls with eosinophils, absence of vasculitis, and, frequently, peripheral eosinophils.[4,9] Patients presenting with this syndrome frequently have postprandial nausea and vomiting, abdominal pain, diarrhea, occasional steatorrhea, and failure to thrive (young infants) or weight loss (adults). There appears to be a subset of patients with allergic eosinophilic gastroenteritis who have symptoms secondary to food. These patients generally have the mucosal form of this disease with IgE-staining cells in jejunal tissue, elevated IgE in duodenal fluids, atopic disease, elevated serum IgE concentrations, positive prick skin tests to a variety of foods and inhalants, peripheral blood eosinophils, iron deficiency anemia, and hypoalbuminemia (Fig. 13-4).

The diagnosis of this entity is based on an appropriate history and a gastrointestinal biopsy demonstrating a characteristic eosinophilic infiltration (Fig. 13-5). Multiple sites (up to eight) may need to be biopsied to effectively exclude eosinophilic gastroenteritis, because the eosinophilic infiltrates may be quite patchy. Patients with the mucosal form of the disease may have atopic symptoms, including food allergy, elevated serum IgE concentrations, positive skin tests or radioallergosorbent tests (RASTs), and

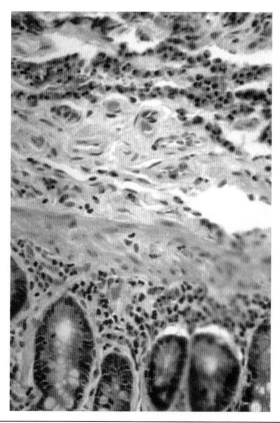

**Figure 13-4.** Photomicrograph demonstrating a jejunal mucosal biopsy with findings typical of eosinophilic gastroenteritis. (From Mitros FA (ed): Atlas of Gastrointestinal Pathology. New York, Gower Medical Publishing 1988, p 5.11.)

peripheral eosinophilia. Other laboratory studies consistent with this disease include Charcot-Leyden crystals in the stool, anemia, hypoalbuminemia, and abnormal D-xylose tests. An elimination diet for as long as 12 weeks may be necessary before complete resolution of symptoms and normalization of intestinal histology.

## NON–IMMUNOGLOBULIN E–MEDIATED FOOD HYPERSENSITIVITY

*Dietary protein enterocolitis* (also known as protein intolerance) (Box 13-7) is a disorder that presents most commonly in children between 1 day and 1 year of age. The typical symptoms are isolated to the gastrointestinal tract and consist of typically recurrent vomiting and/or diarrhea. The symptoms can be severe enough to cause dehydration. Cow's milk or soy protein (particularly in infant formulas) are most often responsible for this syndrome, although egg sensitivity has been reported in older patients. The children will often have stools that contain occult blood, polymorphonuclear neutrophils, and eosinophils and are frequently positive for reducing substances (indicating malabsorbed sugars). Prick skin tests for the putative food protein are characteristically negative. Jejunal biopsies classically reveal flattened villi, edema, and increased numbers of lymphocytes, eosinophils, and mast cells (Figs. 13-6 and 13-7). A food challenge with the responsible protein generally results in vomiting or diarrhea within minutes to several hours, occasionally leading to shock.[4,10] It is not uncommon to find children who are intolerant to both cow's milk and soy protein. This disorder tends to subside by 18 to 24 months of age. Elimination of the offending allergen generally results in improvement or resolution of the symptoms within 72 hours, although secondary disaccharidase deficiency may persist longer. Oral food challenges, which should be done in a medical setting because they can induce severe vomiting, diarrhea, dehydration, or hypotension, consist of administering 0.6 g/kg body weight of the suspected food allergen.

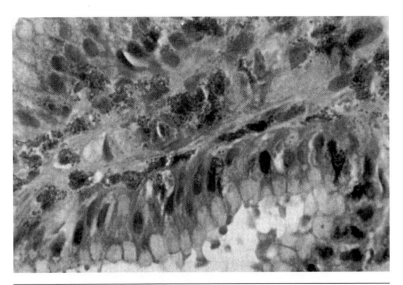

**Figure 13-5.** Photomicrograph of a small-bowel biopsy specimen with dense infiltration of eosinophils in the lamina propria. (From Metcalfe DD, Sampson HA, Simon RA, et al (eds): Food Allergy: Adverse Reactions to Foods and Food Additives, 2nd ed. Cambridge, MA, Blackwell Science, 1997, p 272.)

*Dietary protein proctitis* generally presents in the first few months of life and is often secondary to cow's milk or soy protein hypersensitivity.[11] Infants with this disorder often do not appear ill and have normally formed stools. Generally, this problem is discovered because of the presence of blood (gross or occult) in the stools. Gastrointestinal lesions are confined to the small bowel and consist of mucosal edema, with eosinophils in the epithelium and lumina propria. If lesions are severe with crypt destruction, polymorphonuclear neutrophils are also prominent.[12] It is thought, but without proof from well-controlled studies, that cow's milk and soy protein–induced colitis resolves after 6 months to 2 years of allergen avoidance. Elimination of the offending food allergen leads to resolution of hematochezia within 72 hours, but the mucosal lesions may take up to 1 month to disappear and range from patchy mucosal injection to severe friability with small aphthoid ulcerations and bleeding.

*Celiac disease* is an extensive enteropathy leading to malabsorption. Total villous atrophy and an extensive cellular infiltrate are associated with sensitivity to gliadin, the alcohol-soluble portion of gluten found in wheat oat, rye, and barley (Fig. 13-8). The general incidence is thought to be 1 in 4000 but has been reported

---

**BOX 13-7**
**Dietary Protein Enterocolitis (Protein Intolerance)**

**Manifestations**
Diarrhea with bleeding
Anemia
Emesis
Abdominal distention
Failure to thrive
Hypotension
Fecal leukocytes
Normal immunoglobulin E
Food challenge: Vomiting in 3–4 hr; diarrhea in 5–8 hr

**Age at Onset**
1 day to 1 yr

**Implicated Proteins**
Cow's milk, soy, rice, poultry, fish

**Pathology**
Patchy villous injury and colitis

**Treatment**
80% or more of cases respond to hydrolyzed casein formula, and symptoms clear in 3–10 days
Up to 20% of cases require L-amino acid formula or temporary intravenous therapy

**Natural History**
In general: With treatment, 50% of cases resolve by 18 mo; 90% of cases resolve by 36 mo
Cow's milk: With treatment, 50% of cases resolve by 18 mo; 90% of cases resolve by 36 mo
Soy: Illness is often more persistent

From Sampson HA, Anderson JA: Summary and recommendations: Classification of gastrointestinal manifestations due to immunologic reactions to food in infants and young children. J Pediatr Gastroenterol Nutr 2000;30(suppl 1):588.

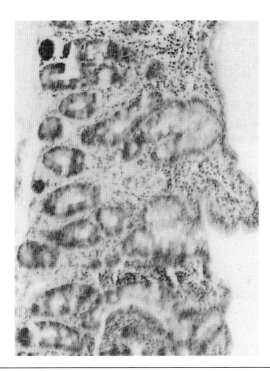

**Figure 13-6.** Small-bowel biopsy section from a 9-month-old boy suffering from recurrent, profuse diarrhea due to cow's milk enteropathy. Although the mechanism for the flattening of the jejunal mucosa and other histopathologic changes is not known, there is strong evidence suggesting immune system involvement.

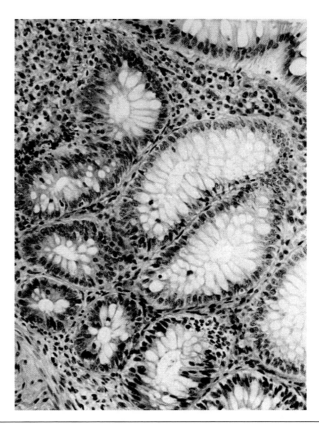

**Figure 13-7.** Photomicrograph of colonic biopsy specimen from a 6-week-old infant with soy protein–induced enterocolitis. (From Metcalfe DD, Sampson HA, Simon RA, et al (eds): Food Allergy: Adverse Reactions to Foods and Food Additives, 2nd ed. Cambridge, MA, Blackwell Science, 1997, p 272.)

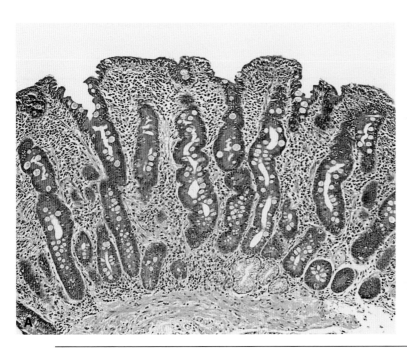

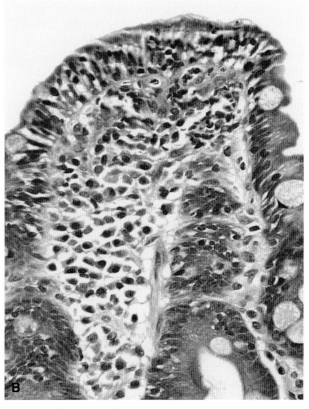

**Figure 13-8.** Digital photomicrographs (*A,* low power; *B,* high power) demonstrating the characteristic villous atrophy and cellular infiltrate of celiac disease. (Images provided by Dr. Marcia Gottfried, Department of Pathology, Duke University Medical Center, Durham, North Carolina.)

as high as 1 in 500 in Ireland. Patients have an apparent genetic predisposition to this disease—approximately 90% of patients are HLA-B8 positive, and nearly 80% have the HLA-DW3 antigen. Patients often have presenting symptoms of diarrhea or frank steatorrhea; abdominal distention and flatulence; weight loss; and, occasionally, nausea and vomiting. Oral ulcers and other extraintestinal symptoms secondary to malabsorption are not common.

## DIAGNOSING ADVERSE FOOD REACTIONS

As with all medical disorders, the diagnostic approach to the patient with a suspected adverse food reaction begins with the medical history and physical examination. Based on the information derived from these initial steps, various laboratory studies may be helpful (Box 13-8).[13–15]

The true value of the medical history is largely dependent on the patient's recollection of symptoms and the examiner's ability to differentiate disorders provoked by food hypersensitivity and other etiologies. The history may be directly useful in diagnosing food allergy in acute events (e.g., systemic anaphylaxis following the ingestion of fish). However, in many cases, less than 50% of reported food allergic reactions could be substantiated by double-blind, placebo-controlled food challenge (DBPCFC).[7,16] Several pieces of information[1] are important to establish that a food allergic reaction occurred (Box 13-9): the food suspected of having provoked the reaction,[2] the quantity of the food ingested,[3] the length of time between ingestion and development of symptoms,[4] a description of the symptoms provoked,[5] whether similar symptoms developed on other occasions when the food was eaten,[6] whether other factors (e.g., exercise) are necessary,[7] and the length of time since the last reaction. Any food may cause an allergic reaction, although only a few foods account for 90% of the reactions. In children, these foods are egg, milk, peanuts, soy, and wheat (plus fish in Scandinavian countries). In chronic disorders like atopic dermatitis, the history is often an unreliable indicator of the offending allergen.

Frequently, a diet diary has been utilized as an adjunct to the medical history. Patients are asked to keep a chronologic record of all foods ingested over a specified period and to record any symptoms they experience during this time. The diary can then be reviewed at a patient visit to determine if there is any relationship between the foods ingested and the symptoms experienced. Uncommonly, this method detects an unrecognized association between a food and a patient's symptoms. In contrast to the medical history, one can collect information on a prospective basis that is not so dependent on a patient's or parent's memory.

An elimination diet is frequently used both in diagnosis and management of adverse food reactions. If a certain food or foods are suspected of provoking a reaction, they are completely eliminated from the diet. The success of an elimination diet depends on several factors, including the correct identification of the allergen(s) involved, the ability of the patient to maintain a diet completely free of all forms of the possible offending allergen, and the assumption that other factors will not provoke similar symptoms during the study period. The likelihood of meeting all of these requirements is often slim, and elimination diets are rarely diagnostic of food allergy, particularly in chronic disorders such as atopic dermatitis or asthma. For example, in a young infant reacting to cow's milk formula, resolution of symptoms following substitution of a soy formula or casein hydrolysate (Alimentum®, Nutramigen®) is highly suggestive of cow's milk allergy but also could suggest lactose intolerance. Avoidance of suspected food allergens prior to any food challenge is recommended so the reactions during the challenge may be heightened.

Allergy prick skin tests are highly reproducible[17] and often utilized to screen patients with suspected IgE-mediated food allergies. The glycerinated food extracts (1:10 or 1:20)[7] and appropriate positive (histamine) and negative (saline) controls are applied by either the prick or puncture technique. A food allergen eliciting a wheal (not including erythema) at least 3 mm larger than the negative control is considered positive; anything else is considered negative. There are two important pieces of information from allergy prick skin test. First, a positive skin test to a food indicates the *possibility* that the patient has symptomatic reactivity to that specific food. (Overall, the positive predictive accuracy is less than 50%.) Second, a negative skin test confirms the absence of an IgE-mediated reaction. (Overall, the negative predictive accuracy is greater than 95%.) Both of these statements are justified if appropriate and good-quality food extracts are utilized.

---

**BOX 13-8**
**Methods Used in the Evaluation of Food Allergic Reactions**

Medical history
Diet diary
Elimination diet
Prick skin testing (PST)
Radioallergosorbent tests (RAST)
Basophil histamine release assay (BHR)
Intestinal mast cell histamine release (IMCHR)
Double-blind placebo-controlled food challenge (DBPCFC)
   (open or single blind)

---

**BOX 13-9**
**Historical Criteria Helpful in the Diagnosis of Food Allergy**

1. The food suspected to have provoked the reaction

2. The quantity of the food ingested

3. The length of time between ingestion and development of symptoms

4. A description of the symptoms provoked

5. Whether similar symptoms developed on other occasions when the food was eaten

6. Whether other factors (e.g., exercise) are necessary to provoke the reaction

7. The length of time since the last reaction

The prick skin test should be considered an excellent means of excluding IgE-mediated food allergies but is only "suggestive" of the presence of clinical food allergies. There are some minor exceptions to the general statement[1]: IgE-mediated sensitivity to several fruits and vegetables (e.g., apples, oranges, bananas, pears, melons, potatoes, carrots, celery) is frequently not detected with commercial reagents, presumably secondary to the instablilty of the responsible allergen in the food[2]; children younger than 1 year may have IgE-mediated food allergy without a positive skin test; and children younger than 2 years may have smaller wheals, possibly due to the lack of skin reactivity.[3] Conversely, a positive skin test to a food ingested in isolation that provokes a serious systemic anaphylactic reaction may be considered diagnostic.

An intradermal skin test is a more sensitive tool than the prick skin test but is much less specific when compared with a DBPCFC. In this study, no patient who had a negative prick skin test but a positive intradermal skin to a specific food had a positive DBPCFC to that food.[18] In addition, intradermal skin testing increases the risk of inducing a systemic reaction compared with prick skin testing.

Radioallergosorbent tests and similar in vitro assays (including enzyme-linked immunosorbent assays) are utilized for the identification of food-specific IgE antibodies. These tests are often used to screen for IgE-mediated food allergies. While generally considered slightly less sensitive than skin tests, one study comparing Phadebos RAST® with DBPCFCs found prick skin tests and RASTs to have similar sensitivity and specificity when a Phadebos score of 3 or greater was considered positive.[19] In this study, if a score of 2 was considered positive, there was a slight improvement in sensitivity while the specificity decreased significantly. In general, in vitro measurements of serum food-specific IgE performed in high-quality laboratories provide information similar to prick skin tests. The newest generation of in vitro studies for specific IgE includes the CAP-RAST (CAP-FEIA®). For patients with suspected food allergy, there are now accepted levels of specific IgE that are more than 95% predictive of a patient being allergic to that food.[15] This test is best used for patients with possible allergic reactions to milk, eggs, and peanuts (and possibly wheat, soy, and fish) (Table 13-1).

The double-blind placebo-controlled food challenge has been labeled the "gold standard" for the diagnosis of food allergy.[4] This test has been utilized successfully by many investigators in both children and adults for the past several years to examine a wide variety of food-related complaints. The foods to be tested in the oral challenge are based on history and/or prick skin test (RAST) results.

A DBPCFC is the best means of controlling for the variability of chronic disorders (e.g., chronic urticaria, atopic dermatitis), any potential temporal effects, and acute exacerbations secondary to reducing or discontinuing medications. Particularly, psychogenic factors and observer bias are eliminated. False-negative challenges are rare in a DBPCFC but may occur when a patient receives insufficient material during the challenge to provoke the reaction or the lyophilization of the food antigen has altered the relevant allergenic epitopes (e.g., fish). Overall, the DBPCFC has proven to be the most accurate means of diagnosing food allergy at the present time.

Open food challenges (or single-blind challenges) may be utilized in many cases to diagnosis patients with food allergy. There are many different schemes available for the administration of food for an oral challenge. A protocol for an open oral challenge is shown in Table 13-2. Box 13-10 lists vehicles in which food challenges may be hidden.

## PRACTICAL APPROACH TO DIAGNOSING FOOD ALLERGY

The diagnosis of food allergy remains a clinical exercise that utilizes a careful history, selective prick skin tests or RASTs (if

**TABLE 13-1**
**Food-Specific IgE Concentrations Predictive of Clinical Reactivity**

| Allergen | Decision Point (KU/L) | Sensitivity | Specificity | PPV | NPV |
|---|---|---|---|---|---|
| Egg | 7 | 61 | 95 | 98 | 38 |
| Infants ≤ 2 yr | 2 | | | 95 | |
| Milk | 15 | 57 | 94 | 95 | 53 |
| Infants ≤ 2 yr | 5 | | | 95 | |
| Peanut | 14 | 57 | 100 | 100 | 36 |
| Fish | 20 | 25 | 100 | 100 | 89 |
| Soybean | 30 | 44 | 94 | 73 | 82 |
| Wheat | 26 | 61 | 92 | 74 | 87 |
| Tree nuts | ~15 | — | — | ~95 | |

NPV, negative predictive value; PPV, positive predictive value.
Data from Boyano MT, Garcia-Ara C, Diaz-Penal M, et al: Validity of specific IgE antibodies in children with egg allergy. Clin Exp Allergy 2001;31(9):1464–1469 and Garcia-Ara C, Munoz-Lopez F, Reche-Frutos M, et al: Specific IgE levels in the diagnosis of immediate hypersensitivity to cows' milk protein in the infant. J Allergy Clin Immunol 2001;107(1):185–190.

**TABLE 13-2**
Example of Open Oral Peanut Challenge
with Peanut Butter

| Time, min | Dose | Amount and Route |
|-----------|------|------------------|
| 0 | 1st | 0.03125 tsp* PB, touch lip |
| 15 | 2nd | 0.03125 tsp PB, inside buccal |
| 25 | 3rd | 0.03125 tsp PB, on tongue |
| 35 | 4th | 0.0625[†] tsp PB, ingested |
| 45 | 5th | 0.25 tsp PB, ingested |
| 55 | 6th | 0.25 tsp PB, ingested |
| 65 | 7th | 1 tsp PB, ingested |
| 75 | 8th | Remaining PB up to a total of 2 T |

*0.03125 tsp is the size of three kernels of rice.
[†]0.0625 tsp is the size of a kernel of corn.
PB, peanut butter.

an IgE-mediated disorder is suspected), appropriate exclusion diet, and blinded provocation (Boxes 13-11, 13-12, and 13-13). Other diagnostic tests that do not appear to be of significant value include food-specific IgG or IgG4 antibody levels, food antigen–antibody complexes, evidence of lymphocyte activation[3] (e.g., uptake, interleukin-2 production, leukocyte inhibitory factor), and sublingual or intracutaneous provocation. Blinded challenges may not be necessary in suspected gastrointestinal disorders where laboratory values and biopsies before and after challenge are often used.

An exclusion diet eliminating all foods suspected by history or prick skin testing (or RASTs) for IgE-mediated disorders should be conducted for at least 2 weeks. Table 13-3 lists potential cross-reacting allergens that should be considered. Some gastrointestinal disorders may need to have the exclusion diet extended for up to 12 weeks following appropriate biopsies. If no improvement is noted following the diet, it is unlikely that food allergy is involved. In the case of some chronic diseases, such as atopic dermatitis or chronic asthma, other precipitating factors may make it difficult to discriminate the effects of the food allergen from other provocative factors.

**BOX 13-10**
**Vehicles in Which Food Challenges May Be Hidden***

Infant formulas
Ices; vanilla-flavored element formulas
Apple sauce
Milkshakes
Popsicles
Capsules (opaque, gelatin)

*Patients should not be allergic to the vehicle used for the challenge.

**BOX 13-12**
**Diagnostic Approach: IgE-Mediated Food Allergy**

Test for specific IgE antibody
    Negative: Reintroduce food*
    Positive: Start elimination diet

Elimination diet
    No resolution: Reintroduce food*
    Resolution
        Open/single-blind challenges to "screen"
        DBPCFC for equivocal open challenges

*Unless convincing history warrants supervised challenge.
DBPCFC, double-blind placebo-controlled food challenge; IgE, immunoglobulin E.

**BOX 13-11**
**Diagnostic Approach: Non–IgE-Mediated Disease**

Includes disease with unknown mechanisms
    Food additive allergy
Elimination diets (may need elemental diet)
Oral challenges
    Timing/dose/approach individualized for disorder
        Enterocolitis syndrome can elicit shock
        Enteropathy/eosinophilic gastroenteritis-prolonged
            feedings to develop symptoms
DBPCFCs preferred
May require ancillary testing (endoscopy/biopsy)

DBPCFC, double-blind placebo-controlled food challenge; IgE, immunoglobulin E.

**BOX 13-13**
**Food Allergy Prevention**

Aimed at "high-risk" newborn
    Positive family history: Biparental or parent/sibling
Breastfeeding generally protective of allergy
Wean/supplement with extensively hydrolyzed hypo-allergenic protein hydrolysate
Delay introduction of solid foods >6 mo
    Cow milk/dairy: 6–12 mo
    Egg: 12–24 mo
    Peanut, tree nut, seafood: >24–48 mo

Open or single-blind challenges in a clinic setting may be helpful to screen suspected food allergens. The presumptive diagnosis of food allergy based on a patient's history and prick skin tests or RAST results is no longer acceptable. There are exceptions to this, such as with patients who have severe anaphylaxis following the isolated ingestion of a specific food. It is important that the medical care provider make an unequivocal diagnosis of food allergy. If the present practice continues, more than one quarter of the population worldwide will continue to alter their eating habits based on misconceptions of food allergy.

## *TREATMENT*

Once the diagnosis of food allergy is established, the only proven therapy is the strict *elimination* of the food from the patient's diet. Elimination diets may lead to malnutrition or eating disorders, especially if these diets exclude a large number of foods or are utilized for extended periods. Studies have shown that symptomatic food sensitivity generally is lost over time, except for sensitivity to peanuts, tree nuts, and seafood.

Symptomatic food sensitivity is usually very specific, so patients rarely react to more than one member of a botanical family or animal species. Certain factors place some individuals at increased risk for more severe anaphylactic reactions: (1) history of a previous anaphylactic reaction; (2) history of asthma, especially if poorly controlled; (3) allergy to peanuts, nuts, fish, and shellfish; (4) the need for beta-blockers or angiotensin-converting enzyme (ACE) inhibitors; and (5) possibly being female.

## Medications

Several medications have been used in an attempt to protect patients with food hypersensitivity, including oral cromolyn, $H_1$ and $H_2$ antihistamines, ketotifin, corticosteroids, and prostaglandin synthetase inhibitors.

Some of these medications may modify food allergy symptoms, but overall they have minimal efficacy or unacceptable side effects. The use of epinephrine is vitally important in acute anaphylaxis. The importance of prompt epinephrine administration when symptoms of systemic reactions to foods develop cannot be overemphasized. Epi-Pen (0.3 mg) and Epi-Pen, Jr.® (0.15 mg) can be given intramuscularly or subcutaneously (most recent studies suggest that intramuscularly is better) at an epinephrine dose of 0.01 mg/kg to a maximum of 0.3 mg.

## Immunotherapy

Recent blinded, placebo-controlled studies of rush immunotherapy for the treatment of peanut hypersensitivity demonstrated efficacy in a small number of patients.[20] The adverse reaction rates were significant and preclude general clinical application at this time.

Newer types of vaccines for immunotherapy specifically for food-induced anaphylaxis are being developed and include[21] humanized anti-IgE monoclonal antibody therapy,[2] plasmid-DNA immunotherapy,[3] peptide fragments ("overlapping" peptides),[4] cytokine-modulated immunotherapy,[5] immunostimulatory sequence–modulated immunotherapy,[6] bacteria-encapsulated allergen immunotherapy,[7] and "engineered" recombinant protein immunotherapy.

Additionally, recent studies with humanized, monoclonal antibody anti-IgE have been utilized in phase I trials for patients with peanut allergy.[22] This type of therapy appears to be a promising option for patients with a history of food-induced anaphylaxis or with a food allergy that puts them at risk for a future systemic anaphylactic reaction.

## Patient Education

Patient education and support are essential with food allergies. In particular, adults and older children prone to anaphylaxis (and their parents) must be informed in a direct but sympathetic way that these reactions are potentially fatal.

When eating away from home, food-sensitive individuals should feel comfortable to request information about the contents of prepared foods. The American Academy of Pediatrics Committee of School Health has recommended that schools be equipped to treat anaphylaxis in allergic students. Children older than 7 years usually can be taught to inject themselves with epinephrine. The physician must be willing to explain and, with the parents, help instruct school personnel about these issues. In the home, consider the need to eliminate the incriminated allergen, or if this is not practical, place warning stickers on foods with the offending antigens.

A variety of groups can help provide support, advocacy, and education, including The Food Allergy and Anaphylaxis Network (10400 Easton Place, Suite 107, Fairfax, VA 22030-5647; www.foodallergy.org), the National Allergy and Asthma Network (3554 Chain Bridge Road, Suite 200, Fairfax, VA 22030-2709), and the Asthma and Allergy Foundation of America (1125 15th Street, NW, Suite 502, Washington, DC 20005).

## TABLE 13-3
### Allergen Cross-Reactivity: Summary

| If Allergic to | Risk of Reaction to | Risk |
| --- | --- | --- |
| A legume | Other legumes | 5–10% |
| A tree nut | Other tree nuts | 40% |
| A fish | Other fish | 50% |
| A shellfish | Other shellfish | 50–75% |
| A grain | Other grains | 20% |
| Egg | Chicken | 5% |
| Cow's milk | Beef | 10% |
| Cow's milk | Goat's milk | >90% |
| Cow's milk | Mare's milk | 4% |
| Pollen | Fruits/vegetables | 50% |
| Melon | Other fruits (melon, banana, avacado) | 90% |
| Latex | Fruits | 35% |
| Fruits | Latex | 10% |

## PROGNOSIS

For many young children diagnosed with anaphylaxis to foods such as milk, egg, wheat, and soybeans, there is a good possibility that the clinical sensitivity may be outgrown after several years.[9,23,24] Children who develop their food sensitivity after 3 years of age are less likely to lose their food reactions over a several-year period. Patients who develop very mild reactions (skin symptoms only) to peanuts early in life (first 12 to 24 months) may outgrow their symptoms.[25,26] Allergies to foods such as tree nuts, fish, and seafood are generally not outgrown no matter at what age they develop. Individuals with these allergies appear likely to retain their allergic sensitivity for a lifetime. Consequently, several groups are evaluating new strategies to "desensitize" patients to these foods.

# REFERENCES

1. Anderson J, Sogn D: Adverse Reactions to Foods. American Academy of Allergy and Immunology Committee on Adverse Reactions to Foods and the National Institute of Allergy and Infectious Disease. Washington, DC, National Institute of Allergy & Infectious Disease, 1984.
2. Sampson HA, Burks AW: Mechanisms of food allergy. Ann Rev Nutr 1996; 16:161–177.
3. Sampson HA: Food allergy. JAMA 1997;278:888–894.
4. Sampson HA, Anderson JA: Summary and recommendations: Classification of gastrointestinal manifestations due to immunologic reactions to foods in infants and young children. J Pediatr Gastroenterol Nutr 2000;30(suppl): S87–S94.
5. Bock SA: Natural history of severe reactions to foods in young children. J Pediatr 1985;107:676–680.
6. Bock SA, Atkins FM: Patterns of food hypersensitivity during sixteen years of double-blind, placebo-controlled food challenges. J Pediatr 1990;117:561–567.
7. Sampson HA: Adverse reactions to foods. In Middleton E, Reed C, Ellis E, et al (eds): Allergy: Principles and Practice. St. Louis, Mosby-Year Book, 1998, pp 1162–1182.
8. Eigenmann PA, Sicherer SH, Borkowski TA, et al: Prevalence of IgE-mediated food allergy among children with atopic dermatitis. Pediatrics 1998;101:E8.
9. Bock SA: Prospective appraisal of complaints of adverse reactions to foods in children during the first 3 years of life. Pediatrics 1987;79:683–688.
10. Goldman AS, Anderson DW, Sellers WA, et al: Milk allergy: I. Oral challenge with milk and isolated milk proteins in allergic children. Pediatrics 1963;32: 425–443.
11. Crowe SE, Perdue MH: Gastrointestinal food hypersensitivity: Basic mechanisms of pathophysiology. Gastroenterology 1992;103:1075–1095.
12. Jenkins HR, Pincott JR, Soothill JF, et al: Food allergy: The major cause of infantile colitis. Arch Dis Child 1984;59:326–329.
13. Burks AW, Sampson HA: Diagnostic approaches to the patient with suspected food allergies. J Pediatr 1992;121:S64.
14. Schwartz HJ: Food allergy: Adverse reactions to foods and food additives. In Metcalfe DD, Sampson HA, Simon RA (eds): Asthma and Food Additives. Cambridge, MA, Blackwell Science, 1997, pp 411–418.
15. Sampson HA: Utility of food-specific IgE concentrations in predicting symptomatic food allergy. J Allergy Clin Immunol 2001;107:891–896.
16. Sampson HA: Food allergy. J Allergy Clin Immunol 1989;84(6, pt 2): 1062–1067.
17. Bock SA, Lee WY, Remigio L, et al: Appraisal of skin tests with food extracts for diagnosis of food hypersensitivity. Clin Allergy 1978;8:559–564.
18. Bock SA, Buckley J, Holst A, et al: Proper use of skin tests with food extracts in diagnosis of hypersensitivity to food in children. Clin Allergy 1977;7: 375–383.
19. Sampson HA, Albergo R: Comparison of results of skin tests, RAST, and double-blind, placebo-controlled food challenges in children with atopic dermatitis. J Allergy Clin Immunol 1984;74:26–33.
20. Oppenheimer JJ, Nelson HS, Bock SA, et al: Treatment of peanut allergy with rush immunotherapy. J Allergy Clin Immunol 1992;90:256–262.
21. Burks AW, Bannon GA, Lehrer SB: Classic spcific immunotherapy and new perspectives in specific immunotherapy for food allergy. Allergy 2001;67: 121–124.
22. Leung DYM, Sampson HA, Yunginger JW, et al: Effect of anti-IgE therapy in patients with peanut allergy. N Engl J Med 2003;348:986–993.
23. Bock SA: The natural history of food sensitivity. J Allergy Clin Immunol 1982;69:173–177.
24. Bock SA, Atkins FM: Patterns of food hypersensitivity during sixteen years of double-blind, placebo-controlled food challenges. J Pediatr 1990;117:561–567.
25. Skolnick HS, Conover-Walker MK, Koerner CB, et al: The natural history of peanut allergy. J Allergy Clin Immunol 2001;107:367–374.
26. Hourihane JO, Roberts SA, Warner JO: Resolution of peanut allergy: Case-control study. BMJ 1998;316:1271–1275.

*Vincent S. Beltrani*

# *14* Contact Dermatitis

*Contact dermatitis* (CD) is the objective inflammation or subjective dysesthesia of the skin induced by contact with an exogenous substance. It is a very common problem, constituting 7.8 million physician visits a year, and can be a significant impediment to an individual's quality of life. When CD occurs in association with occupational exposure, the financial impact on both patients and employers can be considerable.

The spectrum of skin reactions resulting from touching exogenous agents varies from subjective burning to complete exfoliation (Box 14-1).

The clinical response to the offending agent can result from an immunologic or a nonimmunoloigc mechanism. *Allergic CD* (ACD) is recognized as the prototypic delayed hypersensitivity immunologic reaction, and *irritant CD* (ICD) is a nonimmunologic reaction.

It is estimated that there are more than 85,000 agents that can elicit skin reactions in the environment. When these agents come in contact with the skin, the majority of them are more likely to induce an irritant reaction; there are approximately 2800 others that are allergens and can cause a contact hypersensitivity reaction (in sensitized individuals; Box 14-2).

## CLINICAL MANIFESTATIONS

The distinction between ICD and ACD has become increasingly blurred. The difference is best demonstrated in extreme examples and is more indistinct with milder reactions. Morphologic guidelines for distinguishing the two diseases have been offered but are not useful for mild to moderate reactions.[1]

### *IRRITANT CONTACT DERMATITIS (ICD)*

ICD is considered the more common type of CD. Clinically, it is a very polymorphous syndrome, since each irritant demonstrates uniqueness to both chemicals and individuals. Because ICD is not an immunologic reaction, it does not require prior sensitization to the causative substance.

Irritants are more likely to cause symptoms and signs within minutes to hours (whereas allergens take days). Common "irritants" are listed in Box 14-3.

Irritant reactions are usually cytotoxic events resulting from varying degrees of epidermal damage induced by the noxious substance. The inflammatory response is both dose dependent and time dependent. The clinical presentation of ICD is restricted to the skin site directly in contact with the offending agent. Little to no reaction is noted beyond the site of contact (Fig. 14-1). Several different clinical manifestations of ICD have been described.[2]

---

**BOX 14-1**
**"Contact" Reactions That Can Occur on the Skin**

Dysesthesia (e.g., stinging, burning)
Pruritus
Irritant contact dermatitis
Allergic contact (spongiotic) dermatitis (type IV hypersensitivity)
(Contact) urticaria (type I hypersensitivity)
Acneiform eruptions
Hypopigmentation and/or hyperpigmentation
Photosensitivity reactions
Purpura
Atrophy
Dermal reactions

---

**BOX 14-2**
**Classes of Putative Agents That Can Cause Contact Dermatitis**

Water, solvents
Plants (e.g., *Rhus* [poison ivy], alstromeria)
Metals (e.g., nickel, chromium, cobalt)
Commercial chemicals (48,253)
Food additives (8627)
Cosmetics (3410)
Pesticides (3350)
Drugs (1815)

---

*Acute ICD* is usually the result of accidental contact with a potent irritant (acids and alkalis). The patient experiences rather sudden burning, stinging, and pain at the site(s) of contact. Objectively, one can see erythema, edema, bulla, and possible necrosis (see Fig. 14-1). Borders are sharply demarcated. The prognosis is good.[3]

*Acute delayed ICD* is characteristic for certain irritants, such as tretinoin (Retin A®), anthralin (Fig. 14-2), jellyfish, and others. Clinically, it resembles acute ICD, except that the visible inflammation and subjective discomfort appear 8 to 24 hours or more after exposure.

*Irritant reaction ICD* is recognized as the scaling, redness, tiny vesicles, pustules, and erosions in individuals exposed to wet work (Fig. 14-3), such as hairdressers and food handlers. It usually begins under rings, then may spread over the fingers to the hands and the forearms. It is commonly seen in infants as a "diaper" rash.

Fortunately, this condition resolves spontaneously, as a result of "hardeneing" of the skin, but sometimes it progresses to cumulative irritant dermatitis.

*Cumulative ICD* is a consequence of multiple subthreshold damages to the skin to weak irritants when the time between exposures is too short for complete restoration of skin barrier

---

### BOX 14-3
### Important Cutaneous Irritants

| | |
|---|---|
| Soaps, detergents | Dust, dirt, sewage |
| Janitorial cleaning agents | Cement, mortar, plaster |
| Disinfectants | Fiberglass |
| Solvents, degreasers | Acids, alkalis |
| Oils, greases | Insects, fruits, vegetables |
| Plastic resins | Grasses, weeds, shrubs |
| Paints, inks, varnishes | Shampoos |
| Glues, adhesives | Permanent wave solutions |
| Gasoline, diesel and jet fuels | Pesticides, herbicides, fungicides |
| Metalworking fluids | Fertilizers |

---

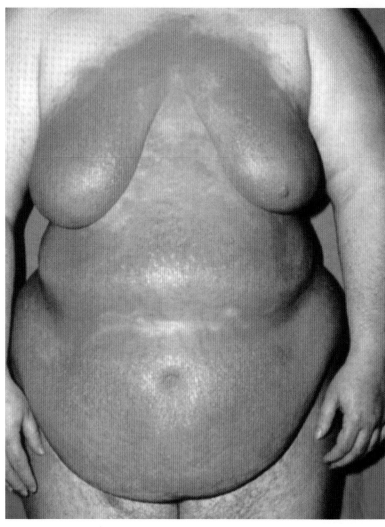

**Figure 14-2.** Delayed irritation contact dermatitis appeared 24 hours after the application of anthralin as treatment of psoriasis.

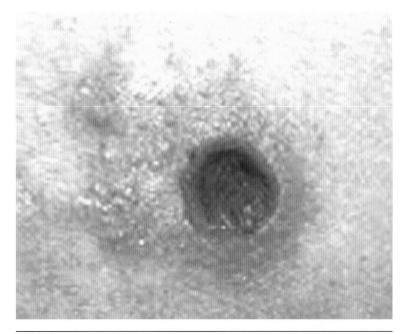

**Figure 14-1.** Positive acute irritant contact patch test caused by monoethanolamine, a caustic agent.

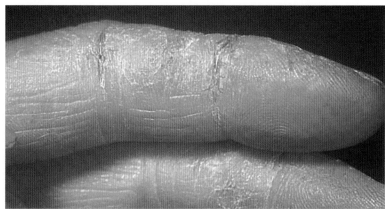

**Figure 14-3.** "Dishpan hands" due to wet work plus detergent.

function. Symptoms include itching and pain due to cracking of hyperkeratotic skin. The skin appears dry, erythematous, vesicular, lichenified, and hyperkeratotoic. Xerotic dermatitis is the most frequent type of cumulative toxic dermatitis (Fig. 14-4).

*Asteatotic eczema* is seen mainly in elderly individuals with a history of frequent showering or bathing without moisturizing (especially in the winter months). Patients suffer from intensive itching, and the skin appears dry, scaly, and fissured with erythematous islands of eczema (Fig. 14-5). Lesions are diffuse with irregular reticulation, especially on the extremities. When fissures appear in the dry, reddened areas, they are called eczema craquelé (Fig. 14-6).

*Traumatic ICD* develops after acute skin trauma, such as burns, lacerations, and acute ICD. These eczematous lesions heal very slowly, persisting for many weeks.

*Pustular and acneiform ICD* is a result of exposure to certain irritants, such as croton oil, mineral oil, tars, greases (chlorinated hydrocarbons), and naphthalene. The pustules are sterile and transient. This acne is resistant to treatment and requires avoidance of the acneiforming agents.

*Nonerythematous ICD* is defined as a subclinical form of ICD with changes in the epidermal barrier function without a clinical correlate.

*Subjective ICD* is another subjective experience with no clinical signs. Patients feel a stinging or burning after contact with certain chemicals, such as lactic acid, menthol, and alcohol. This subjective ICD is modified by external factors (e.g., type of irritant, exposure, mechanical pressure, temperature, humidity).

## ALLERGIC CONTACT DERMATITIS

ACD is the immunologic, antigen-induced cutaneous reaction resulting from contact with a hapten on previously sensitized skin. These eczematous reactions can be identified clinically and histologically as acute, subacute, and chronic.

The "eczema" of ACD is caused by specific cytokines released from sensitized Th1 cells after being activated by its sensitizing hapten (antigen). The sequence of events for the "delayed" reaction is shown in Figure 14-7. The initial reaction has a longer latent period, whereas each subsequent exposure occurs more rapidly (an anamnestic response).

*Acute ACD* is best exemplified by the most common ACD reaction; namely, *Rhus dermatitis* or poison ivy. The dermatitis begins with itching and redness, which evolves to streaks of erythema or papulovesicles in linear arrangements.

The oleoresin (urushiol) of the sap of *Rhus* plants contains catechols, which are the sensitizing chemicals. *Rhus* dermatitis may be acquired without touching the plants through exposure to the oleoresin-contaminated fur of animals, garden utensils, golf sticks and balls, or other items. Scratching, which releases the vesicle fluid (serum), does not spread the rash.

These *Rhus* plants belong to the family of plants known as the *Anacardiaceae* (see Table 14-1 and Figs. 14-9 and 14-10). Cross-reaction may occur with related plants. Eruptions undistinguishable from those caused by poison ivy (see Fig. 14-11) can occur in sensitized individuals when in contact with the cross-reactors listed in Box 14-4.

Although patch testing with *Rhus* oleoresin should not be done routinely, patch testing (see later) remains the gold standard and, when used properly, provides support for the diagnosis of ACD. The North American Contact Dermatitis Group (NACDG)

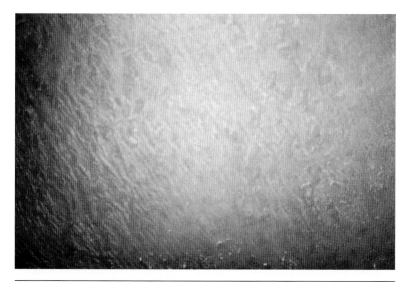

**Figure 14-4.** Dry, scaly skin (Xerosis), usually seen in winter in elderly individuals.

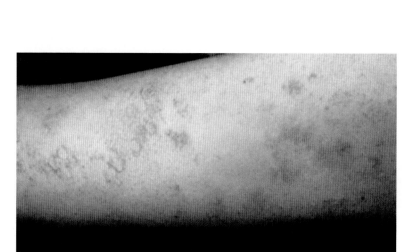

**Figure 14-5.** Asteototic eczema.

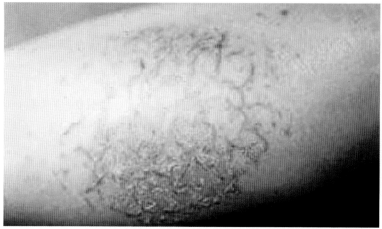

**Figure 14-6.** Eczema craquelé.

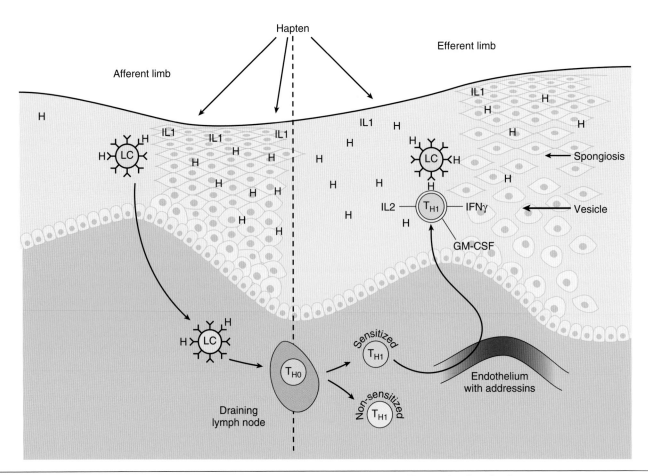

**Figure 14-7.** The immune pathogenic response of allergic contact dermatitis. Afferent limb: The hapten must penetrate the stratum corneum, activating the underlying keratinocytes, which release cytokines. Haptenated Langerhans' cells (LCs) migrate to the draining lymph nodes (within 24 hours). The haptens are then presented to Th0-cells in the lymph nodes and 1 of 100 to 500 become sensitized Th1-cells. Efferent limb: The sensitized Th1 cells, which possess skin-specific homing receptors, enter the circulation and are then attracted to antigen-presenting LCs at the site of antigen entrance. When the antigen is presented to the sensitized Th1 cell, it releases its cytokines, which produce the spongiosis (of eczema) within 12 to 36 hours. (From Kalish RS: Recent developments in the pathogenesis of allergic contact dermatitis. Arch Dermatol 1991;127:1558–1563.)

**TABLE 14-1**
**Characteristics of *Rhus* "Poison" Plants**

| Name | Habitat | Leaves | Growth Features |
|---|---|---|---|
| Common poison ivy (*Rhus radicans*) | United States, except the extreme southwest; throughout Canada | Group of three leaflets, edges smooth or notched, green in summer, reddish in fall | As woody, ropelike vine; as trailing shrub on ground, or erect without support |
| Oakleaf poison ivy (*Rhus diversiloba*) | Southeastern United States, from New Jersey to eastern Texas | Group of three leaflets; center leaf resembles oak leaf | Low-growing shrub |
| Western poison oak (*Rhus toxicodendron*) | Pacific coast from southern California to Canada | Group of three leaflets; center oak leaf and side leaflets of irregular shapes | Upright shrub, can grow into large spreading clumps 6 ft tall; in forests, becomes vine up to 30 ft tall |
| Poison sumac (*Rhus vernix*) | Damp, swampy areas throughout the United States, particularly east of the Mississippi | Seven to 13 leaflets, arranged as pairs along a central midrib with a single leaflet at the end | Coarse, woodish shrubs, or as tree; never as a vine |

regularly publishes the results of its multicenter patch testing group, the purpose of which is to guide physicians in choosing which chemicals to use for patch testing and which to include or exclude from topical formulation. They recently concluded that the usefulness of patch testing is enhanced with the number of allergens tested.[4,5] The results of patch testing in 3120 patients are listed (according to frequency of positive results) in Table 14-2. The average age of the patient population was 47 years (range, 4 to 96 years), and 62% were female.

Nickel is a ubiquitous contact allergen. The almost continuous exposure to nickel is reflected in the increasing number of patients who are sensitized to it. Nickel produces more cases of ACD than all the other metals combined.[6] Women are more commonly

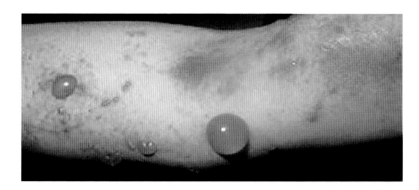

**Figure 14-8.** Acute *Rhus* dermatitis (poison ivy). Note the linear configuration (Koebner's phenomenon) exemplifying that the eczema (vesiculobulla) appears only at sites of deposition of *Rhus* antigen. Because poison ivy, sumac, and oak all contain the identical *Rhus* antigen, they produce identical eruptions.

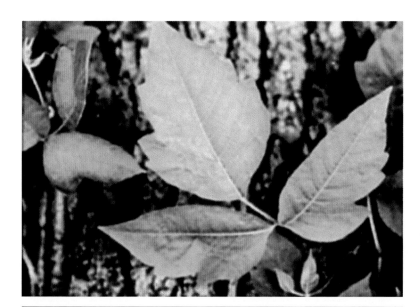

**Figure 14-9.** Poison ivy vine climbing a tree trunk. Remember the saying "Leaves three, leave them be."

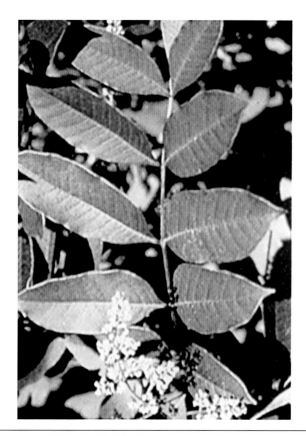

**Figure 14-10.** Poison sumac leaves.

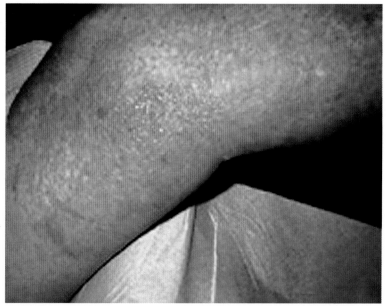

**Figure 14-11.** Gingko biloba–induced exacerbation of "old" *Rhus* dermatitis.

---

**BOX 14-4**
**Cross-Reactors with *Rhus* Plants**

Cashew nut shell oil
Rind of the mango
"Marking nut tree of India" (causes dhobi itch)
Japanese lacquer tree
Fruit pulp of the gingko tree (present in gingko biloba pills)

sensitized by nonoccupational contacts (jewelry; Figs. 14-12 and 14-13. Men are often sensitized by industrial exposure. Industrial solutions penetrate rubber gloves (heavy-duty vinyl gloves should be used instead). Dietary nickel is a contributing factor to the worsening of dermatitis in some nickel-sensitive persons. Reduction of intake or the use of disulfiram, a nickel chelator, has resulted in clinical improvement in some of these patients.

Hand dermatitis is extremely common (occurring in 10% of women and 4.5% of men), and the differential diagnosis can be challenging. ACD is rarely noted on the palms and occurs most often on the thinner skin between the fingers and the dorsum of the hands. It is the most common type of contact dermatitis in the workplace. Thiurams are the most common sensitizers among the rubber components found in gloves (North American Contact Dermatitis Group results) (see Figs. 14-14 and 14-15).[5]

Hexavalent chromium is the chief allergen in cement, but it is also used in the tanning of leather and rust inhibition in paints and in certain photographic materials (see Fig. 14-16).

Facial ACD is most often the result of an allergen being transferred to the face from other regions of the body. Considering the millions of daily applications of innumerable cosmetics, the incidence of dermatitis from their use is low. Even so, it is not unusual for an individual to use a particular cosmetic for years without reacting and then suddenly acquire an allergic hypersensitivity. Paraphenylenediamine (PPDA), an oxidative-type hair dye, remains a most common cause of facial dermatitis. Thus, performing a patch test before each application of a paraphenylenediamine hair dye is legally a mandatory requirement (Figs. 14-17 and 14-18).

Interestingly, unoxidized paraphenylenediamine and the black end product is not the sensitizer; rather, intermediate partially oxidized quinones are believed to be the sensitizers. Thus, the dye should be freshly prepared prior to "self-testing."[6]

Fragrances, lanolin, emollients, emulsifying agents, or preservatives may be sensitizers in face creams. Fragrance allergy is the most common cause of cosmetic contact dermatitis. Patients typically are sensitized to a fragranced skin-care product and not

## TABLE 14-2
### Positive Patch Test Result (1994–1996) to 20 Most Common Agents

| Test Agent | % Allergic | % Definite Relevance | % Probable Relevance | % Past Relevance |
|---|---|---|---|---|
| Nickel sulphate 2.5% | 14.3 | 5.6 | 39.2 | 40 |
| Neomycin 20% | 11.6 | 11.1 | 30.2 | 36 |
| Balsam of Peru 25% | 10.4 | 5.8 | 70 | 6.2 |
| Formaldehyde aq 1% | 9.2 | 10.1 | 65 | 4.2 |
| Quaternium 15 2% | 9.2 | 18.2 | 67 | 5.6 |
| p-Phenylenediamine 1% | 6.8 | 6.7 | 41 | 14 |
| Thiuram mix 1% | 6.8 | 18.4 | 64 | 6 |
| Carba mix 3% | 5.7 | 15.9 | 56 | 7.4 |
| Wool wax alcohol 30% | 3.3 | 16.7 | 66 | 4.9 |
| Ethylenediamine DHCl 1% | 2.9 | 2.2 | 20 | 22 |
| p-tert-Butylphenol | 2.7 | 10.6 | 48 | 4.7 |
| Benzocaine 5% | 2.6 | 9.9 | 31 | 33 |
| Colophony 20% | 2.6 | 9.9 | 40 | 12 |
| Imidazolidinyl urea 2% aq | 2.6 | 14.6 | 65 | 3.7 |
| Cinnamic aldehyde 1% | 2.4 | 5.3 | 80 | 2.6 |
| Black rubber mix 0.6% | 2.3 | 7 | 50 | 7 |
| Epoxy resin 1% | 2.2 | 16.4 | 46 | 3 |
| Mercapto mix 1% | 2.2 | 17.4 | 66 | 5 |
| Mercaptobenzothiole 1% | 2.1 | 16.9 | 62 | 7 |
| Potassium dichromate 0.25% | 2.0 | 8.1 | 51 | 15 |

aq, aqueous; DHCl, dehydrocholesterol.

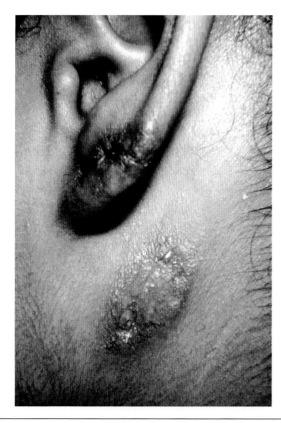

**Figure 14-12.** Nickel allergic contact dermatitis (chronic) from earrings.

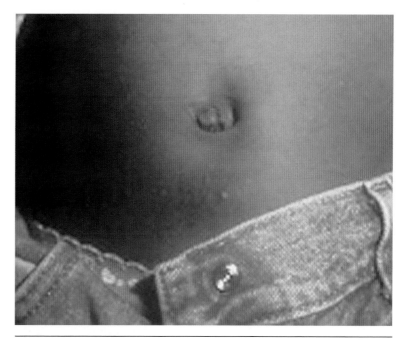

**Figure 14-13.** Nickel allergic contact dermatitis from metal snap in jeans.

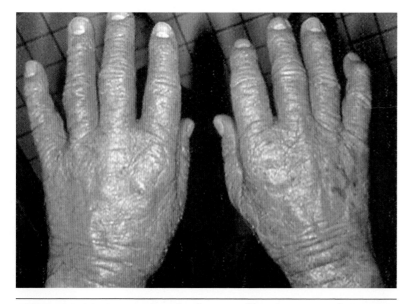

**Figure 14-14.** Occupational subacute allergic contact dermatitis almost always occurs on the dorsum of the hands. Caused by thiuram (in gloves).

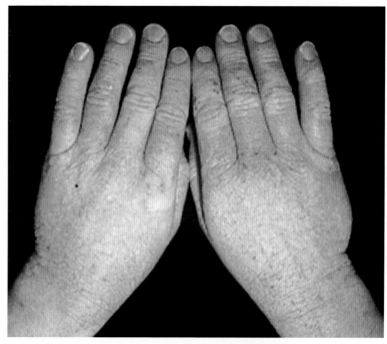

**Figure 14-15.** Chronic chromate allergic contact dermatitis.

to a perfume or cologne used alone.[7] Many occult sources of fragrance exist. Due to the increasing popularity of aromatherapy (a treatment using essential oils), this must be considered as a cause of ACD in patients using aromatherapy.

Lanolin is a natural product that has been a questionable sensitizer. Lanolin sensitivity is rarely seen in noneczematous skin, occasionally seen in atopics, and usually seen in patients with stasis dermatitis and ulcers. Lanolin-sensitive patients can sometimes tolerate one lanolin preparation but not another (Fig. 14-19).[8]

Topical medications are increasingly being recognized as potential causes of ACD. Topical anesthetics, antibiotics, (Figs. 14-20 and 14-21) and corticosteroids should be suspected as the cause of any persistent eczematous eruption. When applied

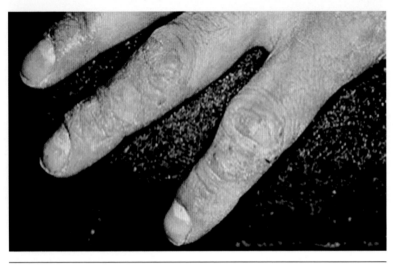

**Figure 14-16.** Occupational chronic chromium allergic contact dermatitis.

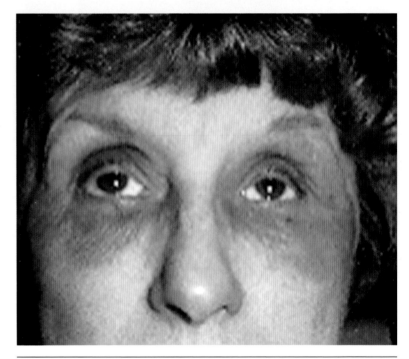

**Figure 14-18.** Facial allergic contact dermatitis noted 36 hours after dyeing hair. The patch test results were positive for *p*-phenylenediamine.

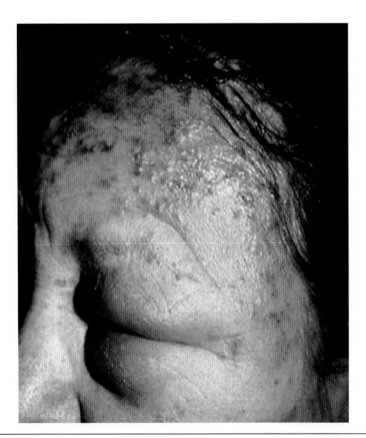

**Figure 14-17.** Facial allergic contact dermatitis (with eyelid edema) 48 hours after applying hair dye (*p*-phenylenediamine) to scalp. Patient had been using the same dye monthly for years.

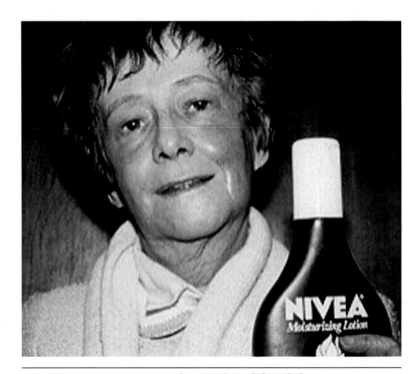

**Figure 14-19.** Lanoline-induced facial dermatitis.

to the skin, neomycin, nitrofurazone, doxepin (Zonalon), and iodochlorhydroxquin (Vioform) are each potent sensitizers (Fig. 14-22). Topical corticosteroids have also been shown to be sensitizers.

Neomycin is the most widely used topical antibiotic and is second to nickel in frequency on the list of most common positive patch test results. Neomycin is particularly sensitizing when used on stasis ulcers, in chronic otitis externa, and on chronic eczematous conditions. Allergic sensitivity to neomycin is not readily suspected, as neomycin ACD is slow to develop, slow to spread, and often dry and scaly rather than eczematous and oozing. The clinical appearance is that of an insidious aggravation of a preexisting dermatitis rather than that of an obvious ACD.[9]

Although neomycin and bacitracin (present in Polysporin) are not related chemically, they often co-react.

Iodine is a primary irritant, but topical inorganic iodine preparations such as Betadine (povidone-iodine) can occasionally sensitize. In patients in whom it has sensitized, it may cross-react with injectable radiopaque iodine (used in contrast media; Fig. 14-21).

Medical adhesive bandages consist of a pressure-sensitive adhesive and a backing that contains an adhesive, which can be a sensitizer. Rubber compounds and rosin are the usual sensitizers in adhesive tapes. Acrylate rosin–based adhesive were developed to avoid allergic reactions. Although allergic reactions to acrylate-based adhesive tapes are rare, they do occur (Fig. 14-24).

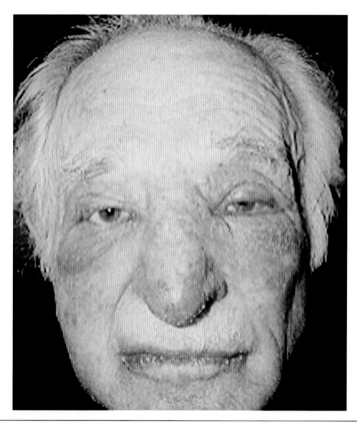

**Figure 14-20.** Zonalon-induced allergic contact dermatitis.

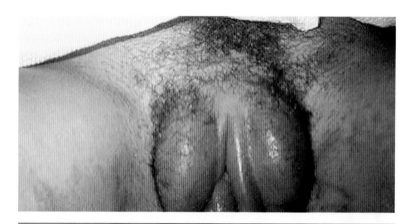

**Figure 14-22.** Acute allergic contact dermatitis caused by the application of Terazol (terconazole) cream for a yeast infection.

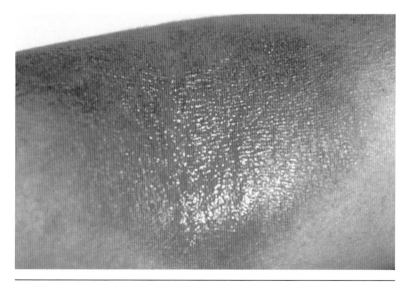

**Figure 14-21.** Acute allergic contact dermatitis caused by Betadine (povidone-iodine) applied to antecubital fossa.

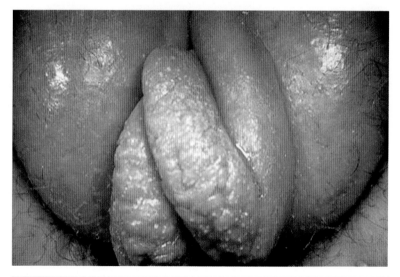

**Figure 14-23.** Allergic contact dermatitis of the labia minora and majora of the patient in Figure 14-22 (enlargement).

# CLINICAL EVALUATION (DIAGNOSIS)

Because avoidance is the best (and perhaps the only truly effective) treatment of CD, accurate diagnosis and successful identification of the inciting agent are critically important. Careful history-taking, a meticulous physical examination, and (if necessary) patch testing are essential to make the diagnosis of CD.

## *HISTORY*

The suspicion of CD is the first step to making that diagnosis. For CD to occur, the site of involvement must have come in direct contact with a putative agent. Initially, the area may itch, burn, or sting. Irritants are thought to cause symptoms and signs within minutes to hours, whereas allergens take days. (Unfortunately, there are exceptions.) The evolution of the lesion depends on multiple factors, including the allergenicity or irritancy of the agent, a history of prior reactions, immune status of the patients (i.e., immunosuppression by disease or medication). Work history must be closely examined. Hobbies and nonwork activities such as gardening, macramé, painting, ceramic work, carpentry, and photography may be sources of exposure to other contactants. Remissions and exacerbations may be related to weekend and vacation activity and work schedule. Occasionally, in sensitized individuals a systemically administered allergen produces a hemotogenous contact-type dermatitis presenting as focal flares at sites of previous dermatitis, but generalized eruptions may occur (see Fig. 14-11).[10] The history should also include response to treatment used to date and its effect.

## *PHYSICAL EXAMINATION*

The key to making the diagnosis of CD is *location, location, location*. Thus, the area of greatest involvement reflects the area of greatest contact with the causative agent, and the regional distribution of the lesion may suggest the cause (Figs. 14-25 and 14-26). Clinically, ACD is usually an eczematous disease. Eczematous lesions manifest as itchy, red, scaly, (see Fig. 14-16) and clustered papules, (see Fig. 14-11) vesicles, (see Fig. 14-17) or bullae (see Fig. 14-8). ICD may present as unspecific damage to the skin but often presents with lesions remarkably similar to those in ACD (Box 14-5).

Regional contact dermatitis often suggests the causative agent. The hands are the most common anatomic site reported to be afflicted with CD (Table 14-3). Occupational dermatoses occur most often on the hands. ACD involving the thinner skin of the

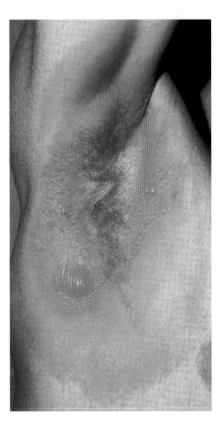

**Figure 14-25.** Formaldehyde-induced allergic contact dermatitis after a patient sweated while wearing a new, crease-resistant shirt. Note sparing of apex of axilla.

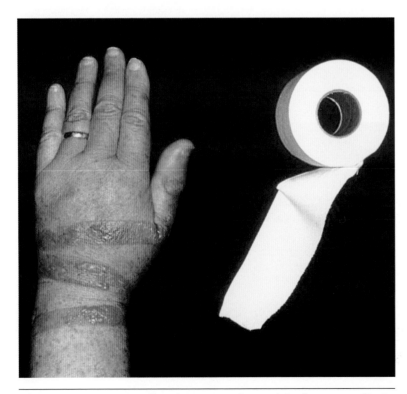

**Figure 14-24.** Acute allergic contact dermatitis due to acrylic in "hypoallergenic" adhesive tape.

---

**BOX 14-5**
### Clinical Types of Irritant Contact Dermatitis

| | |
|---|---|
| Acute | Traumatic |
| Acute delayed | Pustular and acneiform |
| Irritant reaction | Nonerythematous |
| Cumulative | Subjective |
| Asteatotic eczema | |

face (especially of the eyelids) is most often caused by cosmetics, medications, and plants.

## PATCH TESTING

The patch test is the standardized diagnostic procedure of choice for ACD. The paradox of patch testing lies in its deceptive simplicity. While the application of antigens for patch testing is rather simple, antigen selection and patch test interpretation require much experience on the part of the testing physician, especially for final assessment of the relevance of the test results.

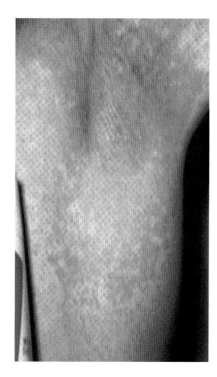

**Figure 14-26.** Deodorant-(fragrance)- induced axillary allergic contact dermatitis. Note entire axillary vault involvement.

The technique of patch testing can be thought of as a five-step procedure (Box 14-6):

a. Who to patch test: The greater the suspicion for ACD, the more frequently the diagnosis will be made. Patch testing is warranted for any patient with a chronic, pruritic, or recurrent eczematous or lichenified dermatitis and for any patient in whom CD is suspected.

b. How to patch test: The technical aspects of patch testing are well described in textbooks[11] and include details for the purchase of antigens and materials for application, forms for record-keeping, preparation of patch test sites, application of the antigens, and interpretation of "positive" and "negative" tests. The only available standardized patch test panel in the United States is the thin-layer rapid-use epicutaneous (TRUE) test, which contains 23 standardized antigens and a negative control (Table 14-4). The testing materials are suspended in a vehicle and attached to an adhesive backing, which is applied to the patient's skin back (Figs. 14-27 through 14-30). Other (non–FDA-approved) antigens are available from Trolab,

---

**BOX 14-6**
**The Technique of Patch Testing**

Understanding the pathophysiology of allergic contact dermatitis
Selecting the proper patient to test
Correctly performing the application of the tests
Reading the patch test correctly
Determining relevance and instructing the patient

---

**TABLE 14-3**
**Most Frequently Reported Sites of Contact Dermatitis**

| Site | Frequency, % |
| --- | --- |
| Hands | 37 |
| Face | 21 |
| Arm | 16 |
| Leg | 11 |
| Trunk | 10 |
| Generalized | 9 |
| Foot | 8 |
| Neck | 8 |
| Eyelids | 7 |

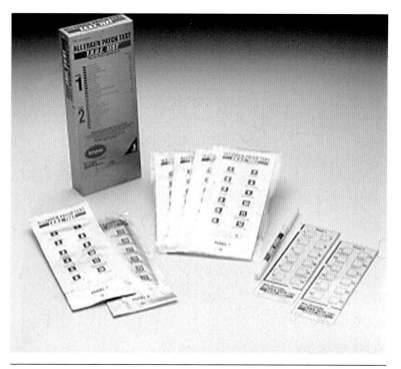

**Figure 14-27.** Thin-layer rapid-use epicutaneous (TRUE) test kit.

**TABLE 14-4**
**TRUE Test Panel of Standard Antigens**

| Substance | Source |
| --- | --- |
| Nickel sulfate | Metal objects |
| Wool alcohols (lanolin) | Ointments, creams, lotions, soaps |
| Neomycin sulfate | Antibiotic creams, lotions, ointments |
| Potassium dichromate | Cement, industrial chemicals |
| Caine mix (benzocaine, tetracaine hydrochloride, dibucaine hydrochloride) | Topical anesthetic medications |
| Fragrance mix | Toiletries, perfumes, flavorings |
| Colophony | Adhesives, sealants, pine oil cleaners |
| Paraben mix | Cosmetics, skin creams, paste bandages |
| Negative control | |
| Balsam of Peru | Resin used in cosmetics, perfumes, flavoring agent in cough syrups, lozenges, chewing gum, and candles |
| Ethylenediamine dihydrochloride | Stabilizer, emulsifier, and preservative in topical fungicides, topical antibiotics, eye drops, and nose drops |
| Cobalt dichloride | Metal-plated objects and costume jewelry |
| p-tert-Butylphenol formaldehyde resin | Waterproof glues, leather goods |
| Epoxy resin | Adhesives, surface coatings, paints |
| Carba mix | Stabilizer in rubber products, pesticides, glues |
| Black rubber mix | Antioxidant and antiozonate in almost all black rubber products (e.g., tires, hoses) |
| Cl + Me–isothiazolinone | Antibacterial preservative in shampoos, creams, lotions, and other skin care products |
| Quaternium-15 | Preservative in shampoos, lotions, soaps, and other skin care products |
| Mercaptobenzothiazole | Vulcanization accelerator used in most rubber products and some adhesives |
| p-Phenylenediamine | Permanent and semipermanent hair dyes |
| Formaldehyde | Building materials and plastics industry |
| Mercapto mix | Accelerators found in rubber products |
| Thimerosal | Mercury-containing preservative in cosmetics, nose drops, and eardrops |
| Thiuram | Antimicrobials and antioxidants found in rubber products |

TRUE, thin-layer rapid-use epicutaneous.

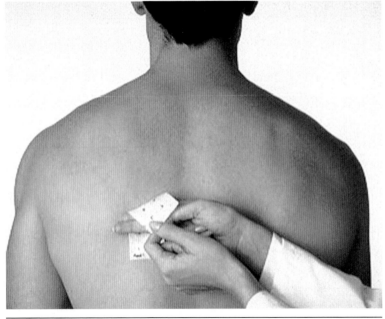

**Figure 14-28.** Application of thin-layer rapid-use epicutaneous (TRUE) test antigens.

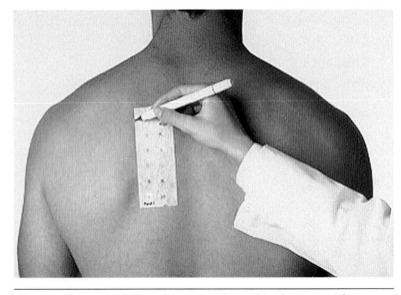

**Figure 14-29.** Marking placement for a thin-layer rapid-use epicutaneous (TRUE) test.

Pharmascience and Chemotechnique, Dormer Labs, Toronto, Canada. These allergens are dispersed in petrolatum and filled in 5-mL syringes, which are applied onto a filter paper disc or an aluminum Finn chamber and applied to the patient's back (Figs. 14-31 through 14-33).

c. When to patch test: Patch testing should be done when there is no "acute" or severe dermatitis, and the patient should not be on systemic immunosuppressants (i.e., corticosteroids, cyclosporine). It is always preferable to test a patient after discontinuation of treatment for at least 1 week. Patch tests should not be applied if the patient is going to perform activity that results in loosening of the patch tests. Patch testing should not be done in a patient who gives a history of an immediate urticaria-type eruption.

d. Reading the patch tests: Patch test must be removed and read at 48 hours, with a second reading 72 hours after initial application. On removal of the patches, the sites should be marked (using a felt-tipped permanent marker). The first reading should be delayed until the pressure marks from the discs disappear (usually in 15 to 30 minutes). A patch test–reading morphology code has been established by the North American Contact Dermatitis Group (Table 14-5; Fig. 14-34A-D). The distinction between irritancy and allergy is not always an easy one and in some cases may be very difficult.

e. Determining clinical relevance: Finally and most importantly, following the identification of an allergen, its clinical relevance must be determined. This is based on the history and the

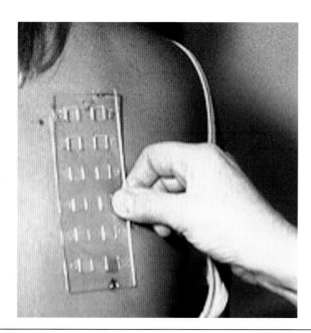

Figure 14-30. Reading thin-layer rapid-use epicutaneous (TRUE) test template antigens of TRUE test antigens.

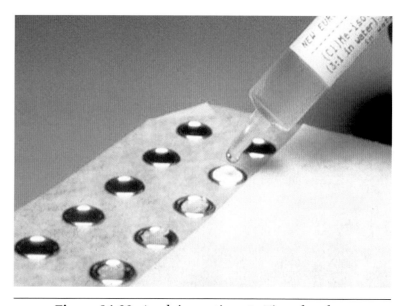

Figure 14-32. Applying antigen to Finn chamber.

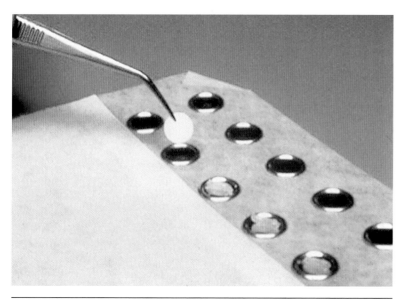

Figure 14-31. Placing filter paper on Finn chamber in preparation for testing.

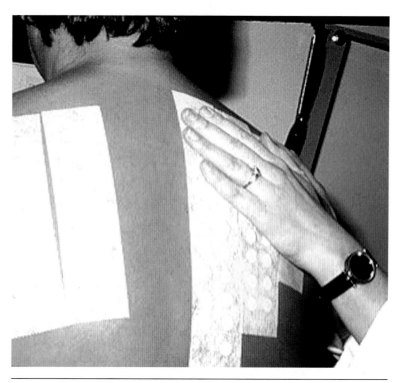

Figure 14-33. Securing patch test.

**TABLE 14-5**
Patch Test Reading Morphology Code

| Patch Test Grading | Clinical Interpretation of Grading |
|---|---|
| 0 = No reaction | No evidence of contact allergy |
| ?(+/−) = Mild erythema | Doubtful existence of contact allergy |
| 1+ = Erythema with edema | Possible contact allergy |
| 2+ = Papular erythema | Probable contact allergy |
| 3+ = Erythema with vesicles | Definite contact allergy |

identification of the source of the antigen in the patient's environment. In addition to explaining exposure to the patient, suggestions should be made for substitutions of products that may be used safely. See "Instructions to Prevent Recurrences."

The diagnosis and management of patients with chronic eczematous rashes can be most challenging. Thus, referral to a facility with special expertise in CD may be advantageous (especially if employment-related compensation or disability issues are involved).[12]

## DIFFERENTIAL DIAGNOSIS OF "ECZEMA"

Contact dermatitis should be included in the differential diagnosis of every eczematous eruption (Box 14-7), especially eczematous lesions that do not respond to appropriate therapy or any skin lesion that exacerbates (as an acute eczema) following topical therapy. There is little doubt that the more often one considers CD, the more often a putative agent will be identified.

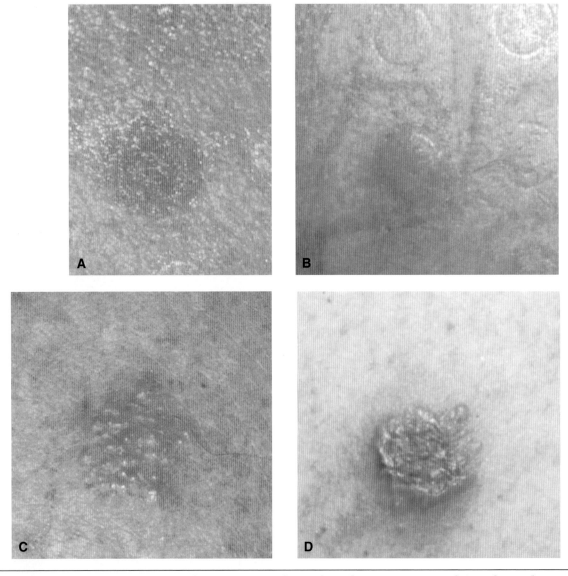

**Figure 14-34.** *A,* ?(+/−) Macular erythema. *B,* 1+ Indurated erythema. *C,* 2+ Papules and vesicles. *D,* 3+ Confluent vesicles.

Unfortunately, the histology (i.e., spongiotic dermatitis) of all eczemas is the same. Thus, whereas a biopsy can confirm spongiosis, it is the history that suggests CD and patch testing that confirms ACD.

# TREATMENT

The identification of the offending agents is the key to success in managing patients with CD. All other measures are directed toward symptom relief with the suppression of the resulting inflammatory reaction.

The aggressiveness of the prescribed treatment should be determined by the limitations on the quality of life caused by the CD. Localized acute CD warrants different treatment than other special circumstances, that is, occupational dermatitis, chronic contact dermatitis (Box 14-8).

## AVOIDANCE

Only after the putative agent is identified can avoidance be instituted (see "Instructions to Prevent Recurrences"). Unless the causative agent is removed, all other modalities of treatment are palliative.

## TOPICAL ANTIPRURITICS

In the acute phase, when itching, edema, and oozing are features, compresses with cold water to which crushed ice has been added are valuable. Cold is usually an effectively antipruritic, whereas the addition of calamine, colloidal oatmeal, or other soothing substances is of questionable value; topical diphenhydramine (Benadryl) should be strictly avoided because of the risk of cutaneous sensitization.

---

**BOX 14-7**
**Differential Diagnosis of "Eczema"**

Contact dermatitis
(allergic or irritant)
Seborrheic dermatitis*
Atopic dermatitis
Nummular eczema
Stasis dermatitis
Dyshidrotic eczema
Asteatotic eczema
Lichen simplex chronicus
Autosensitization or "id"
reactions
Dermatophytosis*
Pityriasis rosea*

Photoallergic dermatitis
Photocontact dermatitis
Polymorphous light
eruption
Drug-induced eczema
Wiskott-Aldrich disease
Acrodermatitis
enteropathica
Vitamin deficiencies
Pellagra
Riboflavin deficiency
Hartnup's disease
Hyper-IgE syndrome

*Histologically spongiotic and not clinically eczematous.
IgE, immunoglobulin E.

---

**BOX 14-8**
**Treatment of Contact Dermatitis**

1. Avoidance

2. Topical antipruritics

3. Topical anti-inflammatory agents

4. Systemic anti-inflammatory agents

5. Instructions to prevent recurrences

---

**BOX 14-9**
**Ranking of Some Brand-Name Topical Steroids***

Group I: Superpotent (anti-inflammatory activity >1500)
Temovate 0.05%
Diprolene 0.05%
Ultravate 0.05%
Psorocon 0.05%

Group II: High potency (anti-inflammatory activity = 100–500)
Lidex 0.05%
Halog 0.05%
Cyclocort 0.05%
Topicort 0.25%
Diprosone 0.05%
Elocon 0.1%
Florone 0.05%
Maxiflor 0.05%
Lotrisone 0.05%

Group III: Midpotency (anti-inflammatory activity = 10–100)
Synalar 0.025%
Kenalog 0.1%
Aristocort 0.1%
Cordran 0.05%
Locoid 0.1%
Cutivate 0.05%
Westcort 0.2%
Cloderm 0.1%
Valisone 0.1%
Benisone 0.028%

Group IV: Low potency (anti-inflammatory activity = 1–10)
Hydrocortisone (1% is OTC; >1% is prescription)
Tridesilon 0.05%
DesOwen 0.05%
Aclovate 0.05%
Decadron 0.1%
Medrol 1%
Metiderm 0.5%

*The individual compound can be moved up in the potency ranking by changing the base from cream to ointment or the concentration of the topical medication.
OTC, over the counter.

## TOPICAL ANTI-INFLAMMATORY AGENTS

Two classes of effective, topical anti-inflammatory agents are available. Topical corticosteroids have a long track record of effectiveness and safety (when used appropriately), and the newer calcineuron inhibitors (tacrolimus [Protopic], pimecrolimus [Elidel]), which are at least as effective as the low to moderately potent corticosteroids. These topical agents can manage cases of CD localized to less than 10% of the patient's body surface area. Low-potency, nonfluorinated corticosteroids or calcineuron inhibitors are recommended for the thinner skin (i.e., face, eyelids, genital areas), and the higher-potency corticosteroids are indicated for other skin, especially if the lesions are lichenified and the condition is "chronic" (Box 14-9).

The amount of medication to apply remains a most perplexing issue in the management of skin disease. A guide for proper application of creams is noted in Figure 14-35.

Another guide is referred to as the "Kleenex test": When a treated site is lightly dabbed with tissue paper, it should not reveal any "grease." If there is any on the tissue, too much medication has been applied.

### A PARENT'S GUIDE TO THE USE OF TOPICAL TREATMENT

**Use the adult *Fingertip Unit* (FTU) as your guide**

 One adult *Fingertip Unit* (FTU)

The diagrams of the child (below) show how many adult *Fingertip Units* of cream or ointment are required to cover each area of the child's body.

| Age | Face & Neck | Arm & Hand | Leg & Foot | Trunk (Front) | Trunk (Back) inc. Buttocks |
|---|---|---|---|---|---|
| | Number of FTUs | | | | |
| 3-6 mth | 1 | 1 | 1½ | 1 | 1½ |
| 1-2 y | 1½ | 1½ | 2 | 2 | 3 |
| 3-5 y | 1½ | 2 | 3 | 3 | 3½ |
| 6-10 y | 2 | 2½ | 4½ | 3½ | 5 |

Reprinted with permission from Long CC, Mills CM, Finlay AY. A practical guide to topical therapy in children. *Br J Dermatol.* 1998;138(2):293-296.

**Figure 14-35.** A parent's guide to the use of topical treatment. (From Long CC, Millis CM, Finlay AY: A practical guide to topical therapy in children. Br J Dermatol 1998;138(2):293–296.)

## SYSTEMIC ANTI-INFLAMMATORY AGENTS

Systemic anti-inflammatory agents are indicated for those more uncomfortable patients. Immunosuppression is usually most appropriate during the acute eruptive stages. Acute poison ivy is the most common example of an acute, distressing allergic contact dermatitis. Prednisone (0.5 to 1.0 mg/kg/day) is the treatment of choice. Generally, this dosage should be tapered (by half, and then discontinued) after the acute phase has resolved. The total treatment time is usually 10 to 14 days. Tapering the treatment too soon often results in a rebound of the initial dermatitis. More gradual tapering is not necessary, and steroid side effects, although possible, are very rare with this duration of treatment.

Oral cyclosporine at a dose of 3 mg/kg/day should be considered for patients with more chronic (6 weeks or longer) ACD and for diabetics.

Oral antihistamines, while very effective for contact urticaria, offer minimal relief from the pruritus of ACD.

## INSTRUCTIONS TO PREVENT RECURRENCES

The patient must be instructed to avoid the cause of the CD once it is identified. Cross-reacting agents should be included in the list of avoidances. A Mayo Clinic database (the Contact Allergen Replacement Database [CARD]) that helps patients avoid antigens identified by patch test is available via the Internet (to members of the American Contact Dermatitis Society; www.contactderm.org).

Other sources of information regarding contact allergens are as follows:
1. Cosmetic, Toiletries and Fragrances Association, Inc. (CFTA): Provides a Cosmetic Ingredient Dictionary
2. Material Safety Data Sheets (MSDS):
   a. Available by law to all employees
   b. Most helpful for occupational dermatoses
   c. Lists all potentially hazardous and toxic substances
   d. Does not provide a complete ingredients list

## SUMMARY

Contact dermatitis represents a spectrum of inflammatory skin reactions induced by exposure to external agents. It is a common skin disorder and should be considered in the differential diagnosis of every eczematous eruption. Identifying the putative agent is essential for the appropriate management. Patch testing is the gold standard for diagnosing ACD. When avoidance of the causative substance is not attained, the condition may become chronic and disabling and result in major impairment to one's quality of life.

## REFERENCES

1. Rietschel RL: Irritant dermatitis: Diagnosis and treatment. In Menne T, Maibach HI (eds): Exogenous Dermatoses: Environmental Dermatitis. Boca Raton, FL, CRC Press, 1991, pp 375–379.
2. Berardesca E, Distante F: Mechanisms of skin irritation. In Elsner P, Maibach HI (eds): Irritant Dermatitis: New Clinical and Experimental Aspects. Basel, Karger, 1995, pp 1–8.
3. Elsner P: Irritant dermatitis in the workplace. Dermatol Clin 1994;3:461–467.
4. Kalish RS: Recent developments in the pathogenesis of allergic contact dermatitis. Arch Dermatol 1991;127:1558–1563.

5. Marks JG, Belsito DV, DeLeo VA, et al: North American Contact Dermatitis Group patch test results for the detection of delayed-type hypersensitivity to topical allergens. J Am Acad Dermatol 1998;38:911–918.

6. Rietschel R, Fowler J: Fisher's Contact Dermatitis, 5th ed. Philadelphia, Lippincott Williams & Wilkins, 2001, p 636.

7. Am J Clin Dermatol 1997;8:239–242.

8. Rietschel R, Fowler J: Fisher's Contact Dermatitis, 5th ed. Philadelphia, Lippincott Williams & Wilkins, 2001, p 126.

9. Epstein S: Dermal contact dermatitis from neomycin: observations on forty cases. Ann Allergy 1958;16:268–280.

10. Fisher AA: Systemic contact-type dermatitis. In Rietschel R, Fowler J (eds): Fisher's Contact Dermatitis, 5th ed. Philadelphia, Lippincott Williams & Wilkins, 2001, p 89.

11. Marks JG, DeLeo VA (eds): Contact and Occupational Dermatology, 2nd ed. St Louis, Mosby, 1997, pp 61–132.

12. Blauvelt A, Hwang ST, Udey MC: Allergic and immunologic disease of the skin. J Allergy Clin Immunol 2003;111:S560–S570.

*Vincent S. Beltrani*

# *15* Atopic Dermatitis

## INTRODUCTION

Atopic dermatitis (AD) is the cutaneous syndrome of the *atopic triad;* it is often associated with allergic asthma and allergic rhinitis but can occur alone. Among the descriptive labels assigned to this itchy, chronic, inflammatory skin condition (including atopic eczema, infantile eczema, and neurodermatitis) is *"asthma of the skin,"* implying its link to the pulmonary hyperreactive entity.

Although the first documented description of this itchy rash was by Willan in 1808, it was not until 1935 that Wise and Sulzberger introduced the term *atopic eczema,* which is still the preferred nomenclature for many Europeans. Each of the earlier labels describes a feature of the clinical spectrum of AD. However, as Leung[1] clearly emphasizes, "an understanding of the immunologic basis of AD is the key to the important clinical implications in our approach to the diagnosis and management of AD." The significance of the immunologic aspects was not appreciated until the past decade.

Without the recognized immunologic aberrations that are unique to AD, its clinical "eczema" could not be differentiated from any other eczematous eruption.

It is "atopy" that identifies this syndrome. Atopy is the expression of an array of polygenic and phenotypic immunologic aberrations in which a spectrum of inflammatory reactions can occur in various organ systems (e.g., nose, lungs, and/or skin) induced by the response of specific T-lymphocytes associated with elevated serum immunoglobulin E (IgE) levels and eosinophilia. Of note is that those effector T-lymphocytes can be activated by both immunologic and nonimmunologic secretagogues, and it is the atopic's propensity for a helper T (Th)2-cell dominance, which differentiates atopics from nonatopics.[2]

## EPIDEMIOLOGY (PREVALENCE)

Atopic dermatitis is quite common. Eighty percent of patients with this disease develop it before the age of 5 years (Table 15-1). The lifetime prevalence in younger schoolchildren in the United States and Europe is conservatively estimated to be between 10% and 20%. In adults, the reported prevalence is 2% to 10%, with a higher prevalence in the cold northern regions. Several population-based studies consider that at least 80% of the AD population has mild eczema (Fig. 15-1), which has a more favorable prognosis. Yet, there is an anamnestic feature, because 80% of "occupational"

dermatoses occur in symptom-free workers with a past history of AD. An increased incidence of AD and atopic respiratory diseases began in the early 1960s, and it is believed that the peak incidence of AD cases may have been reached in some societies. The peak prevalence of AD seems to have occurred primarily in rapidly industrialized societies. Risk factors that influence the incidence of AD are listed in Box 15-1.[3]

## PATHOGENESIS (ETIOLOGY)

The etiology and progression of AD are multifactorial, with no single dominant factor. The spectrum of clinical findings and immunologic behavior of the syndrome can be ascribed to the pathogenic factors listed in Box 15-2. However, *genetics* and *environment* are definitely key players that generate the gamut of recognized epiphenomena.

### GENETICS

There is little doubt that several genes are involved in the development of AD as well as allergic diseases. The complex interactions among those genes are considered necessary for the expression of atopy. The gene predisposing to atopy was found on chromosome 11q13. Chromosome 3q21 is the major locus for susceptibility to

**TABLE 15-1**
**Age of Onset for Atopic Dermatitis**

| Age, yr | Percent |
|---------|---------|
| < 1 | 58 |
| 1–5 | 26 |
| 6–15 | 8 |
| 16–25 | 8 |
| 26–40 | 3 |
| Total | 100 |

From two Scandinavian studies of a total of 411 patients by Hellerstrom, Norrlind, and Nexmand.

AD. Chromosome 5q31-33 has been recognized as the determinant of the all-important (atopic) Th2 cytokines (i.e., interleukin [IL]-3, IL-4, IL-5, IL-13, granulocyte-macrophage colony-stimulating factor).

While not yet identified, it must be assumed that the characteristic signs and symptoms of pruritus, xerosis, and vascular behavior noted in AD are also genetically influenced.

## ENVIRONMENT

Environmental factors trigger the course of AD, with exaggerated responses to common stimuli that do not occur in nonatopic individuals. In atopic individuals, the combination of the genetic predisposition and environmental exposures results in the spectrum of immunologic aberrations (Box 15-3). It is thus not surprising that, as a result of all the possible genetic combinations and permutations, combined with the interaction of phenotypic

(environmental) vicissitudes, each atopic individual possesses a unique "atopic fingerprint" and thus presents with diverse clinical manifestations of the gamut of atopic signs and symptoms. At present, we can associate AD with possible genetic traits and their consequential immunologic aberrations.

# PRURITUS

The itching of AD is also multifactorial, being caused by xerosis (dryness), inflammation, and probably (genetically induced) disturbed regulation of itch sensation in the central nervous system.[3] The itch of AD should be regarded more than the result of a "lowered threshold." It has been appropriately described as an innate perception of mild mechanical stimulation as "itch"

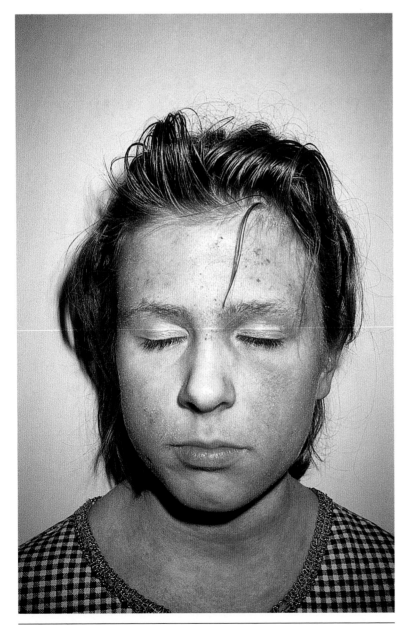

**Figure 15-1.** Typical facial atopic dermatitis with characteristic sparing of nasal skin (the "headlight" sign).

---

**BOX 15-1**
**Risk Factors That Increase the Incidence of Atopic Dermatitis**

**Parental history of atopy or AD:** The strongest risk factor. Maternal atopy>>>paternal atopy.

**Female-to-Male:** 1.13:1.

**Social class:** Upper (35%) >> lower (14%).

**Family structure:** Prevalence of AD is inversely related to sib-ship size. Strongest predictors of AD were lower number of older sibs.

**Hygiene hypothesis:** The relative freedom from infections caused by viruses, bacteria, and helminths during infancy.

**Migration:** Moving to an urban setting increases the risk of developing atopy.

**Maternal smoking:** Smoking during pregnancy and lactation increases risk of atopy.

**Questionable factors:** Prolonged gestational age, increased intake of polyunsaturated fat, hard water, and month of birth.

AD, atopic dermatitis.

---

**BOX 15-2**
**Pathogenic Factors**

Genetics, environment
Immunologic aberrations
Pruritus
Xerosis
Pharmacologic and vascular abnormalities
Thermal sweating abnormalities
Epidermal deficient antimicrobial and "barrier" activity

and not as touch. They also elicit **alloknesis**—the ability of the surrounding skin to react to initial light stimuli with more itch.

There are no specialized receptors for itch in the skin. Instead, there are polymodal receptors (i.e., activated by chemicals, temperature, touch) present on dendritic processes in the epidermis and around the dermoepidermal junction. In inflamed skin, pruritogenic mediators (e.g., histamine, IL-2, proteases, neuropeptides) released from effector cells (Th2-lymphocytes, mast cells, and eosinophils) evoke itching by direct action on the receptors. Prostaglandins, although not intrinsically pruritogenic, enhance itch due to other pruritic mediators, such as histamine. Mediators associated with the itch of AD are listed in Table 15-2. It appears that the severe itch of atopics is not caused exclusively by histamine, and its basis remains unknown.[4,5]

## XEROSIS (DRY SKIN)

"Dry skin" is considered to be the most common skin finding of atopic individuals. This xerotic skin not only acts as a "trigger" of pruritus but also contributes to the impaired epidermal barrier function noted in AD, which may be important in the development of AD. The dry skin of AD is characterized by a diminished water permeability barrier and inherent deficient water-holding properties (increased transepidermal water loss [TEWL]). Involved and noninvolved xerotic skin of patients with AD has a decrease in ceramide content compared with healthy skin.[6] This ceramide deficiency is noted in other xerotic and asteototic conditions.

---

**BOX 15-3**
## Some Immunologic Aberrations Noted in Atopic Dermatitis

Increased number of (IL-4– and IL-5–secreting) Th2-lymphocytes resulting in
    Increased IgE levels with specific IgE antibodies
    Eosinophilia with its associated
        Increased eosinophilic cationic protein
        Increased eosinophilic major basic protein
        Increased eosinophil-derived neurotoxin levels
        Increased urinary eosinophil protein X
Decreased number of (IFN-γ–secreting) Th1-lymphocytes
Increased basophil (and mast cell) spontaneous histamine release
Increased expression of CD23 on mononuclear cells
Chronic macrophage activation with
    Increased secretion of GM-CSF
    Increased secretion of PGE$_2$
    Increased secretion of IL-10
Increased serum sIL-2 receptor levels
T-cell skin homing receptors (cutaneous lymphocyte associated antigen) rather than lung-homing receptors
Increased number of high-affinity IgE-bearing Langerhans' cells

GM-CSF, granulocyte-macrophage colony-stimulating factor; IFN, interferon; Ig, immunoglobulin; IL, interleukin; PGE, prostaglandin; Th, helper-T cell.

---

## PHARMACOLOGICAL AND VASCULAR ABNORMALITIES

The small blood vessels in AD have a tendency toward vasoconstriction (Box 15-4):[7] Whereas none of these findings are pathognomonic, they are primarily noted in AD and are seen less regularly with other atopic disorders.

## THERMAL SWEATING ABNORMALITIES

Atopic patients have an abnormal pattern of thermoregulation, which may reflect an intrinsic disturbance of the parasympathetic system, which influences the pathogenesis of AD.[8] Heat- and exercise-induced sweating are very common triggers of itch that exacerbate AD. Heat- and exercise-induced cholinergic urticaria is thought to occur almost exclusively in atopic patients.[9]

## EPIDERMAL ANTIMICROBIAL PEPTIDE DEFICIENCY

Patients with AD have an increased tendency to develop bacterial and fungal infections. *Staphyloccocus aureus* is found in more than 90% of AD skin lesions. The colonization of *S. aureus* on inflamed AD skin without clinical impetiginization can be high, and besides impetiginization, *S. aureus* can exacerbate or maintain skin inflammation in AD by acting as a superantigen (stimulating marked activation of T cells and macrophages). Even patients without overt infection show a reduction in the severity of skin lesions when treated with antistaphylococcal antibiotics.[10]

In 2002, the increased susceptibility of patients with AD to skin infection with *S. aureus* was ascribed to an inherent deficiency in the expression of antimicrobial peptides (cathelicidins and β-defensins).[11] It is also known that the ceramide deficiency (see previous) results in a deficiency of sphingomyelin (a "natural" skin surface antibiotic), making the dry skin more susceptible to infection.

# DIAGNOSIS

The diagnosis of AD can be made by the clinical recognition of three essential criteria (Box 15-5). Each of the essential features of AD has particular aspects that differentiate the syndrome from other similar or related entities. Each criterion is addressed individually, and the clinical implications thereof are discussed.

## ATOPY

It would indeed be difficult to make the diagnosis of AD without atopy!

The simple definition of *atopy* is a personal or familial history of AD, asthma, or allergic rhinitis. The presence of an elevated IgE level or positive skin prick or radioallergosorbent test (RAST) adds some objective evidence of atopy. However, these criteria are but epiphenomena of what atopy really is.

Thus, it is the Th1/Th2 lymphocyte transient reversal, with its specific, resultant cytokinal profiles, that is unique in the patient with AD (Fig. 15-2). The Th1/Th2 ratio is crucial to effective immunity, and many factors influence the ratio of Th1 cell to Th2 cells, thus explaining many of the findings in AD (Box 15-6).

## Increased Allergen-Specific IgE Antibody Response to Common Antigens

Elevated IgE levels with increased specific IgE antibodies have been noted in 43% to 82% of patients with AD.[12,13] In fact, the highest serum IgE levels (greater than 1000) are noted when AD coexists with respiratory atopic disease (Fig. 15-3).

IgE is a B-cell product induced by IL-4 and/or IL-13 stimulation. In atopic individuals, excessive amounts of IL-4 and IL-13 are released from activated Th2 cells and mast cells.

The presence of IgE antibodies can be objectively identified in the atopic by a skin prick test or serologic IgE antibody test, which identifies the afferent arm of a potential immunologic reaction. A reactive shock organ (skin, lung, or nose) contributes

**TABLE 15-2**
**Agents Producing Itch After Intradermal Injection in Healthy Volunteers**

|  | Itch Response* | Mechanism |
|---|---|---|
| **Amines** | | |
| Histamine | +++ | Direct |
| Serotonin | + | Histamine release? |
| **Proteases and kinins** | | |
| Trypsin | +++ | Histamine release? |
| Chymase | +++ | Histamine release? |
| Papain | +++ | Direct† |
| Kallikrein | +++ | Direct† |
| Bradykinin | + | Histamine release |
| **Arachidonic acid metabolites** | | |
| Prostaglandins | (+) | Potentiate itch‡ |
| HETEs | 0 | |
| LTs | 0 | |
| **Neuropeptides** | | |
| Substance P | +++ | Histamine release |
| VIP | +++ | Histamine release |
| Neurotensin | + | Histamine release |
| Secretin | + | Histamine release |
| CGRP | 0 | |
| **Opioids** | | Potentiate itch‡ |
| Morphine | + | |
| β-Endorphin | + | |
| met-Enkepalin | + | |

*0, no itch; (+), very mild itch; +, mild itch; +++, marked itch.
†Painful, pricking itch, not inhibited by antihistamines, no triple response.
‡Weak or no pruritogenic effect, but potentiation of histamine itch.
CGRP, calcitonin gene-related peptide; HETE, hydroxyeicosatetraenoic acid; LT, leukotriene; VIP, vasoactive intestinal polypeptide.

---

**BOX 15-4**
**Vascular Abnormalities of Atopic Dermatitis**

Pallor of the skin
Low finger temperature
Pronounced vasoconstriction on exposure to cold
White dermatographism
Abnormal (paradoxic) reactions to histamine in affected skin
White reactions to nicotinic acid esters
Delayed blanch with acetylcholine

**BOX 15-5**
**The Essential Criteria for the Diagnosis of Atopic Dermatitis**

Atopy
Pruritus
Eczema

the efferent arm, which is required for a clinical immunologic "immediate-type" reaction. Approximately 85% of AD patients have a positive skin and/or serologic IgE antibody test result for inhalants and/or food allergens. However, a direct relationship between the positive skin test reactivity to implicated allergens and the clinical course of AD has been difficult to establish consistently.[14] In fact, many of the positive skin tests, especially for foods, often do not correlate with double-blind provocative oral food challenges.

## Eosinophilia

Abnormal accumulation of eosinophils in blood or tissue can have profound clinical effects because of their proinflammatory capability. The most common cause of eosinophilia (moderate to severe: 1500 to more than 5000 cells per cubic millimeter) worldwide is helminthic infections. In industrialized nations, eosinophilia (mild to moderate: 350 to 1500 cells per cubic millimeter) is most commonly seen in atopics, the result of stem-cell activation by IL-5 released from their Th2 lymphocytes. Tissue eosinophilia has been recognized as the effector cell of the allergen-induced late-phase response of immediate hypersensitivity reactions. Eosinophil major basic protein (EMB) is extensively deposited in the skin of AD patients, and its concentration correlates with disease activity. Therapeutically, the beneficial effects of glucocorticosteroids are associated with a reduction of the eosinophilia.[15]

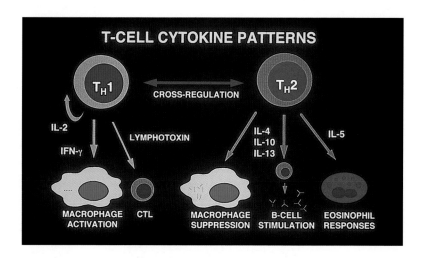

**Figure 15-2.** T-helper (Th) cell paradigm. CTL, cytotoxic T-lymphocyte; IFN, interferon; IL, interleukin.

---

**BOX 15-6**

**Factors That Influence the Differentiation of Th-lymphocytes**

Host genetic background
Activity of costimulatory environmental molecules and hormones
Antigen dose
The cytokine profile evoked by antigen
Antigen-presenting cells and cytokines they produce

## PRURITUS

*Pruritus* could be considered the "primary lesion" of AD, and the diagnosis of AD should not be made if there is no history of itching. The pruritus is variable, fluctuating from mild to extremely intense.

Virtually anything can make the patient with AD itch. The most common triggers of itch in AD are found in Table 15-3.[16,17]

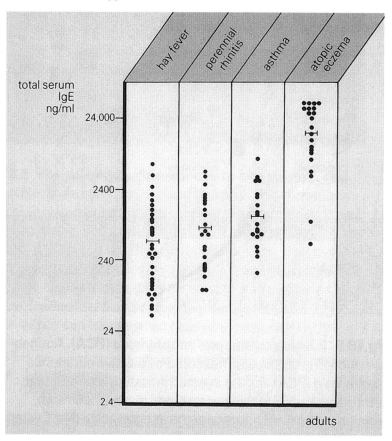

**Figure 15-3.** Serum immunoglobulin (Ig) E level in atopic diathesis

---

**TABLE 15-3**

**The Most Common Provokers of Itch in Patients with Atopic Dermatitis**

| Provoker | Prevalence, % |
|---|---|
| Heat and perspiration | 96 |
| Irritants (e.g., wool) | 91 |
| Emotional stress | 81 |
| Certain foods (vasodilatory>>allergic) | 49 |
| Alcohol | 44 |
| Viral infections (e.g., upper respiratory infections) | 36 |
| House dust mite ("contact") | 35 |

Data from Wahlgren CF: Itch and atopic dermatitis: Clinical and experimental studies. Acta Derm Venereol Suppl (Stockh) 1991;165:1–53 and Beltrani VS: The role of house dust mites in atopic dermatitis. Dermatol Clin North Am 2003;(21)3:177–182.

However, the full spectrum of identifiable triggers of itch in AD are listed in Box 15-7.[18,19]

In no dermatosis is the relationship of physical and emotional components so closely interwoven and so complex as in AD. Patients can (and frequently) easily induce a flare-up of their eczema by scratching. Anything that increases blood flow through the skin (such as heat, alcohol, febrile illness, and the normal hemodynamic diurnal variation) generates itching in the atopic patient.[20] Avoiding the triggers of itch in patients with AD is the key to successful management.

## ECZEMA

*Eczema* is a clinical symptom. Histologically, all eczemas are spongiotic dermatitis, but not all spongiotic dermatoses are clinically eczematous (Fig. 15-4). Spongiosis is the result of T-lymphocyte activation and the proinflammatory mediators released from the diverse T cells, and the varied inciting secretagogues produce the spectrum of clinical presentations. The bulla and vesiculobullous lesions of the Th1-driven acute allergic contact dermatitis are never seen in the papulovesicular Th2-driven lesions of AD. The eczema of AD is almost exclusively isomorphic: It is not an itch that erupts on its own but an itch that erupts when scratched (or rubbed).

The characteristic clinical features of the eczema of AD are as follow:

1. It occurs predominantly at an early age (usually between 2 and 5 months of age; see Table 15-1). There is a correlation between the age of onset of AD and its severity. The earlier the onset, the more severe the course.[21]
2. The age-related distribution demonstrates the condition's isomorphic feature (Fig. 15-5). Generalized, symmetric

---

**BOX 15-7**
**The Full Spectrum of "Triggers" of Itch in Atopic Dermatitis**

Scratching
Xerosis

Irritants
    Lipid solvents (e.g., soaps, detergents)
    Disinfectants (e.g., bleaches, cleaning chemicals)
    Coarse bedding
    Occupational and/or hobby irritants
    Household fluids (e.g., juices from fresh fruits, vegetables, meats)
    Wool
    Perfumes

Contact allergens
    Furry animals (cat more than dog)
    House dust mites
    Pollens (seasonal)
    Molds
    Human dander ("dandruff")

Microbial agents
    Viral (including upper respiratory infections)
    *Staphyloccocus aureus* (as pathogen, or "super-antigen")
    *Pityrosporon* yeast
    *Candida* (rarely)
    *Dermatophytes* (rarely)

Foods
    Vasodilatory (alcohol, spicey) >> Contactants > allergens

Psyche
    Stress
    Anxiety
    Chronic disease
    Sleep deprivation
    Other

Climate
    Especially heat and sweating
    Cold, dry weather
    Extremes or sudden changes of temperature and humidity

Hormones
    Puberty
    Menstrual cycle

---

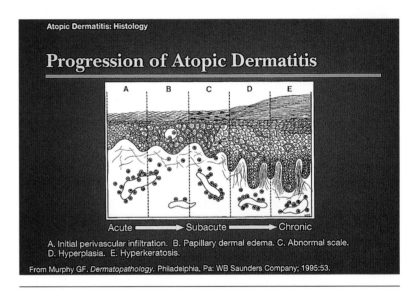

**Figure 15-4.** The histology of eczema.

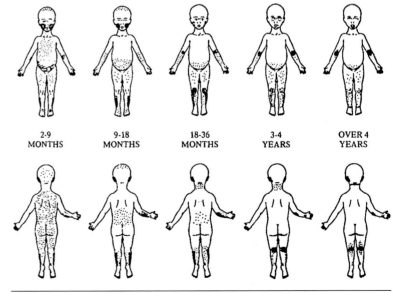

**Figure 15-5.** Distribution of atopic dermatitis in relation to age.

involvement of AD is seen most often with acute exacerbations (Fig. 15-6). Typically, in the subacute or chronic stages, the lesions tend to be more localized to areas of the body that are accessible to scratching (Figs. 15-7 through 15-13). In the later stages, it is common to see all stages of eczema (i.e., acute, subacute, and chronic) plus areas of postinflammatory hypopigmentation and hyperpigmentation. Conceptually, when an atopic individual has a chronic or relapsing pruritic eczematous eruption, even if it is restricted almost exclusively to a single site (e.g., eyelids, nipples, lips), this is still part of the spectrum of AD (Fig. 15-14). ("Hot and sweaty" fossa and folds are most frequently involved; see Figs. 15-8 and 15-9.) Excoriations (Figs. 15-15 and 15-16) are a "secondary" sign of the intense scratching of patients with AD, unlike the histamine-induced itch of urticaria, in which excoriations are almost never seen.

3. Atopic dermatitis is a chronic and relapsing eczema. Although the natural course of AD can be highly variable, most cases resolve by 2 years of age, and in the remaining patients,

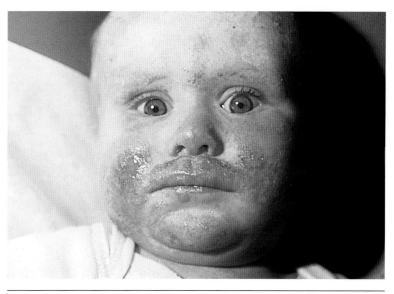

**Figure 15-7.** "Classic" facial eczema in an infant (from rubbing the face on the bed linens; note sparing of nose).

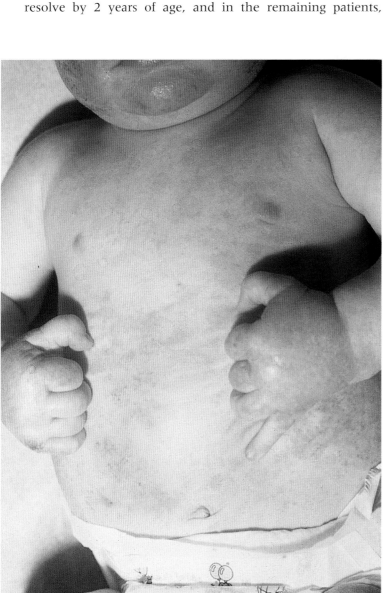

**Figure 15-6.** Scratching child with generalized pruritus and atopic dermatitis.

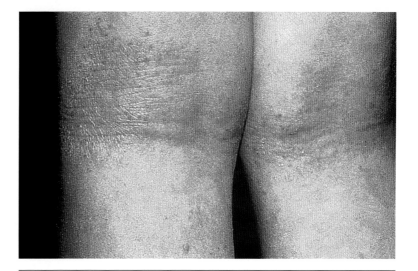

**Figure 15-8.** Popliteal (subacute) eczema, the result of scratching hot sweaty skin.

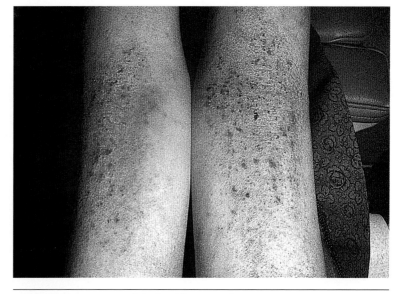

**Figure 15-9.** Antecubital (subacute/chronic) eczema. A very accessible site for scratching.

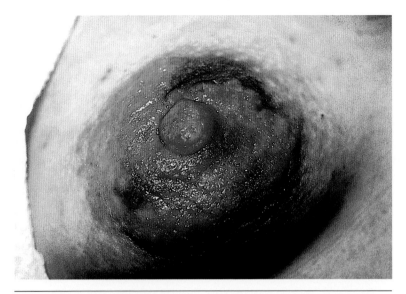

**Figure 15-10.** Nipple (acute) eczema in an atopic adolescent.

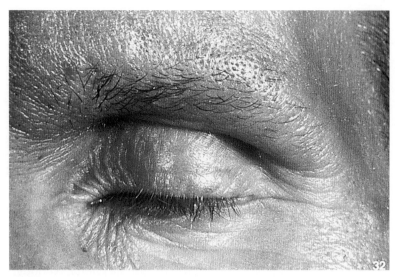

**Figure 15-13.** This patient with atopic dermatitis has rubbed off the eyebrows because of intense pruritus (Hertoe's Sign). This patient was frequently evaluated for hypothyroidism.

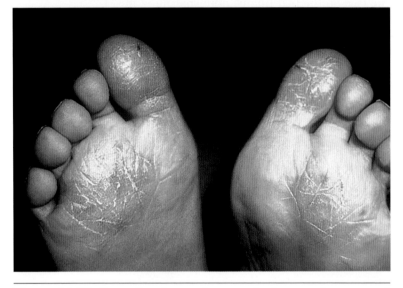

**Figure 15-11.** Juvenile plantar dermatosis, frequently managed as "athlete's foot," is the plantar eczema of atopics. Sparing of interdigital spaces and intense pruritus should strongly suggest the atopic etiology. Often, this (with and without palmar involvement) is the only skin finding.

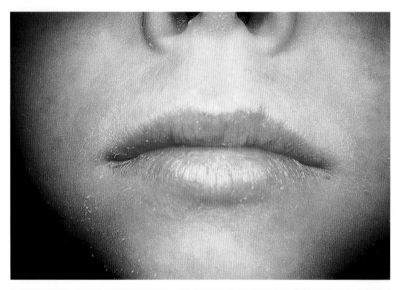

**Figure 15-14.** Atopic (subacute) cheilitis in a teenager who constantly licked her dry lips.

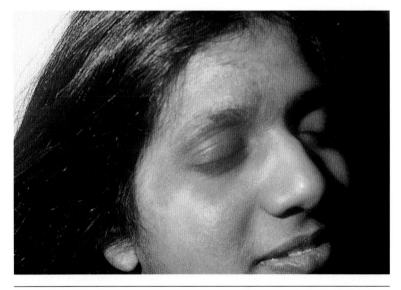

**Figure 15-12.** Eyelid (chronic) dermatitis in an adult atopic with postinflammatory hyperpigmentation. This woman admitted to constantly rubbing her itchy eyes.

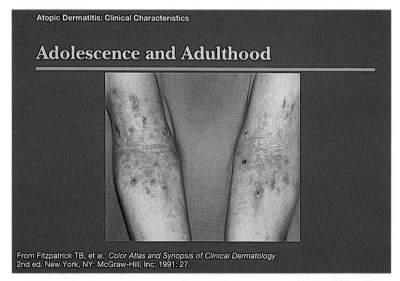

Atopic Dermatitis: Clinical Characteristics

**Adolescence and Adulthood**

From Fitzpatrick TB, et al. *Color Atlas and Synopsis of Clinical Dermatology.* 2nd ed. New York, NY: McGraw-Hill, Inc; 1991: 27.

**Figure 15-15.** Deep excoriations from intense scratching of chronic, lichenified antecubital fossa.

improvement by puberty is common. In a study by Wurthrich,[22] 11.3% of patients were considered "cured," and a "persistence" rate of 63% was noted. Twenty-six percent of patients "cleared" by puberty, but 20% of them reported episodic exacerbations later in life. (The author also reported that 60% of patients with a history of AD manifested respiratory allergies by 23 years of age.)

# THE COMPLETE SPECTRUM OF AD

Were eczema the only skin finding in patients with AD, *atopic eczema,* a label preferred by some in Europe, would be appropriate; however, there are other noneczematous findings that are frequently seen in patients with AD. These (probably genotypic) noneczematous findings have been called "minor" or nonessential factors for the diagnosis of AD. These are findings also seen in nonatopic individuals, but are more frequently noted in atopics (Box 15-8; Figs. 15-17 to 15-22).

**BOX 15-8**
### "Minor" or Unessential Features of Atopic Dermatitis

Xerosis ("dry skin")
Keratosis pilaris ("chicken" skin; see Fig. 15–18)
Perifollicular accentuation (see Fig. 15–19)
Allergic "shiners" (see Fig. 15–17)
Dennie-Morgan lines (see Fig. 15–17)
Pityriasis alba (see Figs. 15–20 and 15–21)
Anterior neck fold
Palmar and/or plantar hyperlinearity (see Fig. 15–22)
Periocular milia
Anterior capsular cataracts
Keratoconus

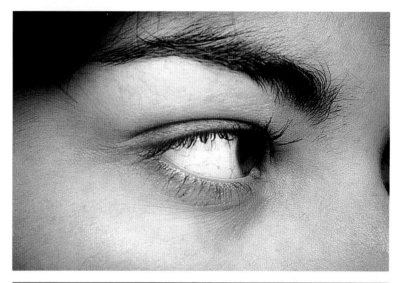

**Figure 15-17.** Allergic "shiners" are symmetrical, asymptomatic blue-gray darkenings of periorbital skin, noted in 60% of atopics with or without atopic dermatitis and in 38% of nonatopics. Dennie-Morgan lines are symmetrical folds below margins of eyelids, noted in 60% to 80% of atopics.

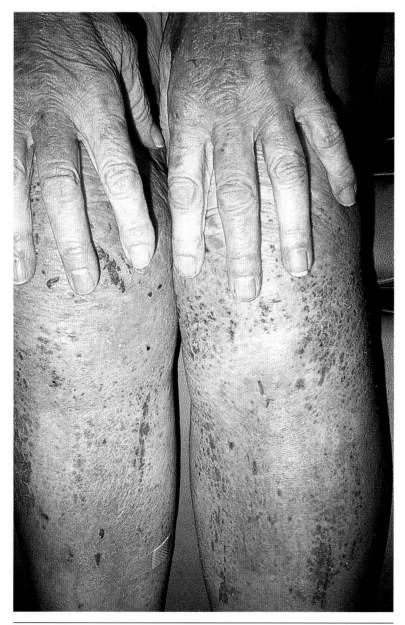

**Figure 15-16.** Generalized excoriations in an adult with generalized atopic dermatitis since infancy.

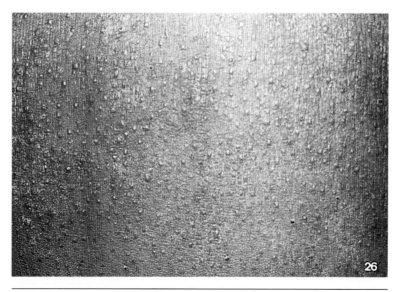

**Figure 15-18.** Keratosis pilaris ("chicken" skin), a defect of follicular keratinization. This most often occurs on the extensor aspect of upper arms, thighs, buttocks, and cheeks and is noted in 55% of atopics and 15% of nonatopics.

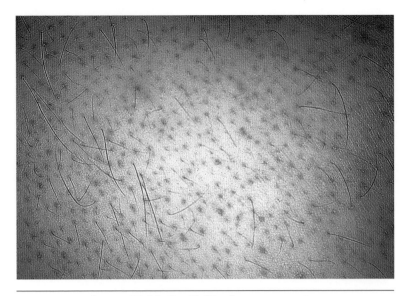

**Figure 15-19.** Perifollicular accentuation.

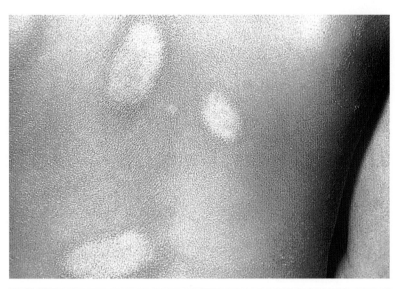

**Figure 15-21.** Pityriasis alba in a white male.

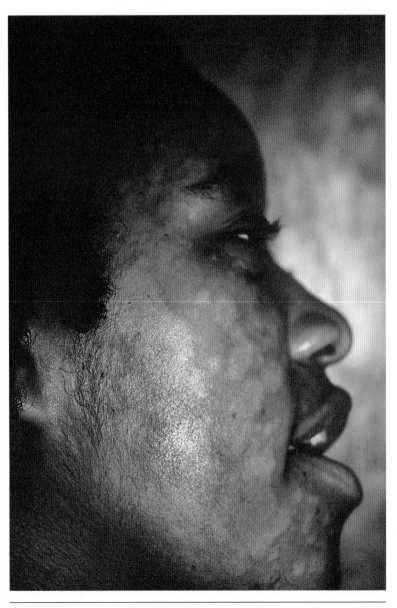

**Figure 15-20.** Pityriasis alba in a young African-American girl.

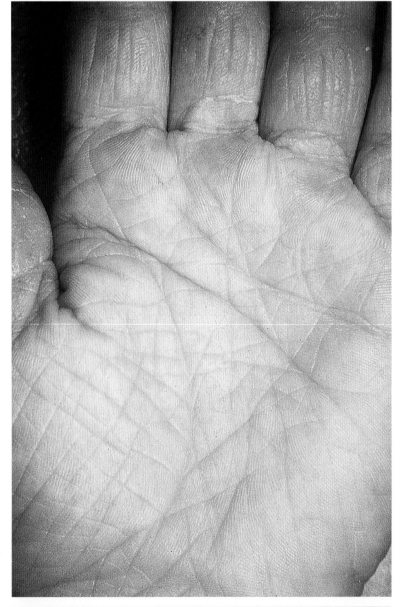

**Figure 15-22.** Hyperlinearity of palms in a patient with atopic dermatitis.

## COMPLICATIONS OF ATOPIC DERMATITIS

All the complications of AD can be attributed to the immunologic aberrations noted in the disorder. These include 1) impetiginization (caused by the epidermal antimicrobial peptide deficiency; Fig. 15-23A); 2) "super-antigenicity" (caused by epidermal antimicrobial peptide deficiency; see Fig. 15-23B); and 3) increased susceptibility to some cutaneous viral infections (due to Th1/Th2 reversal; Figs. 15-24 through 15-27).

## DIFFERENTIAL DIAGNOSIS

Eczema occurs in many disorders. When the very pruritic rash is noted during infancy and childhood, AD must be the first consid-

eration. However, its association with other persistent symptoms (e.g., systemic infections, diarrhea, chronic candidiasis of the nails), other diagnoses must be considered (Box 15-9).

The differential diagnosis of adults with eczemas is often more challenging (Box 15-10). Because special tests may be required for confirmation of the "other" eczemas, consultation with appropriate specialists (e.g., pediatrician, dermatologist) is warranted. Skin biopsies may be required, and proper interpretation by a dermatopathologist is recommended. Patch testing of any indolent

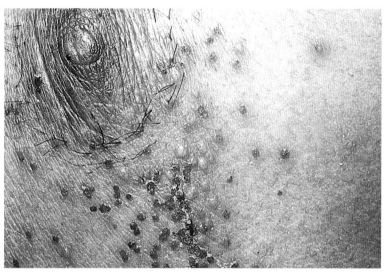

**Figure 15-25.** Herpes simplex infection in a patient with atopic dermatitis. Casual contact with herpes labialis resulted in these pustules, crusting, and punched-out lesions, which responded nicely to systemic antiviral therapy.

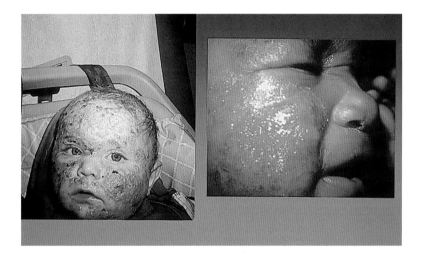

**Figure 15-23.** *A,* Impetiginized atopic dermatitis (caused by *Staphyloccocus aureus*). *B,* Super-antiginized atopic dermatitis (caused by endotoxins).

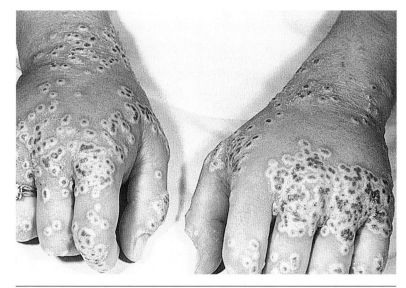

**Figure 15-24.** Vaccinia (smallpox) infection in a patient with atopic dermatitis. This youngster's sibling was vaccinated, and casual contact resulted in the inoculation of the virus into the patient's impaired epidermal barrier.

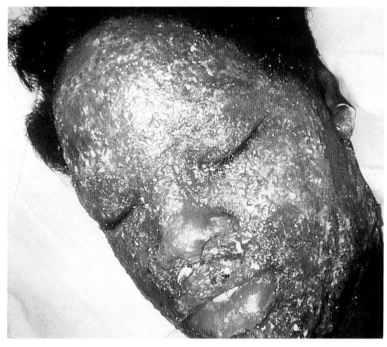

**Figure 15-26.** Kaposi herpetiform eruption (generalized herpes simplex) in a patient with atopic dermatitis. Prior to effective systemic antiviral therapy, this condition frequently resulted in a fatal outcome. Early recognition and initiation of appropriate therapy has made this a relatively benign complication today.

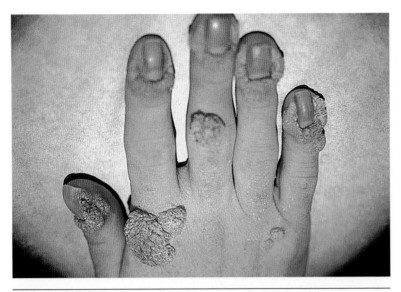

**Figure 15-27.** Multiple warts in a youngster with atopic dermatitis. While warts are not more frequent in atopic individuals, multiple, extensive, indolent infections are seen more often in atopic individuals.

---

**BOX 15-9**
**Differential Diagnosis of Pediatric Eczemas**

Atopic dermatitis
Acrodermatitis enteropathica
Agammaglobulinemia
Ataxia-telangiectasia
Hartnup's disease
Hyper-IgE syndrome
Netherton's syndrome
Phenylketonurea
Scabies
Seborrheic dermatitis
Wiskott-Aldrich syndrome

Ig, immunoglobulin.

---

**BOX 15-10**
**Differential Diagnosis of Adult Eczemas**

Allergic contact dermatitis
Cutaneous T-cell lymphoma
Glucagonoma syndrome
Irritant contact dermatitis
Pellagra
Pityriasis rubra pilaris
Psoriasiform eruptions
Scabies
Seborrheic dermatitis

---

eczematous eruption must be included in the algorithm of management for eczematous contact dermatitis (see Chapter 14).

The diagnosis of AD remains essentially a clinical one. The history and physical examination should lead to the diagnosis in almost all the cases. It is only when the essential criteria are not fulfilled and atypical ancillary findings are noted that specific testing is indicated. Results of serum total IgE levels, allergy skin prick, or serologic-specific IgE antibody tests offer a guide but are not absolute for specific environmental management of the great majority of patients with AD.

Food allergy should be considered especially in infants and children with moderate to severe generalized AD. Sicherer and Sampson report that only 33% of their (select) population group has proven food-affected AD.[23] Most commonly, milk, egg, soy, wheat, peanut, nuts, fish, and shellfish are the responsible foods, and milk-, egg-, soy-, and wheat-provoked AD frequently resolve after infancy. Food allergy is noted in fewer than 2% of adults with severe AD.

The new serum IgE antibody test, (Pharmacia CAP System) is the most reliable serum test, with a predictive value (greater than 95% reaction rate) for children (especially for egg, milk, peanut, and codfish). Elimination diets should be imposed only for foods with class III or class IV positive IgE antibodies to foods. A double-blinded oral food challenge is the definitive diagnostic test and should be supervised by a physician experienced in managing anaphylactic reactions.

Patch testing, especially for patients who note a flare-up with the application of any topical medication (especially non-fluorinated topical corticosteroids), should be considered in select patients (see Chapter 14). Skin biopsies are indicated to establish the specific diagnosis, especially in adult atopics with atypical findings.

# MANAGEMENT

To avoid disappointment by the patient and disillusionment by the health care provider, it should be clearly understood that AD cannot be cured by any medication. The clinician should stress that AD usually resolves spontaneously in 60% to 70% of children by puberty (although relapses may occur), and that management (and any therapy) can only offer some degree of comfort. *Primum non nocere* (first do no harm) should be emphasized.

Repeated reminders for avoiding all the potential triggers of itch (see previous section) should be the major therapeutic goal in the care of patients with AD. Despite the proliferation of therapeutic options available for the management of AD, the choice of treatment should be supported by evidence-based data.

The success of any therapeutic is wholly dependent on its use for the appropriate diagnosis. For example, anti-inflammatory agents are only effective for inflamed dermatoses—they are not required for xerosis ("dry skin"). Lubricants will do little for inflamed skin. Antifungal agents are indicated only for documented fungal infections.

## EMOLLIENTS

Although there is a virtual absence of clinically useful randomized clinical trial data on emollient use in the management of AD, most experts stress their importance, especially when used in conjunction with topical corticosteroids. The intent of emollients and moisturizers is to hydrate the skin, which enhances medication penetration and the barrier function (see previous section). Vaseline remains the standard to accomplish those goals; unfortunately, it is not very acceptable cosmetically. There is little evidence that the addition of other ingredients (e.g., aloe, vitamins) have any beneficial effect. Preparations with fragrances should be avoided.

An 8% ceramide-containing cream (e.g. Triceram cream) has been shown to repair the damaged barrier function and enhance the water-holding function in addition to providing a significant clinical improvement of xerosis.

## TOPICAL CORTICOSTEROIDS

Topical corticosteroids have been the cornerstone of treatment for AD for decades. However, monotherapy with topical corticosteroids is not likely to control AD. Adjuvant skin care in combination with patient/parent education is also very important.

Based on the best evidence-based data, once- or twice-daily topical corticosteroids are justified as first-line therapy in all patients with AD. The potency of the corticosteroid selected should be based on several factors (Box 15-11). The younger the patient, the milder the choice of therapy. Facial, genital, and intertriginous areas should be treated with very mild corticosteroids (1% or 2.5% hydrocortisone). Hands and feet require higher-potency topical corticosteroids (0.1% triamcinalone ointment). Similarly, lichenified plaques warrant higher-potency preparations. Box 15-12 ranks selected topical steroids from superpotent (Group I) to less potent (Group IV). Potency of corticosteroids used to treat the acute dermatitis may not be the same as the preparations required for maintenance.

Research of medication compliance in several chronic conditions suggests that between 30% and 40% of medication is not used as prescribed. The successful management of dermatologic conditions is often hindered by intentional or subconscious noncompliance. Aesthetic appeal of a product is probably the most important aspect of a topical therapy to a patient. No matter how effective a formulation, if patients find it irritating, disagreeable, or difficult to use, the efficacy of that product is compromised. In AD, ointments are usually more effective than creams, lotions, or gels; however, always take aesthetic appeal into consideration.

Patients who have chronically used topical corticosteroids without success will not be good candidates of their continued use. Many of these patients will benefit from corticosteroids in conjunction with the newer immunomodulators.

---

**BOX 15-11**

**Factors to Consider When Choosing a Topical Corticosteroid for Atopic Dermatitis**

Disease severity
  Body surface area involved
  Extent of involvement
  Disease chronicity
  Other skin characteristics
  Patient's age

Site of involvement
  Facial, genital, intertriginous
  Hands, feet
  Lichenified plaques

History of prior therapies
  Preparation used
  Pattern of use
  Compliance

---

**BOX 15-12**

**Ranking of Selected Brand-Name Topical Steroids***

Group I: Superpotent (anti-inflammatory activity > 1500)
  Temovate 0.05%
  Diprolene 0.05%
  Ultravate 0.05%
  Psorocon 0.05%

Group II: High potency (anti-inflammatory activity = 100–500)
  Lidex 0.05%
  Halog 0.05%
  Cyclocort 0.05%
  Topicort 0.25%
  Diprosone 0.05%
  Elocon 0.1%
  Florone 0.05%
  Maxiflor 0.05%
  Lotrisone 0.05%

Group III: Midpotency (anti-inflammatory activity = 10–100)
  Synalar 0.025%
  Kenalog 0.1%
  Aristocort 0.1%
  Cordran 0.05%
  Locoid 0.1%
  Cutivate 0.05%
  Westcort 0.2%
  Cloderm 0.1%
  Valisone 0.1%
  Benisone 0.028%

Group IV: Low potency (anti-inflammatory activity = 1–10)
  Hydrocortisone (1% is OTC; >1% is prescription)
  Tridesilon 0.05%
  DesOwen 0.05%
  Aclovate 0.05%
  Decadron 0.1%
  Medrol 1%
  Metiderm 0.5%

*The individual compound can be moved up or down in the potency ranking by changing the base or the concentration of the topical medication.
OTC, over the counter.

## TOPICAL IMMUNOMODULATORS

Since the year 2000, topical immunomodulators (caclineuron inhibitors) have been gaining a firm footing in the management algorithm of AD and offer an additional treatment option, either as monotherapy or in combination with topical corticosteroids. Their safety profile and enhanced efficacy; particularly for eczema involving the head and neck, and the fact that they suppress inflammation through pathways independent of those utilized by glucocorticoids is most appealing. There is some concern based on animal studies that there may be increased risk of neoplasias with prolonged use of these medications.

Tacrolimus (Protopic) ointment in concentrations of 0.03% and 0.1% was approved by the Food and Drug Administration in December 2000. Pimecrolimus (Elidel) cream 1% was approved in 2002. Both are calcineuron inhibitors that have been shown to be efficacious for mild to moderately severe AD for both short-term and long-term therapy (up to 3 years of use), with no increased infections. The most common adverse effects (with tacrolimus slightly more often than with pimecrolimus) were local application site events, included skin burning (up to 23%), pruritus (22%), and erythema (8%).

Patients using the immunomodulators experienced fewer flare-ups and reduced the need for topical corticosteroids by more than 50%. At present, some clinicians use topical immuno-modulators initially, and most continue to use topical corticosteroids. However, as soon as the case is refractory and requires long-term treatment, the trend is to introduce topical modulators.

A recommended algorithm for the management of AD can be found in Figure 15-28.

## ANTIMICROBIALS

The relationship between skin colonization and secondary infection with *S. aureus* and AD activity remains unclear. It is well known that *S. aureus* is abundant in AD, both in clinically involved and uninvolved areas, and the density increases with the severity of the lesion. Few doubt the need for antibiotic therapy for the obviously infected lesion, but management of nonclinically infected skin is less certain.

For localized infection, topical mupirocin (Bactroban) usually suffices. Systemic antibiotics are necessary for patients with multifocal infections or impetigo. Oral cefuroxime 15 mg/kg twice a day for 10 days is the preferred systemic antibiotic. If there is no clinical improvement in patients after 2 weeks of antibiotic therapy, a culture for bacterial sensitivities should be taken.

## ANTIHISTAMINES

Antihistamines have long been prescribed for AD because it is believed that they will block histamine receptor type 1 ($H_1$)-induced pruritus; however, as noted previously, histamine is but one of many mediators that can induce pruritus in AD. Sedating antihistamines may offer some relief by their sedative effect; however, this author prefers using more effective sedatives (e.g., chloral hydrate, Zolpidem) for more effective sedation for adult patients. Studies comparing sedative and nonsedative antihistamines with placebo for the itch of AD do not show a clear benefit for the active drugs.

Topical doxepin (Zonalon) has been effective in relieving some of the pruritus of AD; however, it was most effective in those patients who experienced sedation, and there was a 13% incidence of allergic contact dermatitis in those using the drug.

## SYSTEMIC THERAPEUTIC OPTIONS

For severe AD, especially when other treatments fail, systemic corticosteroids (e.g., prednisone 0.05 to 1.0 mg/kg/day to a maximum of 60 mg per day; methylprednisolone 0.04 to 0.08 mg/kg/day) are recommended for short-term management of disease activity. Long-term administration of systemic corticosteroids for AD should be avoided. Cyclosporine (0.3 to 0.5 mg/kg/day) is an excellent alternative for the short-term treatment of refractory disease, especially if repeated courses of prednisone are considered.

Patients with AD requiring systemic therapy should be referred to physicians with expertise in managing such difficult cases.

## PHOTOTHERAPY

When topical agents fail in the treatment of moderately severe and severe AD, phototherapy can be a useful modality. The preferred form of phototherapy is narrowband ultraviolet B (available in selected medical centers). Photochemotherapy, which combines methoxsalen with ultraviolet A light, has proven efficacious in the treatment of AD. The administration of phototherapy should be restricted to specialists. Remember, the more complex the intervention, the more precarious the risk-to-benefit ratio.

# PSYCHOLOGICAL ASPECTS OF ATOPIC DERMATITIS AND ITS IMPACT ON QUALITY OF LIFE

Quantitiative psychometric measurements assessing quality of life repeatedly rate AD the most miserable of dermatologic disorders, having the greatest impact on a child's quality of life. The impact of AD is not limited simply to the patient's physical, psychological, and social well-being but also negatively impacts the parents' quality of life and family dynamics.

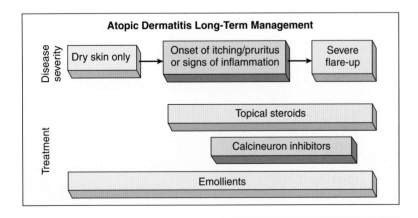

**Figure 15-28.** An algorithm for the management of atopic dermatitis.

## PLANT DEFENSE RELATED FUNCTION

The latex allergen Hev b 2 with β-1,3-glucanase property catalyzes the hydrolytic cleavage of polymers of β-1,3-glucans, the essential cell wall component of most fungi. Hence, this protein appears to be involved in plant protection against fungal infection by degrading the cell walls of fungal pathogens. Chitinases are proteins common in a wide variety of seed-producing plants. The recently characterized latex allergen Hev b 11 shows endochitinase activity and may be involved in hydrolytic cleavage of chitin, the major structural component of the cell wall of many fungi as well as the exoskeleton of insects. The cross-reactivity among the class 1 endochitinases from avocado, banana, chestnut, and latex has been associated with latex-fruit syndrome.[17-19] Hevamine, a basic protein from the lutoid fraction functions as a defense-related bifunctional enzyme with chitinase and lysozyme activity. Hevamine catalyzes the cleavage of β-1,4-glycosidic bonds of chitin and the sugar moieties of the cell surface peptidoglycans.

## COMMON ENZYMES AND STRUCTURAL PROTEINS OF HEVEA LATEX

The proline-rich Hev b 5 with a predominantly random secondary structure shows a 46% amino acid sequence homology to an acidic protein from kiwi.[9] The latex profilin Hev b 8 is an actin-binding protein and appears to involve in the organization of actin network of the plant cytoskeleton. The latex enolase Hev b 9 is a key enzyme of the glycolytic pathway, and Hev b 10 with MnSOD activity protects the plant against highly toxic oxygen radicals produced during the phagocytic processing of foreign organisms.

# MANUFACTURING OF LATEX PRODUCTS

The majority (88%) of latex is acid coagulated at a pH of approximately 4.5 and made into dry sheets or crumb rubber.[7] This is used

**TABLE 16-3**
Immunological Characterization of *Hevea brasiliensis* Latex Allergens

| Allergens | Allergen Name | Molecular Weight, kDa | Accession Number | Function | Significance as Allergens |
|---|---|---|---|---|---|
| Hev b 1 | Elongation factor | 14.6 tetramer –58 | X56535 | Rubber biosynthesis | Major |
| Hev b 2 | 1,3-glucanase | 34/36 | U22147 | Defense protein | Major |
| Hev b 3 | Elongation factor | 23 | AF 051317 AJ223388 | Rubber biosynthesis | Major |
| Hev b 4 | Microhelix complex | 50–57 dimer 100–115 | NA | Defense protein | Major |
| Hev b 5 | | 16 | U51361 — U42640 — | | Major |
| Hev b 6.01 | Prohevein | 20 | M36986 | Defense protein | Major |
| Hev b 6.02 | Hevein | 4.7 | M36986 | Defense protein | Major |
| Hev b 6.03 | C-terminal hevein | 14 | M36986 | Defense protein | Major |
| Hev b 7 | Patatin homolog | 42.9 | AJ220388 | Defense protein Inhibit rubber biosynthesis | Minor |
| Hev b 8 | Latex profiling | 14 | Y15402 | Structural protein | Minor |
| Hev b 9 | Latex enolase | 51 | AJ132580 | — | Minor |
| Hev b 10 | Mn superoxide dismutase | 26 | L11707 AJ249148 | — | Minor |
| Hev b 11 | Class 1 chitinase | 33 | AJ238579 | Defense protein | Minor |
| Hev b 12 | Lipid transfer protein | 9.3 | AY057860 | Defense protein | Major |
| Hev b 13 | Latex esterase | 42 | P83269 | — | Major |

NA, not available.

to manufacture thousands of products, such as injection-molded diaphragms, tennis balls, or rubber tires. Sulfur heat vulcanization of these types of products at extreme temperatures and prolonged times to cross-link the isoprene likely results in low quantities of allergen protein being retained in the finished product. Thus, the majority of latex products made by this method likely represent a low risk of causing allergic reactions in latex-allergic subjects. This is born out by the relatively low percentage of allergic reactions reported to the United States Food and Drug Administration from this type of natural rubber (Table 16-4).

Only 12% of latex is used in an uncoagulated state.[7] It is treated with either 0.7% ammonia (high-ammoniated latex) or

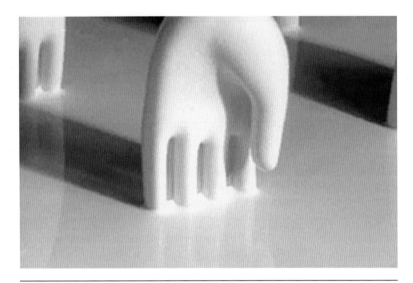

**Figure 16-3.** Latex gloves are made by a dipping method with insertion of a porcelain former crated with a coagulant on the surface. The latex forms a thin film, which is then cross-worked by sulfur heat vulcanization. (Courtesy of Kathy Nightingale, Creative Education Options LLC; Latex Allergy CD ROM, Kevin J. Kelly, MD, 2000, Hartland, Wisconsin.)

a combination of 0.2% ammonia with thiuram chemical (low-ammoniated latex) at the time of collection. This latex is used to manufacture products like condoms and gloves by a "dipping" method (Fig. 16-3). Although only a small proportion of products are made by this method, the majority of the type I immediate hypersensitivity reactions reported to the Food and Drug Administration derive from these products (Fig. 16-4). The medical literature and clinical allergy practice also show that most individual allergic reactions are associated with contact to a latex product made by a dipping method. These observations suggest that a threshold content of latex allergen that is capable of inducing an allergic reaction can be identified.[20] In turn, that will allow the manufacturing industry to set a maximum allowable allergen content in finished products before distribution for use by the public. Unfortunately, it is unlikely that the latex-sensitized individual will be able to safely use these products, since the allergen content achievable is not zero.

Latex is harvested from trees at a plantation, preserved in low or high ammonia concentrations, gathered by workers, transported to a collecting station, centrifuged to concentrate the latex, and then stored until ready for use (see Fig. 16-4A though D). The yield of latex from a particular tree depends on the season, frequency of tapping a tree, age of the tree, hormone treatments such as ethepon to enhance the latex yield, and other factors. Pressure to produce more latex products with the introduction of universal medical precautions led to a marked reduction in storage time from 6 months to as low as a few weeks (Paul Caccioli, PhD, personal communication). In addition, more frequent tapping of trees and the use of yield-enhancing chemicals may have adversely enhanced the allergen content of latex. These latter two procedures are known to induce production of defense proteins, which may have had the inadvertent consequence of producing disproportionately more allergenic proteins. This may have resulted in a higher allergen content of finished products in the past decades. Scientific experiments to confirm that these known effects of chemicals and tapping frequency actually result in higher allergen content of a finished latex product have not been accomplished to date.

**TABLE 16-4**
**Examples of Common Products Made from Natural Rubber Latex**

| Products Made by Dipping or Films of Latex (more allergic) | Products Made with Coagulated Latex (less allergic) |
| --- | --- |
| Gloves—surgeon, examination, household | Tires |
| Balloons | Erasers |
| Condoms | Tennis balls |
| Bladder catheters | Hot water bottles |
| Barium enema retention catheter | Multiple-dose medication bottle tops |
| Dental dams | Molded toys |
| Rubber bands | Carpet pads |

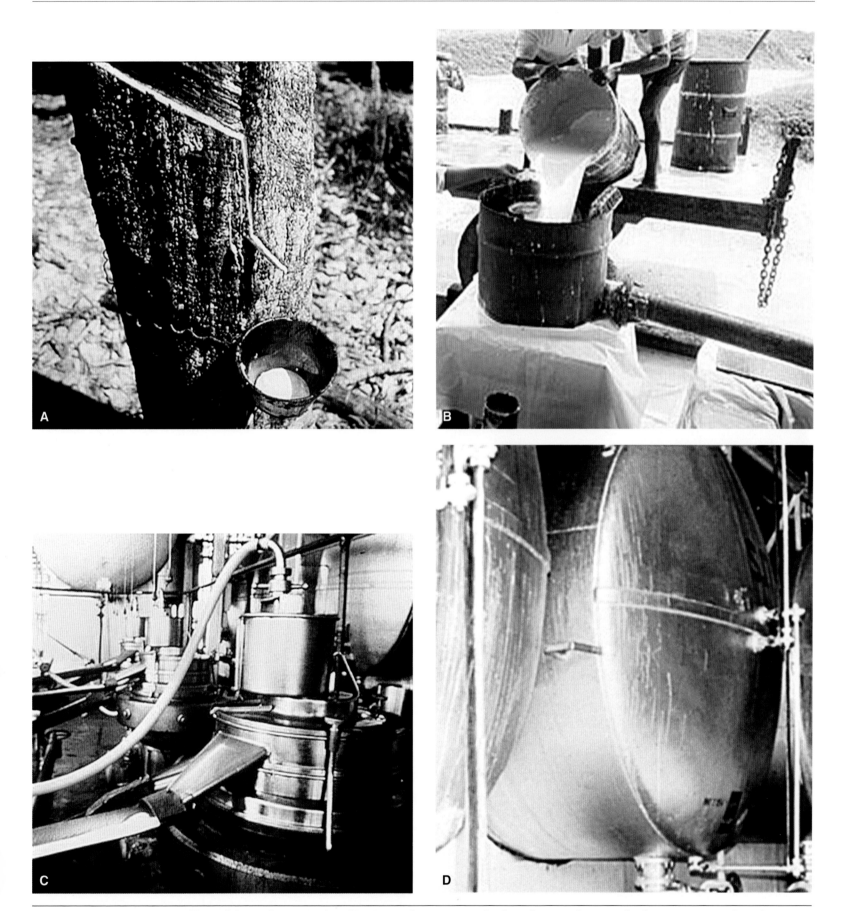

**Figure 16-4.** *A,* Latex is collected from the *Hevea brasiliensis* tree by injuring the lactifer circulation. The latex is secreted and collected in a pail with ammonia and thiuram to prevent coagulation. *B,* The latex is brought to a collecting station and combined from the trees. *C,* The latex is centrifuged to concentrate rubber particles. *D,* The latex is then stored in larger warehouse tanks until used. (Courtesy of Kathy Nightingale, Creative Education Options LLC; Latex Allergy CD ROM, Kevin J. Kelly, MD, 2000, Hartland, Wisconsin.)

The actual manufacturing process has numerous steps that may affect the final latex allergen content of a finished product. During a dipped manufacturing process, specific formers (e.g., porcelain hand forms) are coated with a coagulant such as calcium carbonate and then dipped into liquid latex for a specific length of time to produce a product of the correct thickness. Multiple chemical accelerators and antioxidants are added to the latex to ensure the correct consistency to produce a satisfactory finished product. Heating, coupled with the chemical accelerators, convert the liquid film of latex into a solid layer coating the porcelain form but with incomplete cross-linking of the polyisoprene. Subsequently, the latex gloves are leached (washed) to remove proteins and residual chemicals. This leaching is incomplete and results in persistent levels of protein and chemicals that may lead to adverse health effects in subjects who contact the finished product. The gloves are then sulfur heat vulcanized at a relatively low temperature (100°C) compared with coagulated rubber products, so as to complete the cross-linking. Often, a slurry of cornstarch powder is applied to reduce the tackiness of the gloves. In other cases, halogenation with chlorine may be used to produce powder-free products. The cornstarch powder rarely causes allergic reactions alone but may efficiently promote protein adherence. The source of protein comes from the product itself but also from the cornstarch slurry baths that may be contaminated with excess protein from the latex products that pass through them. This powder, when dry, may aerosolize with subsequent induction of allergic symptoms in hypersensitive subjects (Fig. 16-5A and B). In the late 1980s and 1990s, allergen content of latex gloves was markedly different among manufacturers but is likely caused by multiple factors. Today, the least allergen release is found in nonpowdered, chlorinated, or highly washed gloves (Table 16-5). Aeroallergen levels relate to the use of cornstarch powder carrying allergen into the air.[21-24]

# CLINICAL ISSUES IN LATEX ALLERGY

The clinician is faced with a number of concerns when confronted with a patient who is at high risk of latex sensitization or has

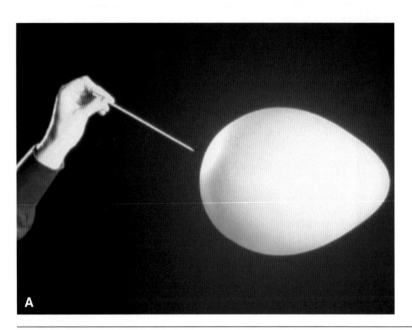
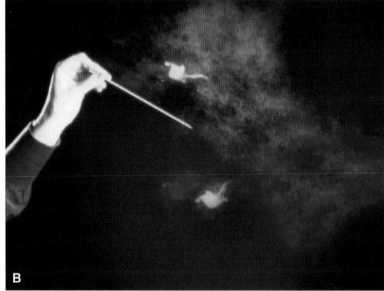

**Figure 16-5.** *A,* A balloon is a dipped latex product often coated with cornstarch powder. *B,* Breaking the balloon shows that cornstarch powder easily aerosolizes and may cause allergen reactions by inhalation.

**TABLE 16-5**

Harvesting and Manufacturing Procedures That May Affect Latex Allergen Content in Finished Natural Rubber Products

| Latex Allergen Enhancement | Latex Allergen Reduction |
| --- | --- |
| Frequent tapping of rubber tree | Reduced tapping frequency |
| Hormone treatment (e.g., ethepon) | High-temperature vulcanization |
| Defense protein induction | Prolonged vulcanization time |
| Low-temperature vulcanization | No powder |
| Dipping process | Pre- and postvulcanization leaching |
| Storage time shortened | Acid coagulation |
| Cornstarch donning powder | Halogenation |

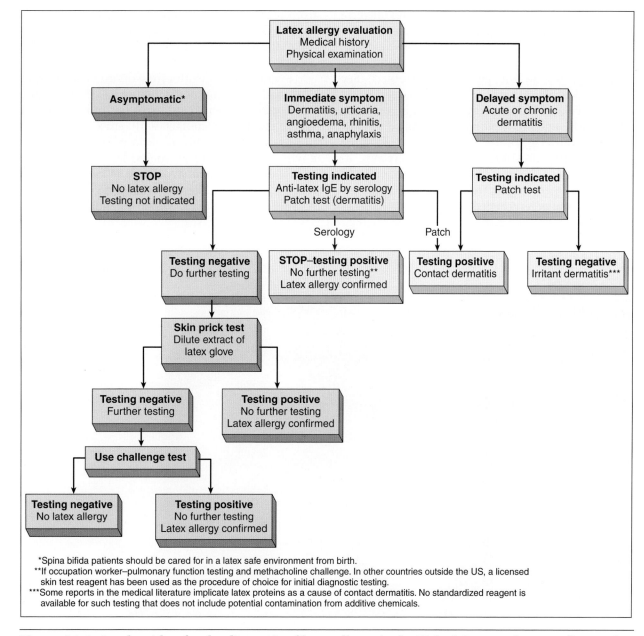

**Latex allergy evaluation**
Medical history
Physical examination

**Asymptomatic***

**Immediate symptom**
Dermatitis, urticaria,
angioedema, rhinitis,
asthma, anaphylaxis

**Delayed symptom**
Acute or chronic
dermatitis

**STOP**
No latex allergy
Testing not indicated

**Testing indicated**
Anti-latex IgE by serology
Patch test (dermatitis)

**Testing indicated**
Patch test

Serology                    Patch

**Testing negative**
Do further testing

**STOP–testing positive**
No further testing**
Latex allergy confirmed

**Testing positive**
Contact dermatitis

**Testing negative**
Irritant dermatitis***

**Skin prick test**
Dilute extract of
latex glove

**Testing negative**
Further testing

**Testing positive**
No further testing
Latex allergy confirmed

**Use challenge test**

**Testing negative**
No latex allergy

**Testing positive**
No further testing
Latex allergy confirmed

*Spina bifida patients should be cared for in a latex safe environment from birth.
**If occupation worker–pulmonary function testing and methacholine challenge. In other countries outside the US, a licensed
  skin test reagent has been used as the procedure of choice for initial diagnostic testing.
***Some reports in the medical literature implicate latex proteins as a cause of contact dermatitis. No standardized reagent is
  available for such testing that does not include potential contamination from additive chemicals.

**Figure 16-6.** An algorithm for the diagnosis of latex allergy in the United States, where no diagnostic skin test reagent is cleared for use by the Food and Drug Administration.

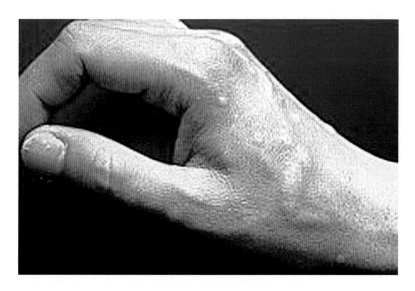

**Figure 16-7.** Acute urticaria from direct contact with a latex glove.

already started to manifest signs and symptoms of latex adverse reactions. The medical history, physical examination, risk factor assessment, diagnostic tools, treatment, work-related consequences, home or school issues, as well as prevention issues all must be considered in providing care to the latex-allergic subject. See Figure 16-6 for a diagnostic algorithm.[25]

Patients with IgE-mediated latex allergy most frequently complain of urticaria at the site of contact with a latex-dipped product such as a glove or condom (Fig. 16-7). Localized or generalized angioedema, rhinitis, pruritis, flushing, tearing, anaphylaxis, or death may accompany these symptoms. Some subjects have acute episodes of bronchospasm with contact from latex, either directly or after inhalation of latex allergen carried on cornstarch particles from products using this powder for lubrication. Products such as balloons and gloves use this powder for reduced friction on either inflation or donning of the respective products (Figs. 16-8A and B and 16-9A and B).

Evaluation of health care workers with latex allergy by inhalation challenge with methacholine has shown that more than 50% have bronchial reactivity.[23] This has ramifications in work settings where inhalation contact with latex may occur. Clinicians are most familiar with this scenario when medical personnel work in environments where powdered latex gloves are used for patient care. Despite personal avoidance of latex products, these workers may experience allergic reactions when other workers use powdered latex gloves. These individuals with latex allergy and

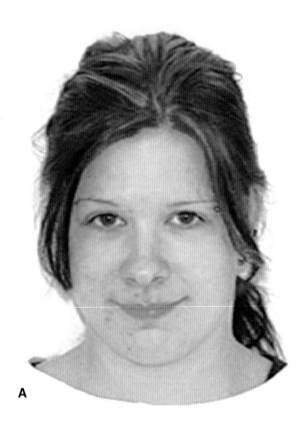

A

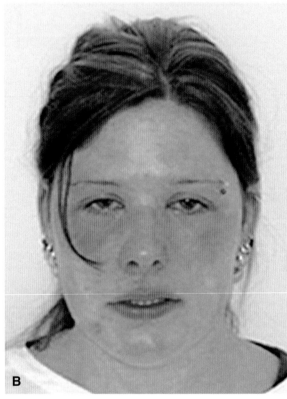

B

**Figure 16-8.** *A*, Patient with systemic IgE-mediated latex allergy prechallenge. *B*, Patient with ocular itching, facial angioema, and tearing 20 minutes after an inhalation challenge with latex. (Courtesy of Dr. Henning Allmers.)

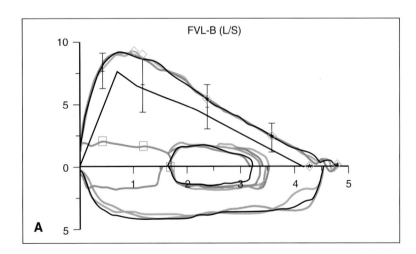

A

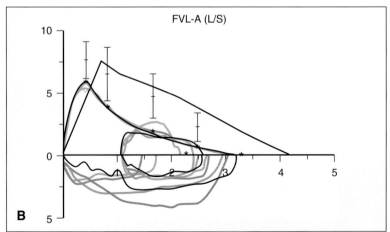

B

**Figure 16-9.** *A*, Pulmonary function of a patient with latex asthma before a challenge (FVL-B) to latex. *B*, Flow volume loop after inhalation challenge (FVL-A) with latex. (Courtesy of Dr. Henning Allmers.)

occupational asthma follow the general historic findings of other IgE-mediated occupational asthma findings associated with western red cedar or snow crab exposure (see Chapter 6). There may be progressive disease, often associated with exposure to the offending occupational allergen. Unfortunately, a number of latex-allergic individuals will continue to have asthma despite removal of the inciting allergen of latex.

The medical history in latex allergy requires knowledge of personal risk factors for the development of the disease. Certain medical conditions predispose these subjects to development of latex allergy through a combination of genetic (atopy), medical condition (spina bifida), and environmental (occupation and personal exposure) situations.[2,4,12,21,23,26–33] In addition, the clinician must be aware that allergic reactions in certain clinical settings often indicate the possibility of latex allergy as the cause. Anaphylaxis during or shortly after administration of barium by a latex balloon–tipped catheter or placement of a bladder catheter or unexplained anaphylaxis during surgical operations should raise the physician's suspicions that latex allergy may be implicated (Fig. 16-10). Other situations where latex material comes in contact with mucous membranes (e.g., dental work) or vascular systems (Fig. 16-11) and results in angioedema or other allergic manifestations are compelling and raise questions of the possibility of latex allergy.

In situations where latex materials are not constantly in contact with the skin, it seems that dermatitis is not a prominent problem. However, when the patient frequently wears latex materials, dermatitis is often found. The majority of health care worker with latex allergy report dermatitis at the site of latex glove contact. This dermatitis is often irritant in nature, which breaks down the skin barrier and may allow access of proteins to the immune system. This in turn may lead to the development of

IgE-mediated latex allergy. Because 30% of health care workers without latex allergy may have irritant dermatitis, its presence is not diagnostic. Frequent hand washing, multiple glove changes, glove powder, and failure to completely dry the skin may contribute to this common dermatitis. Irritant dermatitis can be easily recognized by the findings of dry, cracked skin surface; itching; and erythema that is *not* accompanied by vesicles, blistering, or weeping of the skin. This dermatitis may respond to cotton glove liners, reduction of powder use, thorough hand drying, non–petroleum-based barrier creams that cause latex to degrade, as well as moisturizers.

Others may develop contact dermatitis; a type IV cell-mediated immune response (Fig. 16-12). This dermatitis is distinguished from irritant dermatitis because of its vesicular, weeping appearance coupled with dermatitis extending away from the site of direct contact with latex materials. This is due to the fact that lymphocytes and Langerhans cells may home to remote sites away from the site of contact but are activated on contact with the offending allergen. Contact dermatitis from latex additive chemicals is most commonly induced by thiuram and mercapto-benzothiazole derivatives. This may be diagnosed by the use of standard patch testing (see Chapter 14). Recently, reports of contact dermatitis from latex protein have been described. No standardized reagent for the patch testing of latex proteins is available that would allow a systematic and safe evaluation of a patient. It is critical that the physician understand that dermatitis may or may not be present in a patient with latex allergy. Neither the presence nor absence of dermatitis is diagnostic of type I IgE-mediated allergy to latex but often may accompany it.

A number of other factors enhance the risk of developing latex allergy. These include the need for multiple surgeries or chronic mechanical ventilation, ventriculoperitoneal shunts in children,

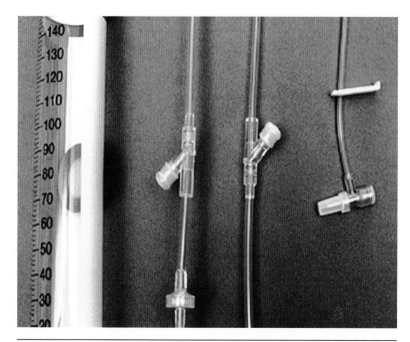

Figure 16-10. The buretrol system was implicated in latex-induced anaphylaxis in patients with spina bifida. Note that there are inline valves in the buretrol and the intravenous line. The injection ports are common but the valves are not.

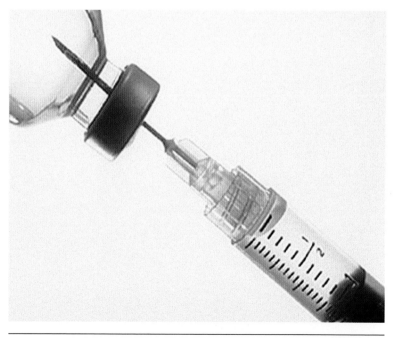

Figure 16-11. Concern has been raised about transfer of latex allergen in multidose vials to medication. Although allergic reactions are detectable, they are rarely reported. (Courtesy of Kathy Nightingale, Creative Education Options LLC; Latex Allergy CD ROM, Kevin J. Kelly, MD, 2000, Hartland, Wisconsin.)

and hospitalization of premature infants. They all have remarkably similar profiles of exposure to latex, especially latex examination gloves.

Considerable concern and confusion has been raised about the prevalence of latex allergy in the general population.[32,35,36] A modestly high prevalence of the disease would be a cause for concern because of the risks this would present to millions of people with even casual contact with latex, especially routine medical care. This has not seemed to be the case, as clinical allergic reactions to latex in the general population remain exceedingly unusual. Thus, it is important that only the clinically allergic or individuals at risk for reactions be identified. This requires a clear definition of latex allergy be agreed on. The presence of circulating IgE in the serum alone is not sufficient to make a diagnosis of latex allergy. Medical history and physical examination coupled with laboratory confirmation are necessary to confirm a diagnosis, when possible. Insufficiently sensitive and specific diagnostic reagents have hindered this endeavor. This may lead to some subjects who have latex hypersensitivity remaining undiagnosed while some without this allergy may be overdiagnosed. The clinician must use clinical judgment when the tests are asynchronous to the history and exam.[8,31,34–37]

In the daily activities of medicine, clinicians rarely find symptoms of latex allergy in their general practice. One study of more than 3000 selected (seen in clinic for a medical problem) subjects who underwent skin testing for latex allergy in an allergy/dermatology clinic in Finland showed skin test reactivity of approximately 1.1%.[38] Another large study from Italy of more than 1000 subjects confirms that skin tests infrequently show positive results (<1%) in a randomly selected population of children.[39] Even more important, all the skin test–reactive children in this study had no discernable clinical history of allergic reactions to latex. A smaller case series in children showed reactivity to latex in approximately 3% of the population by skin test. Unfortunately, the sample size of the study is too small to draw conclusions.[33]

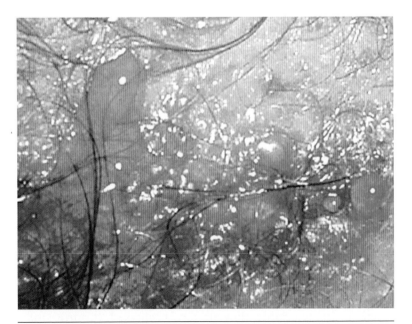

**Figure 16-12.** Irritant dermatitis with dry, cracked skin surface but no vesicles, blistering, or extension beyond the contact with a glove.

In sharp contrast, two blood donor studies using serologic testing alone found circulating antilatex IgE antibodies in 6% of the population.[34,35] Given the current sensitivity and specificity of available serologic testing, without the addition of confirmatory medical histories or skin tests, standard statistical calculation confirms that the rate of false-positive serum tests is likely to be significant in populations where there is a low prevalence of disease.[31] In fact, screening the general population for latex allergy by a blood test is not recommended for this reason, except in research settings.[37]

# DIAGNOSTIC TESTING IN LATEX ALLERGY

Testing for latex allergy has been hindered in the United States by lack of a standard reagent approved by the Food and Drug Administration. Despite a multicenter skin test study that confirmed one nonammoniated reagent to be reliable and safe, no licensed product has been forthcoming.[40,41] In contrast, Europe and Canada have utilized latex reagents for almost a decade. These reagents include latex from Stallergenes (France), Lofarma (Italy), and Bencard (Canada), which is no longer available. The French and Italian products are ammoniated latex extracts. In Finland, one group of researchers using a finished product (high-allergen latex glove) as source material showed high reliability in skin testing as well. Unfortunately, a standardized finished product for such testing is not available to the clinician. Attempts to use finished materials in an office practice of allergy may result in false-negative reactions because the source product is low in allergen or even leads to adverse reactions because of excessively high allergen content. To combat the latter problem, most practicing allergists have used sequential multiple dilutions to avoid the risk of systemic reactions. Initial reports of adverse reactions to skin testing from our clinic may have slowed the enthusiasm for skin testing.[36] The Mayo Clinic demonstrated that adverse reactions to skin testing for latex allergy are more frequent when compared with diagnostic skin testing for common environmental allergies.[42,43] The rate of systemic reaction for latex skin testing at the Mayo Clinic was 152 to 200 per 10,000 skin tests. This elevated rate is not unexpected, as latex allergen is known to result in life-threatening anaphylactic reactions in sensitized patients, whereas common environmental allergens rarely result in anaphylaxis. This risk should not deter the release and use of latex skin test reagents. Inability to confirm a diagnosis of latex allergy because of unavailability of skin testing reagents may present more risk to a patient who would continue latex exposures (e.g., health care work) that result in life-threatening reactions or asthma.

The second available method to detect latex-specific IgE is serologic testing. The three commercially available tests include the CAP radioallergosorbet test fluorescent enzyme linked immunoassay (FEIA) from Pharmacia, Uppsala, Sweden; AlaSTAT from Diagnostics Products Corporation (DPC) Los Angeles, California; and HY-TEC-EIA from Hycor Biomedical, Irvine, California. The sensitivity of the CAP and AlaSTAT is similar, with approximately 25% false-negative tests. The HY-TEC has a 27% false-positive result. These tests are very useful when coupled with a medical history but do not demonstrate complete diagnostic reliability. Serologic testing in some research centers has shown high sensitivity and specificity as well. Most recent analysis suggests that the diagnostic sensitivity of the CAP system may be lower because of the lack of Hev b 5 and, potentially, Hev b 13. Pharmacia now makes a new CAP with enriched allergen with added Hev b 5.

Research findings indicate that specific challenges by glove provocation, hooded exposure chamber, and nasal provocation may result in improved diagnostic sensitivity. Currently, these are impractical, given the lack of standard reagents or gloves for such challenges. The clinician must use judgment in discerning the proper diagnosis and therapy of a patient with a positive history and negative serologic test, because 25% of subjects with latex allergy have a negative serum test. Other tests, including flow cytometry, cell proliferation, and patch testing, have been helpful but not always available to the practicing clinician.

# MANAGEMENT OF THE NRL ALLERGIC PATIENT

Successful management of the natural rubber latex (NRL)-allergic patient is critical to avoid untoward allergic reactions and occupational asthma.[44–48] Avoiding contact with NRL products has remained the mainstay of therapy (Box 16-1). Whether a latex-free environment is possible depends on a strict definition. However, it is more practical to speak about a latex-safe environment. Some concern has been raised about patients developing excessive vigilance and phobic reactions when in close proximity to NRL products after stringent warnings to adhere to a latex-free environment. A safe environment is one where there is no NRL direct skin, mucous membrane, or aeroallergen contact by a person with NRL allergy. Currently, NRL products made by a dipping method with a powder donning lubricant are the most

likely to result in serious reactions from either direct contact or aeroallergen inhalation. A few common examples of these include gloves, balloons, and rubber bands. Dust from grinding NRL in a doll manufacturing plant is an uncommon but predictable problem.

In the past, it was highly unlikely that rubber products made after coagulation and extreme processing would induce reactions without direct skin or mucous membrane contact. It has been strongly advocated that long lists of rubber products, without designated allergen content or risk of reactivity, be furnished to patients with examples of alternative substitute products that do not contain NRL. In the future, it makes sense to stratify the risks of these products to allow a patient to have a rational and safe approach to avoidance measures. This will require refinement of the current labeling of NRL medical products that stratifies the labeling of the product into low and high allergen risks. Although NRL medical devices are labeled with content and warnings, no stratification of risk has been made to date. An NRL product heat vulcanized at 600°C for 1 hour will have considerably less allergen content than a product heat vulcanized at 100°C for a few minutes.

NRL-"safe" precautions in the operating room have allowed for uncomplicated anesthesia for the majority of patients with NRL allergy (see Box 16-1). Premedication with antihistamines and corticosteroids may be used, but there is no documentation that this improves patient outcome. Occasionally, NRL-safe precautions have failed to prevent an allergic reaction in some individuals. However, it is not clear whether the institution reporting the reactions was actually using latex avoidance. Clearly, some of those institutions were still using powdered latex gloves, except during an individual case. Because the level of aeroallergen in operating rooms declines when there is no activity, it has been suggested that operating on latex-allergic patients as the first case of the day to avoid aeroallergen exposure is safe. However, a prospective study demon-strated that NRL aeroallergen can be detected in the operating room even when no surgery was being performed in that room, although they were found at lower levels than on surgery days. Presumably, residual allergen from prior glove use or recirculation from ventilation systems may be the cause of these reactions. Thus, avoidance of NRL allergen must include a complete institutional buying change to powder-free gloves that do not release NRL aeroallergen. Many institutions have been unsuccessful in adopting such a policy due to price constraints and individual preference of workers for specific glove types. Placing NRL allergic patients' needs first for safety purposes will require these changes in health care.

In addition to the operating room, safe care for NRL patients in an ambulance, emergency room, laboratory, radiology, general ward, intensive care unit, post anesthesia care unit, and clinic is required. Medical literature repeatedly demonstrates that powdered NRL gloves are the major contributor of transferable allergen. Strict avoidance of the use of powdered NRL gloves is necessary in all these areas, as it is impossible to predict when an NRL-allergic patient may present for care. Not only should the patient wear proper identification about the NRL allergy, but the room or area in which they receive care should be clearly marked to prevent accidental exposure (e.g., by bringing a powdered NRL balloon into the room). Policies and procedures for caring for such patients are necessary. Central purchasing should control ordering practices and maintain lists of alternative products. Fortunately, mandatory content and warning labels on packaging of medical

---

**BOX 16-1**

**Latex-Safe Precautions in Hospital and Clinical Settings in Documented or Suspected Latex Allergy**

Only nonlatex glove use

Allergy alert band for the patient

"Latex-safe precautions" on door to patient room

Check all medical devices for latex content

No latex contact to skin or mucosal surfaces of patient (no source for inhalation)

No intravenous valves inline

Inject medication via stopcock devices instead of injector ports on tubing

Operating room—Schedule as the first case of the day if powdered gloves in prior use in operating room

Multiple-dose vials—Take top off or change needle after drawing up medication

Premedication—Not necessary when strict latex-safe precautions used

Ideal—Latex gloves used should be powder free and low in allergen for nonlatex allergic patients

Ban powdered latex products manufactured by dipping process from building (e.g., balloons)

devices has made central lists of NRL-containing products unnecessary and cumbersome. Consumer products are not labeled at present, and some vigilance is necessary to avoid accidental exposures. With these measures, NRL allergy will diminish in frequency and severity in the future.

# REFERENCES

1. Nutter AF: Contact urticaria to rubber. Br J Derm 1979;101:597–598.
2. Turjanmaa K, Laurila K, Makinen-Kiljunen S, et al: Rubber contact urticaria. Contact Dermatitis 1988;19:362–367.
3. Ownby D, Tomlanovich M, Sammons N, McCullough J: Anaphylaxis associated with latex allergy during barium enema examinations. Am J Roentgenol 1991;156:903–908.
4. Slater J: Rubber anaphylaxis. N Engl J Med 1989;17:1126–1130.
5. Sussman G, Tarlo S, Dolovich J: The spectrum of IgE-mediated responses to latex. JAMA 1991;265:2844–2847.
6. Feczko PJ, Simms SM, Bakirci N: Fatal hypersensitivity during a barium enema. Am J Roentgenol 1989;153:275–276.
7. Subramaniam A: The chemistry of natural rubber latex. In: Fink JN (ed). Immun Allergy Clin North Am. Philadelphia: WB Saunders Company, 1995:1–20.
8. Kurup VP, Alenius H, Kelly KJ, et al: A two-dimensional electrophoretic analysis of latex particles reacting with IgE and IgG antibodies from patients with latex allergy. Int Arch Allergy Immunol 1996;109:58–67.
9. Akasawa A, Hsieh LS, Martin BM, et al: A novel acidic allergen, Hev b 5, in latex. Purification, cloning and characterization. J Biol Chem 1996;271:25389–25393.
10. Alenius H, Kalkkinen N, Reunala T, et al: The main IgE binding epitopes of a major latex allergens, prohevein is present in its 43 amino acid fragment hevein. J Immunol 1996;156:1618–1625.
11. Alenius H, Kurup V, Kelly K, et al: Latex allergy: Frequent occurrence of IgE antibodies to a cluster of 11 latex proteins in patients with spina bifida and histories of anaphylaxis. J Lab Clin Med 1994;123:712–720.
12. Alenius H, Palosuo T, Kelly K, et al: IgE reactivity to 14-kD and 27-kD natural rubber proteins in latex-allergic children with spina bifida and other congential anomalies. Int Arch Allergy Immunol 1993;102:61–66.
13. Archer BL, Barnard D, Cockbain EG, et al: Structure, composition and biochemistry of Hevea latex. In Bateman L (ed): The Chemistry and Physics of Rubber-like Substances. New York, John Wiley & Sons, 1963, p 41.
14. Banerjee B, Wang X, Kelly KJ, et al: IgE from latex-allergic patients binds to cloned and expressed b cell epitopes of prohevein. J Immunol 1997;159:5724–5732.
15. Beezhold DH, Sussman GL, Kostyal DA, Chang N: Identification of a 46-kD latex protein allergen in health care workers. Clin Exp Immunol 1994;98:408–413.
16. Breiteneder H: The allergens of *Hevea brasiliensis*. ACI International 1998;10:101–109.
17. Beezhold DH, Sussman GL, Liss GM, Chang NS: Latex allergy can induce clinical reactions to specific foods. Clin Exp Immunol 1996;26:416–422.
18. Blanco C, Carrillo T, Castillo R, et al: Latex allergy: Clinical features and cross reactivity with fruits. Ann Allergy 1994;73:309–314.
19. Brehler R, Theissen U, Mohr C, Luger T: "Latex-fruit syndrome." Frequency of cross-reacting IgE antibodies. Allergy 1997;52:404–410.
20. Baur X, Chen Z, Allmers H: Can a threshold limit value for natural rubber latex airborne allergens be defined? J Allergy Clin Immunol 1998;101:24–27.
21. Baur X, Ammon J, Chen Z, et al: Health risk in hospitals through airborne allergens for patients presensitized to latex. Lancet 1993;342:1148–1150.
22. Swanson MC, Olson DW: Latex allergen affinity for starch powders applied to natural rubber gloves and released as an aerosol: From Dust to Don: Can J Allergy Clin Immunol 2000;5(3):328–335.
23. Vandenplas O, Delwiche JP, Evrared G, et al: Prevalence of occupational asthma due to latex among hospital personnel. Am J Respir Crit Care Med 1995;151:54–60.
24. Heilman DK, Jones RT, Swanson MC, Yuninger JW: A prospective, controlled study showing that rubber gloves are the major contributor to latex aeroallergen levels in the operating room. J Allergy Clin Immunol 1996;98(2):325–330.
25. Kelly KJ, Kurup VP, Reijula K, Fink JN: The diagnosis of natural rubber latex allergy. J Allergy Clin Immunol 1994;93(5):813–816.
26. Kelly KJ, Pearson ML, Kurup VP, et al: Anaphylactic reactions in patients with spina bifida during general anesthesia: Epidemiologic features, risk factors, and latex hypersensitivity. J Allergy Clin Immunol 1994;94(1):53–61.
27. Allmers H, Brehler R, Chen Z, et al: Reduction of latex aeroallergens and latex-specific IgE antibodies in sensitized workers after removal of powdered natural rubber latex gloves in a hospital. J Allergy Clin Immunol 1998;102(5):841–846.
28. Brugnami G, Marabini A, Siracuse A, Abbritti G: Work-related late asthmatic response induced by latex allergy. J Allergy Clin Immunol 1995;96(4):457–464.
29. Charous BL, Schuenemann PJ, Swanson MC: Passive dispersion of latex aeroallergen in a health care facility. Ann Allergy Asthma Immunol 2000;85:285–290.
30. Liss GM, Sussman GL, Deal K, et al: Latex allergy: Epidemiological study of 1351 hospital workers. Occup Environ Med 1997;54:335–342.
31. Liss GM, Sussman GL: Latex sensitization: Occupational versus general population prevalence rates. Am J Ind Med 1999;35:196–200.
32. Tarlo S, Sussman G, Holness D: Latex sensitivity in dental students and staff: A cross-sectional study. J Allergy Clin Immunol 1997;99:396–401.
33. Shield S, Blaiss M: Prevalence of latex sensitivity in children evaluated for inhalant allergy. Allergy Proc 1992;13:129–130.
34. Ownby DR, Ownby HE, McCullough J, Shafer AW: The prevalence of anti-latex IgE antibodies in 1000 volunteer blood donors. J Allergy Clin Immunol 1996;97(6):1188–1192.
35. Saxon A, Ownby D, Huard T, et al: Prevalence of IgE to natural rubber latex in unselected blood donors and performance characteristics of AlaSTAT testing. Ann Allergy Asthma Immunol 2000;84:199–206.
36. Kelly KJ, Kurup VP, Zacharisen MC, et al: Skin and serologic testing in the diagnosis of latex allergy. J Allergy Clin Immunol 1993;91:1140–1145.
37. Slater J, Mostello L: Routine testing for latex allergy in patients with spina bifida is not recommended. Anesthesiology 1992;74:391.
38. Ylitalo L, Turjanmaa K, Palosuo T, Reunala T: Natural rubber latex allergy in children who had not undergone surgery and children who had undergone multiple operations. J Allergy Clin Immunol 1997;100(5):606–612.
39. Bernardini R, Novembre E, Inhargiola A, Veltroni M, et al: Prevalence and risk factors of latex sensitization in an unselected pediatric population. J Allergy Clin Immunol 1998;101:621–625.
40. Hamilton RG, Adkinson F, Multicenter Latex Skin Testing Study Task Force: Diagnosis of natural rubber latex allergy: Multicenter latex skin testing efficacy study. J Allergy Clin Immunol 1998;102:482–490.
41. Hamilton RG, Biagini RE, Krieg EF, Multi-Center Latex Skin Testing Study Task Force: Diagnostic performance of FDA-cleared serological assays for natural rubber latex-specific IgE antibody. J Allergy Clin Immunol 1999;103:925–930.
42. Valyasevi MA, Maddox DE, Li JT: Systemic reactions to allergy skin tests. Ann Allergy Asthma Immunol 1999;83:132–136.
43. Yuninger JW: Diagnostic skin testing for natural rubber latex allergy. J Allergy Clin Immunol 1998;102:351–352.
44. Federal Register: Natural Rubber-Containing Medical Devices. User Labeling. Vol. 62, no. 189. September 30, 1997, pp 52021–51030.
45. National Institute of Occupational Safety and Health ALERT: Preventing allergic reactions to natural rubber latex in the workplace. Cincinatti, Ohio. Vol. 6. DHHS Publication #97-135. 1997, pp 1–11.
46. Schwartz HJ: Latex: A potential hidden "food" allergen in fast food restaurants. J Allergy Immunol 1995;95(1):139–140.
47. Sussman GL, Lem D, Liss G, Beezhold D: Latex allergy in housekeeping personnel. Ann Allergy Asthma Immunol 1995;74:415–418.
48. U.S.FDA: Surgeons and Examination Gloves: Reclassification. Federal Register. Vol. 64 (#146), 1999, pp 41710–41743.

*Leslie C. Grammer and Rachel E. Story*

# *17* Drug Allergy

Immunologically mediated adverse drug reactions or drug allergy and/or hypersensitivity account for 6% to 10% of all adverse drug effects. Table 17-1 provides a general overview of adverse drug reactions. There are a number of specific characteristics that are generally helpful in distinguishing drug allergy from other adverse drug reactions. They tend to occur in only a small fraction of patients, are reproducible with minute amounts of the drug, can mimic other allergic reactions, and do not resemble other known pharmacologic effects. These distinguishing characteristics are listed in Box 17-1.

Many drug hypersensitivity reactions can be classified according to the revised Gell and Coombs schema. Table 17-2 is a synopsis of the clinical manifestations and mechanism of each reaction type. Penicillin has been associated with all of them. These mechanisms are schematically depicted in Figure 17-1. In the type I, or anaphylactic, mechanism, allergen is recognized by immunoglobulin (Ig) E bound by receptors to mast cells or basophils. The cross-linking of IgE by allergen results in cellular release of mediators, such as histamine, leukotrienes, and prostaglandins. The cytotoxic, or type II, mechanism involves antibody recognition of cell-bound antigen; this antibody fixes complement, which causes cell damage. Antigen-antibody lattices or complexes are formed in the type III, or Arthus, mechanism; complement is fixed, and some components of the complement cascade act as chemoattractants to cells that mediate inflammation. Sensitized T-lymphocytes recognize antigen presented by macrophages in the delayed hypersensitivity, or type IV, mechanism. This recognition results in T-cell activation and release of cytokines, which then mediate inflammation, primarily by recruitment of nonsensitized cells. The Type IVa1 delayed-type hypersensitivity reaction is responsible for contact dermatitis that occurs when antigen is presented to sensitized CD4+ cells that release cytokines and attract other

**TABLE 17-1**
**Classification of Adverse Drug Reactions**

| Reaction | Example |
|---|---|
| **Predictable Adverse Reactions Occurring in Normal Patients** | Hepatic failure with acetaminophen |
| Overdosage or toxicity | Urinary retention with anticholinergic medications |
| Side effects | *Clostridium difficile* colitis with use of ampicillin |
| Secondary or indirect effects | Erythromycin increasing theophylline blood levels |
| Drug-drug interaction | |
| **Unpredictable Adverse Reactions** | |
| Allergy and hypersensitivity reactions (IgE-mediated) | Anaphylaxis from β-lactam antibiotic |
| Pseudoallergic reactions (non–IgE-mediated events that mimic IgE-mediated events) | Anaphylaxis with radiocontrast dye |
| Intolerance | Tinnitis after a single aspirin |
| Idiosyncratic reactions | Hemolytic anemia in patients with G6PD deficiency exposed to primaquine |

Adapted from Abraham D, Saltoun CA: Overview of adverse drug reaction. In Grammer LC, Greenberger PA (eds): Drug Allergy and Protocols for Management of Drug Allergies. Providence, OceanSide Publications, 2003, with permission.

cells, producing tissue inflammation. The Type IVb delayed-type hypersensitivity reaction is responsible for toxic epidermal necrolysis and occurs when cytotoxic CD8+ lymphocytes recognize fragments of antigen on the surface of target cells and exhibit a drug-specific cytotoxicity against dermal cells. In addition to those drug hypersensitivities that are classifiable according to the Gell and Coombs schema, there are other adverse reactions that appear to be immunologically mediated that do not fit into this schema. Examples include pulmonary infiltrates from nitrofurantoin and interstitial nephritis from methicillin. Furthermore, there are also adverse drug reactions that closely mimic the manifestations of immunologically mediated reactions, but no immunologic mechanism can be demonstrated. An example would be the anaphylactoid reactions to opiates that have been described in certain cases.

# EPIDEMIOLOGY

The frequency of adverse drug reactions is not precisely known. In studies of hospitalized patients on medical floors, the estimates of prevalence of adverse drug reactions range from 15% to 30%.[1] Of all adverse reactions, approximately 6% to 10% are believed to represent drug hypersensitivity.[2] In 1998, drug hypersensitivity reactions accounted for 137,000 to 230,000 hospital admissions in the Unites States, with a cost estimated between 275 and 600

**TABLE 17-2**
**Examples of Drug Allergy Categorized According to the Revised Gell and Coombs Reaction Classification**

| Reaction Type Clinical Presentation | Revised Gell and Coombs Reaction Type | Mechanism |
|---|---|---|
| Anaphylaxis, bronchospasm, urticaria, angioedema | Type I: Anaphylactic | Antigen cross-links IgE on cell surface, resulting in mediator release |
| Hemolytic anemia due to binding of drug to red cells, thrombocytopenia, interstitial nephritis | Type IIa: Cytotoxic | Cell-bound antigen reacts with IgG or IgM antibody, thus activating complement and producing cell injury |
| | Type IIb: Cell stimulating | IgG cell-stimulating antibody interacts with cell surface receptors involved in cell signaling |
| Serum sickness, drug fever | Type III Immune complex | Formation of antigen-antibody complexes that activate complement, resulting in recruitment of macrophages and leukocytes that cause tissue damage |
| Contact dermatitis with topical application | Type IVa1: Cell mediation hypersensitivity | Antigen is presented to sensitized CD4+ T-lymphocytes (Th1 cells) that release cytokines that attract other cells, which cause tissue inflammation |
| Delayed allergic reactions | Type IVa2: Cell mediated hypersensitivity | Antigen is primarily presented to sensitized CD4+ T-lymphocytes (Th2 cells); sensitized CD8+ T-lymphocytes (Th2 cells) also may be involved |
| Toxic epidermal necrolysis (TEN) | Type IVb: Tissue injury by cytotoxic T-lymphocytes | Cytotoxic CD8+ T-lymphocytes recognize fragments of antigen on the surface of target cells |

Ig, immunoglobulin; Th, T-helper.

million dollars annually.[3] It has been estimated that the risk of allergic reaction is about 1% to 3% for most drugs. In practice, penicillins and sulfonamides account for a significant proportion of drug allergy. Although apparently not immunologically mediated, aspirin and other nonsteroidal anti-inflammatory drugs (NSAIDs) are also frequent causes of adverse reactions that mimic drug allergy: urticaria, angioedema, and bronchospasm. The term *pseudoallergy* is often applied to these reactions. Drugs that have been implicated frequently in allergic drug reactions are listed in Box 17-2.

## IMMUNOGENICITY OF DRUGS

Molecular weight of at least 3 to 5 kDa and multivalency are generally required for a compound to be immunogenic. Therefore, with the exception of a few protein drugs, such as insulin or streptokinase, very few drugs are complete antigens. The vast majority of drugs are organic chemicals with molecular weights less than 1 kDa that function as univalent ligands. Based on the classic reports of Landsteiner in the 1920s, it is generally acknowledged that low-molecular-weight drugs (haptens) are not immunogenic unless they are bound to a high-molecular-weight (>5 kDa) substance, usually a protein (carrier).

β-Lactam antibiotics are reactive with proteins and can directly haptenize carrier proteins. Most drugs, however, are not chemically reactive with proteins. It is probable that the haptens from most drugs are reactive metabolites of the parent compound that then bind to carrier proteins; certainly, this is the case with metabolites of penicillin. Studies of human IgE to sulfonamides have demonstrated the N4-sulfonamidoyl determinant to be the major sulfonamide haptenic determinant.[4] For most other allergenic drugs, the formation of reactive metabolites and their conjugation with carrier proteins is somewhat speculative. In the absence of the relevant drug haptens, immunologic assessment is, of course, impossible.

## CLINICAL PRESENTATION

The clinical presentations of drug allergy can take many different forms, and they are generally not pathognomonic for drug hypersensitivity. That is, similar clinical presentations can be the result of exposure to other allergens, or they can be associated with other nonimmunologic diseases. Dermatologic manifestations are the most common manifestation of drug allergy. However, many other organ systems can be involved, either alone or in combination, in a patient with drug allergy. It should be appreciated that in many reactions that are believed to be drug allergy, a definitive immunologic mechanism has not been established. A list of the clinical presentations of drug allergy is given in Box 17-3.

Anaphylaxis, a potentially life-threatening condition, can include any or all of the following: hypotension, bronchospasm, laryngeal edema, angioedema, and generalized urticaria. If the antigen has been ingested, gastrointestinal symptoms, such as nausea, vomiting, diarrhea, or cramping, may be prominent.

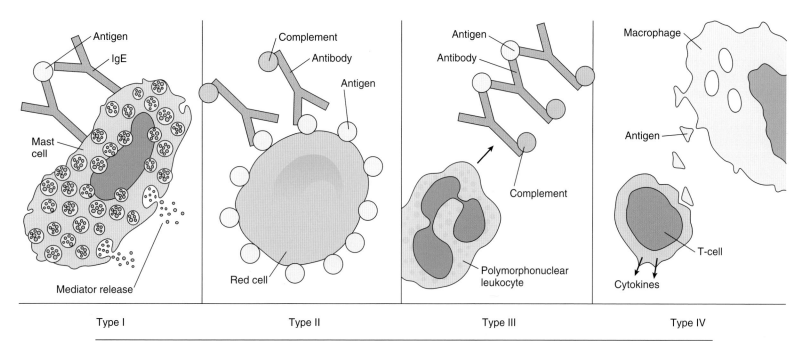

**Figure 17-1.** Schematic representation of the mechanisms underlying the four Gell and Coombs reaction types. The type I, or anaphylactic reaction, arises when a drug allergen cross-links immunoglobulin (Ig) E molecules on the surface of mast cells, precipitating the release of inflammatory mediators. The type II, or cytotoxic, reaction occurs when antibodies bind to cell-bound antigens. The antibodies fix complement, which causes cell lysis. The type III reaction, or Arthus phenomenon, involves formation of antigen-antibody complexes that fix complement, several components of which are chemoattractants to cells that cause inflammation. The type IV reaction, delayed hypersensitivity, occurs when sensitized T cells recognize antigens presented by macrophages. This process activates the T cells, resulting in the release of cytokines.

Symptoms usually begin within 30 minutes of drug exposure and generally subside within 24 hours. Penicillin is one drug for which frequency of anaphylactic reactions is reported; the estimates range from 0.01% to 0.05% per treatment course.[5] Other drugs that have been implicated frequently in anaphylactic symptoms include radiocontrast material, plasma expanders, and NSAIDs, such as aspirin. None of these agents is thought to cause anaphylaxis via an lgE-mediated mechanism.

Serum sickness–like reactions usually occur 1 to 3 weeks after drug exposure. Because of this latent period, it is imperative to question a patient about any drugs that may have been ingested in the previous month. The symptoms may include fever, urticaria and/or angioedema, arthralgias, joint effusion, lymphadenopathy, and, occasionally, neuritis (brachial plexus). Renal disease is usually not detected in humans, although it is prominent in animal models. Symptoms may last from several days to several weeks. Other multisystemic clinical presentations of drug allergy include drug fever, drug-induced lupus erythematosus, and vasculitis.

Of all the organ systems affected by drug allergies, the most frequently involved is the skin (Box 17-4). Although exanthematous eruptions are the most common manifestations, drug allergy can result in almost any type of cutaneous eruption. Other common dermatologic manifestations include urticaria, angioedema, and (from topical medications) contact dermatitis. Less common presentations include fixed drug eruptions from medications such as phenolphthalein, photosensitivity from drugs such as doxycycline, and erythema multiforme from penicillins and sulfa drugs. On rare occasions, dermatologic manifestations occur that are severe enough to be potentially life threatening. These include exfoliative dermatitis and Stevens-Johnson syndrome, a fulminant variant of erythema multiforme with cutaneous and mucous membrane involvement. Uncommon dermatologic presentations of drug allergy include purpura, erythema nodosum, and TEN (toxic epidermal necrolysis), or Lyell's syndrome. Various other dermatologic manifestations are shown in Figures 17-2 through 17-5.

Though the skin is most commonly involved, drug allergy can involve other single-organ systems. Examples would be the pulmonary reactions induced by nitrofurantoin, thrombocytopenia

---

**BOX 17-2**
**Listing of Drug Groups Most Frequently Implicated in Allergic and Pseudoallergic Drug Reactions**

Allopurinol
Anesthetic agents (muscle relaxants, thiopental)
Antiarrythmic agents (quinidine, procainamide)
Anticonvulsants (hydantoin, tegretol)
Antihypertensive agents (hydralazine, methyldopa, angiotensin-converting enzyme inhibitors)
Antimalarials
Antipsychotic tranquilizers (phenothiazines, tricyclics)
Antisera and vaccines (antitoxins, monoclonal antibodies)
Antituberculosis drugs (isoniazide, rifampin)
Aspirin and nonsteroidal anti-inflammatory drugs
Cisplatin
Enzymes (chymopapin, L-asparaginase, streptokinase)
Grisefulvin
Heavy metals (gold)
Narcotics (codiene, morphine)
Nitrofurans
Organ extracts (adrenocorticotropic hormone, insulin)
Penicillamine
Penicillins and cephalosporins
Phenolphthalein
Radiocontrast media
Sedative-hypnotics (barbiturates)
Sulfonamides

Adapted from Ditto AM: Drug allergy. In Grammer LC, Greenberger PA (eds): Patterson's Allergic Diseases, Philadelphia, Lippincott Williams & Wilkins, 2002, pp 295–360; with permission.

---

**BOX 17-3**
**Listing of Various Single-Organ and Multisystem Manifestations of Drug Allergy**

**Single-organ system involvement**
Dermatologic manifestations (see Box 17-4)
Respiratory or pulmonary manifestations
   Asthma
   Acute infiltrative reactions (probably allergic)
   Hypersensitivity pneumonia
   Pulmonary infiltrates with eosinophilia
   Nitrofurantoin reactions
   Noncardiac pulmonary edema
Hematologic manifestations
   Eosinophilia
   Drug-induced immune cytopenias
      Thrombocytopenia
      Hemolytic anemia
      Agranulocytosis
Hepatic manifestation
   Cholestasis
   Hepatocellular damage
   Mixed pattern
Renal manifestations
   Glomerulonephritis
   Nephrotic syndrome
   Acute interstitial nephritis
Lymphoid system manifestations
   Pseudolymphoma
   Infectious mononucleosis-like syndrome

**Multisystem involvement**
Immediate generalized reactions
   Anaphylaxis
   Anaphylactoid reactions
Serum sickness
Drug fever
Drug-induced autoimmunity (lupus erythematosus)
Vasculitis

Adapted from Ditto AM: Drug allergy. In Grammer LC, Greenberger PA (eds): Patterson's Allergic Diseases. Philadelphia, Lippincott Williams & Wilkins, 2002, pp 295–360; with permission.

induced by sulfonamides, hepatitis induced by halothane, and acute interstitial nephritis induced by methicillin.

# NEW AGENTS

In recent years, several new classes of drugs have come into widespread use and deserve special consideration. These classes include

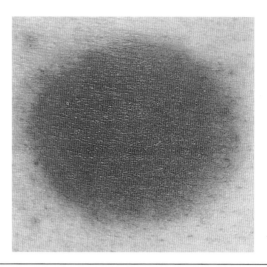

**Figure 17-3.** Single, well-demarcated, red-dish lesion of a fixed drug eruption. The chief feature of such reactions is that they occur in the same site each time the particular allergen is ingested. Lesions develop within hours of ingestion and subside rapidly, often leaving the skin characteristically hyperpigmented. (Reprinted from du Vivier A: Drug and toxic eruptions of the skin. In Atlas of Clinical Dermatology, Philadelphia, W.B. Saunders, 1986, pp 14.1–14.20; with permission.)

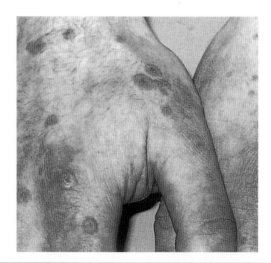

**Figure 17-4.** Iris-type lesions of erythema multiforme. These lesions typically occur on the extremities, particularly the hands, forearms, and feet. They can be precipitated by exposure to a number of agents, including sulfonamides, barbituates, and phenylbutazone. (Reprinted from du Vivier A: Drug and toxic eruptions of the skin. In Atlas of Clinical Dermatology, Philadelphia, W.B. Saunders, 1986, pp 14.1–14.20; with permission.)

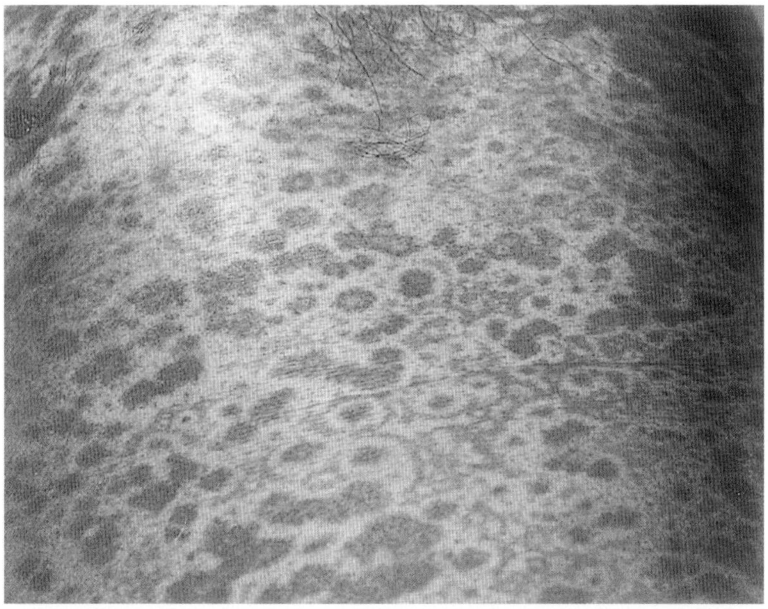

**Figure 17-2.** Drug eruption caused, in this case, by allergy to ampicillin. These lesions are usually puritic and confluent and tend to show widespread distribution. (Reprinted from du Vivier A: Drug and toxic eruptions of the skin. In Atlas of Clinical Dermatology, Philadelphia, W.B. Saunders, 1986, pp 14.1–14.20; with permission.)

monoclonal antibodies, cytokines, cyclo-oxygenase-2 (COX-2) inhibitors, and angiotensin-converting enzyme inhibitors (ACEs).

Monoclonal antibodies are used to treat many disorders, including lymphoma, breast cancer, inflammatory bowel disease, and rheumatoid arthritis. Many monoclonal antibodies are chimerized with murine proteins and lead to hypersensitivity reactions. For example, rituximab (Rituxan) is a chimeric antibody with a small murine component that binds CD20 on B-lymphocytes and is used in the treatment non-Hodgkin's lymphoma. Frequently, there are reactions during infusions, including fever, rigors, diaphoresis, flushing hypotension, bronchospasm, dyspnea, and a sensation of tongue and throat swelling. These infusion reactions are common with other monoclonal antibodies and are easily treated by reducing the infusion rate and, in some patients, pretreatment with antihistamines, acetaminophen, and corticosteroids. There are also rare reports of allergic reactions including anaphylaxis, angioedema, serum sickness, immune-mediated thrombocytopenia, and anemia.[6] Cytokine-release syndrome (or cytokine storm) occurs when binding of the monocolonal antibody–target cell complex via the Fc receptor activates macrophages in the liver, spleen, or lung. This activation leads to increasing concentrations of tumor necrosis factor alpha and interleukin-6 proportional to the number of malignant lymphocytes.[7]

Treatment with cytokines such as interferon (INF)-β for multiple sclerosis, and INF-α for hepatitis C has become widespread in recent years. INF-β for the treatment of multiple sclerosis is commonly associated with flulike symptoms and local injection site reactions. There are case reports of capillary leak syndrome, anaphylaxis, and a thrombotic thrombocytopenic purpura–like syndrome in patients receiving INF-β. INF-β–neutralizing antibodies can develop and decrease the effectiveness of treatment. Reports of the prevalence of neutralizing antibodies in patients receiving INF-α for the treatment of hepatitis C vary from 1.2% to 20.2%.[8]

Aspirin (ASA) and nonselective NSAIDs are inhibitors of cyclo-oxygenase-1 capable of producing nonimmunologic-mediated bronchoconstriction, urticaria, and anaphylaxis. The selective cyclo-oxygenase-2 inhibitors celoecoxib (Celebrex) and refecoxib (Vioxx) have been tolerated in aspirin-intolerant asthma patients, patients with history of angioedema with aspirin, and patients with adverse respiratory and cutaneous reactions to NSAIDs.[9] There have been reports of patients with NSAID-triggered urticaria developing urticaria following COX-2 exposure.

Angiotensin-converting enzyme inhibitors are associated with angioedema in 0.1% to 0.5% of patients who use them, and symptoms occur within 1 month of therapy in the majority of patients.[10] Because there appears to be cross-reactivity among ACE inhibitors, the entire class is contraindicated in a patient who has developed angioedema. Angiotensin II antagonists (ARB) are used as alternatives to ACE inhibitors and are not contraindicated in those with ACE inhibitor–induced angioedema. However, there are reports of patients with angioedema secondary to ACE inhibitors who subsequently developed angioedema while taking an angiotensin II antagonist. Thus, caution must be exercised when giving angiotensin II antagonists to patients with a history of angioedema from ACE inhibitors.

# DIAGNOSIS

Occasionally, diagnosis of drug allergy is fairly straightforward, but this is not usually the case. As indicated in Box 17-5, the most important diagnostic tool is the history. First, it is imperative to have a complete and accurate list of all the drugs taken by the patient over the previous month. If a physician does not specifically ask about such nonprescription drugs as aspirin, the patient may not volunteer this information. Second, it is necessary to study the patient's manifestations to see if they are consistent with known drug allergies. As discussed above, it is important to recognize the protean nature of drug allergy and that it is not confined to rashes. Finally, it is important to consider the temporal relationship between exposure(s) to the drug and onset of clinical manifestations. If a patient is receiving a drug for the first time, allergy generally does not occur until several days have passed. However, it usually occurs within several months. That is, if a patient has been receiving a drug on a daily basis for over a year, that drug is not likely to be the cause of drug allergy. If a patient has received a drug in the past, sensitization may already have

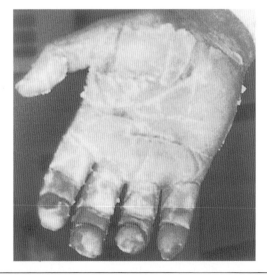

**Figure 17-5.** Exfoliative dermatitis of the hand in a patient with Stevens-Johnson syndrome secondary to administration of allopurinol.

---

**BOX 17-5**
**Guidelines for the Diagnosis of Drug Allergy**

**History**
Careful, complete drug history
Clinical manifestations consistent with drug allergy; a temporal relationship between drug exposure and onset of clinical manifestations consistent with drug allergy

**In vitro Testing**
Research tool
Generally no clinical value

**In vivo Testing**
Clinically indicated in selected cases
Cutaneous testing
Provocative test dosing

occurred, and drug allergy may appear immediately upon readministration.

There are numerous in vitro tests that have been utilized in the investigation of drug allergy. Among these are histamine release, drug-specific IgE radioallergosorbent tests (RASTs), immunoassays for specific IgG or IgM, lymphocyte reactivity as measured by lymphokine production or lymphocyte transformation, and agglutination and lysis of blood cells in the presence of the suspected drug and the patient's serum. With the exception of the last, which may be clinically useful in the evaluation of immunologically mediated cytopenias, in vitro tests are rarely of clinical value, even though they may be valuable research tools. Studies indicate that elevated levels of perforin, granzyme B, tumor necrosis factor-$\alpha$, and Fas-L are found with delayed cutaneous reactions to drugs.[11] It is possible that these markers may be used in the future to monitor cytotoxic T-cell response in delayed drug reactions.

In vivo testing for drug allergy—that is, cutaneous testing or provocative test dosing—may be clinically indicated in selected cases. It must be recognized that a serious limitation of cutaneous testing is the dearth of appropriate multivalent test reagents or drug metabolites. This is primarily because the antigenic determinants responsible for drug allergy are unknown for most drugs. If a patient has a history compatible with drug allergy, cutaneous tests are negative, and there is a clear indication for a drug reaction, provocative test dosing may be considered. In this method of testing, the initial dose is one that would not cause a serious reaction. Subsequent doses represent incremental increases. An example is given in Table 17-3. At each dose increment, it is imperative to ascertain whether or not any symptoms have occurred before proceeding to the subsequent dose.

It is important to appreciate the difference between provocative test dosing and desensitization. The former describes the incremental administration of a drug to which a patient probably does not have an IgE-mediated allergy, even though the history is somewhat suggestive of an allergic reaction. On the other hand, if true IgE-mediated allergy exists, the incremental administration of the drug is termed *desensitization*, as it converts the patient from a state of sensitivity to that of nonsensitivity to the drug. The

mechanism is not entirely clear, but it may be the result of graded antigen binding of specific IgE or of controlled mediator release. An example of a desensitization schedule for penicillin in a pregnant woman with syphilis is given in Table 17-4. In a sense, desensitization is a treatment for drug allergy; however, as it is so closely associated with cutaneous testing and test dosing, it is also considered to be diagnostic. Box 17-6 indicates agents for which desensitization can be carried out. Prior to cutaneous testing, test

---

**TABLE 17-4**

**Schedule for Penicillin (PCN) Desensitization in a Pregnant Woman with Syphilis***

| Concentration[†] | Dose |
|---|---|
| 1 U/mL PCN | 0.1 U SC |
| 10 U/mL PCN | 1.0 U SC |
| 100 U/mL PCN | 10 U SC |
| 1000 U/mL PCN | 100 U SC |
| 10,000 U/mL PCN | 1000 U SC |
| 100,000 U/mL PCN | 10,000 U SC |
| 1,000,000 U/mL PCN | 100,000 U SC |
| | 200,000 U IM |
| | 2.1 million U IM |

*Although the protocols may be similar, it is important to appreciate the difference between provocative test dosing and desensitization. The former is a diagnostic technique; the latter, a treatment.
[†]The SC route should be used because ID tests with >10,000 U/mL PCN cause irritant reactions.
SC, subcutaneous; ID, intradermal; IM, intramuscular.
Adapted from Vemuri P, Tripathi A: Penicillin and other β-lactam antibiotics. In Grammer LC, Greenberger PA (eds): Drug Allergy and Protocols for Management of Drug Allergies. Providence, OceanSide Publication, 2003, pp 1–4; with permission.

---

**TABLE 17-3**

**Typical Protocol for Provoactive Test Dosing in a Patient with History of Penicillin Allergy***

If a patient has negative prick and intradermal tests to Penicilloyl-polylysine (Pre-Pen), the major determinant, and to the minor determinant mixture (if available) or to penicillin G potassium, you may test dose as follows:

| Route | Amount |
|---|---|
| IV | 1/1000 of full dose |
| IV | 1/100 of full dose |
| IV | 1/10 of full dose |
| IV | Full dose |

*Following each dose increment, it is necessary to assess the patient and determine whether any symptoms of allergy have developed.

---

**BOX 17-6**
**Agents for Which Drug Desensitization Protocols Are Published**

Allopurinol
Aminoglycosides
Aspirin
Dapsone
Furosemide
Heterologous antisera
Insulin
Measles mumps rubella (MMR) vaccine
Penicillin
Sulfa
Tetanus toxoid
Vancomycin

dosing, or desensitization, it is important that there be a clear indication for the drug; that the risks and benefits of drug administration are explained to the patient; and that the medical records document indications, informed consent, and administration schedule.

# TREATMENT AND PREVENTION

If drug allergy is suspected, it is important to discontinue the offending drug. Patients often receive multiple drugs, and it may be impossible to determine which is the offending agent. It is generally appropriate to discontinue all nonessential drugs and to replace any necessary drugs with non–cross-reacting substitutes. In some very rare circumstances, it may be necessary to continue administering a drug to which the patient is allergic. An example would be continuing sulfa for an AIDS patient with toxoplasmosis brain abscess and sulfa allergy. This would be done only with informed consent and careful consideration of the risks and benefits. Corticosteroids may be required to allow continued administration of an essential, nonreplaceable drug to which a patient is allergic.

Treatment of cutaneous eruptions depends on the severity. If the cutaneous manifestations are mild, antihistamines alone generally suffice. However, if the cutaneous eruption is severe or progressive, prednisone, 60 mg daily or twice a day, is administered until there is improvement; on improvement, prednisone dosage should be tapered rapidly.

Treatment of anaphylaxis due to drug allergy is comparable to that of anaphylaxis from other causes. The initial treatment for adults consists of subcutaneous or intramuscular 1:1000 epinephrine, 0.3 mL; this may be repeated twice at 15-minute intervals. Depending on the manifestations of anaphylaxis, additional therapy may be indicated. For example, patients who are hypotensive may require fluids and vasopressors; patients who have bronchospasm may require an aerosolized beta-2 agonist and/or intravenous aminophylline 6 mg/kg over 30 minutes. Those who have laryngeal edema may require tracheostomy.

If a patient has a truly essential indication for radiocontrast media (RCM), pretreatment has been useful in reducing the number of repeat anaphylactoid reactions. Low-osmolality contrast material also reduces the risk. Pretreatment medications include prednisone 60 mg at 13 hours, 7 hours, and 1 hour before RCM; diphenhydramine hydrochloride 50 mg 1 hour before; and albuterol 4 mg 1 hour before.[12] Albuterol may be contraindicated if the patient has coronary artery disease or an arrhythmia. It is, of course, necessary to document the risks and benefits of the RCM and the patient's informed consent.

Prevention of drug allergy is obviously a desirable goal. Several important prevention guidelines are listed in Box 17-7. First, there is the obvious principle of prescribing drugs only when clearly indicated. Next, patients should be carefully questioned about previous drug reactions so that they are not given drugs to which they may be allergic. There are some agents, such as foreign antisera, to which many are allergic; cutaneous testing must be performed prior to administration. If a patient experiences an allergic reaction, the patient or responsible person should be informed so that he or she can avoid the drug in the future. The medical record should reflect this information and, in selected patients, Medic-Alert tags may be appropriate.

Finally, adverse reactions such as drug allergies should be reported to the relevant agency, especially in the case of drugs that are relatively new. In the United States, physicians are urged to call or write to pharmaceutical manufacturers and the Food and Drug Administration (FDA) via MedWatch (FDA Medical Products Reporting Program, FDA, 5600 Fishers Lane, Rockville, MD 20852-9787). Voluntary reporting forms (form 3500) can be obtained from the FDA and the *Physician's Desk Reference* and on-line at www.accessdata.FDA.gov/scripts/medwatch. Mandatory reporting is not available on-line. MedWatch can be called (24 hours/day) at 800-332-1088. In emergent situations, the FDA may be contacted by calling 301-443-1240.

---

**BOX 17-7**
**Key Measures for the Prevention of Drug Allergy**

Prescribe drugs only if essential

Prior to prescribing drugs, obtain a thorough, careful drug history; drugs to which patients have had reactions or cross-reacting drugs should not be prescribed

Perform cutaneous tests prior to administration of foreign antisera

If an allergic drug reaction occurs, fully inform the patient; medical records should reflect the incident

Report adverse drug reactions, such as drug allergy, to the Food and Drug Administration; this is especially important for newly introduced drugs

# REFERENCES

1. Jick H: Adverse drug reactions: The magnitude of the problem. J Allergy Clin Immunol 1985;74:555–558.
2. Ditto AM: Drug Allergy. In Grammer LC, Greenberger PA (eds): Patterson's Allergic Diseases, Philidelphia, Lippincott Williams & Wilkins, 2002, pp 295–360.
3. Adkinson NF, Essayan D, Guchalla R, et al: Health and Environmental Sciences Institute Task Force Report: Future research needs for the prevention and management of immune mediated drug hypersensitivity reactions. J Allergy Clin Immunol 2002;109(3):S461–S478.
4. Carrington DM, Earl HS, Sullivan TJ: Studies of human IgE to a sulfonamide determinate. J Allergy Clin Immunol 1987;79:442–447.
5. Idsoe O, Gunthe T, Silcox RR, et al: Nature and extent of penicillin side reactions with particular reference to fatalities from anaphylactic shock. Bull World Health Org 1968;38:195.
6. Rotskoff B, Saltoun CA: Monoclonal antibodies. In Grammer LC, Greenberger PA (eds): Drug Allergy and Protocols for Management of Drug Allergies. Providence, OceanSide Publications, 2003.
7. Cobleigh MA, Vogel CL, Tripathy D, et al: Multinational study of the efficacy and safety of humanized HER2 monoclonal antibody in woman who have HER2-overexpressing metastatic breast cancer that has progressed after chemotherapy for metastatic disease. J Clin Oncol 1999;17;2639–2648.
8. Antonelli G, Giannelli G, Currenti M, et al: Antibodies to interferon (INF) in hepatitis C patients relapsing while continuing recombinant INF-α2 therapy. Clin Exp Immunol 1996;104:384–387.
9. Flais M, Ditto AM: Aspirin, non-selective and selective non-steroidal anti-inflammatory drugs. In Grammer LC, Greenberger PA (eds): Drug Allergy and Protocols for Management of Drug Allergies. Providence, OceanSide Publications, 2003, pp 31–32.
10. Posadas SJ, Padial A, Torres MJ, et al: Delayed reactions to drugs show levels of perforin, grazyme B, and Fas-L to be related to disease severity. J Allergy Clin Immunol 2002;109:155–161.

*Michael D. Tharp, Macy I. Levine, and Philip Fireman*

# *18* Urticaria and Angioedema

Urticaria, commonly called hives, is characterized by pale or erythematous localized swellings of the skin that vary in size and shape, without surface scaling. Sometimes surrounded by a red halo, these lesions can coalesce and are always associated with itching. Angioedema, also known as giant urticaria, is manifested by a more generalized swelling of the skin due to deep dermal and subcutaneous edema. Thus, these lesions have poorly defined borders and often retain normal skin color. Angioedema commonly affects the eyelids, lips, tongue, genitalia, hands, feet, and, on occasion, the larynx, gastrointestinal tract, or urinary bladder.

Urticaria and angioedema are very common conditions in the general population, occurring in as many as 20% to 25% of all people at some time during their lives.[1] In one study of a large number of patients, 49% had both conditions, 40% had urticaria alone, and 11% had angioedema alone.[2] These conditions may be classified as acute—symptoms lasting up to 6 weeks—and chronic—the presence of hives or angioedema occurring on most days for longer than 6 weeks. Acute and chronic conditions are discussed together, because they generally have similar causes and treatment.[3]

Frequently, patients with urticaria or angioedema seek the attention of a physician who specializes in the treatment of allergic or skin diseases. Clinicians must be aware that some primary skin disorders and systemic diseases with cutaneous manifestations may mimic these lesions, and a portion of this chapter is dedicated to the differential diagnosis of these conditions.

## EPIDEMIOLOGY

Urticaria and angioedema may arise in all age groups. Acute disease appears to be more common in young adults and children, at times arising from the triggering of cutaneous mast cells through antigen-specific immunoglobulin (Ig) E antibodies. The chronic form of urticaria or angioedema occurs much more frequently in adults, particularly in middle-aged women. Available data on the natural history of these cutaneous reactions among large groups of patients indicate that a majority of individuals with urticaria alone are free of lesions after 1 year, although a few continue to experience their eruption for a number of years. Similarly, approximately one half of patients with acquired angioedema alone continue to experience the disorder for more than 1 year. A personal or family history of atopy may be more common in patients with acute urticaria, but this association does not appear to be a factor in patients with chronic urticaria or angioedema.

## *CLINICAL PRESENTATION*

Because they are so common, the lesions of urticaria are often correctly diagnosed by the patient. Classically, this cutaneous eruption appears as round to oval white or erythematous wheals (Fig. 18-1). Surrounding erythema may or may not be present. Lesion size ranges from a few millimeters to several centimeters in diameter (Fig. 18-2). Less commonly, urticarial lesions may assume annular, arcuate, or serpiginous configurations (Fig. 18-3).

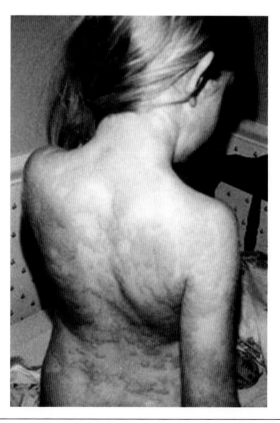

**Figure 18-1.** Urticarial lesions of various sizes ranging from 1 mm to several centimeters in diameter. Individual erythematous lesions may coalesce, as shown here.

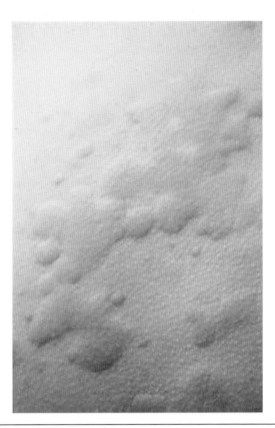

**Figure 18-2.** A close-up photograph of typical urticarial lesions, which may show considerable size variation.

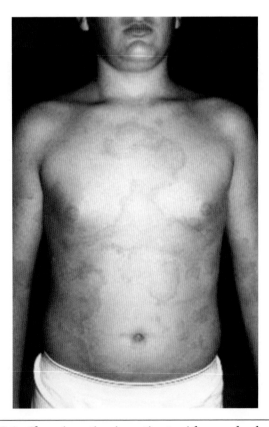

**Figure 18-3.** Chronic urticaria patient with annular lesions on the upper and mid-thorax and arcuate lesions in the abdominal area. Typical serpiginous lesions are seen in the right upper abdominal quadrant.

The clinical expression of urticarial lesions results primarily from upper dermal inflammation and edema. This appears clinically as

- Normal skin surface markings (absence of scaling)
- Normal pigmentation
- Erythema, which is indicative of vasodilatation

Urticarial lesions are usually pruritic and generally last less than 24 hours. In contrast to urticaria, angioedema reactions occur deep in the dermis and may involve subcutaneous tissue (Fig. 18-4A and B). These lesions appear as large, slightly erythematous areas with normal epidermal surface markings and poorly defined borders. Often, these subcutaneous swellings are asymptomatic but may be slightly painful. Typically, lesions of angioedema are asymmetrical.

## ETIOLOGY

Numerous agents have been implicated in the provocation of urticaria or angioedema, and these include medications, foreign sera, foods, food additives, infections, insect bites and stings, contactants, inhalants, and physical agents (e.g., heat, cold, pressure, vibration, water, light). A subset of patients with chronic urticaria have been demonstrated to have circulating IgG antibodies to IgE receptors and/or IgE on the mast cell surface, which has led to the term *autoimmune urticaria*.[4,5] Studies have shown that approximately 30% of chronic idiopathic urticaria patients have these circulating antibodies. Although the cause and effect of these IgG antibodies in urticaria remains uncertain, it appears that binding of IgG to IgE on the mast cell or to its IgE receptors results in complement activation and the generation of anaphylatoxins C3a, C4a, and C5a.[6] It has been hypothesized that C5a may be responsible for mast cell stimulation in this patient group. Urticaria patients with such circulating anti-IgE and IgE receptor antibodies have a strong association with human leukocyte antigen DR4 and human leukocyte antigen DQ8 and a higher incidence of autoimmune diseases, including thyroid disease, vitiligo, insulin-dependent diabetes mellitus, rheumatoid arthritis, and pernicious anemia. Leznoff and Sussman[7] and Leznoff and colleagues[8] found

---

**BOX 18-1**
**Potential Causes of Urticarial Reactions**

Foods
Medications
Sera
Infections
Insect bites and stings
Contactants and inhalants
Antibodies to IgE and IgE receptor
Physical agents (heat, cold, pressure, vibration, water, and light)
Psychological factors (stress)
Exercise

Ig, immunoglobulin.

that a significant number of patients with chronic idiopathic urticaria had thyroid microsomal antibodies and thyroglobulin antibodies and suggested the presence of thyroid autoimmunity. Emotional stress also may exacerbate these reactions. In addition, urticarial reaction patterns have been associated with certain genetic disorders, pregnancy, connective tissue diseases, and neoplasm (Box 18-1).

Although the origin of acute urticaria can sometimes be detected, an etiologic agent or precipitating cause is often difficult to establish in chronic disease. The association of urticaria with underlying systemic diseases is relatively uncommon, although this cutaneous reaction pattern has been linked to some disorders (Box 18-2).

As is true for urticarial reactions, a definitive cause is usually not determined for many of the patients with chronic angioedema.

> **BOX 18-2**
> **Systemic Diseases Associated with Urticarial Eruptions**
>
> Systemic lupus erythematosus
> Serum sickness, cryoglobulinemia
> Juvenile rheumatoid arthritis
> Hyperthyroidism, hypothyroidism
> Neoplasms
> Mastocytosis

However, hereditary angioedema must be considered in any patient with recurrent lesions, and this disorder is discussed later.

# PATHOLOGY

## HISTOLOGIC CHANGES

Classically, cutaneous biopsies of urticarial lesions have revealed surprisingly few histopathologic alterations. Dilatation and engorgement of superficial vessels and lymphatics in association with dermal edema is a prominent feature, and, typically, a sparse to moderate perivascular mononuclear infiltrate with few eosinophils is also seen (Fig. 18-5A).[9] Cases of this type of inflammatory cell infiltrate have been termed *lymphocyte predominant urticaria*. However, a greater spectrum of histopathologic changes may be observed in lesional skin of urticarial patients. Skin biopsy specimens may demonstrate a perivascular infiltrate consisting of neutrophils and eosinophils in addition to mononuclear cells, with no evidence of vasculitis (see Fig. 18-5B). Such cases have been labeled polymorphonuclear predominant urticaria.[9] Rarely, a true vasculitis can be observed in lesional skin specimens, which is characterized by a neutrophil-rich, perivascular infiltrate associated with leukocytoclasis and fibrin-like deposition around dermal vessels (see Fig. 18-5C). Direct immunofluorescence studies of such lesions demonstrate the presence of immunoglobulins, C3, and/or fibrin, suggesting the presence of immune complex disease (see Fig. 18-5D).

Whereas the histopathologic alterations in lesions of angioedema have not been as extensively investigated, vasodilation

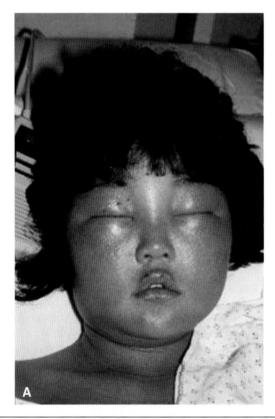 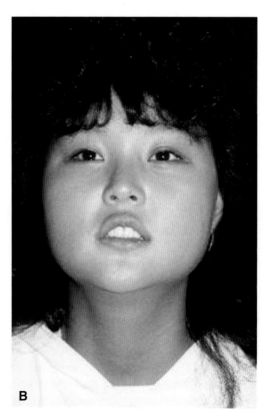

**Figure 18-4.** *A,* Angioedema involving the periorbital areas bilaterally due to recurrent allergen exposure. *B,* The patient's normal facial appearance following resolution of the reaction.

and edema associated with a mixed cellular infiltrate appear to be common features. In contrast to the superficial dermal changes of urticaria, these alterations are observed primarily in the deep dermis and subcutaneous tissue.

## PATHOGENESIS

Numerous clinical and pathophysiologic studies suggest a primary role for the tissue mast cell in the expression of urticaria and/or angioedema.[6] Mast cell stimulation may result from a number of different immune and non–immune-mediated mechanisms, which are listed in Box 18-3. One or a combination of these factors may be important in triggering an urticarial reaction. The early vascular changes observed in these cutaneous eruptions can be readily attributed to the release of the preformed mediator, histamine, but may also involve the elaboration of mast cell–derived prostaglandin D2 and leukotrienes. Tissue mast cells may also release several different chemotactic factors (histamine, neutrophil chemotactic factor, eosinophil chemotactic factors of anaphylaxis, tumor necrosis factor-α, and possibly leukotriene B4) that result in the influx of inflammatory cells to the primary site of mast cell activation. It is likely that the infiltration of activated leukocytes into the area leads to the release of additional cell-derived inflammatory mediators, resulting in local tissue injury and possibly provoking a second wave of tissue mast cell activation.[10,11]

Although theoretically this series of events could explain in total the pathogenesis of urticaria and/or angioedema, evidence suggests that the local release of neuropeptides from sensory nerve

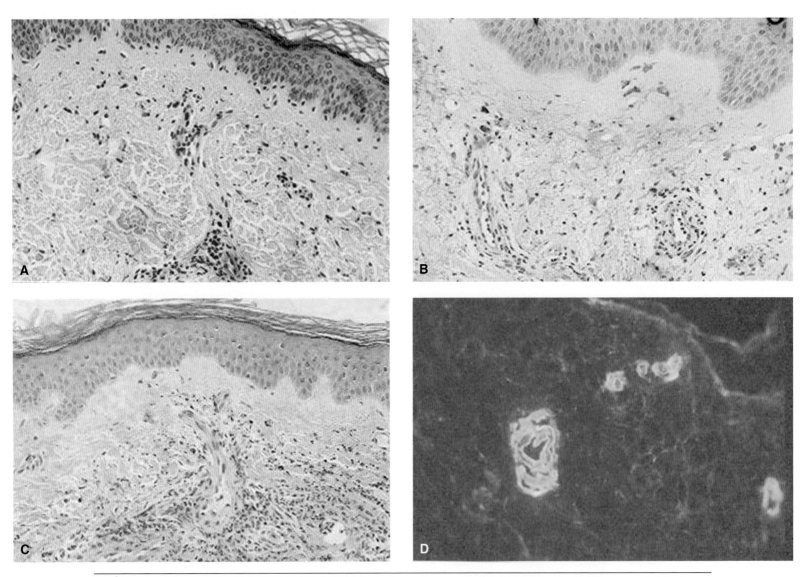

**Figure 18-5.** Photomicrographs of the spectrum of histologic changes in patients with urticarial lesions. *A,* Typical urticaria with dermal edema and a sparse perivascular, mononuclear cell infiltrate. *B,* Less commonly, one sees the accumulation of dermal plasma cells and the infiltration of neutrophils around vessels without evidence of vasculitis in the lesional skin of some patients with urticaria. *C,* In urticarial vasculitis, intense perivascular neutrophil accumulation with damage to neutrophils (cytoclasis) and endothelial cells is the characteristic histologic feature. *D,* Immunofluorescent staining documents the presence of complement (C3) and immunoglobulin (Ig) G and IgM deposition around vessels in early lesions of urticarial vasculitis. This histology was described by Jones and colleagues in 1983.[9]

endings may play a role in the expression of these cutaneous eruptions, especially in patients with chronic disease.[12] A number of different neuropeptides, including substance P, vasoactive intestinal polypeptide, calcitonin gene-related peptide, and neuropeptide Y, have been identified by immunocytochemical methods in sensory nerves in the dermis. When released in human skin, these substances induce a wheal-and-flare reaction. A model for potential interaction of sensory nerves with dermal mast cells is illustrated in Figure 18-6. When cutaneous sensory nerves are activated by some stimulus, both orthrodromic (forward) and antidromic (retrograde) action potentials may be generated. These retrograde impulses may subsequently lead to the release of one or more neuropeptides in the dermis.

Taken together, it can be postulated that skin mast cell mediator release leads to vasodilatation, plasma extravasation, inflammatory cell chemotaxis, and sensory-nerve stimulation. The subsequent generation of antidromic and sensory-nerve potentials could, in turn, lead to the local release of neuropeptides, which also induce vasodilatation and edema formation by their direct effects on endothelial cells, as well as cause additional mast cell stimulation. Ultimately, the number and type of infiltrating leukocytes may dictate the severity and duration of the inflammatory reaction. Because leukocytes are known to stimulate mast cell mediator release, it is conceivable that these cells may perpetuate the initial reaction. Furthermore, the elaboration of leukocyte-derived lysosomal enzymes and other inflammatory mediators in the local environment may lead to additional sensory nerve stimulation and subsequent neuropeptide release. Thus, from our understanding to date, it appears that the clinical expression of urticaria or angioedema results from a combination of

pathophysiologic events. To varying degrees, this may include mast cell activation, the elaboration of mediators, the local release of sensory nerve peptide, and the infiltration of different groups of inflammatory cells.

# DIAGNOSIS AND EVALUATION

## *DIFFERENTIAL DIAGNOSIS*

Although the lesions of urticaria and angioedema are often easily recognized, there are instances in which other cutaneous disorders may mimic these eruptions. In these cases, careful consideration of all diagnostic possibilities is essential.[13]

## *PRURITIC URTICARIAL PAPULES AND PLAQUES OF PREGNANCY*

The term *pruritic urticarial papules and plaques of pregnancy* (PUPPP) refers to an intense pruritic eruption that is occasionally observed in pregnant women.[14] Characteristically, patients with this disorder develop erythematous, urticarial plaques and papules during the last trimester of pregnancy (Fig. 18-7). Classically, these lesions begin centrally over the abdomen and extend to involve the thighs, buttocks, and distal extremities. The facial area is usually spared. In some patients, only the lower extremities are involved. Although the pathophysiologic mechanism for this disorder is unknown, skin biopsies of lesional tissue show histologic changes similar to those observed in other urticarial reactions and therefore suggest an important role for the mast cell. The maternal cutaneous lesions usually resolve shortly after delivery, and no associated abnormalities or adverse reactions have been reported in infants from mothers with PUPPP. Patients who develop PUPPP with their initial pregnancy are not necessarily at risk for recurrence of this disorder with subsequent pregnancies.

## *IDIOPATHIC URTICARIAL VASCULITIS*

Another disorder that may present with urticaria-like lesions is the syndrome called *idiopathic urticarial vasculitis*.[15] This disorder is more prevalent in women than in men and is associated with recurrent urticaria-like lesions. The hands, elbows, ankles, and knees are most frequently involved, and the patient often experiences pain or tenderness of cutaneous lesions in conjunction with pruritus (Fig. 18-8*A* and *B*). Joint pain and stiffness are also common and usually parallel skin disease activity. Gastrointestinal symptoms, including abdominal pain, nausea, vomiting, and diarrhea, have been temporally associated with skin and joint involvement. Other symptoms encountered less frequently in patients with urticarial vasculitis include recurrent headaches, eye pain, and chest pain.

In addition to arthritis, other clinical signs of systemic involvement in these patients include generalized lymphadenopathy, bronchospasm, uveitis, episcleritis, and, more rarely, neurologic findings such as pseudotumor cerebri, meningitis, and mononeuritis.

The diagnosis of idiopathic urticarial vasculitis is established by the histologic changes in the skin biopsy. In the majority of

---

**BOX 18-3**
**Potential Mechanisms of Mast Cell Activation in Clinical Urticaria**

**Immunologic Mechanisms**
Antigen reaction with specific mast cell membrane IgE antibody
Complement anaphylatoxin (C3a and C5a) stimulation of specific mast cell–associated receptors
Eosinophil-derived major basic protein activation of mast cells
Leukocyte-derived histamine releasing factor(s), stimulation of mast cells
Antibodies to IgE and IgE receptors

**Nonimmunologic Factors That Stimulate Mast Cells**
Neuropeptides (substance P, calcitonin gene–related peptide, vasoactive intestinal polypeptide, neurokinin Y)
Hormones (gastrin, estrogen, ACTH)
Medications (aspirin, nonsteroidal anti-inflammatory agents, codeine, curare, succinylcholine, polymyxin B, thiamine)
Physical stimuli (heat, cold, pressure, light)
Venoms
Radiocontrast media

ACTH, adrenocorticotropic hormone; Ig, immunoglobulin.

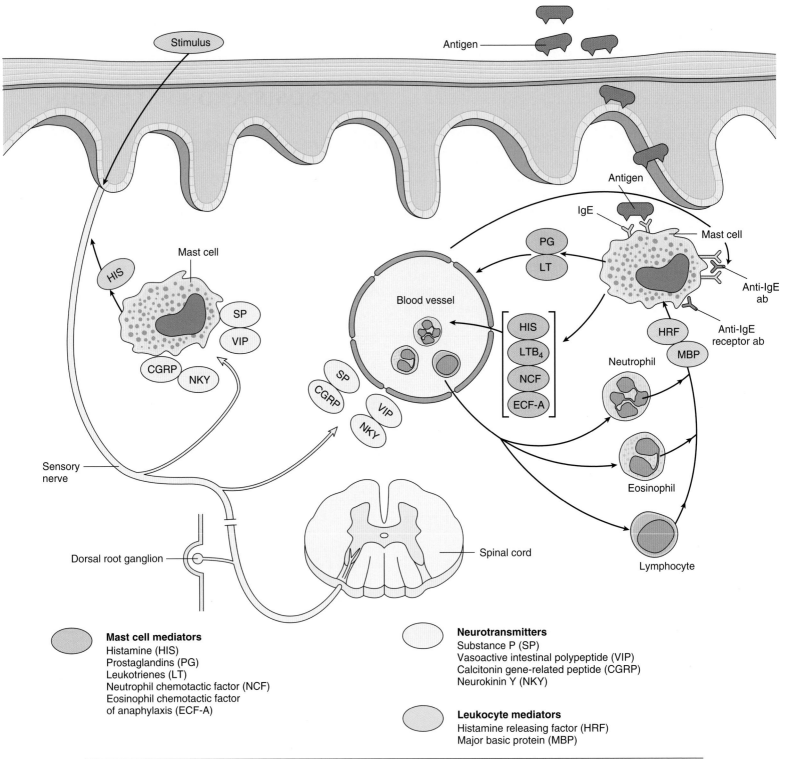

**Mast cell mediators**
Histamine (HIS)
Prostaglandins (PG)
Leukotrienes (LT)
Neutrophil chemotactic factor (NCF)
Eosinophil chemotactic factor
of anaphylaxis (ECF-A)

**Neurotransmitters**
Substance P (SP)
Vasoactive intestinal polypeptide (VIP)
Calcitonin gene-related peptide (CGRP)
Neurokinin Y (NKY)

**Leukocyte mediators**
Histamine releasing factor (HRF)
Major basic protein (MBP)

**Figure 18-6.** Pathogenesis of chronic urticaria. Mast cell stimulation and mediator release may be initiated through antigen or antibodies cross-linking surface-bound immunoglobulin (Ig) E or IgE receptors or by histamine-releasing factors elaborated from leukocytes that have been activated by foreign proteins or other immune stimuli. Mast cell–derived histamine, prostaglandin $D_2$, and leukotrienes all have direct dilating effects on blood vessels, thus provoking dermal edema. These mediators also show chemotactic properties that attract leukocytes into tissues. Mast cell–derived neutrophilic and eosinophilic chemotactic factors also encourage local leukocyte infiltration. Histamine, prostaglandin $D_2$, and possible leukocyte-derived mediators are capable of stimulating sensory nerves in the skin. Whereas orthrodromic neuroimpulses would be expected to transmit signals to the central nervous system via the spinal cord, antidromic or retrograde neurotransmission is also theoretically possible, and these impulses may lead to the release of neuropeptides in the skin. Neuropeptides such as substance P, calcitonin gene–related peptide, vasoactive intestinal polypeptide, and neurokinin Y are capable of causing additional vasodilatation and possibly mast cell degranulation.

patients, the hallmarks of necrotizing vasculitis are evident in cutaneous lesions and indicative of immune complex–mediated disease. Direct immunofluorescence studies of lesional skin from some, but not all, patients with this syndrome show complement and/or immunoglobulins within dermal vessels and/or along the dermoepidermal junction (see Fig. 18-5D). Approximately 50% to 60% of patients with urticarial vasculitis have detectable hypocomplementemia, most having depressed levels of the early classical pathway components (C2 and C4). In addition, low-molecular-weight (7S) Clq precipitins have been reported in the sera of some urticarial vasculitis patients. Presumably, urticaria-like lesions develop as a result of immune complex deposition in the skin leading to complement activation and the formation of the anaphylatoxins C3a and C5a. These activated complement components in turn stimulate mast cells to release histamine and other mediators. A few patients with this disorder develop renal disease, ranging in severity from a focal necrotizing glomer-ulonephritis to a diffuse proliferative process. More recent reports also indicate that some patients with urticarial vasculitis may have an accelerated course of chronic obstructive pulmonary disease. Additional tests (antinuclear antibodies, antibodies to double-stranded DNA, cryoglobulins, circulating rheumatoid factors, false-positive Venereal Disease Research Laboratory testing, hepatitis B surface antigen) that are frequently employed for the diagnosis of connective tissue diseases or immune complex–mediated disorders are usually either negative or of low titer in patients with urticarial vasculitis, limiting their diagnostic value in this context.

## SYSTEMIC LUPUS ERYTHEMATOSUS AND OTHER DISORDERS

Urticarial lesions have been reported to occur in the rare patient with systemic lupus erythematosus.[16] In some cases, these lesions have the typical histologic changes of urticaria, while in others, there is evidence of leukocytoclastic vasculitis. Some patients with essential mixed cryoglobulinemia may also present initially with urticaria-like lesions following cold exposure. However, the presence of palpable purpuric lesions (vasculitis), Raynaud's phenomenon, and cutaneous ulcerations helps to distinguish these patients from those with uncomplicated chronic urticaria.

Most patients with serum sickness develop an urticarial re-action pattern early in the course of disease. Histologically, these lesions may demonstrate changes typical of urticaria or may show more significant inflammation in the form of vasculitis. Urticarial-like papules and plaques also have been reported in children with juvenile rheumatoid arthritis, but, unlike common hives, these lesions are characteristically nonpruritic. Lesions of acute and chronic urticaria also have been reported in patients with hypothyroidism, hyperthyroidism, and occult lymphomas. Patients with mastocytosis may have dermatographism or a spontaneous urticaria-like eruption in foci of cutaneous mast cell infiltrates (Fig. 18-9).[17] Unlike urticaria, lesions of mastocytosis are persis-tent and readily identified by their tan (in children) or reddish-brown (in adults) color. This condition has been called *urticaria pigmentosa* because of the appearance.

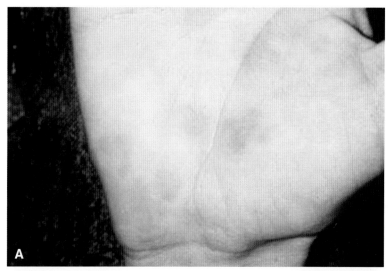

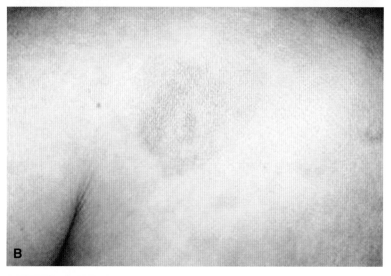

**Figure 18-8.** Lesions of urticarial vasculitis. *A,* Palmar involvement frequently occurs in these patients, and this may mimic the lesions of erythema multiforme. *B,* Evidence of purpura may be seen in resolving urticarial vasculitis lesions.

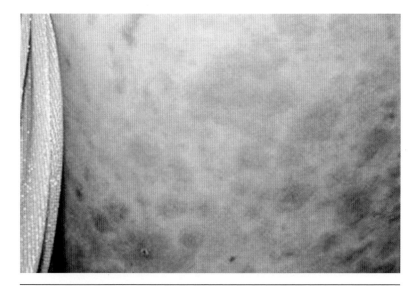

**Figure 18-7.** Urticaria-like eruption of pruritic urticarial papules and plaques of pregnancy. Characteristically, these erythematous lesions begin on the abdomen of patients during the last trimester of pregnancy and may extend to the proximal extremities.

Recurrent episodes of urticaria and angioedema have also been described in adolescents with the rare hereditary disorder originally described by Muckle and Wells.[18] These children experience recurrent urticarial eruptions accompanied by chills and malaise. Progressive nerve deafness and amyloidosis of the kidney develop after a variable period. Schnitzler's syndrome represents a rare disorder characterized by nonpruritic urticarial papules and a monoclonal gammopathy.[19] Patients also may experience a number of other signs and symptoms, including angioedema, fever, bone pain, weight loss, hepatosplenomegaly, and lymphadenopathy. In addition to an IgM monoclonal gammopathy, these patients also may have an elevated erythrocyte sedimentation rate and increased serum fibrinogen levels. Biopsies of lesional skin may show varying degrees of neutrophilic infiltrates with or without vasculitis.

Several other well-defined cutaneous diseases also should be considered in the differential diagnosis of urticaria or angioedema (Box 18-4). The annular and arcuate morphology of some urticarial lesions must be distinguished from a group of disorders termed the figurative erythemas. This group includes erythema annulare centrifugum (Fig. 18-10A), erythema chronicum migrans, and erythema marginatum. In contrast to urticaria, usually these eruptions are nonpruritic. Erythema annulare centrifugum, which most closely resembles an urticarial reaction pattern, can be identified by a characteristic scaling ring that trails its advancing red border. Individual lesions of erythema multiforme may also assume an urticarial morphology. However, the more typical target-like lesions are usually also present (see Fig. 18-10B).

Early in their course, some of the primary blistering disorders may appear urticarial. In particular, the autoimmune blistering diseases such as dermatitis herpetiformis (see Fig. 18-10C) and bullous pemphigoid[20] may present as pruritic papules. Similarly, herpes simplex and herpes zoster may begin as pruritic, slightly painful urticarial lesions, and in some instances, the full clinical expression of grouped vesicles may not occur (see Fig. 18-10D). Lesion arrangement (grouped) and, a focal anatomic distribution, however, provide important clinical characteristics for differentiating herpetic lesions from typical lesions of urticaria (see Fig. 18-10E).

## HEREDITARY ANGIOEDEMA

In patients with recurrent angioedema (Fig. 18-11), several disorders should be considered in the differential diagnosis, including hereditary angioedema (HAE), acquired deficiency of the inhibitor of complement (C)1 esterase, and angioedema-eosinophilia syndrome. Hereditary angioedema is an autosomal disorder characterized by episodic, nonpruritic, and painless subcutaneous swellings lasting for several hours to days.[21] The lesions are often triggered by local trauma or emotional stress and are usually asymmetrical. Unlike acquired angioedema, an urticarial reaction pattern is not present in patients with this disorder. Also, a history of recurrent nausea, vomiting, and abdominal colicky pain resulting from localized intestinal edema is common in this patient population.

The onset of HAE usually begins in childhood or young adulthood. There is often a positive history of other family members with similar complaints. It is important to differentiate HAE from other causes of angioedema, because patients with this disorder may be at greater risk for laryngeal edema leading to sudden death. The underlying mechanism for HAE is a genetically determined partial deficiency of an alpha2-glycoprotein, termed C1 esterase inhibitor (C1 INH). This serum protein normally inactivates the first component of complement. The absence of C1 INH results in excessive consumption of the complement component, C4. Thus, patients with HAE have chronically depressed serum levels of C4, and during acute attacks, both C4 and C2 levels are depressed. In approximately 85% of the patients, C1 INH levels are low, whereas in the remaining 15%, the protein is present in normal amounts. In this latter group, the inhibitory activity of C1

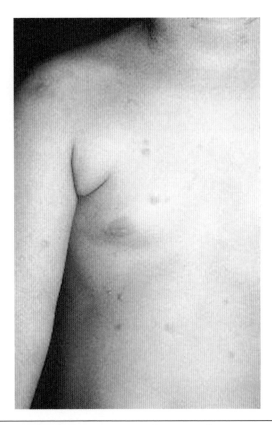

**Figure 18-9.** Urticarial reaction in lesions of mastocytosis. The stroking of mastocytosis skin lesions results in an urticarial response (Darier's sign). These yellow-tan papules are commonly described as urticaria pigmentosa.

---

**BOX 18-4**
**Differential Diagnosis of Urticaria**

Urticaria of pregnancy (PUPPP)
Urticarial vasculitis
Figurative erythemas
Erythema multiforme
Dermatitis herpetiformis
Bullous pemphigoid
Herpes simplex, herpes zoster
Mastocytosis

PUPPP, pruritic urticarial papules and plaques of pregnancy.

INH is abnormal; thus, a functional C1 INH assay is necessary to correctly identify this subset of HAE.

The underlying mechanisms for hereditary angioedema appear to involve both the activation of the complement and plasma kinin–forming pathways. In the absence of C1 INH activity, the stimulation of the complement cascade proceeds essentially uninhibited following minor stimuli. Generation of the anaphylatoxins, C3a and C5a, under such circumstances would be expected to provoke mast cell and basophil mediator release. C1 INH also inhibits kallikrein, Hageman factor fragments, and plasmin. Following tissue trauma, kallikrein is readily generated from high-molecular prekallikrein in a patient with HAE, and as a result

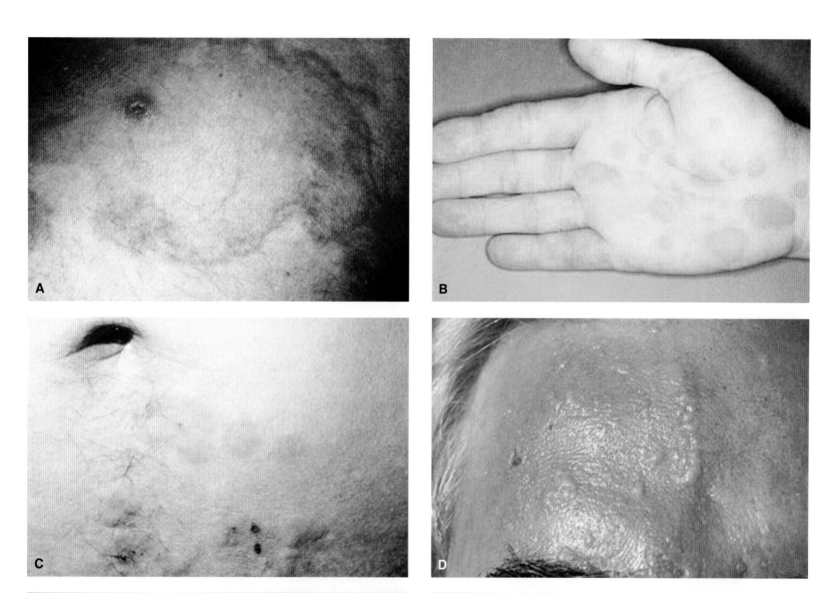

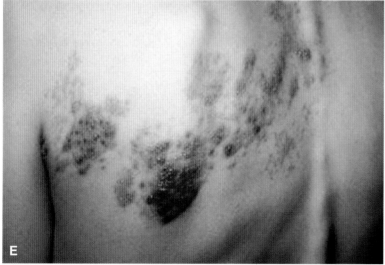

**Figure 18-10.** Cutaneous disorders that may appear as urticaria. *A,* Erythema annulare centrifugum. *B,* Erythema multiforme involving the palm. Both of these belong to the group of disorders known as the figurative erythemas. *C,* Dermatitis herpetiformis. An urticaria-like eruption may be seen in early lesions of this blistering disease. *D,* Edematous plaques, which may appear urticarial in herpes zoster. *E,* More typically grouped lesions of herpes zoster.

of inadequate C1 INH activity, it stimulates kininogen, leading to the generation of bradykinin, a potent vasoactive polypeptide (Fig. 18-12). Subcutaneous injections of either C1 or kallikrein result in angioedematous lesions in patients with HAE, suggesting a role for other complement factors and the plasma kinin–forming pathway. Both HAE variations respond to stanazolol or danazol therapy.

## ACQUIRED COMPLEMENT 1 ESTERASE INHIBITOR DEFICIENCY

Occasionally, certain neoplastic disorders, including lymphomas and multiple myeloma, as well as pulmonary and colon carcinomas, have been associated with a clinical syndrome similar to HAE.[22] However, unlike patients with HAE, these often have urticarial lesions accompanying the angioedema. Referred to as acquired deficiency of serum C1 INH, this disorder can be detected through its association with a decrease of C4 and C2 levels as well as C1 inhibitor. In contrast to HAE patients, however, levels of C1q are depressed in patients with acquired C1 INH deficiency.

## ANGIOEDEMA-EOSINOPHILIA SYNDROME

Recently, a most unusual disorder characterized by recurrent episodes of angioedema and urticaria in association with fever, prominent weight gain, and peripheral blood eosinophilia was described. Characteristically, these patients develop angioedema that persists for up to 7 to 10 days and is associated with a 7- to 9-kg (15- to 20-pound) weight gain. The most striking laboratory abnormality is a marked increase in peripheral blood eosinophils (ranging from 2760 to 95,0404 mm$^3$). Cutaneous biopsies from lesional tissue demonstrate dermal edema and perivascular lymphocytic infiltrates with scattered eosinophils. Despite few demonstrable tissue eosinophils, immunofluorescence staining for eosinophil granule–derived major basic protein has been uniformly positive in each skin biopsy specimen. Extensive study of each case for an underlying parasitic infection and/or antigen stimulus has shown negative results. The prognosis for these patients appears good in that they respond to systemic corticosteroid therapy. Two subjects have had this disorder for at least 10 years without significant disseminated disease or complications.

There are several disorders that may mimic lesions of angioedema. These include panniculitis, localized cellulitis, thrombophlebitis, lymphangitis, and cheilitis granulomatosa (Box 18-5).

## PATIENT EVALUATION

Once the clinical diagnosis of urticaria or angioedema has been established and other conditions have been excluded, careful attention to both the morphology and the anatomic distribution of lesions may provide insight into potential etiologic factors. Small

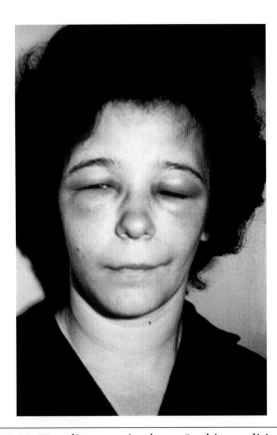

**Figure 18-11.** Hereditary angioedema. In this condition, the swellings frequently involve the face, including the oropharynx. The edema is typically nonerythematous and nonpruritic. These lesions can be extensive, involving the deep dermal and subcutaneous tissues.

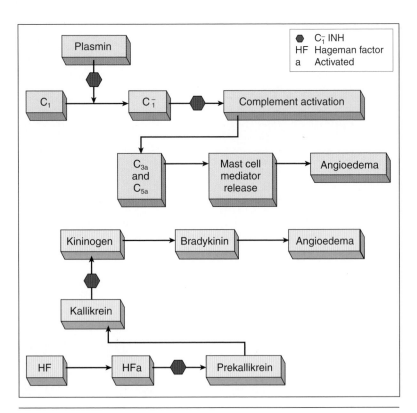

**Figure 18-12.** Pathogenesis of hereditary angioedema. Deficiency in the first component of complement (C1) esterase inhibitor (C1-INH) leads to uninhibited complement activation and anaphylatoxin (C3a, C5a) formation, which, in turn, stimulates mast cell mediator release. In addition, Hageman Factor activation also proceeds in the absence of C1-INH activity, which may result in the formation of the vasodilating agent bradykinin.

(1- to 3-mm) wheals with large surrounding areas of erythema suggest a diagnosis of cholinergic urticaria (Fig. 18-13). Focal urticarial lesions with geometric shapes (linear, angular, straight edged) indicate the presence of external influences, as may be seen in pressure urticaria or dermatographism (Fig. 18-14*A*). Similarly, urticarial lesions localized to exposed areas suggest the possibility of solar (see Fig. 18-14*B*) or cold-induced reactions (see Fig. 18-14*C*).

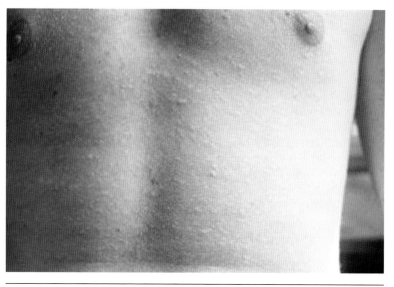

**Figure 18-13.** Typical lesions of cholinergic urticaria. Papules 1 to 3 mm in diameter with surrounding erythema are commonly seen, especially after exercise or increased body temperature.

---

**BOX 18-5**
## Differential Diagnosis of Angioedema

Hereditary angioedema (HAE)
Acquired C1 inhibitor deficiency
Angioedema-eosinophilia syndrome
Panniculitis, cellulitis
Thrombophlebitis, lymphangitis
Cheilitis granulomatosa

---

C1, first component of complement.

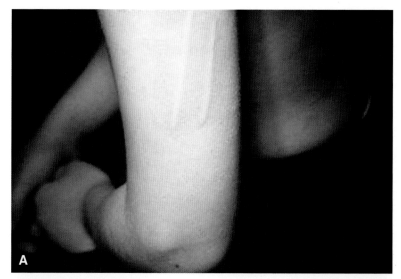

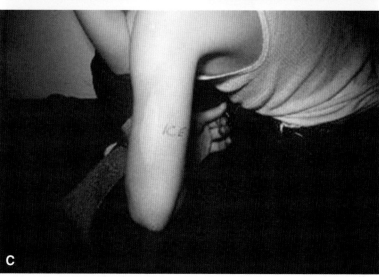

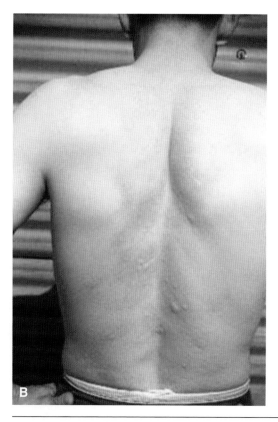

**Figure 18-14.** Physical urticarias. *A,* Pressure urticaria. This photograph demonstrates a typical response 20 minutes after applying pressure by firmly stroking the skin with a tongue depressor. *B,* Solar urticaria. This photograph was taken after 30 minutes of unprotected sunlight exposure. *C,* Cold urticaria. An urticarial response minutes after removal of ice applied to the skin for 5 minutes.

In patients with distal extremity involvement alone, the diagnosis of papular urticaria or urticarial vasculitis should be considered (see Fig. 18-8), whereas small urticarial papules with a follicular-like arrangement suggest the possibility of aquagenic urticaria.

In general, when the history and physical examination fail to uncover potential etiologic factors, a skin biopsy is warranted in cases of chronic urticaria. Patients with polymorphonuclear predominant urticaria often have skin lesions that burn and sting as well as itch. Patients who frequently present with this histologic change will be resistant to antihistamine therapy alone. Extensive laboratory studies, such as a complete blood count, erythrocyte sedimentation rate, urinalysis, serum chemical analyses, allergy testing, as well as sinus and dental radiographs, are rarely useful. Figure 18-15 outlines a clinical algorithm for the diagnosis and management of unresponsive chronic urticaria or angioedema.

# TREATMENT

The most effective approach to the treatment of urticaria or angioedema is the identification and elimination of the causative agents. In patients with medication- or food-induced eruptions, for example, avoidance of these substances is curative. In cases of physical urticaria, an explanation of the disease process and its initiating factors permits patients to modify their lifestyle. Those with cold urticaria should be warned of the potential danger of diving into or swimming in cool or cold water and should never swim alone. Commonsense measures, such as wearing warm socks and gloves and protecting one's face from cold air, can markedly reduce the frequency of symptomatic episodes. Patients with solar urticaria should be instructed on the use of combined ultraviolet B and ultraviolet A sunscreens and should be advised

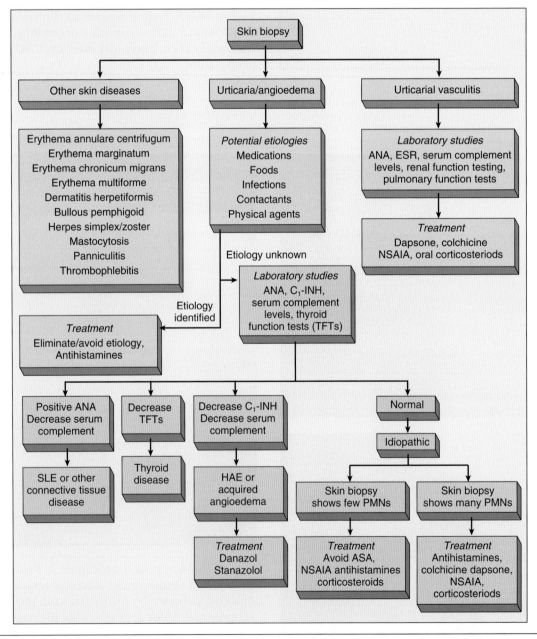

**Figure 18-15.** Algorithm for the diagnosis and treatment of chronic urticaria and angioedema. ANA, anti-nuclear antibody; C1, first component of complement; ESR, erythrocyte sedimentation rate; HAE, hereditary angioedema; C1 INH, C1 esterase inhibitor; NSAIA, nonsteroidal anti-inflammatory agent; PMN, polymorphonuclear neutrophils; SLE, systemic lupus erythematosus.

against direct sun exposure. In addition, a gradual increase in exposure to natural or artificial light may effectively induce tolerance to light in patients with solar urticaria. Chloroquine also may be effective in controlling some solar urticaria patients. Obviously, patients who have underlying infections or other systemic disorders should be treated with modalities directed specifically at these diseases.[23]

Unfortunately, in more than 75% of the patients with chronic urticaria or angioedema, no etiologic factors can be identified. Nevertheless, because of the pruritus and undesirable cosmetic features associated with these skin eruptions, some form of therapy is usually necessary. In the following sections, a rational, although empiric, approach to the treatment of chronic urticaria or angioedema is presented.

## AVOIDANCE OF ASPIRIN AND NONSTEROIDAL ANTI-INFLAMMATORY AGENTS

Some patients with chronic urticaria and angioedema may experience an exacerbation of their clinical symptoms on ingestion of aspirin and related drugs. Therefore, avoidance of aspirin and nonsteroidal anti-inflammatory agents is recommended empirically. In those cases in which aspirin sensitivity is evident, patients should also avoid exposure to azo dyes and benzoates.

## ANTIHISTAMINES

Because the cutaneous mast cell and its released mediators play a central role in urticarial reactions, therapy directed at blocking the effects of mast cell–derived histamine is indicated as first-line therapy. Histamine receptor 1 ($H_1$) antagonists, both first- and second-generation antihistamines, have proven to be effective in controlling many, but not all, cases of urticaria. Although most first-generation $H_1$ antihistamines have similar properties, individual patients may note a superior therapeutic response to one class or one particular agent, such as dyphenhydramine or hydroxyzine. Cyproheptadine has been suggested to be more effective than other $H_1$ antagonists in controlling cases of cholinergic urticaria. In some instances, a combination of two different $H_1$ antihistamines may prove to be superior to either alone.[24] In this latter case, it is recommended that agents representing two different classes of $H_1$ antagonists be employed for maximal therapeutic benefit. The second-generation, less-sedating antihistamines, fexofenadine, loratadine, and desloratadine, as well as ceterizine, appear to be as effective as other $H_1$ antagonists in controlling lesions of chronic urticaria, and because of their longer half-life, require less-frequent dosing. Because histamine mediates its effects through both $H_1$ and histamine receptor 2 ($H_2$), $H_2$ antagonists such as cimetidine and ranitidine have been used in combination with $H_1$ antihistamines in the management of chronic urticaria.[24,25] Although the efficacy of this combination remains in question, the addition of an $H_2$ antagonist to an $H_1$ antihistamine may be worthwhile in selected patients who are unresponsive to $H_1$ treatment alone.

## TRICYCLIC ANTIDEPRESSANTS

If chronic urticaria is unresponsive to $H_1$ antihistamine therapy, the use of tricyclic antidepressant agents, which are known to be potent $H_1$ antagonists, may be considered. Doxepin, a heterocyclic variation of amitriptyline, has been demonstrated in vitro to be nearly 800-fold more active at the $H_1$ receptor site on a molar basis than the $H_1$ antagonist diphenhydramine and has been useful in treating acute and chronic urticaria.[26] Doxepin has been reported in a double-blind study to be superior to hydroxyzine and cyproheptadine in the treatment of cold-induced urticaria.

## ADRENERGIC AGENTS

The use of intramuscular epinephrine by injection may be helpful for the treatment of acute urticaria and angioedema. Because the clinical effects of this medication last only a few hours, it is imperative that the patient also be treated with another medication, such as an $H_1$ antihistamine. Oral terbutaline and ephedrine also may be beneficial for the control of urticaria and angioedema in some patients when combined with antihistamine therapy.

## SYSTEMIC CORTICOSTEROIDS

The use of systemic corticosteroids is sometimes indicated in patients experiencing acute urticarial reactions, especially if associated with extensive angioedema or anaphylaxis. Corticosteroids may also be effective in controlling severe exacerbations in patients with idiopathic chronic urticaria. However, they are to be avoided on a long-term basis in the management of cases of chronic urticaria. In general, only a 3- to 5-day course of corticosteroids should be employed while introducing an alternative treatment regimen. An exception to this statement pertains to the treatment of patients with urticarial vasculitis or the angioedema-eosinophilia syndrome, who may require daily or alternate-day systemic steroid therapy.

## OTHER TREATMENTS

Thyroxine has been reported to be effective in treating cases of hypothyroid and euthyroid chronic urticaria in which there is evidence of circulating antithyroid antibodies. The calcium channel blocker nifedipine has been reported effective in the treatment of chronic urticaria when combined with $H_1$ antihistamines. Colchicine and dapsone in combination with $H_1$ antihistamines have proven effective for controlling polymorphonuclear predominant urticaria cases. A subset of these patients may be poorly responsive to combination therapy and require treatment with cyclosporine A and/or plasmapheresis to control their symptoms.[27]

# CONCLUSIONS

Urticaria and angioedema represent cutaneous reaction patterns for which multiple etiologic factors have been identified. Initial evaluation of patients with urticaria or angioedema should focus on a thorough history and physical examination. When the cutaneous diagnosis is in question, a skin biopsy should be performed. Additional diagnostic testing is dictated by the information gained from the initial patient examination. Treatment of urticaria and angioedema is directed toward eliminating the etiologic agents when possible. In instances where such factors cannot be identified or eliminated, empiric therapy should include the avoidance of aspirin and related drugs and the use of $H_1$ (and possibly $H_2$) antagonists. Initially, oral corticosteroids for several days may be necessary to control patient symptoms, but these should not be used chronically. As our understanding of the forces responsible for the expression of urticaria or angioedema improve, more effective approaches to treatment should emerge.

# REFERENCES

1. Swinny B: The atopic factor in urticaria. Southern Med J 1941;24:855.
2. Champion RH, Roberts SO, Carpenter RG, Roger JH: Urticaria and angioedema. A review of 554 patients. Br J Dermatol 1969;81:588–597.
3. Tharp MD, Levine MI, Fireman P: Urticaria. In Fireman P, Slavin R (eds): Atlas of Allergies. Vol. 16. New York, Gower Medical Publishing, 1990, pp 2–15.
4. Sabroe RA, Francis DM, Barr RM, et al: Anti-Fc(espsilon)RI auto antibodies and basophis histamine releasability in chronic idiopathic urticaria. J Allergy Clin Immunol 1998;102(4, pt 1):651–658.
5. Fiebiger E, Hammerschmid F, Stingl G, Maurer D: Anti-FceRIa autoantibodies in autoimmune-mediated disorders. Identification of a structure-function relationship. J Clin Invest 1998;101:243–251.
6. Kaplan A: Urticaria and angioedema. In Middleton's Allergy Principles and Practice 6th edition vol. 2. Philadelphia, Mosby, 2003, pp 1552–1553.
7. Leznoff A, Sussman GL: Syndrome of idiopathic chronic urticaria and angioedema with thyroid autoimmunity: A study of 90 patients. J Allergy Clin Immunol 1989;84:66–71.
8. Leznoff A, Josse RG, Denburg J, Dolovich J: Association of chronic urticaria and angioedema with thyroid autoimmunity. Arch Dermatol 1983;119(8):636–640.
9. Jones RR, Bhogal B, Dash A, Schifferli J: Urticaria and vasculitis: A continuum of histological and immuno-pathological changes. Br J Dermatol 1983;108(6):695–703.
10. Kaplan AP: Chemokines, chemokine receptors, and allergy. Int Arch Allergy Immunol 2001;124:423.
11. Zavadak D, Tharp MD: Chronic urticaria as a manifestation of the late phase reaction. Immunol Allergy Clin North Am 1995;15:745–759.
12. Foreman JC: Neuropeptides and the pathogenesis of allergy. Allergy 1987;42:1–11.
13. Cooper KD: Urticaria and angioedema: Diagnosis and evaluation. J Am Acad Dermatol 1991;25:166–176.
14. Yancey KB, Hall RP, Lawley TJ: Pruritic urticarial papules and plaques of pregnancy. Clinical experience in twenty-five patients. J Am Acad Dermatol 1984;10(3):473–480.
15. Monroe EW, Schulz CI, Maize JC, Jordon RE: Vasculitis in chronic urticaria. An immunopathologic study. J Invest Dermatol 1981;76:103–107.
16. Becker LC: Allergy in systemic lupus erythematosus. Johns Hopkins Med J 1973;133:38–44.
17. Soter N: The skin in mastocytosis. J Invest Dermatol 1991;96:325–395.
18. Muckle TJ, Wells M: Urticaria, deafness, and amyloidosis: A new heredofamilial syndrome. Q J Med 1962;31:235–248.
19. Janier M, Bonvalet D, Blanc MF, et al: Chronic urticaria and macroglobulinemia (Schnitzler's syndrome): Report of two cases. J Am Acad Dermatol 1989;20(2, pt 1):206–211.
20. Hadi SM, Barnetson RS, Gawkrodger DJ, et al: Clinical, histological and immunological studies in 50 patients with bullous pemphigoid. Dermatologica 1988;176(1):6–17.
21. Donaldson VH, Evans RR: A biochemical abnormality in hereditary angioneurotic edema. Am J Med 1963;35–37.
22. Markovic SN, Inwards DJ, Frigas EA, Payliky RP: Acquired C1 esterase inhibitor deficiency. Ann Intern Med 2000;132:144–150.
23. Kennard CD, Ellis CN: Pharmacologic therapy for urticaria. J Am Acad Dermatol 1991;25:176–187.
24. Monroe EW, Cohen SH, Kalbfleisch J, Schulz CI: Combined $H_1$ and $H_2$ antihistamine therapy in chronic urticaria. Arch Dermatol 1981;117:404–407.
25. Phanuphak P, Schucket A, Kohler PF: Treatment of chronic idiopathic urticaria with combined $H_1$ and $H_2$ blockers. Clin Allergy 1978;8:429–433.
26. Bernstein JE: Effect of doxepin hydrochloride an acute and chronic urticaria. J Invest Dermatol 1982;78:353.
27. Grattan CE, Francis DM, Slater NG, et al: Plasmapheresis for severe, unremitting, chronic urticaria. Lancet 1992;339(8801):1078–1080.

*Thomas A. Medsger, Jr., and Tharaknath Rao*

# *19* Rheumatologic Diseases

In this chapter, we describe the six most common "connective tissue diseases" (Fig. 19-1). These condition have a number of features in common, and in each condition demonstrated immunologic abnormalities and immune mechanisms are believed to participate in disease pathogenesis.

## RHEUMATOID ARTHRITIS

Rheumatoid arthritis (RA) is a systemic, chronic inflammatory disease characterized by symmetric polyarthritis often leading to progressive joint damage and deformity.[1]

### *EPIDEMIOLOGY*

Rheumatoid arthritis has a worldwide distribution and affects twice as many women as men. Peak onset occurs between the 4th and 6th decades. Prevalence estimates in North America range from 0.3% to 1.5%, and rates as high as 6% have been described in some Native American populations. Absence of identifiable disease clustering in space or time and the failure to identify infectious or environmental associations supports a role for genetic factors in disease causation. A strong tendency to familial aggregation, significantly increased concordance among monozygotic twins (12% to 15%) versus dizygotic twins (4%), and greater prevalence in certain inbred populations (e.g., the Pima and Chippewa Native Americans) supports involvement of susceptibility genes. The presence of human leukocyte antigen (HLA)-DR4 alleles, particularly the DRB1 subtype alleles *0401 and *0404, is recognized to be associated with both increased disease severity and radiographic damage.

### *PATHOGENESIS*

The synovium is the primary site for immune activation and inflammation in RA.[2] The earliest recognizable changes are edema and fibrin exudation, resulting from microvascular damage, hyperplasia of the superficial lining layer, and infiltration with lymphocytes and macrophages. T-lymphocytes predominate over B cells, with the majority belonging to the memory phenotype. Plasma cells are frequently encountered in the more advanced stages of inflammation. Characteristic events in the synovial sublining layer include (1) endothelial activation and adhesion molecule expression, (2) neoangiogenesis with the formation of high endothelial venules suited to providing oxygen and nutrition and facilitating leukocyte egress, and (3) tissue fibrosis. The destructive phase that is responsible for cartilage and bone damage is driven by the formation of a histologically distinct, locally invasive mass of synovial tissue known as pannus (Fig. 19-2). Soluble factors (chemokines and cytokines) play a central role in disease pathogenesis at all stages of inflammation.[3] Tumor necrosis factor-α, interleukin (IL)-1, IL-6, 1L-8, granulocyte-macrophate-colony stimulating factor, IL-12, IL-15 and IL-18 (monocyte and fibroblast derived), interferon-γ, IL-2, and IL-17 (T cell–derived) promote the inflammatory response, whereas IL-10 and IL-4 exhibit anti-inflammatory functions (Fig. 19-3).

Rheumatoid factors (RFs) are autoantibodies directed against antigenic determinants present on immunoglobulin (Ig) G Fc fragments and are found in the serum of about 80% of RA patients. RFs are also encountered in numerous other diseases (Table 19-1) and occasionally in healthy individuals. RFs in RA tend to be non–isotype specific (the most common isotype being

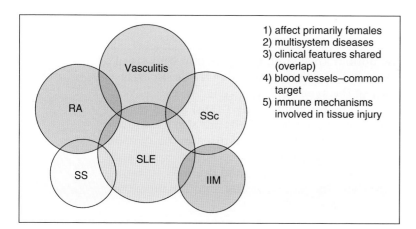

**Figure 19-1.** Diagrammatic representation of the connective tissue diseases. Vasculitis. IIM, idiopathic inflammatory myopathy; RA, rheumatoid arthritis; SLE, systemic lupus erythematosus; SS, Sjögren's syndrome; SSc, systemic sclerosis.

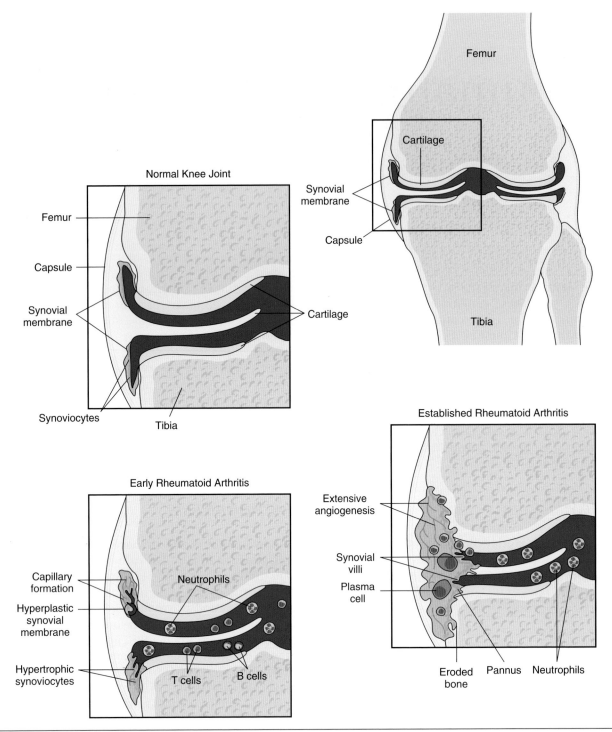

**Figure 19-2.** Pathogenesis of rheumatoid arthritis. In the normal knee joint, the synovium consists of a synovial membrane (usually one or two cells thick) and underlying loose connective tissue. In early rheumatoid arthritis, there is hyperplasia and hypertrophy of the synovial lining cells. An extensive network of new blood vessels is formed in the synovium. T cells (predominantly CD4+) and B cells (some of which become plasma cells) infiltrate the synovial membrane. These cells are also found in the synovial fluid, along with large numbers of neutrophils. In the early stages of disease, the synovial membrane begins to invade the cartilage. In established rheumatoid arthritis, the synovial membrane becomes transformed into inflammatory tissue, the pannus. This tissue invades and destroys adjacent cartilage and bone. (Modified from Choy EHS, Panayi GS: Cytokine pathways and joint inflammation in rheumatoid arthritis. N Engl J Med 2001;344(12):907–916; with permission.)

IgM) and exhibit both high affinity and specificity for human IgG. The IgG isotype is commonly encountered in patients with severe disease, and the IgA isotype appears to associate with extra-articular involvement.

Protein epitopes generated by citrullination or deamination of arginine residues have recently emerged as specific targets that are recognized by rheumatoid autoantibodies. Antiperinuclear factor, antikeratin antibodies, and anti-Sa autoantibodies belong to this class and collectively appear to exhibit both high sensitivity (40% to 70%) and specificity (92% to 99%) in RA.

## CLINICAL MANIFESTATIONS

Most patients experience insidious onset of joint pain and swelling associated with morning stiffness that mainly involves small

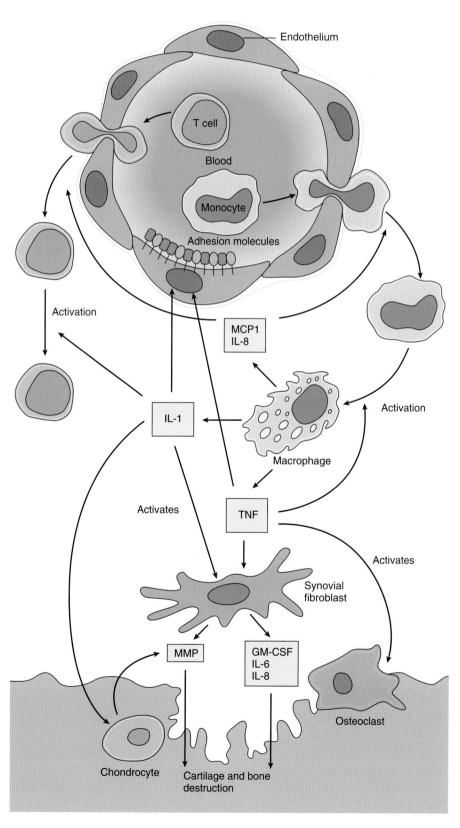

**Figure 19-3.** Soluble factors in pathogenesis of rheumatoid arthritis. Monocytes are attracted to rheumatoid joint, where they differentiate into macrophages and become activated. They secrete tumor necrosis factor (TNF) and interleukin (IL)-1. TNF increases expression of adhesion molecules on endothelial cells, which recruit more cells. Chemokines, such as monocyte chemotactic protein 1 (MCP 1) and IL-8, are secreted by macrophages and attract more cells into the joint. IL-1 and TNF induce synovial fibroblasts to express cytokines (such as IL-6), chemokines (such as IL-8), growth factors (such as granulocyte-macrophage colony-stimulating factor; GM-CSF), and matrix metalloproteinases (MMPs), which contribute to cartilage and bone destruction. TNF stimulates osteoclast activation and differentiation. Also, IL-1 mediates cartilage degradation directly by inducing the expression of MMPs by chondrocytes. (Modified from Pope RM: Apoptosis as a therapeutic tool in rheumatoid arthritis. Nat Rev Immunol 2002;2:527–535; with permission).

peripheral joints, particularly the metacarpophalangeal and proximal interphalangeal joints. Symmetric involvement becomes evident as the disease progresses.

The clinical course of RA varies from mild, often self-limited or episodic synovitis to life-threatening progressive multisystem disease. Older age at onset usually predicts more severe disease. Although synovitis generally follows a fluctuating pattern, structural damage progression occurs as a linear function of the amount of prior synovitis. More than 70% of patients display plain radiographic evidence of joint destruction within the first 2 years. Erosive change can be detected as early as 4 months after onset using more sensitive imaging modalities such as magnetic resonance imaging.

## Articular Features

Signs relating to synovitis, such as warmth and swelling, are best appreciated in superficial joints with distensible capsules. A decrease in the range of joint motion secondary to pain or distention with fluid is a frequent accompaniment. Prolonged subjective stiffness following an extended period of joint immobilization is a consistent feature in almost all types of inflammatory arthritis and tends to correlate well with the degree of synovial inflammation. This stiffness is most often experienced in the mornings and typically lasts longer than 1 hour.

The spectrum of structural damage in RA includes cartilage loss, focal erosions of marginal and subchondral bone, and juxta-articular osteoporosis.[4] The consequences are joint space narrowing (Fig. 19-4), painful joint deformities, joint instability, and increased fracture risk, all of which contribute to significant functional disability. Joint deformities arise from pannus-mediated bone and cartilage destruction, alterations (contracture, lengthening, or disruption) in supporting and stabilizing periarticular soft tissue structures (ligaments, tendons, and fibrous tissue), or as a consequence of joint contracture that accompanies prolonged voluntary joint immobilization as an attempt to minimize pain.

Cervical spine disease involves the spinal diarthrodal joints and manifests as neck stiffness accompanied by decreased movement. Cervical myelopathy can result from C1–C2 instability precipitated by erosion of the odontoid process or transverse cervical ligament laxity or rupture, possibly secondary to tenosynovitis of adjacent structures. Apophyseal joint arthritis can also contribute to neck instability.

Rheumatoid hand disease shows a predilection for the metacarpophalangeal and proximal interphalangeal joints and tends to spare the distal interphalangial joints. Metacarpophalangeal involvement leading to volar subluxation and ulnar deviation produces a characteristic abnormality (Fig. 19-5). The loss of collateral ligament support at the proximal interphalangeal joint predisposes to development of two classic deformities—the swan neck and the boutonnière deformity, characterized by proximal interphalangeal joint hyperextension and fixed flexion, respectively. Tenosynovitis of the finger flexor tendons is common; the affected fingers may lock painfully in flexion during use ("trigger finger"). Wrist involvement often presents as loss of active extension, leading to carpal supination-subluxation followed by volar and ulnar subluxation of the carpus, sometimes accompanied by wrist collapse. Entrapment neuropathies of the median and ulnar nerves at the wrist can occur secondary to synovitis and swelling.

Knee synovitis and resultant effusion can result in the formation of a popliteal (Baker's) cyst. This fluid-filled cyst usually arises from the posteromedial aspect of the joint capsule and enlarges as a result of an internal ball-valve mechanism that prevents decompression. Symptoms can occur from pressure effects, especially with knee flexion, inflammation within the cyst, or rupture of the cyst into the calf, producing signs that mimic thrombophlebitis (Fig. 19-6).

Foot and ankle disease characteristically affects the metatarsophalangeal, talonavicular, and subtalar joints. Metatarsophalangeal involvement leads to metatarsal head subluxation with "cock up" deformities of the toes, a common cause of painful gait in RA.

---

**TABLE 19-1**
**Diseases Commonly Associated with Rheumatoid Factor**

| Category | Diseases |
| --- | --- |
| Rheumatic diseases | Rheumatoid arthritis, systemic lupus erythematosus, systemic sclerosis, mixed connective tissue disease, Sjögren's syndrome |
| Viral infections | AIDS, mononucleosis, hepatitis, influenza, and many others; after vaccination (may yield falsely elevated titers of antiviral antibodies) |
| Parasitic infections | Trypanosomiasis, kala-azar, malaria, schistosomiasis, filariasis, and others |
| Chronic bacterial infections | Tuberculosis, leprosy, yaws, syphilis, brucellosis, subacute bacterial endocarditis, salmonellosis |
| Neoplasms | After irradiation or chemotherapy |
| Other hyperglobulinemic states | Hypergammaglobulinemic purpura, cryoglobulinemia, chronic liver disease, sarcoidosis, other chronic pulmonary diseases |

From Carson DA: Rheumatoid factor. In Kelley WN, Harris ED Jr., Ruddy S, et al (eds): Textbook of Rheumatology, 4th ed. Vol. 1. Philadelphia, WB Saunders, 1993, p 155; with permission.

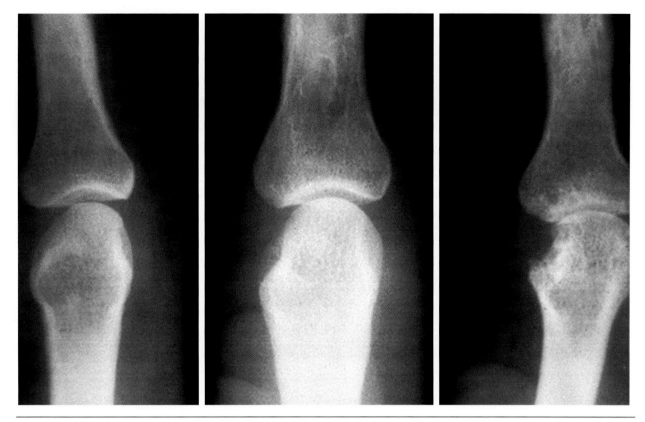

**Figure 19-4.** Progressive metacarpophalangeal joint radiographic changes in rheumatoid arthritis. *A,* soft tissue swelling. *B,* Minimal joint space narrowing. *C,* Joint space narrowing and marginal erosion. (From 1972–1999 American College of Rheumatology Clinical Slide Collection; with permission.)

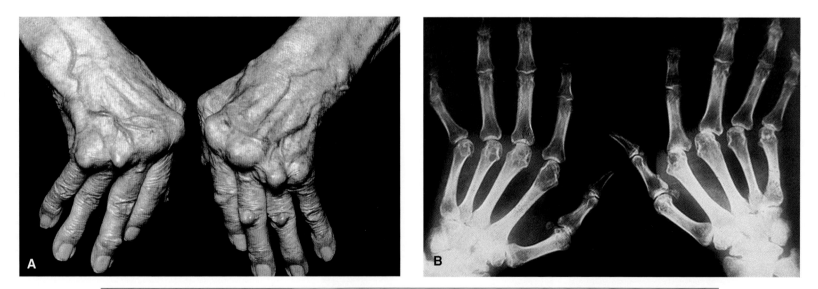

**Figure 19-5.** Chronic clinical and radiographic changes in the hands in rheumatoid arthritis. *Left,* Ulnar deviation, metacarpophalangeal joint subluxation, intrinsic muscle atrophy, and rheumatoid nodules. *Right,* Marked narrowing, subluxation, and ulnar deviation involving the metacarpophalangeal joints. The proximal interphalangeal joints and carpal spaces are also narrowed, and carpal and ulnar styloid erosions are present. (From 1972–1999 American College of Rheumatology Clinical Slide Collection; with permission.)

Talonavicular and subtalar joint involvement result in pronation and eversion foot deformities and flat foot formation. Posterior tibial nerve compression in the tarsal tunnel from synovitis results in paresthesias involving the sole, further interfering with ambulation.

## Extra-articular Features

Rheumatoid arthritis can affect many organ systems and lead to a variety of extra-articular manifestations (Table 19-2).[4] In most instances, this involvement can be traced to circulating RF and formation of intravascular complement-fixing immune complexes. In general, the extent and severity of extra-articular involvement correlates with articular disease duration and severity.

Rheumatoid nodules are subcutaneous nodules of varying consistency that appear over extensor surfaces such as the olecranon process and the proximal ulna and occur in 20% to 35% of patients with definite RA (Fig. 19-7). Patients with rheumatoid nodules are almost always circulating RF positive, and nodules are rare in the absence of obvious arthritis. The inciting event for nodule formation is believed to be vasculitis. Histologically, the mature rheumatoid nodule demonstrates a central area of fibrinoid necrosis surrounded by a corona of palisading fibroblasts and histiocytes that in turn is enclosed in a collagenous capsule. Nodules can also occur at sites other than skin, such as the heart, lungs, bone, sclera, larynx, and central nervous system, occasionally producing clinical consequences (Fig. 19-8).

Vasculitis of small blood vessels is a crucial event in the development of synovitis. Overt vasculitis can also occur in patients with severe RF-positive, erosive, nodular disease, with a greater tendency to affect men over women. Manifestations can include digital vasculitis, cutaneous vasculitis producing palpable purpura

**TABLE 19-2**
**Extra-articular Involvement in Rheumatoid Arthritis**

| Organ System | Involvement |
|---|---|
| Skin | Rheumatoid nodules, vasculitis |
| Ocular | Keratoconjunctivitis sicca, iritis, episcleritis |
| Oral | Salivary gland inflammation (sicca symptoms) |
| Respiratory | Pulmonary fibrosis, pleural effusion, cricoarytenoid inflammation |
| Cardiac | Pericardial inflammation, valvular nodule formation, myocarditis |
| Neurologic | Mononeuritis, nerve entrapment, cervical instability |
| Hepatic | Increased aminotransferase concentrations |
| Hematologic | Anaemia, thrombocytosis, leucocytosis, lymphadenopathy |
| | Felty's syndrome: Splenomegaly, thrombocytopenia |
| Vascular | Vasculitis |

Reproduced from Lee DM, Weinblatt ME: Rheumatoid arthritis. Lancet 2001;358:903–911.

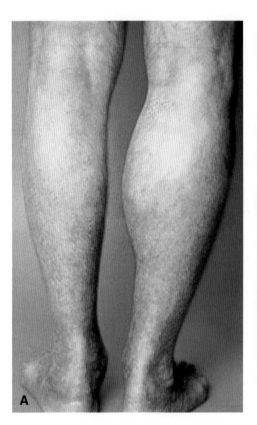
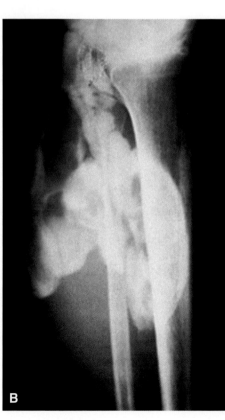

**Figure 19-6.** A popliteal (Baker's) cyst in rheumatoid arthritis. *Left,* Pronounced swelling in the posteromedial calf. *Right,* Arthrogram showing cyst extending into the gastrocnemio-semimembranosus bursa with extension and/or rupture distally into the calf. (From 1972–1999 American College of Rheumatology Clinical Slide Collection; with permission.)

and skin ulcerations, visceral involvement and ischemic peripheral neuropathy. Vascular immune complex deposition, frequently reflected by circulating complement component depletion, underlies the vessel wall inflammation. The histologic picture is characterized by panarterial inflammation leading to fibrinoid necrosis, luminal thrombus formation, and obliterative endarteritis. Rheumatoid vasculitis spares the central nervous system and the kidney.

Pulmonary disease in RA can involve both the upper and lower respiratory tract. The spectrum of lower respiratory involvement includes pleuritis, parenchymal involvement in the form of interstitial fibrosis and nodular lung disease, bronchiolitis, and pulmonary arteritis leading to pulmonary hypertension and small airways disease. Pulmonary nodules in RA patients tend to occur singly or in clusters that coalesce; they can cavitate, leading to bronchopleural fistula formation.

Cardiac involvement in RA can result from myocardial or endocardial (heart valve) granuloma formation or vasculitis. Consequences of granuloma formation can include myocarditis, valvular incompetence, or conduction defects. Pericarditis is common in RF-positive patients and often leads to exudative, fibrinous pericardial effusions.

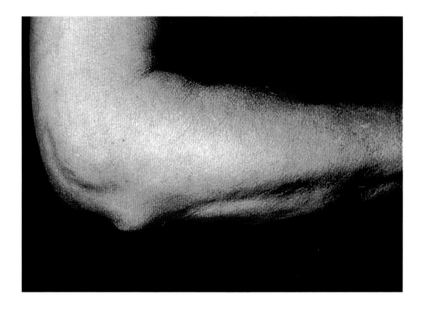

**Figure 19-7.** Subcutaneous nodule over olecranon in rheumatoid arthritis. (From 1972–1999 American College of Rheumatology Clinical Slide Collection; with permission.)

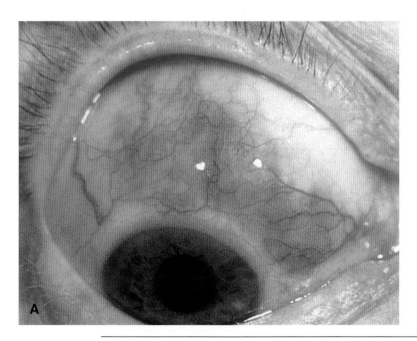
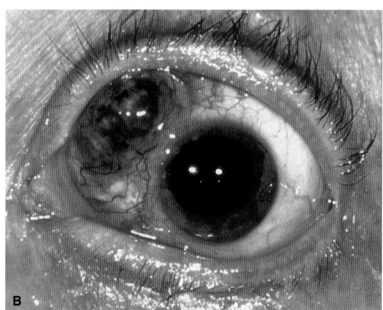

**Figure 19-8.** Scleromalacia leading to scleromalacia perforans and herniation in rheumatoid arthritis. *Left*, Rheumatoid nodule formation in the sclera. *Right*, Marked scleral thinning leading to herniation of the darker pigmented uveal tissue. (From 1972–1999 American College of Rheumatology Clinical Slide Collection; used with permission.)

## DIAGNOSIS AND TREATMENT

Rheumatoid arthritis is a pleomorphic disease with wide variability in disease expression. The 1987 American College of Rheumatology criteria (Table 19-3) serve as a frame of reference for diagnosis. The adoption of validated clinical outcome measurements for assessing disease activity and therapeutic outcomes represents a key advance in RA management. The ultimate goals in managing RA include pain reduction, joint damage prevention, and limitation of disability. An evolving understanding of the pathogenesis of joint damage in RA underlies the growing recent emphasis on early diagnosis and timely intervention. This has led to the earlier "therapeutic pyramid" approach, which advocated initial conservative management with nonsteroidal anti-inflammatory drugs until definitive evidence of erosive damage became manifest, being supplanted by a more aggressive treatment approach involving earlier disease-modifying antirheumatic drug introduction to prevent subsequent damage.[5]

Nonsteroidal anti-inflammatory drugs, intra-articular glucocorticoid injections and low-dose oral corticosteroids are commonly used for symptomatic disease control. Current guidelines encourage the initiation of disease-modifying antirheumatic drugs within the first 3 months of diagnosis in most patients (Fig. 19-9).[6] Disease-modifying antirheumatic drug initiation can involve a "step-up" approach with initial monotherapy followed by the addition of other agents depending on the therapeutic response; alternatively, it can utilize a combination regimen at the outset with "step-down" elimination as disease control improves (see Fig. 19-9). Periodic laboratory assessments for toxicity, depending on the specific type of disease-modifying antirheumatic drug therapy selected, are required. Regular radiographic evaluation for structural damage during the course of treatment is also recommended to monitor the adequacy of intervention. An improved understanding of the key role played by the proinflammatory cytokines tumor necrosis factor-α and IL-1 in disease pathogenesis has led to the development of genetically engineered biologic agents directed at selectively blocking these mediators.[7,8] To date, the tumor necrosis factor-α antagonists (Etanercept, Infliximab, and Adalimumab) have demonstrated the greatest clinical efficacy in addition to a definite positive impact on structural preservation and physical functioning. Importantly, effective management of RA also includes patient education and introduction of nonpharmacologic modalities such as physical and occupational therapy early in the course of disease, as these have been shown to translate into improved patient outcomes.

# SYSTEMIC LUPUS ERYTHEMATOSUS

Systemic lupus erythematosus (SLE, or lupus) is a chronic relapsing multisystem disorder that manifests clinically with a diverse array of both constitutional and organ-related symptoms and findings ranging in severity from trivial to life threatening.[9]

## EPIDEMIOLOGY

Lupus predominantly affects young women in their reproductive years (ages 15 to 45). The overall female-to-male ratio is 6 to

---

**TABLE 19-3**
**American College of Rheumatology Classification Criteria for Rheumatoid Arthritis***

| Criterion | Definition |
| --- | --- |
| Morning stiffness | Morning stiffness in and around the joints lasting at least 1 hr before maximal improvement |
| Arthritis of three or more joint areas | At least three joint areas simultaneously having soft tissue swelling or fluid (not bony overgrowth alone) observed by a physician (the 14 possible joint areas are [right or left] PIP, MCP, wrist, elbow, knee, ankle, and MTP joints) |
| Arthritis of hand joints | At least one joint area swollen as above in wrist, MCP, or PIP joint |
| Symmetric arthritis | Simultaneous involvement of the same joint areas (as in criterion 2) on both sides of the body (bilateral involvement of PIP, MCP, or MTP joints is acceptable without absolute symmetry) |
| Rheumatoid nodules | Subcutaneous nodules over bony prominences or extensor surfaces, or in juxta-articular regions, observed by a physician |
| Serum rheumatoid factor | Demonstration of abnormal amounts of serum "rheumatoid factor" by any method that has been positive in less than 5% of healthy control subjects |
| Radiographic changes | Changes typical of RA on PA hand and wrist radiographs, which must include erosions or unequivocal bony decalcification localized to or most marked adjacent to the involved joints (osteoarthritis changes alone do not qualify) |

MCP, metacarpophalangeal; MTP, metatarsophalangeal; PA, posteroanterior; PIP, proximal interphalangeal; RA, rheumatoid arthritis.
*For classification purposes, a patient is said to have rheumatoid arthritis if he or she has satisfied at least four of the seven criteria. Criteria 1 through 4 must be present for at least 6 weeks.
From Arnett FC, Edworthy SM, Bloch DA, et al: The American Rheumatism Association 1987 revised criteria for the classification of rheumatoid arthritis. Arthritis Rheum 1988;31:315–324; with permission.

10:1 but is lower (2:1) in childhood and advanced years. The worldwide prevalence of SLE is estimated at 10 to 60 per 100,000 individuals, and reports indicate more than a tripling of incidence during the past 4 decades. A two- to fourfold higher incidence is noted in African-Caribbean, Asian, and Native American women compared with white women.

A strong tendency for familial aggregation, significantly increased disease risk among first-degree relatives of patients, and 10-fold higher concordance in monozygotic versus dizygotic twin pairs all suggest a central role for genetic factors in pathogenesis. Also, SLE clusters with other autoimmune conditions (e.g., thyroiditis, hemolytic anemia, and idiopathic thrombocytopenic purpura) within extended families. On the other hand, the observed discordance for clinical SLE within most monozygotic twin pairs and overall predominant sporadic occurrence of the disease imply a role for environmental factors, several of which have been proposed as disease inducers/ propagators, including ultraviolet B light, sex hormones, and exposure to certain medications.

## PATHOGENESIS

Lupus is believed to occur because of the overproduction of pathogenic antibodies.[10] Serum autoantibodies directed against nuclear antigens (antinuclear antibodies, ANA) develop in more than 95% of patients (Fig. 19-10). These autoantibodies bind to DNA, RNA, protein, and nucleoprotein antigens present within nuclei as components of large protein–nucleic acid complexes (e.g., nucleosomes). Specificities include antibodies to double-stranded DNA, the Smith antigen, ribonucleoprotein, Sjögren's syndrome antigen A (SSA) or (Ro), Sjögren's syndrome antigen B (SSB) or (La), and others. Accumulating evidence points to these

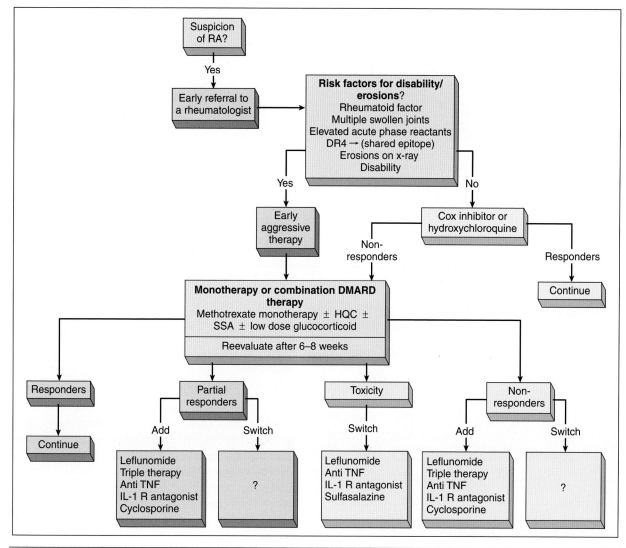

**Figure 19-9.** Decision model for treating patients with rheumatoid arthritis (RA). Assessment of prognostic indicators and prompt initiation of disease-modifying antirheumatic drug (DMARD) therapy are important to maximize the chance for an improved outcome. *Question marks* denote that clinical data are insufficient to support recommendation, but agents listed under "Add" may be used when medications need to be switched. CCP, cyclic citrullinated peptide; HQC, hydroxychloroquine; IL, interleukin; SSA, sulfasalazine; TNF, tumor necrosis factor. (Modified from Goldbach-Mansky R, Lipsky PE: New concepts in the treatment of rheumatoid arthritis. Ann Rev Med 2003;54:197–216; with permission.)

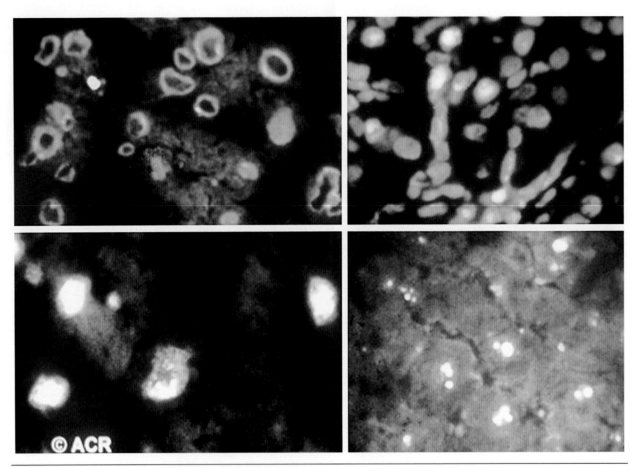

**Figure 19-10.** Antinuclear antibodies, composite (photomicrographs). In clockwise order from top left, the peripheral, diffuse, nucleolar, and speckled immunofluorescence patterns. (From 1972–1999 American College of Rheumatology Clinical Slide Collection; with permission.)

---

**BOX 19-1**
## Immune Abnormalities in Systemic Lupus Erythematosus

### Hyperactivated B Cells
Number of activated B cells producing Ig increased in peripheral blood

B-cell abnormalities are present in unaffected family members and may precede SLE development

Lupus B cells are more prone to polyclonal activation by specific antigens

Raised IL-6 and IL-10 concentrations may promote B-cell hyperactivity

B-cell responses to activating signals are abnormal

### Hyperactivated T Cells
Number of activted T cells increased in peripheral blood

Abnormal early events of T-cell activation

T-cell function skewed toward B-cell help and Ig production

Lupus T cells produce little IL-2 on stimulation

### Abnormal Phagocytic Functions
Phagocytic cells cannot bind or process immune complexes efficiently

Phagocytosis of apoptotic cells impaired

### Abnormal Immunoregulation
Defective clearance of immune complexes and apoptotic materials because of qualitative or quantitative defects of early complement proteins (C2, C4, C1q), Fcγ, CR1, and C1q receptors on cell surfaces

Suppressive activity of suppressor T cells and NK cells on activated T- and B-cell network is inadequate

Idiotypic control of antibody production is dysregulated

Ig, immunoglobulin; IL, interleukin; NK, natural killer; SLE, systemic lupus erythematosus.
Reproduced from Mok CC, Lau CS: Pathogenesis of systemic lupus erythematosus. J Clin Pathol 2003;56:481–490; with permission.

nucleoprotein complexes, rather than their individual components, as the actual targets that drive autoreactivity.

Potential mechanisms that are proposed to explain auto-immunity in SLE include immune dysregulation, abnormal B and helper T cell hyperactivation, accelerated apoptosis resulting in expression of the putative intracellular autoantigens on cell surface blebs, and inadequate clearing of apoptotic cells and immune complexes from the circulation secondary to deficiencies in the early components of complement (Box 19-1). Disease susceptibility and clinical expression are determined by complex interactions involving genetic and environmental factors, including sex and hormonal milieu (Fig. 19-11).

Although highly sensitive for establishing SLE diagnosis, ANA can occur in a variety of other diseases and also sporadically in healthy elderly adults. Antibodies directed against double stranded DNA and Smith antigen, a small nuclear ribonucleoprotein, appear to be unique for SLE. Serum anti–double stranded DNA antibody levels vary over time and tend to correlate with disease activity.

## CLINICAL MANIFESTATIONS

Clinical features of SLE arise from a combination of autoantibody or immune complex–mediated direct tissue injury and consequences of blood vessel inflammation (ischemia, hemorrhage) caused by the vascular deposition of complement fixing immune complexes. Vascular events can range from bland vasculopathy to frank vasculitis.[11]

### Mucocutaneous Involvement

Mucocutaneous involvement in SLE is extremely common. Skin manifestations, in addition to aiding with diagnosis, often provide an excellent window for assessing disease activity per se. The frequently photosensitive, butterfly-shaped malar rash occurs in 30% to 60% of patients and exhibits the strongest association with SLE (Fig. 19-12). The superficial, nonscarring, annular lesions of subacute cutaneous lupus are associated with the presence of circulating anti-Ro (SSA) autoantibodies and often involve

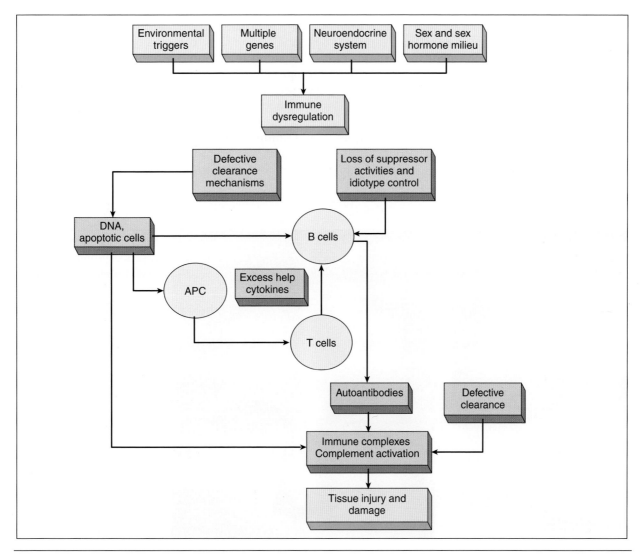

**Figure 19-11.** The pathogenesis of systemic lupus erythematosus. APC, antigen-presenting cells. (Reproduced from Mok CC, Lau CS: Pathogenesis of systemic lupus erythematosus. J Clin Pathol 2003;56:481–490; with permission.)

sun-exposed areas of skin (Fig. 19-13). Discoid lupus occurs in 15% to 30% of SLE patients and has the worst impact on skin, resulting in circumscribed scaly plaque-like lesions and scarring. Alopecia may be diffuse or patchy, reversible or permanent, especially when it is secondary to scarring discoid scalp lesions. Mucosal lesions can affect the nose, anogenital area, and, most commonly, mouth. Oral ulcers in SLE are typically painless and commonly involve the hard palate. Skin manifestations attributable to vascular involvement include livedo reticularis, palpable purpura, digital or nailfold ulcers, periungual erythema, and urticaria. Photosensitivity is a recurring feature in several different forms of cutaneous lupus and likely reflects the propensity of ultraviolet light to augment apoptosis in exposed dermal-epidermal elements and consequently activate regional inflammatory pathways.

## Musculoskeletal Involvement

Nonerosive and nondeforming arthritis may involve both large and small extremity joints and frequently presents as migratory arthralgia with minimal or no swelling. A more unusual nonerosive variant termed *Jaccoud's arthropathy* leads to reducible rheumatoid-like joint changes, producing ulnar deviation at the metacarpophalangeal joints. Deformity also results from involvement of para-articular soft tissues such as joint capsules, ligaments, and tendons. Soft tissue involvement in the form of tenosynovitis and bursitis is common.

## Hematologic Involvement

Although common, lupus-related hematologic abnormalities rarely constitute the presenting feature. Anemia of chronic disease occurs more commonly than Coombs-positive hemolytic anemia.

The latter is characterized by antibody-mediated cell lysis. Leukopenia occurs in more than 50% of patients secondary to circulating lymphocyte depletion and, in the absence of concurrent immunosuppressive therapy, indicates ongoing immunologic activity. Thrombocytopenia is common, especially in association with the antiphospholipid syndrome. Fulminant thrombotic thrombocytopenic purpura is a rare but serious complication.

## Renal Involvement

Renal involvement in lupus is frequent. With sensitive histologic techniques, abnormalities can be discerned in virtually all SLE renal biopsy specimens. Clinical indicators include proteinuria, cells and cellular casts in urine specimens, and reduced creatinine clearance. Histologically, immune complex deposition in the glomerular mesangium and subendothelial and subepithelial sides of the glomerular basement membrane is observed, along with reactive expansion of the mesangial cellular and matrix components, microvascular occlusion and necrosis, and, eventually, fibrosis. The World Health Organization classifies lupus nephritis into six classes based on the type and degree of glomerular involvement on biopsy. Type IV or diffuse proliferative glomerulonephritis carries the highest risk of progression to renal failure (Fig. 19-14) and is most consistently associated with deposition of Ig and complement components in the glomeruli (Fig. 19-15) and circulating anti–double-stranded DNA antibodies.[12] Other adverse prognostic markers include concomitant hypertension, decreased serum albumin, low serum complement levels, and absolute lymphopenia. Relapses or flares are common in lupus nephritis and occur in as many as one third of patients following cessation of immunosuppressive therapy. Renal involvement can also occur as a result of arterial and venous thrombosis associated with the presence of antiphospholipid antibodies.

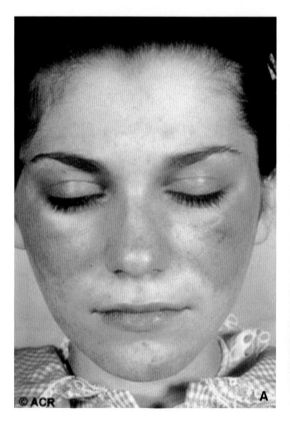 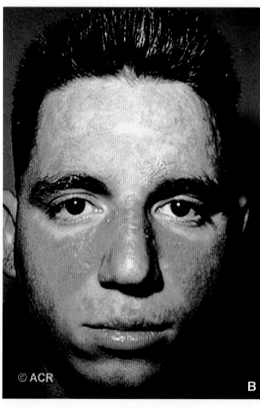

**Figure 19-12.** Facial rash of systemic lupus erythematosus. A confluent erythematous eruption over the bridge of the nose and cheeks creates the typical "butterfly" distribution. (From 1972–1999 American College of Rheumatology Clinical Slide Collection; with permission.)

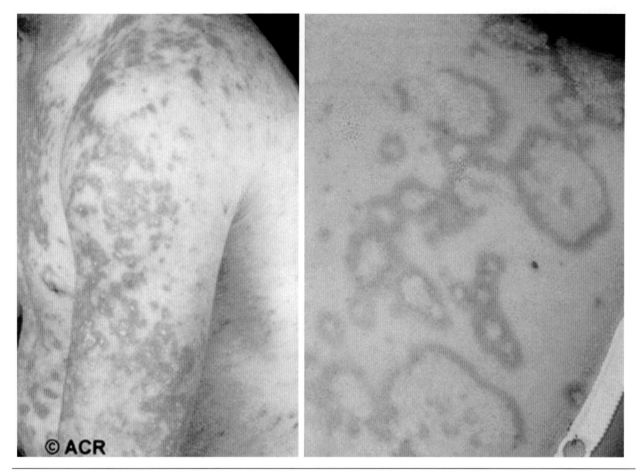

**Figure 19-13.** The rash of subacute cutaneous lupus erythematosus. *Left,* Papulosquamous lesions resembling psoriasis. *Right,* Annular polycyclic lesions with an erythematous border and central clearing. (From 1972–1999 American College of Rheumatology Clinical Slide Collection; with permission.)

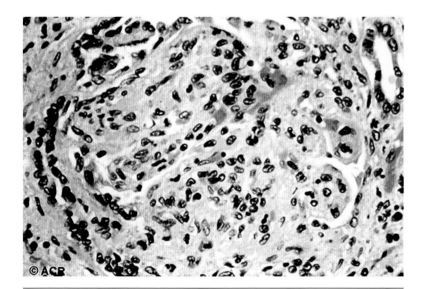

**Figure 19-14.** Photomicrograph of diffuse proliferative lupus glomerulonephritis. The architecture of the glomerulus is largely obliterated with marked hypercellularity and loss of capillary lumina. (From 1972–1999 American College of Rheumatology Clinical Slide Collection; with permission.)

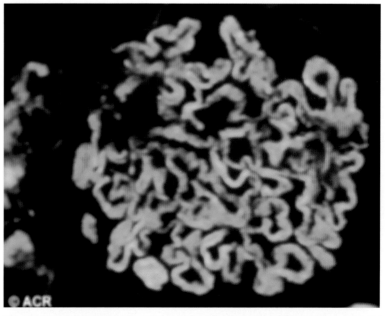

**Figure 19-15.** Glomerular immunoglobulin G deposition in lupus nephritis. The basement membrane is partly outlined by irregular "lumpy and bumpy" deposits of antigen-antibody complex, stained using fluorescein-conjugated rabbit antiserum against human immunoglobulin G. (From 1972–1999 American College of Rheumatology Clinical Slide Collection; with permission.)

## Cardiopulmonary Involvement

Lupus not infrequently involves the respiratory system, producing a wide array of clinical manifestations. Autoantibody/immune complex–mediated injury of the alveolar capillaries underlies two potentially life-threatening but uncommon complications—acute lupus pneumonitis and alveolar hemorrhage. Rarely, a more chronic process characterized by diffuse interstitial involvement progressing into fibrosis and restrictive lung disease occurs. Pleural disease presenting as pleuritis with chest pain or pleural effusion is common. Shrinking lung syndrome is a rare complication that is felt to arise from diaphragmatic muscle or phrenic nerve involvement. Pulmonary hypertension in SLE has a strong association with Raynaud's phenomenon and tends to be gradually progressive, closely resembling primary idiopathic pulmonary hypertension. Pulmonary embolism and pulmonary hypertension can result from pulmonary vascular occlusion in the setting of the antiphospholipid antibody syndrome.

Pericarditis occurs in approximately 25% of SLE patients, not infrequently causing a rapidly accumulating effusion that necessitates emergent intervention. Lupus-related valvulopathies include Libman-Sacks lesions and valve leaflet abnormalities arising from inflammation, fibrosis, or fibrinoid degeneration. Libman-Sacks lesions are sterile, verrucous, platelet-fibrin vegetations typically involving the mitral and aortic valves and frequently occurring in association with the antiphospholipid antibody syndrome. Primary myocardial involvement in SLE is uncommon and can present as congestive heart failure (CHF). Endothelial activation from circulating immune complexes is believed to be an important factor contributing to the premature occurrence of atherosclerosis in SLE—a complication that has been the focus of considerable recent attention.

## Neuropsychiatric Involvement

Neuropsychiatric manifestations occur in 15% to 75% of patients with SLE and can involve the central, peripheral, and autonomic nervous systems. Bland vasculopathy is the most frequent histologic finding, and true vasculitis of the central nervous system is decidedly rare (Fig. 19-16). Clinical manifestations include psychiatric syndromes, focal or generalized seizures, movement disorders (notably chorea), stroke syndromes, aseptic meningitis, myelopathy, transverse myelitis, and peripheral or cranial neuropathies.[13] Diffuse neurologic dysfunction can manifest as cognitive defects, including memory and attention deficits, as well as fluctuating acute confusional states. Cerebral thromboembolic events not uncommonly underlie stroke syndromes, especially in patients with antiphospholipid antibodies. The optic nerve represents the most common cranial nerve involved in SLE.

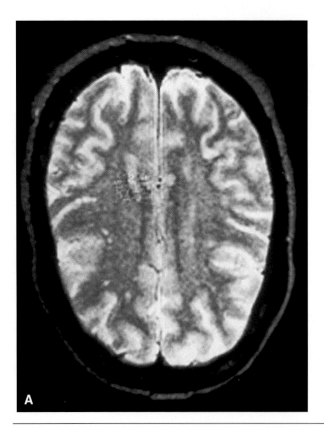
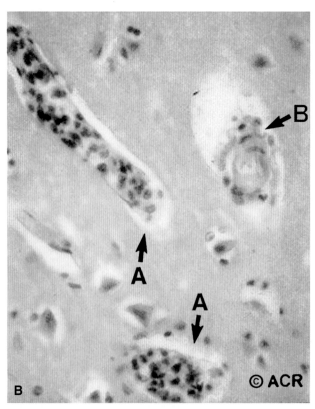

**Figure 19-16.** Magnetic resonance image of the brain in systemic lupus erythematosus.
*Left,* $T_2$-weighted axial image revealing numerous tiny punctate areas of increased signal *(white)* in the white matter of the cerebral hemispheres that represent microinfarcts or cerebral vasculitis.
*Right,* Photomicrograph showing small vessel occlusion by leukoaggregation *(A)* and a fibrin thrombus *(B)* without evidence of vasculitis. (From 1972–1999 American College of Rheumatology Clinical Slide Collection; with permission.)

## DIAGNOSIS

The diversity in clinical presentation and fluctuating disease course frequently make the diagnosis of lupus challenging. The presence of circulating ANA is a unifying laboratory abnormality and is detected in 97% of patients with SLE at some time during their illness. Numerous laboratory abnormalities can be associated with SLE; these are listed in Box 19-1. The American College of Rheumatology classification criteria, last revised in 1997, incorporate major clinical disease manifestations and relevant laboratory parameters and facilitate diagnosis and patient evaluation (see Table 19-4). Current guidelines require that at least 4 of the 11 criteria be present but not necessarily simultaneously. The detection of microscopic hematuria and cellular casts on microscopic urine analysis represents a powerful tool for diagnosing glomerulonephritis, and semiquantitative assessment offers a sensitive means of monitoring nephritis activity. Detection of these findings should prompt renal biopsy prior to initiating definitive treatment to distinguish active immune-mediated nephritis from chronic, irreversible injury.

Brain imaging is a key diagnostic modality in patients with neuropsychiatric SLE. Magnetic resonance imaging is preferred and not uncommonly reveals small, punctate white-matter lesions (Box 19-2). Less common findings may include cortical atrophy, periventricular white-matter changes, ventricular dilatation, diffuse white-matter abnormalities, and gross infarcts.

## MANAGEMENT

Preventative strategies in patients with SLE include avoidance of excessive sun exposure through the use of sunscreens and appropriate clothing, stress reduction, smoking cessation, screening for incipient atherosclerotic disease, aggressive management of hyperlipidemia with statins and low-dose aspirin, and renin-angiotensin pathway inhibition in patients with renal involvement.

Pharmacologic management of SLE is dictated by disease severity and the presence of treatable organ-threatening manifestations.[14] Cutaneous, musculoskeletal, and constitutional symptoms often respond well to treatment with antimalarial drugs (chloroquine, hydroxychloroquine, or quinacrine). Nonsteroidal anti-inflammatory drugs improve fever, musculoskeletal and serositis pain, and constitutional symptoms. Topical steroids, sunscreens, and special ultraviolet-retardant clothing help with skin rash. Non–organ threatening disease rarely calls for prednisone at doses greater than 15 mg/day. Serious lupus that threatens organ function is often managed with a 4- to 6-week course of high-dose oral prednisone (1 mg/kg/day or equivalent). Lung, central nervous system, and renal disease may additionally require monthly intravenous pulse cyclophosphamide (CYC) administration (750 mg/m$^2$/cycle). Once remission is achieved, "step down" to a less toxic drug to maintain immunosuppression is reasonable, thus minimizing cumulative CYC-associated toxicity. Methotrexate, azathioprine, mycophenolate mofetil, and leflunomide are some of the immunosuppressive agents that can be used in this situation, in addition to primary management of less-severe disease or for their steroid-sparing benefits. High-dose (pulse) steroids, such as Solumedrol 1000 mg administered intravenously daily for 1 to 3 days, are often used to jump-start immunosuppressive treatment when organ benefits is severely threatened. A variety of agents targeting specific inflammatory mediators or costimulatory pathways involved in inflammation are currently under evaluation.[15] Lastly, the recognition and management of reversible risk factors that lead to hypertension, premature cardiovascular disease, and osteoporosis, many of which relate to moderate- to high-dose corticosteroid use, deserve special attention.

# SYSTEMIC SCLEROSIS

Systemic sclerosis (SSc) is characterized by hardening or thickening (sclero-) of the skin (-derma), blood vessels, joints/tendons,

---

**TABLE 19-4**

**American College of Rheumatology 1997 Updated Criteria for Classification of Systemic Lupus Erythematosus***

| Type of Criteria | Criteria |
|---|---|
| Skin criteria | Butterfly rash (lupus rash over the cheeks and nose)<br>Discoid rash (a thick, disclike rash, usually in sun-exposed areas)<br>Sun sensitivity (rash after being exposed to ultraviolet light)<br>Oral ulcerations (recurrent sores in the mouth or nose) |
| Systemic criteria | Arthritis (inflammation of at least two peripheral joints)<br>Serositis (pleurisy, pericarditis)<br>Renal disorder (proteinuria, cellular casts)<br>Neurologic disorder (seizure or psychosis) |
| Laboratory criteria | Hemolytic anemia, leukopenia, or thrombocytopenia<br>Antiphospholipid antibodies, lupus anticoagulant, anti-DNA, anti-Sm on a false-positive syphilis test<br>Positive antinuclear antibody |

*For classification purposes, 4 of the 11 criteria must be present at some time during the illness.
Reproduced from Hochberg MC: Updating the American College of Rheumatology revised criteria for the classification of systemic lupus erythematosus. Arthritis Rheum 1997;40:1725; with permission.

> **BOX 19-2**
> ## Classification of Scleroderma
>
> **I. Systemic (systemic sclerosis)**
> With diffuse cutaneous scleroderma: Symmetric widespread skin fibrosis, affecting the distal and proximal extremities and often the trunk and face; tendency to rapid progression of skin changes; and early appearance of visceral involvement
> With limited cutaneous scleroderma: Symmetric restricted skin fibrosis affecting the distal extremities (often confined to the fingers) and face; prolonged delay in appearance of distinctive internal manifestations (e.g., pulmonary arterial hypertension); and prominence of calcinosis and telangiectasias
> With "overlap": Having either diffuse or limited skin fibrosis and typical features of one or more of the other connective tissue diseases
>
> **II. Localized**
> Morphea: Single or multiple plaques of skin fibrosis
> Linear scleroderma: Single or multiple bands of skin fibrosis; includes scleroderma *en coup de sabre* (with or without facial hemiatrophy)
> Eosinophilic fasciitis: Fascial and deep subcutaneous fibrosis
> Eosinophilia-myalgia syndrome
> Toxic oil syndrome

From Medsger TA Jr.: Systemic sclerosis (scleroderma): Clinical aspects. In Koopman WJ (ed): Arthritis and Allied Conditions, 14th ed. Philadelphia, Lippincott Williams & Wilkins, 2001, p 1590; with permission.

skeletal muscle, and internal organs, most notably the gastrointestinal tract, lung, heart, and kidney. The disease is classified according to the degree and extent of skin thickening, as illustrated in Box 19-2, and may overlap with polymyositis/dermatomyositis or Sjögren's syndrome and on occasion with SLE but rarely with RA.[16]

## EPIDEMIOLOGY

The annual incidence of SSc is more than 20 new cases per million population. Incidence increases steadily with age, reaching a peak at 55 to 64 years.[17] The female-to-male ratio is 3:1, and the disease is more frequent in African-Americans than in whites, especially in patients 15 to 45 years of age. Systemic sclerosis is rare in childhood. Several environmental "triggers" for scleroderma-like syndromes have been reported, including inhalation of silica dust, polyvinyl chloride, and other aromatic amines.

## PATHOGENESIS

The current working hypothesis is that systemic sclerosis results from abnormalities in blood vessels, the immune system, and fibroblasts (Fig. 19-17).[18] There is abundant evidence of widespread endothelial damage, possibly mediated by activated circulating T cells. The results are increased vascular permeability and activation of endothelial cells, which then participate in attracting other mononuclear cells and contribute to vasospasm (release of endothelin-1) and reduced blood flow and increased thrombogenesis. Perivascular infiltrates contain primarily CD4+, T-helper, and IL-2–dependent lymphocytes, which can become profibrotic with the release of such cytokines as transforming growth factor-β and IL-4. Precise mechanisms of T-cell activation

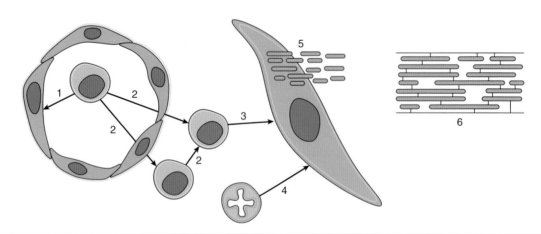

**Figure 19-17.** Pathophysiology of systemic sclerosis with possible sites for therapeutic intervention. Rational therapy would be designed to *(1)* prevent endothelial cell damage; *(2)* alter communication between mononuclear cells; *(3)* prevent mononuclear cell stimulation of fibroblasts; *(4)* prevent mast cell degranulation; *(5)* block fibroblast production and extrusion of procollagen; or *(6)* increase solubilization of preformed collagen. (Reproduced from Koopman WJ (ed): Arthritis and Allied Conditions, 14th ed. Philadelphia, Lippincott Williams & Wilkins, 2001, p 1610; with permission.)

are unknown. The SSc-related serum autoantibodies, which identify nearly 90% of patients, are not found in affected tissues; they are important markers for disease diagnosis but do not have a recognized role in pathogenesis. Scleroderma skin fibroblasts produce increased amounts of collagen and other matrix proteins at a pretranslational level based on detection of increased amounts of corresponding mRNA. An autocrine effect of transforming growth factor-β may contribute to continued fibroblast activation. Again, underlying mechanisms for the upregulation of genes responsible for excessive matrix accumulation are not understood.

## CLINICAL FEATURES

### Blood Vessels

Raynaud's phenomenon is present in more than 95% of patients (Fig. 19-18). It consists of repeated brief (5- to 30-minute) episodes of fingertip blanching or cyanosis on cold exposure or with emotional stress, followed by reactive hyperemia on rewarming. As opposed to Raynaud's disease, where there is no associated systemic disorder, Raynaud's phenomenon is due to a combination of changes, including thickening of the arteriolar wall from subintimal connective tissue proliferation, lumenal narrowing, and vasospasm (Fig. 19-19). Wide-field nailfold capillary microscopy identifies structural abnormalities, including dropout and dilatation. These changes are not unique to SSc, also occurring in patients with other connective tissue diseases (CTDs). Raynaud's phenomenon may be associated with digital tip ischemia, resulting in digital pitting scars, ulcers, or gangrene.

### Skin

Skin thickening is palpable and results in "puffy," indurated fingers or, when more severe, inability to move the skin. This process almost always begins in the fingers and may spread slowly (over months or years) to the dorsum of the hands in limited

cutaneous (lc) SSc or more rapidly to affect the forearms, upper arms, thighs, thorax, and abdomen in diffuse cutaneous (dc) SSc. Hyperpigmentation is common. The "scleroderma facies" is characterized by a "pinched" nose and vertical folds above and below the mouth (Fig. 19-20A), along with numerous telangiectasias in lcSSc (see Fig. 19–20B). Biopsy reveals marked thickening of the dermis with variable collections of mononuclear cells, chiefly T-lymphocytes.

### Joints/Tendons

Symmetrical polyarthrialgias and/or polyarthritis are often present, primarily affecting the small joints of the hands in an RA-like

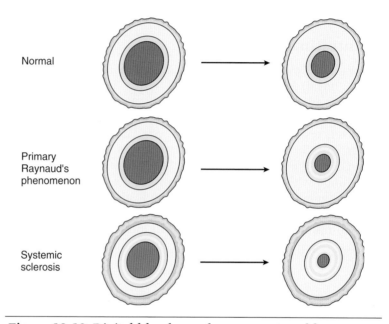

**Figure 19-19.** Digital blood vessel responses to cold exposure.

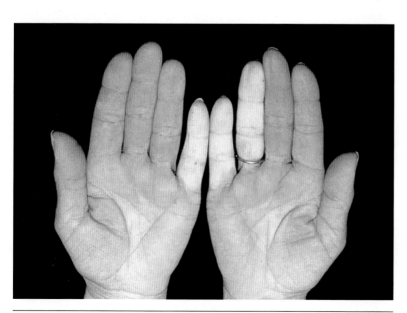

**Figure 19-18.** Raynaud's phenomenon. Note marked pallor of three digits. (From 1972–1999 American College of Rheumatology Clinical Slide Collection; with permission.)

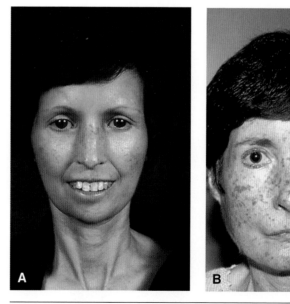

**Figure 19-20.** *A,* Face of a woman with diffuse scleroderma. *B,* Face of a woman with limited scleroderma. Note multiple telangiectasias. (Reproduced from Koopman WJ (ed): Arthritis and Allied Conditions, 14th ed. Philadelphia, Lippincott Williams & Wilkins, 2001, p 1593; with permission.)

distribution. SSc is characterized by a tendency to early joint contractures, which are often due to tendon or tendon sheath fibrosis and shortening. The tendon friction rub, a "leathery"-feeling rub palpable over joints or tendons on motion, is nearly pathognomonic for SSc, especially of the dc subtype.

## Skeletal Muscle

Proximal muscle weakness may be associated with shoulder joint involvement or be a primary myopathy. Most myopathies encountered in SSc patients are noninflammatory and non-progressive, but on occasion there is overlap with polymyositis, in which case the serum creatine kinase is elevated, the electromyogram is abnormal, and the muscle biopsy shows typical polymyositis.

## Intestinal Tract

Three fourths of SSc patients have distal dysphagia for solid foods (bread, meat) and gastroesophageal reflux (heartburn). These symptoms are due to distal esophageal smooth muscle hypomotility and dilatation (Fig. 19-21) and laxity of the gastroesophageal sphincter, respectively. Erosive distal esophagitis can occur from untreated reflux or esophageal stricture from long-standing acid damage to the distal esophagus, but such complications are uncommon with today's potent acid protective regimens.

Hypomotility of the small intestine leads to poor mixing of foods and episodes of small bowel dilatation with functional ileus (pseudo-obstruction) and may result in intestinal malabsorption. Colonic hypomotility may cause constipation/obstipation, and

rectal incompetence leads to lack of sphincter control with rectal seepage of stool. "Watermelon stomach" is a condition in which there are gastric antral venular ectasias that can bleed profusely enough to require transfusion.

## Lung

The two most serious consequences of lung involvement are alveolitis leading to pulmonary interstitial fibrosis and pulmonary arterial hypertension (PAH). Pulmonary fibrosis results in slowly progressive dyspnea over a number of years, audible bibasilar end-inspiratory rales, restrictive physiology on pulmonary function testing (reduced forced vital capacity, parallel reduction in diffusing capacity for carbon monoxide), and a chest radiograph showing lower lobe fibrotic changes that can be confirmed histologically (Fig. 19-22A and B).[19] In contrast, PAH presents with rapidly progressive dyspnea (over 6 to 12 months); a loud pulmonic component of the second heart sound; normal forced vital capacity;

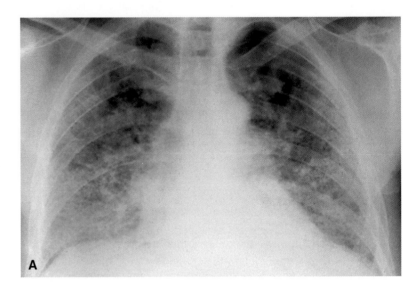

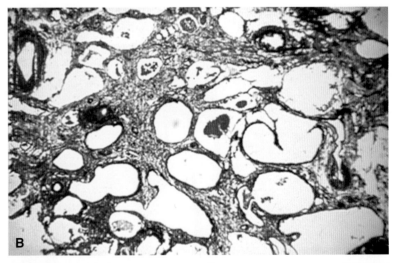

**Figure 19-22.** *A,* Radiograph showing pulmonary fibrosis in scleroderma. (From 1972–1999 American College of Rheumatology Clinical Slide Collection; with permission.) *B,* Histologic appearance of pulmonary fibrosis. There is marked distortion of the pulmonary parenchyma. This trichrome stain shows extensive interstitial collagen deposition *(blue).*

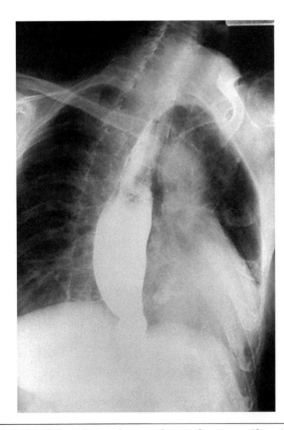

**Figure 19-21.** Dilated esophagus due to hypomotility in scleroderma. (From 1972–1999 American College of Rheumatology Clinical Slide Collection; with permission.)

disproportionately reduced carbon dioxide diffusion in the lungs; clear lung fields radiographically but enlarged pulmonary arteries, sometimes with right ventricular enlargement and histologic evidence of small pulmonary arterial medial hypertrophy; and subinitimal proliferation of connective tissue with near occlusion of the vascular lumen.[20] When advanced, both pulmonary fibrosis and PAH can lead to right-sided CHF with neck vein distention, tricuspid insufficiency, tender hepatomegaly, ascites, and peripheral edema. Pulmonary fibrosis is most common in dcSSc, and PAH in lcSSc. Pleuritis is infrequent clinically, but pleural thickening/fibrosis is found in the majority of SSc patients at autopsy.

### Heart

Severe cardiac involvement is uncommon (less than 5% of patients) and occurs most often in dcSSc patients. The major manifestations are symptomatic pericarditis with or without pericardial effusion, conduction system abnormalities (due to fibrotic replacement) with a variety of arrhythmias, or cardiomyopathy with CHF from fibrous infiltration of the working left ventricular myocardium.

### Kidney

The classic finding is "scleroderma renal crisis," which occurs in as many as 20% of dcSSc patients but rarely in lcSSc patients. This is an acute illness characterized by accelerated arterial hypertension and rapidly progressive oliguric renal failure. Patients typically present with headache, visual disturbances, severe fatigue, or dysphea. Frequent accompanying features are proteinuria, microscopic hematuria, and microangiopathic hemolytic anemia with thrombocytopenia. The hypertension is due to hyperreninemia and, prior to the availability of angiotensin-converting enzyme inhibitors, this complication was almost uniformly fatal.[21] Angiographic and renal biopsy changes are diagnostic of a medium-size (interlobular) and small-vessel angiopathy.

## NATURAL HISTORY OF DISEASE

The most instructive way to describe the natural history of SSc is to consider changes in skin thickness over time (Fig. 19-23). In lcSSc, the early years (or decades) are characterized by Raynaud's phenomenon, digital ischemia, and esophageal disease; only later are there any life-threatening problems, such as PAH. In contrast, most complications in dcSSc occur early (during the first 3 to 4 years), while skin thickening is rapidly progressive. After the peak of skin thickness has been reached (usually within 3 years after disease onset), it is uncommon to develop new internal organ involvement. In our experience, the 10-year cumulative survival in dcSSc is 75% and in lcSSc, 85%.

## DIAGNOSIS

### Clinical and Serologic Classification

Criteria have been developed for description of large series of patients in research studies, as opposed to diagnosis of individual patients. The major criterion is scleroderma skin change proximal to the metacarpophalangeal joints and the minor criteria include

any two of the following: sclerodactyly, digital pitting scars, or bibasilar pulmonary fibrosis on chest roentenogram. These criteria are very sensitive and specific for dcSSc but do not perform well for lcSSc, where as many as 25% of patients may be excluded.

More than 95% of SSc patients have a positive ANA test. There are a number of SSc-related serum autoantibodies. In our experience, seven serum autoantibodies account for 85% to 90% of patients with SSc. Each of these antibodies is associated with certain clinical manifestations.

A combined classification system provides additional insights and identifies unique subsets of patients (Fig. 19-24). It has been proposed that the diagnosis of SSc be extended to include patients who have Raynaud's phenomenon and either nail fold capillary abnormalities or SSc-related serum autoantibodies.

## MANAGEMENT

Measuring outcome in SSc has been hampered by lack of reliable instruments for this purpose. A validated disease severity index was developed in 1999. An activity scale was published in 2002, and the serum levels of various cytokines have been reported to correlate with physician global assessment of disease activity. The patient-completed Health Assessment Questionnaire, developed for RA, has proved to be useful in judging the health status of SSc patients.

### Disease-Modifying Agents

Unfortunately, there are no drugs that have proved effective for SSc in double-blind controlled clinical trials.[22] The primary approach, based on theories of pathogenesis, small patient series, and uncontrolled observations, has been to use immunosuppressive or immunomodulating therapies in dcSSc, including methotrexate, cyclophosphamide, D-penicillamine, cyclosporin A, interferon-γ, and even autologous stem cell transplantation.

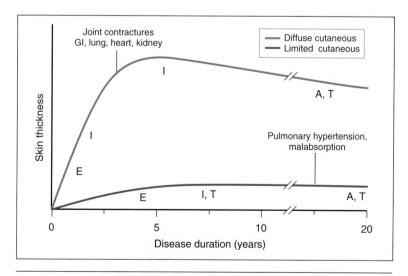

**Figure 19-23.** Natural history of skin thickness and timing of some serious complications during the course of systemic sclerosis with the two major disease variants. A, atrophy; E, edema; I, induration; T, telangiectasia. (Reproduced from Koopman WJ (ed): Arthritis and Allied Conditions, 14th ed. Philadelphia, Lippincott Williams & Wilkins, 2001, p 1594.)

Corticosteroids should be used sparingly, as they are associated with an increased risk of renal crisis. In the future, with increased knowledge of molecular mechanisms, biologic response modifying drugs targeting specific effector substances will undoubtedly be tested.

### Organ-Specific Therapy

Table 19-5 summarizes approaches to disease affecting individual organ systems. Of particular note is that during the past 20 years, mortality and morbidity have been greatly reduced, particularly for peripheral vascular, esophageal, and renal complications.

# IDIOPATHIC INFLAMMATORY MYOPATHIES

## CLASSIFICATION AND DIAGNOSIS

Disease classification in the idiopathic inflammatory myopathies (IIMs) serves to identify clinically homogeneous subsets of patients. Most published methods separate dermatomyositis (DM) from polymyositis (PM), as well as childhood from adult onset, and distinguish myositis associated with malignancy or with other CTDs (overlap syndromes). Supplementation of this clinical classification with myositis-associated antibody test results is also helpful.

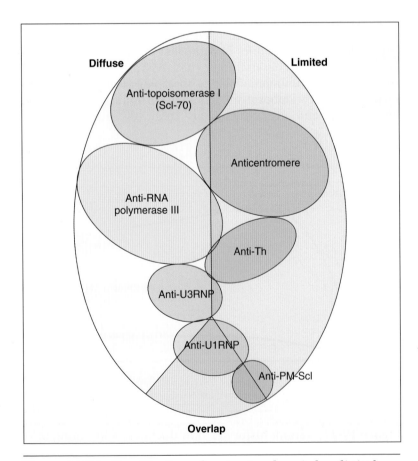

**Figure 19-24.** Classification of systemic sclerosis by clinical subsets and autoantibody types. (Reproduced from Koopman WJ (ed): Arthritis and Allied Conditions, 14th ed. Philadelphia, Lippincott Williams & Wilkins, 2001, p 1592.)

The most widely accepted diagnostic criteria are those proposed by Bohan and Peter in 1975 (Box 19-3). Their sensitivity is 70% for definite and 90% for definite or probable DM or PM; specificity against lupus and scleroderma exceeds 90%.

## EPIDEMIOLOGY

The annual incidence of the IIMs is approximately 10 cases per year per million population at risk. The incidence pattern by age suggests childhood and adult peaks with a paucity of patients diagnosed in adolescence and the young adult years (15 to 24). The overall female-to-male ratio is 2.5:1. African Americans are affected three times more frequently than whites and even more so during young adulthood. No convincing associations between the occurrence of IIMs and genetic or environmental or occupational factors have been recognized.

**TABLE 19-5**
**Organ-Based Therapies for Systemic Sclerosis**

| Organ | Treatments |
|---|---|
| Peripheral vascular | Vasodilators; digital sympathectomy |
| Joints | Exercises, NSAIDs |
| Muscle | Corticosteroids; immunosuppressives |
| Esophagus | Prokinetics, acid-blocking drugs |
| Lung-fibrosis | Corticosteroids; immunosuppressives; vasodilators; endothelin blockers |
| Lung-pulmonary hypertension | Corticosteroids; immunosuppressives |
| Kidney | ACE inhibitors |

ACE, angiotensin-converting enzyme; NSAID, nonsteroidal anti-inflammatory drug.

---

**BOX 19-3**
**Bohan and Peter Diagnostic Criteria For Polymyositis (PM)/dermatomyositis (DM)***

Symmetric proximal muscle weakness on examination
Elevated serum muscle enzymes
Myopathic abnormalities on electromyogram
Typical changes of myositis on muscle biopsy
Typical rash of dermatomyositis

*Definite PM = 4/5 criteria; probably PM = 3/5 criteria. Definite DM = rash + 3/4 other criteria; probable DM rash + 2/4 other criteria.
Modified from Bohan A, Peter JB: Polymyositis and dermatomyositis. N Engl J Med 1975;292:344–347; with permission.

## CLINICAL FEATURES

### Muscle

The classic presentation is insidious (over several weeks or months) painless symmetrical proximal muscle weakness of the neck flexor, shoulder girdle, and hip girdle muscles.[23] An affected person may be unable to raise his or her head from a pillow, lift an object overhead, arise from a low chair or toilet seat without using arms to "push off," or walk up steps without difficulty. Pharyngeal weakness is less common but if present can result in hoarseness, a nasal quality of the voice, and difficulty initiating swallowing (particularly of liquids) with nasal regurgitation and aspiration into the tracheobronchial tree. Respiratory muscle weakness is unusual but can lead to ventilatory insufficiency. Later in the course of disease, visible muscle atrophy is evident.

Objective evidence of myositis includes an elevated serum creatine kinase level and, to a lesser extent, other enzymes in muscle, including aldolase and the transaminases (SGOT, SGPT). The electromyogram is a sensitive but nonspecific diagnostic tool; affected muscles show "myopathic" motor unit potentials (increased spontaneous activity; polyphasic, short-duration, and low-amplitude potentials with muscle contraction). More than 90% of myositis patients have an abnormal electromyogram, and this study is helpful in selecting an appropriate (opposite-side) site for biopsy. The pathognomonic histologic finding is some combination of myofibril degeneration and regeneration along with chronic inflammatory cell infiltration in perivascular and interstitial locations (Fig. 19-25). The infiltrate is predominantly lymphocytic but often also includes histiocytes and plasma cells. More chronic changes consist of increased fibrous tissue between muscle fascicles and fatty replacement of damaged myofibrils. In DM, immunoglobulin and complement components C5 to C9 (membrane attack complex) are deposited in blood vessel walls. Fat-suppressed magnetic resonance imaging is a highly sensitive but expensive method that has been shown to correlate with both clinical evidence of disease activity and inflammatory changes on muscle biopsy.

### Skin

The rash of dermatomyositis is virtually pathognomonic of this condition (Figs. 19-26, 19-27, and 19-28). The upper eyelids; malar areas; bridge of the nose and nasolabial folds; "V" area of the anterior chest and neck; upper back; extensor surfaces of the elbows, knees, metacarpophalangeal and proximal interphalangeal joints; and periungual regions are most commonly affected. The lesions are erythematous (often violaceous) and papular with prominent scaling and chronically become thin and atrophic with numerous telangiectasias. The cutaneous histologic features are similar to those of SLE with vacuolar degeneration and perivascular inflammation at the dermal-epidermal junction, but in DM, immunofluroescence for complement and immunoglobulins is negative.

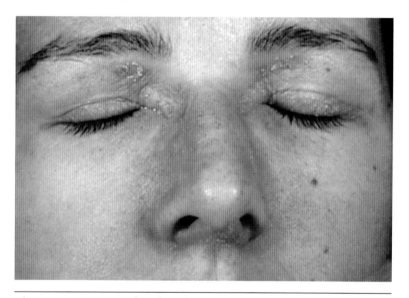

**Figure 19-26.** Periorbital and nasolabial fold erythematous, scaling rash of dermatomyositis.

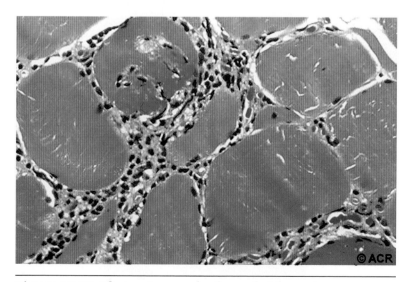

**Figure 19-25.** Photomicrograph of muscle biopsy in dermatomyositis showing diffuse interstitial mononuclear infiltrate and degeneration of a large muscle fiber. (From 1972–1999 American College of Rheumatology Clinical Slide Collection; with permission.)

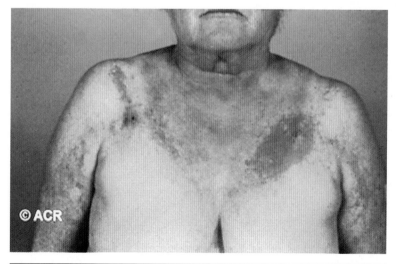

**Figure 19-27.** V-neck and anterior chest rash of dermatomyositis. (From 1972–1999 American College of Rheumatology Clinical Slide Collection; with permission.)

## Joints

Inflammatory polyarthralgias or polyarthritis are common, especially in "overlap" syndromes with other CTDs. The distribution is similar to that found in RA. The arthritis is usually mild and disappears with corticosteroid treatment of myositis but can be severe. Subluxing, deforming, erosive or nonerosive arthropathy can occur, particularly with the antisynthetase antibody syndrome.

## Lung

Pulmonary involvement in myositis may be secondary to respiratory muscle weakness (diaphragm, intercostal muscles) or interstitial lung disease. The latter has the same clinical, physiologic, and histologic characteristics as interstitial lung disease seen in other CTDs but is particularly aggressive in antisynthetase antibody patients, where it may culminate in adult respiratory distress syndrome.

## Heart

Clinically significant cardiac involvement is uncommon. The most frequent findings are electrocardiographic abnormalities, such as conduction defects, but life-threatening arrhythmias may occur due to fibrous replacement of the conduction system. CHF is rare but serious; it may result from inflammation (myocarditis) or fibrosis of the working myocardium.

## Gastrointestinal Tract

Proximal dysphagia in myositis patients is secondary to weak pharyngeal striated musculature and may result in tracheobronchial aspiration with chemical pneumonitis. In contrast, distal dysphagia results from involvement of esophageal smooth muscle similar to the findings in systemic sclerosis. A severe manifestation of childhood-onset DM is gastrointestinal mucosal ulceration and hemorrhage from vasculitis.

## Peripheral Vascular System

Raynaud's phenomenon is frequent in the IIMs and may lead to digital tip ischemia. Soft tissue and intramuscular calcification is an occasionally disabling complication of childhood-onset DM, especially when there has been a prolonged delay in treating active myositis (Fig. 19-29). In men older than 50, DM (but not PM) is associated with malignancy. In the vast majority of instances, the diagnosis of myositis and that of tumor are made within 1 year of each other. Interestingly, primary therapy of the malignancy has been reported to result in regression of DM, suggesting that the latter is a paraneoplastic process.

## Inclusion Body Myositis

Inclusion body myositis is characterized by very slowly progressive (over years) painless proximal and distal muscle weakness, particularly affecting older men.[24] Extramuscular findings, serum autoantibodies, and coexistent malignancy are absent. The serum creatine kinase (CK) level is normal or minimally increased. The electromyogram shows myopathic and neurogenic abnormalities, and muscle biopsy findings include cellular changes similar to those of PM and also vacuoles with basophilic granules and both intranuclear and intracytoplasmic tubulofilamentous inclusions. Typically, inclusion body myositis patients do not respond well to corticosteroids or immunosuppressive drugs.

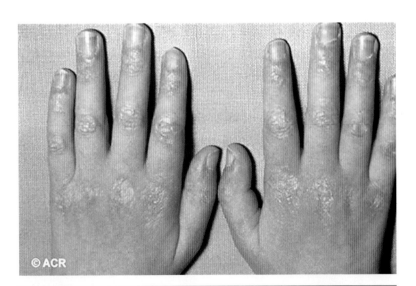

**Figure 19-28.** Gottron's changes over the extensor aspects of hand joints in dermatomyositis. (From 1972–1999 American College of Rheumatology Clinical Slide Collection; with permission.)

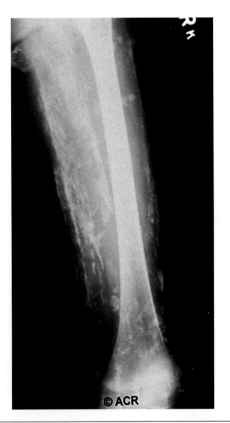

**Figure 19-29.** Radiograph showing calcinosis of subcutaneous tissue, fascia, and muscle of the thigh in dermatomyositis. (From 1972–1999 American College of Rheumatology Clinical Slide Collection; with permission.)

## Antisynthetase Syndrome

Approximately 20% of all IIM patients have serum anti-cytoplasmic antibodies directed against one of several aminoacyl-tRNA synthetase enzymes.[25] The most common is anti-Jo1, which is directed against histidyl-tRNA synethetase. The result is a distinctive clinical syndrome including PM more often than DM, arthralgias or arthritis that may be deforming and rheumatoid-like, Raynaud's phenomenon, "mechanic's hands" (Fig. 19-30), and interstitial lung disease. Subluxation of the distal interphalangeal joint of the thumb (floppy thumb sign; Fig. 19-31) is a distinctive radiographic finding. Other IIM-associated serum antibodies have been identified, and some have characteristic clinical associations. For example, anti-Mi2 is associated with classic DM; anti-U1 RNP identifies "overlap" patients; and in anti-SRP patients, cardiac involvement is more frequent.

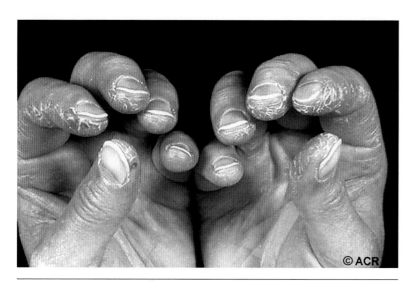

**Figure 19-30.** "Mechanic's hands" in dermatomyositis. There is fissuring and cracking of the finger pad skin. (From 1972–1999 American College of Rheumatology Clinical Slide Collection; with permission.)

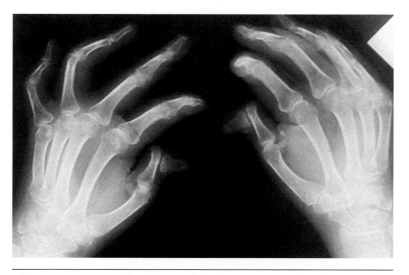

**Figure 19-31.** Hand radiographs of a patient with idiopathic inflammatory myopathy (IIM). There is distal interphalangeal joint subluxation of both thumbs (floppy thumb sign). (Courtesy of C.V. Oddis, University of Pittsburgh, Pittsburgh, PA.)

## PATHOGENESIS

Although the etiology and pathogenesis of the IIMs are unknown, there is considerable evidence that autoimmunity plays an important role.[26] Both cellular and humoral immune mechanisms participate, as summarized in Box 19-4. Immunization of laboratory animals can produce "experimental autoimmune myositis," and there is a mouse model of group B Coxsackievirus–induced chronic myositis.

## NATURAL HISTORY OF DISEASE

Published studies during the corticosteroid era clearly support improved outcome. Today, the expected survival in incident cases of PM or DM (excluding those associated with malignancy) is more than 90% at 5 years after initial diagnosis. Adverse prognostic features include older age, malignancy, pharyngeal involvement with aspiration, delayed initiation of corticosteroid therapy, and complications of corticosteroids and immunosuppressive drugs. The long-term prognosis for muscle strength differs by both disease subtype and serum autoantibody (Fig. 19-32).[27] For example, inclusion body myositis patients have a poor functional outlook because their muscle weakness tends to progress despite therapy, yet their survival is good because of the lack of visceral involvement. Each major exacerbation of myositis most often results in a reduction in muscle strength, but therapy almost never returns the patient to the preceding level of total body muscle mass or strength.

---

**BOX 19-4**
**Immunologic Abnormalities in IIM**

1. Cellular immunity
   a. Activated (DR+) T cells and macrophages in close proximity to myofibrils
   b. T cells cytotoxic to myofibrils
   c. Myofibrils express class I and II antigens
   d. PBMCs proliferate in response to autologous muscle
   e. PBMCs traffic to muscle
   f. Increased expression of T-cell activation in PB

2. Humoral immunity
   a. Increased CD4:CD8 cell ratio in DM, close proximity of CD4+ cells to B cells
   b. Ig and complement deposition in vascular endothelium in DM
   c. Immune dysregulation: hyper-, hypo-, or agamma-globulinemia
   d. Myositis-associated serum autoantibodies

DM, dermatomyositis; Ig, immunoglobulin; IIM, idiopathic inflammatory myopathy; PB, peripheral blood; PBMC, peripheral blood mononuclear cell.
Modified from Medsger TA Jr., Oddis CV: Polymyositis and dermatomyositis. In Belch JJF, Zurier RB (eds.): Connective Tissue Diseases. London, Chapman & Hall Medical, 1995, p 81; with permission.

## MANAGEMENT

There are limitations in our ability to evaluate myositis patients for decisions regarding therapy. The manual assessment of muscle strength is crude, and the serum CK is helpful but sometimes unpredictable as a measure of disease activity. Functional ability may be the most critical indicator of therapeutic response. A preliminary myositis evaluation tool has been developed by consensus but has not yet been widely used.

Corticosteroids are the mainstay of pharmacologic therapy.[28] Typically, prednisone 60 to 80 mg/day or the equivalent, in divided doses, is given until the CK level has fallen into the normal range (usually after 4 to 6 weeks). Thereafter, prednisone is generally reduced every 3 to 4 weeks and consolidated to a single daily dose. When a low maintenance dose of 5 to 10 mg prednisone daily is reached, this dose is continued until the patient has had a minimum of 12 full months of therapy before any consideration of discontinuation. After the 4th month or so, alternate-day steroid administration may be given to minimize toxicity (Fig. 19-33). Corticosteroid myopathy may be superimposed, but in this case, the serum CK should be normal. To prevent corticosteroid-induced osteoporosis, particularly in older individuals, prophylactic calcium (1000 to 1500 mg/day) and vitamin D (800 IU/day) are given from the beginning along with a bisphosphonate.

In patients who do not respond adequately to corticosteroids or are intolerant of them, an immunosuppressive drug is typically added. The most useful agents are methotrexate and azathioprine, but cyclophosphamide or chlorambucil (alkylating agents) and cyclosporin also have been used successfully. Although extremely expensive, intravenous Ig is another treatment that has been reported to benefit patients, but its long-term effectiveness is not well established. Passive range-of-motion exercises to prevent joint contractures should be begun in severely weak patients. As soon as serum muscle enzymes have "normalized" or are stable, an active isometric exercise program, followed by resistive exercises, as tolerated, should be initiated to increase strength and improve endurance.

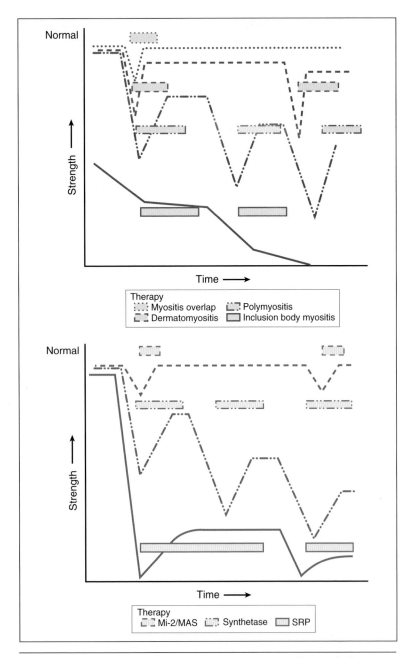

**Figure 19-32.** Generalized myositis courses differ in different idiopathic inflammatory myopathy clinical *(top)* and serologic *(bottom)* subgroups. SRP, signal recognition particle. (Reproduced from Koopman WJ (ed): Arthritis and Allied Conditions, 14th ed. Philadelphia, Lippincott Williams & Wilkins, 2001, p 1575; with permission.)

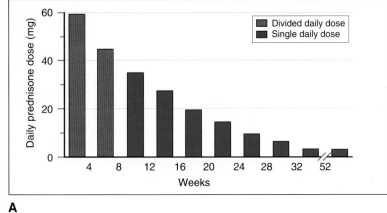

A

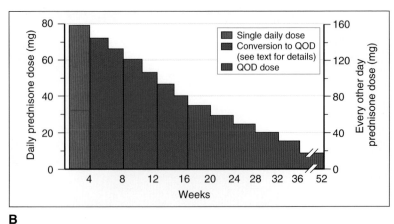

B

**Figure 19-33.** Comparison of two different corticosteroid treatment regimens in the management of myositis. QOD, every other day. (Reproduced from Medsger TA Jr., Oddis CV: Polymyositis and dermatomyositis. In Belch JJF, Zurier RB (eds): Connective Tissue Diseases. London, Chapman & Hall Medical, 1995, p 85; with permission.)

# SJÖGREN'S SYNDROME

## CLASSIFICATION AND DIAGNOSIS

Sjögren's syndrome may occur alone (primary) or in conjunction with another autoimmune disease (secondary) (Box 19-5).[29] A set of criteria for the diagnosis of Sjögren's syndrome has been developed by a European study group and includes dry eyes by history, dry mouth by history, objective evidence of reduced tearing, abnormal lip biopsy, objective evidence of salivary gland enlargement, and presence of one of the following autoantibodies: anti–SSA, anti–SSB, ANA, or rheumatoid factor.[30] A patient with at least three of the six criteria is considered to have Sjögren's disease, provided the findings cannot be explained by another condition, for example, radiation-induced xerostomia.

In addition to its close relationship with the CTDs, Sjögren's syndrome often coexists with other autoimmune disorders. Subclinical autoimmune hypothyroidism (with serum antithyroid antibodies and elevated thyroid-stimulating hormone levels) is present in as many as 50% of Sjögren's patients. Primary biliary cirrhosis is another association, characterized by hepatomegaly, elevated serum alkaline phosphatase, and serum antimitrochondrial antibodies. Liver biopsy shows chronic lymphocytic inflammation of the intrahepatic bile ducts. Among all primary biliary cirrhosis patients, Sjögren's features have been noted in as many as 50%.

Other conditions that can cause partoid gland enlargement and xerostomia, mimicking Sjögren's syndrome, are sarcoidosis, some of the hyperlipoproteinemias, amyloidosis, and HIV infection.

## EPIDEMIOLOGY

The prevalence of primary Sjögren's syndrome is unknown. The female-to-male ratio is 9:1, and the disease is most frequently encountered between the ages of 30 and 60 and is considered rare in childhood. Secondary Sjögren's occurs in 20% to 30% of RA and SSc patients.

## CLINICAL FEATURES

### Dry Eye (Xerophthalmia)

Patients usually complain of a burning foreign-body sensation or a "gritty" or "scratchy" feeling as if there were sand under the eyelids. Light sensitivity is common. Reduced tear production leads to destruction of both corneal and conunctival epithelium. Physical signs include dilatation of the bulbar conjunctival vessels, pericorneal injection, irregularity of the corneal image, and lacrimal gland enlargement.

Objective evidence of inadequate tearing can be obtained by several methods. A simple screening examination is the Schirmer's tear test, in which a strip of filter paper is placed beneath the inferior lid, and the amount of wetting of the strip after 5 minutes is measured (normal is more than 5 mm; Fig. 19-34). Rose Bengal, an analine dye, stains devitalized or damaged corneal epithelium and leaves punctate deposits that can be seen using a slit lamp. A rapid tear film "breakup" time is another common finding in Sjögren's syndrome.

### Dry Mouth (Xerostomia)

This symptom results from decreased saliva production. Patients often complain of difficulty swallowing dry food, fatigue with speaking continuously, abnormal sense of taste, a burning

---

**BOX 19-5**
**Sjögren's Syndrome**

**Definition**
A slowly progressive, inflammatory autoimmune disease affecting primarily the exocrine glands
Lymphocytic infiltrates replace functional epithelium leading to decreased exocrine secretions (exocrinopathy)
Characteristic autoantibodies, Ro(SS-A) and La(SS-B), are produced

**Clinical Features**
Mucosal dryness manifested in keratoconjunctivitis sicca, xerostomia, xerotrachea, and vaginal dryness
Major salivary gland enlargement and atrophic gastritis
Nonerosive polyarthritis; Raynaud's phenomenon without telangiectasia or digital ulceration
Extraglandular disease affecting lungs, kidneys, blood vessels, and muscles
Association with other autoimmune diseases (RA, SLE, systemic sclerosis)
Increased risk of lymphoid malignancy

RA, rheumatoid arthritis; SLE, systemic lupus erythematosus.
From Tzioufas AG, Moutropoulos HM: Sjögren's syndrome. In Hochberg MC, Silman AG, Smolen JS, et al (eds.) Rheumatology, 3rd. ed. Philadelphia, Elsevier Limited, 2003, p 1431; with permission.

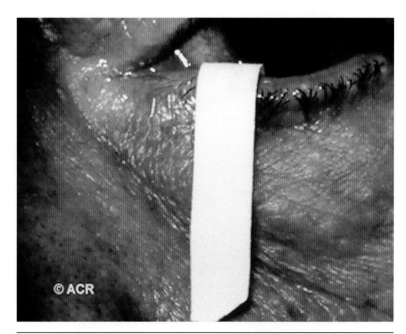

**Figure 19-34.** The Schirmer test in Sjögren's syndrome demonstrates reduced wetting of a filter paper strip confirming reduced tear production. (From 1972–1999 American College of Rheumatology Clinical Slide Collection; with permission.)

sensation in the mouth, an increase in dental caries, and problems wearing complete dentures. Physical examination reveals dry, erythematous, "sticky" oral mucosa, a scant sublingual salivary pool, and papillary atrophy on the dorsum of the tongue (Fig. 19-35). Parotid and submandibular gland enlargement occurs in more than half of patients with primary Sjögren's disease and less commonly in secondary Sjögren's (Fig. 19-36).

Salivary flow rate determined by sialometry is variable among normal persons, and thus, no single value defines Sjögren's disease.

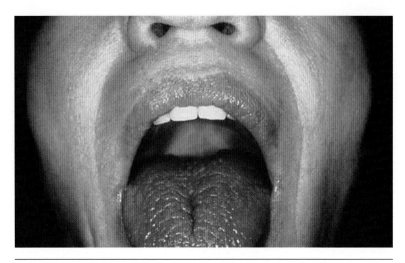

**Figure 19-35.** Dry mouth (xerostomia) in Sjögren's syndrome. (From 1972–1999 American College of Rheumatology Clinical Slide Collection; with permission.)

Sialography with water-soluble media shows dilatation and ectasia of the salivary ductal system (Fig. 19-37). The gold standard is a minor salivary gland biopsy from the inner aspect of the lower lip. The classic findings include lymphocytic replacement of salivary epithelium and the presence of epimyoepithelial islands composed of keratin-containing epithelial cells.[31]

## Other Exocrine Gland Dysfunction

Dryness may affect the nose and upper respiratory tract and lead to hoarseness, recurrent bronchitis, or pneumonia. Dermal and vaginal dryness are common symptoms.

## Extraglandular Manifestations

Constitutional features such as fatigue, low-grade fever, and myalgias are frequently reported. Polyarthralgias, and occasionally true polyarthritis, are common and symmetrically affect the small joints of the hands with prominent morning stiffness. This distribution is reminiscent of RA, but bony erosive changes do not develop. Raynaud's phenomenon is present in one third of patients. Interstitial lung disease similar to that found in other CTDs may occur.

Dysphagia is most often proximal and due to pharyngeal dryness, but distal esophageal hypomotility is occasionally encountered, especially when Sjögren's syndrome occurs in systemic sclerosis patients. Chronic atrophic gastritis may be found. Reduced pancreatic secretory flow may result in loss of pancreatic function and episodes of pancreatitis.

Lymphocyte infiltration in the renal interstitium may result in failure to acidify the urine and distal renal tubular acidosis with hypokalemia and hyperchloremia. Rarely, there is membranous or membranoproliferative glomerulonephritis; when present, it is usually accompanied by cryoglobulinemia and hypocomplementemia.

Vasculitis is a serious but uncommon complication of Sjögren's syndrome occurring in fewer than 5% of patients. Typically, the patient has palpable purpura and peripheral sensory neuropathy

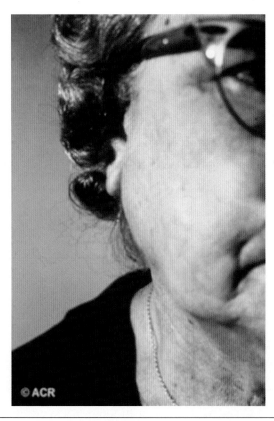

**Figure 19-36.** Parotid gland enlargement in Sjögren's syndrome. (From 1972–1999 American College of Rheumatology Clinical Slide Collection; with permission.)

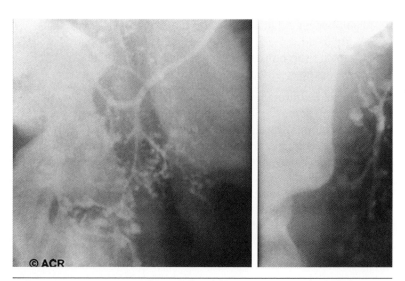

**Figure 19-37.** Localized parotid duct dilatation shown in sialogram in Sjögren's syndrome. (From 1972–1999 American College of Rheumatology Clinical Slide Collection; with permission.)

and the histology is that of leukocytoclastic angiitis hypergamma-globulinemia, positive serum rheumatoid factor, positive anti-SSA antibody, and low serum complement levels are frequent.

Peripheral and central nervous system involvement have been reported, including instances of multifocal, recurrent, and progressive disease. Manifestations include hemiparesis, hemisensory defects, seizures, movement disorders, transverse myelopathy, aseptic meningitis, and encephalopathy. However, the frequency of such findings is controversial in the medical literature.

## LABORATORY ABNORMALITIES

The most frequent findings are mild anemia of chronic disease, leukopenia, elevated erythrocyte sedimentation rate, positive ANA, positive rheumatoid factor, hypergammaglobulinemia, and hypocomplementemia. The most specific tests are anti-SSA or anti–SSB antibodies, but they are detected in only 50% of patients and are also found in some patients whose clinical diagnosis is SLE.[32]

## PATHOGENESIS

The unifying feature of all organs affected by Sjögren's disease is lymphocytic infiltration (Fig. 19-38). The predominant cells in minor labial salivary gland infiltrates are T-helper cells (CD4+). They express the adhesion molecule LFA-1 and other T-cell markers, including CD2 and LFA-3, which mediate an antigen-independent interaction and are upregulated after lymphocyte activation. B cells constitute approximately 20% of all infiltrating cells, and their activation accounts for the production of rheumatoid factor and other Igs.

Viruses such as cytomegalovirus and Epstein-Barr virus have been implicated in triggering Sjögren's disease, and genetic factors are believed to contribute. The expression of neoantigens in infected epithelial cells could be the initiating event, resulting in the ingress of helper/inducer memory T cells and B cells. Ultimately, local tissue destruction and monoclonal B-cell expansion

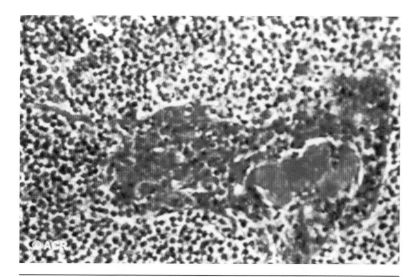

**Figure 19-38.** Photomicrograph of parotid gland in Sjögren's syndrome showing replacement of parenchyma by a diffuse collection of lymphocytes. (From 1972–1999 American College of Rheumatology Clinical Slide Collection; with permission.)

occur. Antibodies are directed against the ribonucleoprotein particles Ro (SSA) and La (SSB). These serum antibodies are associated with earlier disease onset, recurrent parotid gland enlargement, lymphadenopathy, splenomegaly, and vasculitis in primary Sjögren's syndrome.

## NATURAL HISTORY OF DISEASE

B-cell activation is considered the most consistent immuno-regulatory aberration in Sjögren's syndrome patients.[33] It begins as polyclonal activation, evolves to oligoclonal and monoclonal activation, and may ultimately transform to a malignant monoclonal proliferation (lymphoma).[34] The term *pseudolymphoma* is used when there is extraglandular organ infiltration with tumor-like clusters of lymphocytes that do not meet criteria for malignancy. Sjögren's patients have a 40+-fold increased risk of developing lymphoma compared with a demographically matched healthy population. These lymphomas are primarily of B-cell origin, expressing IgM kappa in their cytoplasm. Lymphoma should be suspected in a Sjögren's syndrome patient who develops lymphadenopathy, organomegaly, or unilateral major salivary gland enlargement.

## MANAGEMENT

Lubrication of dry eyes with artificial tears should be done as often as necessary to relieve symptoms. A variety of commercially available preparations differ from one another primarily in viscosity and in the preservative used; patients typically try several before determining which one is most suitable. For overnight use, a gel is sometimes recommended. Punctual occlusion can increase the tear reservoir. Commonsense measures include avoiding wind, low humidity, cigarette smoke, and drugs with anticholinergic side effects. Cyclosporin eyedrops are helpful in some patients.

Treatment of dry mouth is a more difficult problem, as saliva substitutes are not effective. Stimulation of salivary flow by highly flavored sugar-free lozenges (to minimize caries progression), is helpful, and dry food, cigarette smoking, and drugs with anticholinergic effects should be avoided. Good oral hygiene after meals and fluoride treatment or toothpaste retard tooth surface damage. Several oral pilocarpine preparations now available improve dry mouth in some individuals.

Nonsteroidal anti-inflammatory drugs can be used for arthralgias and arthritis. Hydroxychloroquine is helpful for treating both fatigue and the articular manifestations. Systemic corticosteroids and immunosuppressive drugs are generally reserved for severe extraglandular disease, such as interstitial pneumonitis, glomerulonephritis, vasculitis, and neurologic complications.[35] Treatment of lymphoma should be guided by an experienced oncologist.

# VASCULITIS

Primary systemic vasculitis includes a heterogeneous group of idiopathic syndromes in which immunologically mediated blood vessel wall injury results in a variety of clinical consequences, ranging from tissue ischemia secondary to vessel narrowing or intramural thrombus formation to hemorrhage or aneurysm

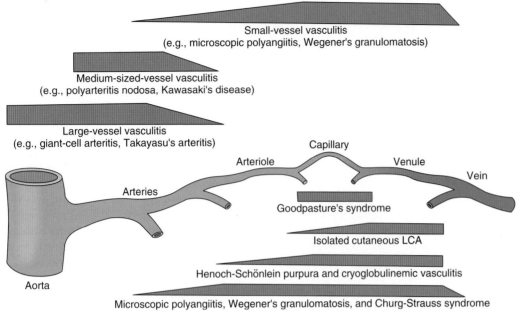

**Figure 19-39.** Preferred sites of vascular involvement by selected vasculitides. LCA, leukocytoclastic angiitis. (Reproduced from Jennette JC, Falk RJ: Small vessel vasculitis. N Engl J Med 1997;337(21):1512–1523; with permission.)

---

**TABLE 19-6**

**Chapel Hill Consensus Conference on the Nomenclature of Systemic Vasculitis—Definitions**

**Large-Vessel Vascullitis**

| | |
|---|---|
| Giant cell (temporal) arteritis | Granulomatous arteritis of the aorta and its major branches, with a predilection for the extracranial branches of the carotid artery. Often involves the temporal artery. Usually occurs in patients older than 50 yr and often is associated with polymyalgia rheumatica. |
| Takayasu arteritis | Granulomatous inflammation of the aorta and its major branches. Usually occurs in patients younger than 50 yr. |

**Medium-Size Vessel Vasculitis**

| | |
|---|---|
| Polyarteritis nodosa (classic polyarteritis nodosa) | Necrotizing inflammation of medium-size or small arteries without glomerulonephritis or vasculitis in arterioles, capillaries, or venules |
| Kawasaki disease | Arteritis involving large, medium-size, and small arteries and associated with mucocutaneous lymph node syndrome. Coronary arteries are often involved. Aorta and veins may be involved. Usually occurs in children. |

**Small-Vessel Vasculitis**

| | |
|---|---|
| Wegener granulomatosis | Granulomatous inflammation involving the respiratory tract and necrotizing vasculitis affecting small to medium-size vessels (e.g., capillaries, venules, arterioles, and arteries). Necrotizing glomerulonephritis is common. |
| Churg-Strauss syndrome | Eosinophil-rich and granulomatous inflammation involving the respiratory tract, and necrotizing vasculitis affecting small to medium-size vessels, and associated with asthma and eosinophilia. |
| Microscopic polyangiitis (microscropic polyarteritis) | Necrotizing vasculitis, with few or no immune deposits, affecting small vessels (i.e., capillaries, venules, or arterioles). Necrotizing arteritis involving small and medium-size arteries may be present. Necrotizing glomerulonephritis is very common. Pulmonary capillaritis often occurs. |
| Henoch-Schönlein purpura | Vasculitis, with IgA dominant immune deposits, affecting small vessels (i.e., capillaries, venules, or arterioles). Typically involves skin, gut, and glomeruli, and is associated with arthralgias or arthritis. |
| Essential cryoglobulinemic vasculitis | Vasculitis, with cryoglobulin immune deposits, affecting small vessels (i.e., capillaries, venules, or arterioles), and associated with cryoglobulins in serum. Skin and glomeruli are often involved. |
| Cutaneous leukocytoclastic vasculitis | Isolated cutaneous leukocytoclastic angiitis without systemic vasculitis or glomerulonephritis. |

Ig, immunoglobulin.
Reproduced from Jennette JC, Falk RJ, Andrassy K, et al: Nomenclature of systemic vasculitides. Proposal of an international consensus conference. Arthritis Rheum 1994;37:187–192; with permission.

formation due to vessel wall injury and weakening.[36] In secondary vasculitic syndromes, vessel inflammation is precipitated by a recognizable trigger in the context of a preexisting primary illness (e.g., drugs, infectious agents, and circulating immune complexes occurring in CTDs [SLE, RF-positive RA]), infections (HIV, hepatitis B and C), or malignancy. Clinical presentation is determined by the type, size, and distribution of the blood vessels involved and specific target organs affected.

Systemic vasculitis is broadly classified into large, medium-size, and small vessel groups (Fig. 19-39).[37,38] Two sets of classification schemes conforming to this general paradigm are commonly used—the American College of Rheumatology criteria (1990), developed to assist with patient classification for clinical studies, and the subsequent Chapel Hill Consensus Conference (1994) definitions that are based on clinical and histopathologic features (Table 19-6).[39]

## EPIDEMIOLOGY

Published studies on the epidemiology of primary systemic vasculitis have emerged mainly from tertiary care/university medical centers rather than being population based and hence are weakened by referral bias owing to poorly defined denominator populations. Estimates of incidence range from 10 to 20 cases per million at risk annually.

## PATHOGENESIS

The initial active recruitment of circulating leukocytes into the vessel wall involves interactions mediated by a complex array of endothelial cell surface receptors known as adhesion molecules.[40] This process is largely directed by endothelial cell–derived chemo-kines (Fig. 19-40). Cytokines and growth factors, also endothelial cell-derived, further serve to amplify the inflammatory response. Angiogenesis, especially in the vascular adventitia, leads to formation of neovasculature expressing high levels of endothelial adhesion molecules, thus contributing fresh portals for further leukocyte incursion. Chronic granulomatous inflammation typifies large-size vessel vasculitis, in contrast to the medium-size and small-size vessel vasculitides in which necrotizing inflammation is prominent.

Antineutrophil cytoplasmic antibodies (ANCA) recognize antigens in neutrophil granules and monocyte lysosomes and are frequently detected in several small-vessel vasculitides—Wegener's granulomatosis, microscopic polyangiitis, and Churg-Strauss syndrome.[41] Two ANCA types are recognized: cANCA, directed against proteinase 3 and responsible for a cytoplasmic immunofluorescent pattern on ethanol-fixed neutrophils, and pANCA, directed against myeloperoxidase, which accounts for perinuclear immunofluorescent staining (Fig. 19-41). ANCA can also occur in a variety of other conditions, including systemic infections and CTDs but does not recognize myeloperoxidase or proteinase 3 antigen specificities. There is considerable evidence supporting an active role of myeloperoxidase and proteinase 3 in either inducing or augmenting vascular inflammation.

The presence of many activated T-lymphocytes and macrophages in the vascular inflammatory infiltrate raises the possibility of specific T-cell–mediated responses directed against intrinsic or exogenously derived vessel wall antigens. For example, hepatitis B infection induces polyarteritis nodosa, in which circulating immune complexes in the early phases of infection trigger formation of vascular lesions. Immune complexes are also causatively implicated in hepatitis C–associated vasculitis with cryoglobulinemia. Other exogenous mechanisms underlying vascular inflammation include direct invasion by microbial infectious agents, especially by rickettsiae and chlamydiae. Molecular mimicry has also been implicated as a potential mechanism in vascular injury.

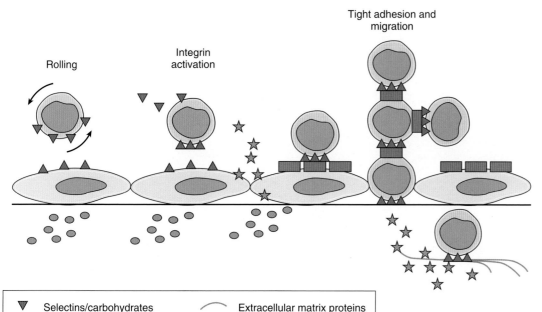

**Figure 19-40.** Sequential steps and principal adhesion molecules involved in leukocyte interactions with endothelial cells required for tissue infiltration. (Reproduced from Cid MC, Vilardell C: Tissue targeting and disease patterns in systemic vasculitis. Best Pract Res Clin Rheumatol 2001;15(2):259–279; with permission.)

## *LARGE VESSEL VASCULITIS*

### Giant Cell Arteritis and Polymyalgia Rheumatica

Giant cell arteritis is the most common form of systemic vasculitis and affects chiefly the older population (older than 50 years) in the western hemisphere. It mainly targets medium- and large-size arteries, often in a segmental or patchy distribution, with a clear preference for specific arteries including extracranial branches of the carotid arteries, vertebral arteries, subclavian arteries, and aorta. Vessel narrowing results from postinflammatory concentric intimal hyperplasia.

Disease onset can vary from abrupt to insidious. Frequently, there is an intense systemic inflammatory syndrome characterized by marked constitutional symptoms, including malaise, fever, myalgia, anorexia, and weight loss. The majority of patients experience polymyalgia rheumatica, an axial arthropathy with marked pain and stiffness of the neck, shoulder girdle, and hip girdle areas and very prominent morning stiffness in those sites. The term *myalgia* is misleading, as there is no disease of the proximal muscles; true weakness is absent, and objective testing, including CK levels, electromyography, and muscle biopsy, is routinely normal. The differential diagnosis of polymyalgia rheumatica includes infection, hypothyroidism, other CTDs, and malignancy. A dramatic symptomatic response to low or moderate doses of glucocorticoids serves as a surrogate criterion in confirming the diagnosis of polymyalgia rheumatica. A rheumatoid-like peripheral arthritis may be present. Symptoms directly relating to vascular inflammation depend on the type of vessel bed affected and the pattern of tissue ischemia.

Headache, often described as new and having an intense, boring, or lancinating character, occurs in two thirds or more of patients. It is often accompanied by scalp tenderness localized to the inflamed temporal or occipital artery regions (Fig. 19-42). Jaw claudication, diplopia, transient ischemic attacks, ischemic optic neuropathy leading to visual loss, and stroke represent consequences related to compromised blood flow. Blindness can result from arteritis involving the ophthalmic or posterior ciliary artery branches. Upper extremity claudication and thoracic aorta aneurysm formation secondary to vessel wall inflammation and weakening can occur.

Key histopathologic findings during the acute phase of inflammation include adventitial inflammation of large arteries, sometimes involving the vasa vasorum, with prominent lymphocytic infiltrates, intimal neovascularization, and marked intimal hyperplasia resulting from myofibroblast proliferation and mucopolysaccharide-deposition (Fig. 19-43). Macrophage derived multinucleated giant cells and granulomas are hallmark findings.

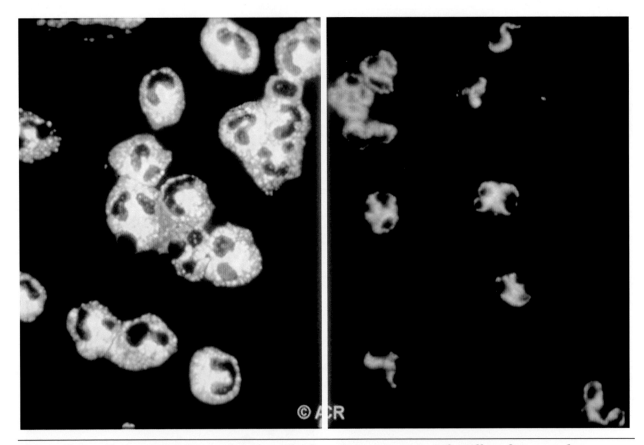

**Figure 19-41.** Antineutrophil cytoplasmic antibody staining patterns. *Left,* Diffuse fine granular, cytoplasmic staining pattern, characteristic of antineutrophil cytoplasmic antibody with cytoplasmic immunofluorescent pattern on ethanol-fixed neutrophils highly specific for Wegener's granulomatosis. *Right,* Perinuclear staining pattern, nonspecific and seen in polyarteritis nodosa, vasculitis associated with connective tissue diseases, and relapsing polychondritis. (From 1972–1999 American College of Rheumatology Clinical Slide Collection; with permission.)

Most patients have anemia and a markedly elevated erythrocyte sedimentation rate, typically, 60 to 110 mm/hour. Another useful systemic inflammatory marker is the plasma IL-6 level. A diagnostic 5- to 6-cm temporal artery biopsy is the best confirmatory test. Biopsy findings include panarteritis with predominant monocyte and lymphocyte infiltrates in about 50% of patients and the classic findings of granulomatous inflammation with multinucleated giant cells in the remainder. A contralateral artery biopsy improves diagnostic yield if a negative biopsy accompanies suspicious clinical signs. Angiography is a valuable tool for studying vessels such as the aorta or its large proximal branches that are not accessible for biopsy.

## Takayasu's Arteritis

Takayasu's arteritis, also known as "pulseless disease," is a chronic inflammatory arteritis that chiefly involves the aorta and its main branches, leading to wall thickening, stenosis, and thrombus formation.[42]

Clinical manifestations range from asymptomatic vascular bruits or reduced/absent peripheral pulses with blood pressure discrepancies detected incidentally on examination to intermittent claudication with use of the extremities or, infrequently, catastrophic cardiovascular and neurologic complications. Systemic inflammatory features include malaise, weight loss, fevers, arthralgia, and myalgia. The chronic phase involves fibrosis of all layers of the vessel wall, leading to patchy stenoses and aneurysm formation. Hypertension is common due to postinflammatory renal artery stenosis. Aortic root involvement resulting in coronary artery ostial narrowing or aortic regurgitation can present as anginal pectoris, CHF, or dilated cardiomyopathy. Neurologic manifestations can result from ischemia or hypertension. Pulmonary artery involvement is common and can lead to pulmonary arterial hypertension.

Although angiography constitutes the gold standard for diagnosis, noninvasive imaging modalities such as magnetic resonance angiography, computed tomography, and digital subtraction angiography may be helpful (Fig. 19-44). Doppler ultrasound can be used to assess the level of vessel wall inflammation. Histologic diagnosis is usually impractical given the type of vessel involvement but can be obtained when primary surgical intervention is required. Histopathologic findings in Takayasu's arteritis mirror those in giant cell arteritis, with the exception that giant cells and granulomas are decidedly rare.

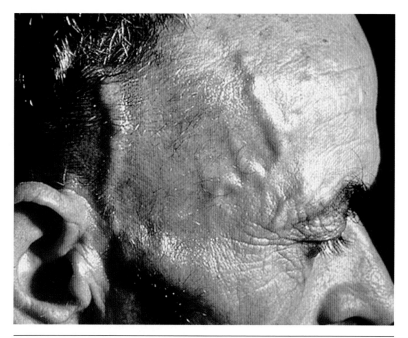

**Figure 19-42.** Temporal artery inflammation leading to tortuous, dilatated branches in giant cell arteritis. (From 1972–1999 American College of Rheumatology Clinical Slide Collection; with permission.)

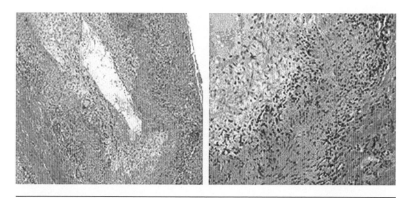

**Figure 19-43.** Giant-cell arteritis of the temporal artery. *Right,* Transmural inflammation of the temporal artery with granulomatous infiltrates in the media and giant cells at the media-intima border. *Left,* Close-up view of a segment of the media with several multinucleated giant cells adjacent to fragments of the internal elastic lamina. (Reproduced from Weyand CM, Goronzy JJ: Medium and large vessel vasculitis N Engl J Med 2003;349(2):160–169; with permission.)

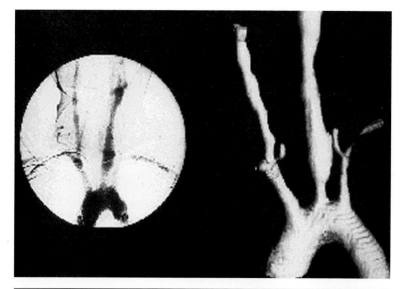

**Figure 19-44.** Magnetic resonance angiography *(left)* and three-dimensional computed tomography *(right)* showing stenosis of left subclavian artery and aneurysm formation of both carotid arteries. (Reproduced from Numano F, Okawara M, Inomata H, Kobayashi Y: Takayasu's arteritis. Lancet 2000;356:1023–1025; with permission.)

## MEDIUM-SIZE VESSEL VASCULITIS

### Polyarteritis Nodosa

Polyarteritis nodosa (PAN) is a necrotizing angiitis that chiefly affects medium-size arteries in a patchy distribution, often leading to aneurysm formation. The cutaneous, gastrointestinal, renal (nonglomerular), cardiac, and peripheral nervous system circulations are most commonly affected.

Onset is typically insidious, with weeks or months of constitutional symptoms punctuated by sudden vascular events from tissue ischemia. Fever, abdominal pain, weight loss, myalgia, and arthralgia represent common systemic symptoms. As many as a third of patients develop cutaneous findings, chiefly palpable purpura, sometimes accompanied by ulcerations. New-onset severe hypertension indicates renal vascular involvement, and severe flank pain may signal renal infarction or spontaneous intrarenal aneurysm rupture. *Mononeuritis multiplex* refers to a type of patchy, asymmetric, often widespread, mixed sensorimotor neuropathy due to ischemic injury to large nerves. The peroneal, median, ulnar, and sural nerves are commonly affected, and nerve involvement is often abrupt and irreversible. Cardiac manifestations include pericarditis, myocardial infarction secondary to coronary vasculitis, conduction system abnormalities, and CHF as a result of myocardial involvement. Mesenteric vasculitis causes dull and constant abdominal pain, often worsened by eating. Testicular pain and swelling can also result from ischemic arteritis.

Laboratory abnormalities in PAN, in addition to those pertaining to target organ involvement, reflect the underlying systemic inflammatory response and include anemia, leukocytosis, and elevated inflammatory markers (erythrocyte sedimentation rate, C-reactive protein). ANCAs are characteristically absent. Hepatitis B antigenemia may be detected.

Polyarteritis nodosa causes necrotizing vessel wall injury known as fibrinoid necrosis, with accumulation of plasma proteins, including coagulation factors, at sites of vascular injury (Fig. 19-45). Other pathologic findings include leukocytoclasis, prominent monocyte and neutrophil infiltration, and superimposed vascular thrombosis. Unfortunately, tissue specimens may yield nonspecific results. Skin and renal biopsies may show nondiagnostic inflammation, and a "blind" muscle biopsy is diagnostic about half the time. Visceral arteriography is the procedure of choice in patients with significant abdominal pain, often revealing widespread aneurysm formation in both the mesenteric and renal circulation (Fig. 19-46). Sural and common peroneal nerve biopsy is frequently rewarding in patients with clinical and electrodiagnostic evidence of neuropathy.

## SMALL VESSEL VASCULITIS

### Microscopic Polyangiitis

Microscopic polyangiitis is a "pauci-immune" necrotizing vasculitis that predominantly affects small-size blood vessels (i.e., capillaries, venules, or arterioles), with a predilection for the renal and pulmonary circulations.

The clinical presentation can range from insidious to rapidly progressive glomerulonephritis and pulmonary hemorrhage; occurring together, these symptoms are known as pulmonary-renal syndrome. Renal disease is almost always present, typically manifesting as renal insufficiency with active urinary sediment (microscopic hematuria with or without red cell casts). The characteristic lesion is a necrotizing glomerulonephritis with segmental necrosis and extravascular crescents, with scanty or no immune deposits visible on immunopathology. Lung involvement (more than 50% of cases) consists of diffuse alveolar hemorrhage with patchy or diffuse alveolar infiltrates on imaging (Fig. 19-47). Dyspnea and hemoptysis can occur but are not uniformly present. Accompanying constitutional symptoms include arthralgia, myalgia, fever, and skin involvement in the form of palpable purpura.

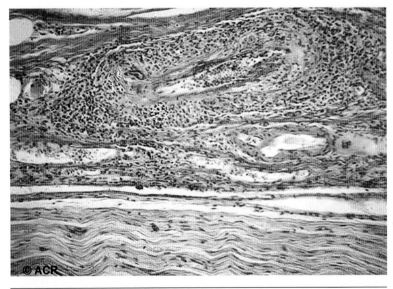

**Figure 19-45.** Sural nerve biopsy in polyarteritis nodosa. Necrotizing arteritis in the perineurium of the sural nerve with extensive inflammatory cell infiltration of the vessel wall. (From 1972–1999 American College of Rheumatology Clinical Slide Collection; with permission.)

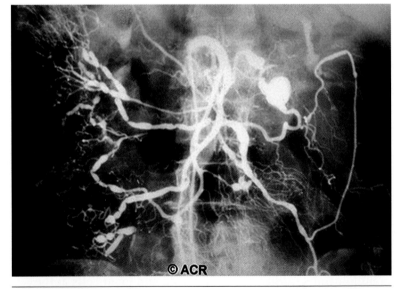

**Figure 19-46.** Mesenteric angiogram in polyarteritis nodosa. The superior mesenteric artery has multiple saccular aneurysms that vary in size and shape. (From 1972–1999 American College of Rheumatology Clinical Slide Collection; with permission.)

The majority of patients with microscopic polyangiitis are myeloperoxidase-ANCA positive, which is helpful in confirming the diagnosis. Histologically, microscopic polyangiitis often produces necrotizing vasculitis that is histologically identical to polyarteritis nodosa.

## Churg-Strauss Syndrome

Churg-Strauss syndrome (CSS) is a small- and medium-size blood vessel vasculitis distinguished by three chief histopathologic findings—necrotizing inflammation, eosinophilic infiltration, and extra-vascular granuloma formation.[43] A prominent atopic history of allergic rhinitis, adult-onset bronchial asthma, and hypereosinophilia consistently accompanies Churg-Strauss syndrome, suggesting more than coincidental development of vasculitis in patients with underlying asthma. Three distinct sequential clinical phases—asthma, tissue eosinophilia, and vasculitis—take place in most patients with Churg-Strauss syndrome.

Eosinophilic tissue infiltration can lead to eosinophilic pneumonia (Loeffler's syndrome) with nonspecific, fleeting pulmonary infiltrates and eosinophilic gastroenteritis. Peripheral nerve involvement occurs in the majority of patients and manifests as mononeuritis multiplex or either symmetric or asymmetric polyneuropathy. Other organs that can be affected include the skin, heart, skeletal muscle, joints, and eye. Skin disease characteristically takes the form of palpable purpura. Cardiac involvement may result in ventricular dysfunction as a consequence of epicardial granulomatous nodule formation, and less frequently secondary to coronary arteritis. Central nervous system and renal involvement are unusual.

Peripheral blood eosinophil counts often exceed 10,000/mm³ and serum IgE levels are characteristically increased. Typical high-yield biopsy sites include peripheral nerve, muscle, and lung when clinical evidence of involvement is present (Fig. 19-48). Subcutaneous extravascular granulomas with eosinophilic cores, which differ from those of sarcoidosis, further increase diagnostic specificity.

## Wegener's Granulomatosis

Wegener's granulomatosis (WG) is a granulomatous necrotizing vasculitis predominantly involving medium- and small-size vessels, with a predilection for the upper and lower respiratory tract and the kidney.

Disease course ranges from indolent to rapidly progressive and, if remission occurs, relapse is not uncommon. WG frequently involves the upper respiratory tract, leading to nasal obstruction, rhinorrhea, serosanguineous nasal discharge, oral and/or nasal ulcers, and nasal septal perforation and collapse, resulting in a "saddle nose" deformity (Fig. 19-49). Sinusitis, accompanied by radiographic evidence of erosive bone change, occurs in the majority of patients. Middle and inner ear involvement leads to otitis media with conductive and sensorineural hearing loss, and laryngotracheal disease characteristically produces subglottic stenosis. Lung involvement is seen in the majority of patients, and common symptoms include cough, dyspnea, hemoptysis, and pleurisy. The most common radiographic findings are pulmonary infiltrates and nodules in as many as one third of patients, even in the absence of respiratory symptoms. Pulmonary nodules are usually peripheral, multiple, bilateral, and frequently cavitate, whereas infiltrates tend to be fleeting in nature. Diffuse pulmonary hemorrhage is associated with a high mortality risk and is fortunately uncommon. Renal involvement usually follows respiratory disease, with clinical presentation ranging from asymptomatic to a fulminant glomerulonephritis. Typical histopathologic findings comprise focal and segmental glomerulonephritis with varying degrees of fibrinoid necrosis and proliferative change. Epithelial crescents and sclerotic lesions often

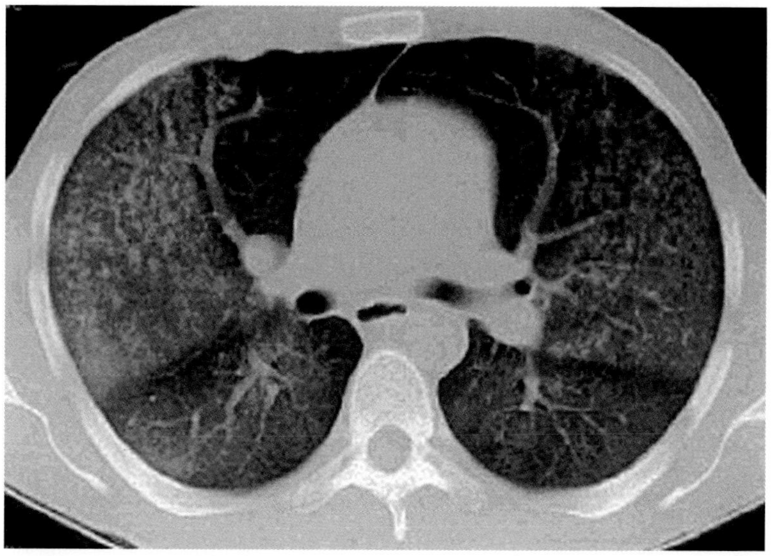

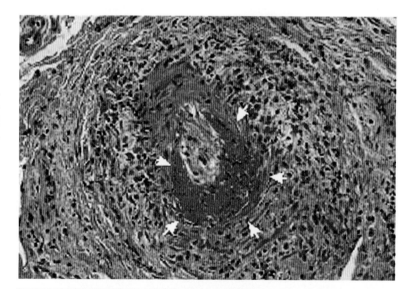

**Figure 19-47.** Computerized tomography of the chest in microscopic polyangiitis showing "ground glass" infiltrates suggestive of alveolar hemorrhage. (Reproduced from Langford CA: Vasculitis. J Allergy Clin Immunol 2003;111:S602–S612; with permission.)

**Figure 19-48.** A small submucosal pulmonary artery in Churg-Strauss vasculitis. There is pronounced, predominantly medial, eosinophilic infiltrate accompanied by fibrinoid necrosis of the inner wall. (Reproduced from Bili A, Condemi J, Bottone SM, Ryan CK: Seven cases of complete and incomplete forms of Churg-Strauss syndrome not related to leukotriene receptor antagonists. J Allergy Clin Immunol 1999;105(5):1060–1065; with permission.)

mark irreversible renal impairment. Immunofluorescence and electron microscopy are negative for immune complex deposits.

Ocular, cutaneous, musculoskeletal, and neurologic manifestations occur in as many as half of all patients with WG. All eye compartments can be affected, leading to nasolacrimal duct obstruction, keratitis, conjunctivitis, scleritis, episcleritis, uveitis, optic neuritis, retinal vessel occlusion, and retro-orbital pseudotumor. Skin findings include ulcers, palpable purpura, subcutaneous nodules, papules, and vesicles. Myalgia, arthralgias, and arthritis are common. Pericarditis, myocarditis, endocarditis, valvulitis, arrhythmia, conduction defects, and coronary vasculitis leading to myocardial ischemia have all been reported. Peripheral neuropathy, often presenting as mononeuritis multiplex, constitutes the most common neurologic manifestation.

Laboratory abnormalities include normocytic normochromic anemia, leukocytosis, thrombocytosis, and elevated erythrocyte sedimentation rate. Serum proteinase 3–ANCA antibodies are highly sensitive (about 90%) and highly specific (more than 90%) for WG, but titers of these antibodies have limited utility in either assessing disease activity or predicting relapse. Computed tomography is the preferred imaging modality for detecting respiratory tract disease. Microscopic urinalysis is valuable, and the presence of red blood cell casts confers a near-100% positive predictive value for active disease.

The triad of necrosis, granulomatous changes, and vasculitis in inflammatory lesions typifies the characteristic histologic changes that occur in WG (Fig. 19-50). Open lung biopsies by far have the highest yield, and nasopharyngeal biopsy is diagnostic in only half of the instances. Renal tissue characteristically shows focal and segmental necrotizing glomerulonephritis without vasculitis or granulomatous change.

## Hypersensitivity Vasculitis

*Hypersensitivity vasculitis* refers a family of vasculitic syndromes in which an aberrant immune response to an extrinsic stimulus is strongly implicated in causation. The distinguishing acute lesion, leukocytoclastic inflammation of dermal postcapillary venules, underlies the characteristic cutaneous manifestation of palpable purpura in dependent body areas (lower legs, feet; Fig. 19-51).[44] These lesions resolve with residual hyperpigmentation. Constitutional symptoms can include generalized arthralgias, fever, and malaise, but true synovitis is uncommon.

Laboratory findings are nonspecific but reflect mildly abnormal inflammatory markers. Histopathology reveals leukocytoclasis, which refers to the presence of residual dark-staining nuclear material from degenerating polymorphonuclear cells in the vessel walls, and fibrinoid necrosis.

A thorough clinical history frequently provides clues about the offending triggering antigen, usually a drug. Other causes of cutaneous vasculitis, as described previously, must be considered in the differential diagnosis. If visceral involvement occurs (e.g., the lung and kidney), microscopic polyangiitis may be the best diagnosis.

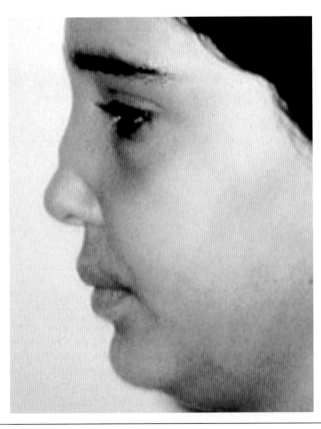

**Figure 19-49.** "Saddle nose" deformity in Wegener's granulomatosis. (From 1972–1999 American College of Rheumatology Clinical Slide Collection; with permission.)

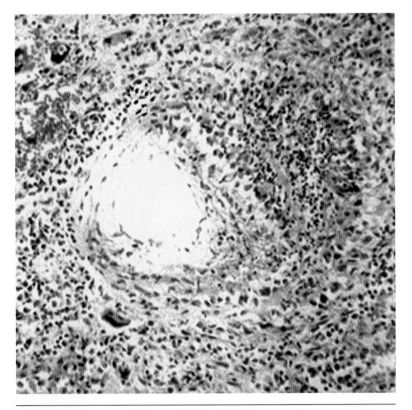

**Figure 19-50.** Lung histopathology in Wegener's granulomatosis. The pulmonary parenchyma has been entirely obliterated by a granulomatous inflammatory reaction bordering large necrotic areas. (From 1972–1999 American College of Rheumatology Clinical Slide Collection; with permission.)

## Henoch-Schönlein Purpura

Henoch-Schönlein purpura (HSP) is a multisystem, small-size vessel vasculitis that primarily involves young children and frequently manifests with a prominent cutaneous component.[44] The disease often follows a respiratory tract infection, and implicated agents include streptococcus, parvovirus, adenovirus, and mycoplasma.

A classic urticarial or palpable purpuric rash involving the extensor surfaces similar to that seen in hypersensitivity vasculitis is a disease hallmark (see Fig. 19-51). The majority of patients (60% to 80%) experience arthralgia of the ankles and knees. Gastrointestinal manifestations occur in about three quarters of patients and range from colicky abdominal pain, nausea, and vomiting to bowel hemorrhage and intussusception. Renal involvement has been reported in 20% to 100% and can also follow repeated attacks of cutaneous purpura, occurring over weeks or months. Hematuria with or without proteinuria is common, although acute nephritis with renal insufficiency and nephrotic range proteinuria may result. All HSP manifestations tend to resolve spontaneously, and renal prognosis is typically excellent. In a minority, especially in older children and adults, renal involvement can progress to chronic renal failure.

A number of IgA-related abnormalities have been described in HSP, including elevated serum IgA levels, circulating IgA immune complexes, and IgA class autoantibodies. Histopathology typically reveals leukocytoclastic vasculitis, with immunofluorescence positive for vascular IgA deposits. The primary renal lesion consists of a proliferative glomerulonephritis, with severity ranging from focal mesangial proliferation to frank crescent formation and mesangial deposition of IgA accompanied by IgG, C3, and fibrin.

## *PRINCIPLES OF MANAGEMENT*

The choice of therapy is largely determined by vasculitis type, disease activity and stage, and the risk-to-benefit ratio associated with the proposed intervention.[45] A major challenge lies in identifying regimens that are efficacious yet minimally toxic. Immunosuppressive therapy for active vasculitis can be envisaged as having two stages—an initial induction phase to achieve disease remission and a maintenance phase to preserve remission and prevent relapse.

The bulk of data on the treatment of systemic vasculitis derive from studies in WG. A treatment strategy that combines low-dose daily CYC with glucocorticoids has been shown to have superior efficacy in patients with immediately life-threatening disease. The high toxicity associated with long-term CYC exposure has led to the emergence of staged regimens that utilize this combination for inducing remission followed by transition to a less-toxic drug (e.g., methotrexate, azathioprine, or mycophenolate mofetil) for remission maintenance. The use of methotrexate with glucocorticoids has been shown to be effective for inducing remission in patients who do not have life-threatening disease. In the absence of prospective long-term studies addressing optimal therapy for microscopic polyangiitis to date, patients with severe active disease (pulmonary hemorrhage, glomerulonephritis) are treated in a manner similar to WG patients.

Efforts to identify an optimally efficacious regimen for PAN led to establishment of the "five factor score" to stage initial disease. Renal insufficiency, proteinuria, gastrointestinal involvement, cardiomyopathy, and central nervous system involvement adversely impact on outcome, and the cumulative occurrence of these factors has been found to correlate with increasing mortality. An initial combined regimen of CYC and glucocorticoids for patients with life-threatening disease or a five factor score indicating poor prognosis is presently recommended. In selected patients with active but nonsevere disease, treatment with prednisone alone with the option to subsequently add CYC for unresponsive or worsening disease deserves consideration. It is important to institute concomitant antiviral treatment for PAN associated with hepatitis B and rapidly withdraw primary immunosuppression once the active vasculitis has subsided.

Glucocorticoids comprise the mainstay of treatment for large-size vessel vasculitis such as Takayasu's arteritis and giant cell arteritis. Other immunosuppressive therapy is considered in patients with persistently active disease despite optimal glucocorticoid treatment or in those unable to tolerate the required glucocorticoid doses, although insufficient evidence to date supports the effectiveness of methotrexate or azathioprine as a steroid-sparing agent.

Henoch-Schönlein purpura and hypersensitivity vasculitis are self-limited illnesses in most cases. Glucocorticoids appear to have a role in improving gastrointestinal and joint symptoms in HSP. Impaired renal function, proteinuria (greater than 1.5 g/day), and hypertension at presentation are adverse prognostic factors in adults with HSP, and aggressive treatment with glucocorticoids and a cytotoxic agent has been shown to positively impact outcome in such cases.

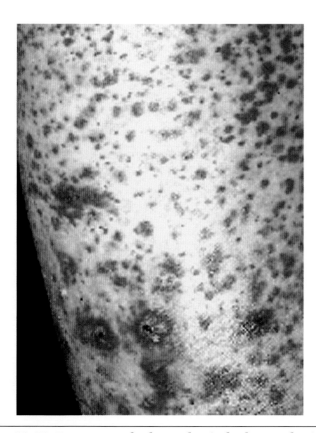

**Figure 19-51.** Purpura on the lower leg in leukocytoclastic angiitis, also seen in Henoch-Schönlein Purpura. (Reproduced from Jennette JC, Falk RJ: Small vessel vasculitis. N Engl J Med 1997;337(21):1512–1523; with permission.)

# REFERENCES

1. Kelley WN, Harris ED Jr, Ruddy S, Sledge CB (eds): Textbook of Rheumatology, 4th ed. Philadelphia, WB Saunders, 1993.

2. Firestein GS: Evolving concepts of rheumatoid arthritis. Nature 2003;423:356–361.

3. Choy EHS, Panayi GS: Cytokine pathways and joint inflammation in rheumatoid arthritis. N Engl J Med 2001;344(12):907–916.

4. Lee DM, Weinblatt ME: Rheumatoid arthritis. Lancet 2001;358:903–911.

5. Smolen JS, Steiner G: Therapeutic strategies for rheumatoid arthritis nature reviews drug discovery. 2003;2:473–488.

6. Goldbach-Mansky R, Lipsky PE: New concepts in the treatment of rheumatoid arthritis. Ann Rev Med 2003;54:197–216.

7. Feldmann M: Development of anti-TNF therapy for rheumatoid arthritis. Nat Rev Immunol 2002;2:364–371.

8. Taylor PC: Anti-cytokines and cytokines in the treatment of rheumatoid arthritis. Curr Pharm Des 2003;9:1095–1106.

9. Kelley WN, Harris ED Jr, Ruddy S, Sledge CB (eds): Textbook of Rheumatology, 4th ed. Philadelphia, WB Saunders, 1993.

10. Mok CC, Lau CS: Pathogenesis of systemic lupus erythematosus. J Clin Pathol 2003;56:481–490.

11. Ruiz-Irastorza G, Khamashta MA, Castellino G, Hughes GRV: Systemic lupus erythematosus. Lancet 2001;357:1027–1032.

12. Kewalramani R, Singh AK: Immunopathogenesis of lupus and lupus nephritis: Recent insights. Curr Opin Nephrol Hypertens 2002;11:273–277.

13. Scolding NJ, Joseph FG: The neuropathology and pathogenesis of systemic lupus erythematosus. Neuropathol Appl Neurobiol 2002;28:173–189.

14. Wallace DJ: Systemic lupus erythematosus. Drugs Today 2002;38(4): 259–263.

15. Wallace DJ: Management of lupus erythematosus: Recent insights. Curr Opin Rheumatol 2002;14(3):212–219.

16. Medsger TA Jr: Classification, prognosis. In Clements PJ, Furst DE (eds): Systemic Sclerosis, 2nd ed. Philadelphia, Lippincott Williams & Wilkins, 2003, pp 17–28.

17. Mayes MD, Reveille JD: Epidemiology, demographics, and genetics. In Clements PJ, Furst DE (eds): Systemic Sclerosis, 2nd ed. Philadelphia, Lippincott Williams & Wilkins, 2003, pp 1–16.

18. Smith EA: Systemic sclerosis: Etiology and pathogenesis. In Hochberg MC, Silman AJ, Smolen JS, et al (eds): Rheumatology, 3rd ed. Sjögren's Syndrome. Philadelphia, Mosby, 2003, pp 1481–1492.

19. Silver RM, Clements PJ: Interstitial lung disease in systemic sclerosis: Optimizing evaluation and management. Scleroderma Care Res 2003;1:3–11.

20. Barst RJ, Seibold JR: Pulmonary arterial hypertension related to systemic sclerosis: A primer for the rheumatologist. Scleroderma Care Res 2003; 1:12–20.

21. Steen VD, Costantino JP, Shapiro AP, Medsger TA Jr: Outcome of renal crisis in systemic sclerosis: Relation to availability of angiotensin converting enzyme (ACE) inhibitors. Ann Intern Med 1990;113:352–357.

22. Denton CP, Black CM: Management of systemic sclerosis. In Hochberg MC, Silman AJ, Smolen JS, et al (eds): Rheumatology, 3rd ed. Sjögren's Syndrome. Philadelphia, Mosby, 2003, pp 1493–1506.

23. Oddis CV, Medsger TA Jr: Inflammatory muscle disease: Clinical features. In Hochberg MC, Silman AJ, Smolen JS, et al (eds): Rheumatology, 3rd ed. London, Elsevier Limited, 2003, pp 1537–1554.

24. Calabrese LH, Mitsumoto H, Chou SM: Inclusion body myositis presenting as treatment resistant polymyositis. Arthritis Rheum 1987;30:397–403.

25. Ohosone Y, Ishida M, Takahashi Y, et al: Spectrum and clinical significance of auto-antibodies against transfer RNA. Arthritis Rheum 1998;41:1625–1631.

26. Nagaraju N, Plotz PH, Miller FW: Etiology and pathogenesis. In Hochberg MC, Silman AJ, Smolen JS, et al (eds): Rheumatology, 3rd ed. London, Elsevier Limited, 2003, pp 1523–1535.

27. Miller FW: Inflammatory myopathies: polymyositis, dermatomyositis, and related conditions. In Koopman WJ (ed): Arthritis and Allied Conditions, 14th ed. Philadelphia, Lippincott Williams & Wilkins, 2001, pp 1562–1589.

28. Catoggio L: Management. In Hochberg MC, Silman AJ, Smolen JS, et al (eds): Rheumatology, 3rd ed. London, Elsevier Limited, 2003, pp 1555–1562.

29. Tzioufas AG, Moutsopoulos HM: Sjogren's syndrome. In Hochberg MC, Silman AJ, Smolen JS, et al (eds): Rheumatology, 3rd ed. Philadelphia, Mosby, 2003, pp 1431–1443.

30. Vitali C, Bmbardieri S, Moutsopoulos HM, et al: Preliminary criteria for the classification of Sjögren's syndrome. Results of a prospective concerted action supported by the European Community. Arthritis Rheum 1992;36:340–348.

31. Daniels TE, Aufdemorte TB, Greenspan JS: Histopatholgy of Sjögren's syndrome. In Talal N, Moutsopoulos HM, Kassan SS (eds): Sjögren's Syndrome: Clinical and Immunological Aspects. Berlin, Springer-Verlag, 1987, pp 266–286.

32. Tzioufas AG, Moutsopoulos HM: Clinical significance of antibodies to Ro/SSA and La/SSB. In Maini R, van Venrooij V (eds): The Manual of Autoantigens-Antibodies. Berlin, Dordrecht-Kluwer, 1996, pp 1–14.

33. Skopouli FN, Dafni U, Ionnidis JP, Moutsopoulos HM: Clinical evolution, and morbidity and mortality of primary Sjögren's syndrome. Semin Arthritis Rheum 2000;29:296–304.

34. Voulgarelis M, Dafni UG, Isenberg DA, Moutsopoulos HM: Malignant lymphoma in primary Sjögren's syndrome: A multicenter, retrospective clinical study by the European Concerted Action on Sjögren's Syndrome. Arthritis Rheum 1999;42:1765–1772.

35. Fox RI, Michelson P: Approaches to the treatment of Sjögren's syndrome. J Rheumatol 2000;61(suppl):15–21.

36. Kelley WN, Harris ED Jr, Ruddy S, Sledge CB (eds): Textbook of Rheumatology, 4th ed. Philadelphia, WB Saunders, 1993.

37. Weyand CM, Goronzy JJ: Medium and large vessel vasculitis. N Engl J Med 2003;349(2):160–169.

38. Jennette JC, Falk RJ: Small vessel vasculitis. N Engl J Med 1997;337(21): 1512–1523.

39. Luqmani RA, Robinson H: Introduction to, and classification of, the systemic vasculitides. Best Pract Res Clin Rheumatol 2001;15(2):187–202.

40. Cid MC, Vilardell C: Tissue targeting and disease patterns in systemic vasculitis. Best Pract Res Clin Rheumatol 2001;15(2):259–279.

41. Hewins P, Savage C: Anti-neutrophil cytoplasm antibody associated vasculitis. Int J Biochem Cell Biol 2003;35:277–282.

42. Numano F, Okawara M, Inomata H, Kobayashi Y: Takayasu's arteritis. Lancet 2000;356:1023–1025.

43. Noth I, Strek ME, Leff AR: Churg Strauss syndrome. Lancet 2003;361:587–594.

44. Stone JH, Nousari HC: "Essential" cutaneous vasculitis: What every rheumatologist should know about vasculitis of the skin. Curr Opin Rheumatol 2001;13:23–34.

45. Langford CA: Management of systemic vasculitis. Best Pract Res Clin Rheumatol 2001;15(2):281–297.

*Philip Fireman*

# *20* Primary Immunodeficiency Diseases

Immunodeficiency diseases range from severe, life-threatening disorders to mild or even asymptomatic conditions. On occasion, they need to be considered in the differential diagnosis of allergic diseases. In these cases, one or more abnormalities of the immune system impair the host's defense mechanisms and result in an increase in susceptibility to infections. Immunodeficiency should be suspected in any patient who has frequent or recurrent infections. Immunodeficiency diseases, however, are relatively uncommon, and many other illnesses may predispose a patient to repeated infections.

Box 20-1 lists and groups these varied conditions according to the mechanisms by which they predispose a patient to repeated infection. If the immune system is intact, some of the listed illnesses, such as dysfunctional cilia syndrome, may actually manifest hypergammaglobulinemia as an increased immune response

to repeated infections. With persistent or recurrent respiratory symptoms, allergy also may be suspected. A thorough patient history and physical examination identify many of these illnesses, and a correct diagnosis can be confirmed by the appropriate laboratory tests. If the clinician has considered and excluded these other, more common clinical syndromes, it is then reasonable to suspect a defect or deficiency of the patient's immune mechanism.

As outlined in Box 20-1, immunodeficiency may be either primary or secondary. Primary immunodeficiencies are divided into four major categories, depending on the portion of the host defense system that is affected.[1] As shown in Box 20-2, these primary immune defects include deficiencies of antibodies (B-lymphocytes), cell-mediated immunity (T-lymphocytes), phagocytic cells, and complement systems. Secondary immunodeficiencies occur in previously healthy individuals who, as a result of some

---

**BOX 20-1**

**Conditions That Increase Host Susceptibility to Infection with Selected Examples**

**Primary Immunodeficiency**
X-linked hypogammaglobulinemia
Severe combined immunodeficiency disease (SCID)
DiGeorge syndrome

**Secondary Immunodeficiency**
AIDS
Lymphoma
Malnutrition
Immunosuppression therapy

**Mucosal Skin Barrier Disorders**
Dysfunctional cilia syndrome
Eczema
Burns
Sinus tract disorders

**Obstructive Disorders**
Cystic fibrosis
Asthma
Eustachian tube obstruction

**Circulatory Disorders**
Sickle cell disease
Diabetes
Congenital heart disease

**Foreign Bodies**
Venous and urinary catheters
Aspirated objects
Artificial heart valves

**Unusual Microbiologic Factors**
Antibiotic overgrowth
Contaminated respiratory equipment
Infectious contact

intercurrent illness or exposure, manifest compromised or defective immune responses.[2] The most severe and devastating of these is AIDS. Although AIDS is, to date, irreversible, other secondary immune defects are reversible if the underlying condition or illness is corrected. The secondary immunodeficiencies are outlined in Box 20-3 and are considerably more common than primary immunodeficiencies.

# EPIDEMIOLOGY

The true prevalence of immunodeficiency is unknown. Good data are difficult to obtain because physicians are not required to report these diagnoses. In addition, as new immunologic technologies are being developed, additional diseases are being diagnosed. It is estimated that one case of primary immunodeficiency occurs in every 10,000 individuals.[3] The genetically determined primary deficiencies are rare. In the United States, it is estimated that X-linked agammaglobulinemia occurs with a frequency of 1:50,000, and severe combined immunodeficiency disease (SCID), with an approximate frequency of 1:200,000 live births. Many primary immunodeficiencies are hereditary and congenital. Consequently, most of these illnesses are recognized in childhood, with individuals younger than 20 years comprising about 80% of the cases. During childhood, there is a 5:1 male-to-female sex predominance for these disorders. This is reversed in adults, with a slight (1:1.4) predominance in females. As better methods of managing and treating these syndromes are developed, it is anticipated that many of these patients will survive into adulthood.

Among the immunodeficiency syndromes, B-cell immunoglobulin or antibody defects are most common. In fact, isolated immunoglobulin (Ig) A deficiency may have an incidence of one per 700 individuals.[4] If IgA deficiency is excluded, B-cell defects make up about 50% of the immunodeficiency syndromes (Fig. 20-1). T-cell deficiencies make up about 30%, with 10% of these conditions being T-cell defects, and 20% being combined T and humoral antibody defects. Therefore, a defect of B-cell function is present in more than 70% of all primary immune defects. Various defects of neutrophil and phagocyte function comprise about 20%, with complement abnormalities being the least common (less than 1%).

**BOX 20-2**
**The Four Major Categories of Primary Immunodeficiency**

Antibody (B-lymphocyte) deficiency
Cell-mediated (T-lymphocyte) deficiency
      T-cell deficiency alone or with B-cell deficiency
Phagocytic deficiency
Complement deficiency

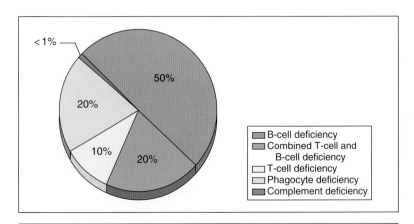

**Figure 20-1.** The relative distribution of the primary immunodeficiency syndromes.

# DEVELOPMENT OF THE IMMUNE SYSTEM

Cellular (T-cell) and humoral (B-cell) immunity develops from fetal pluripotent hematopoietic stem cells (Fig. 20-2). The initial pleuripotent progenitors are detectable at about the 4th week of pregnancy. By 5 to 6 weeks of gestation, these cells appear in the liver, which at this time is the major site of development. Precursor cells are found in the thymus by the 8th week. Stem cells do not appear in the bone marrow until the 12th week of gestation.[5] These same bone marrow stem cells are also the source of polymorphonuclear leukocytes, macrophages, and monocytes, which also participate in host defense. In response to signals from the host's internal environment, these stem cells generate large numbers of lymphocytes that mature into T- and B-lymphocytes

that become capable of antigen responsiveness.[6] The thymus-dependent T-lymphocytes become responsible for cell-mediated immune responses directed against common pathogens, such as viruses and fungi. Patients with T-cell defects have severe infections with organisms such as candida that usually cause mild or limited infections in normal individuals. T-lymphocytes are also important in the expression of tumor cytotoxicity and homograft rejection. T-lymphocytes collaborate in immunoregulation of B-cell function via subpopulations of T-helper (Th; $CD_4$) and T-suppressor ($CD_8$) lymphocytes. Isolated T-cell deficiencies are uncommon.

Also derived from pluripotential stem cells, the B-lymphocytes promote the development of plasma cells. Plasma cells secrete the Igs that have functional capacity for antigen recognition and are defined as antibodies. A lack of one or more of the Ig isotypes (IgG, IgA, IgM) constitutes humoral or serum antibody immunodeficiency, which may or may not be accompanied by decreased

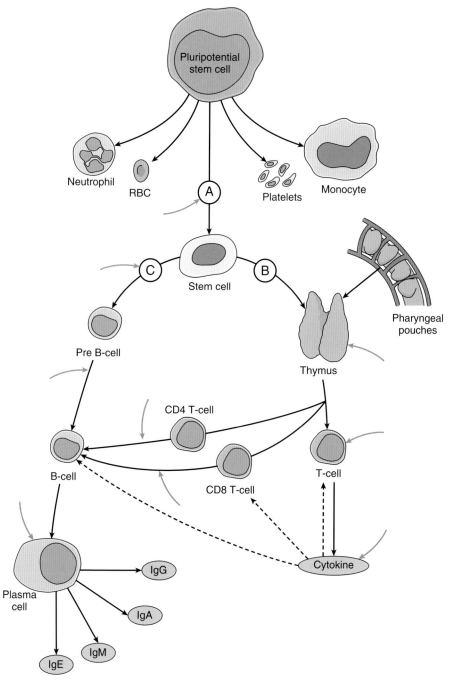

**Figure 20-2.** T- and B-lymphocyte development from stem cells. *Arrows* indicate the various potential sites of abnormal development. Immune cell defects along *pathway A* result in combined T-cell and B-cell immunodeficiencies. Defects at several sites along *pathways B* and *C* result in the various T-cell and B-cell deficiencies. CD4 (Helper) T-cell, CD8 (Suppressor) T-Cell; Ig, immunoglobulin; RBC, red blood cell.

peripheral blood B cells. A few patients with normal numbers of B cells and plasma cells, as well as normal serum Ig levels, are nonetheless immunodeficient because they lack functional antibodies. Primary immunodeficiencies result from abnormalities in expression of B cells with resultant antibody deficiency and/or T cells.

In the developing fetus, T cells begin to appear between the 8th and 10th weeks of gestation and are promptly accompanied by the presence of B cells (Fig. 20-3). Appreciable Ig synthesis directed by these B cells, however, does not usually occur during fetal development; maternal serum IgG does begin to appear in fetal serum by the middle of the second trimester. Through an active placental transport mechanism, maternal IgG continues to increase in fetal serum and at the time of birth achieves a fetal cord serum concentration of 110% that of adults. Maternal serum IgM, IgA, and IgE do not normally cross the placenta. After delivery, the maternal IgG in the infant's serum decreases, being catabolized with a half-life of 3 weeks; it is usually not detectable after 6 months of age. The synthesis of the infant's endogenous serum IgM, IgG, IgA, and IgE increases after birth, as indicated in

Figure 20-3. Therefore, for the first several months of age, the infant's serum IgG is a sum of maternal (exogenous) and infant (endogenous) IgG. Lowest IgG levels occur at 3 to 4 months of age. If the infant's endogenous synthesis of IgG is temporarily delayed, a transient or physiologic hypogammaglobulinemia of infancy can occur, as described later.[7] If there is an intrauterine infection with antigenic stimulation, then appreciable IgM may be synthesized, along with lesser amounts of IgA and IgG, by the fetus prior to delivery. This IgM is detectable in cord blood for serologic diagnosis of intrauterine disease.

# ANTIBODY (B-CELL) DEFICIENCIES

Antibody deficiencies, also called humoral immunodeficiencies, are characterized by low serum levels of one or more Igs and/or impairment of antibody responses to various antigen exposures. This may result from a defect intrinsic to B-cell function or a failure of communication between B and T cells. Cell-mediated

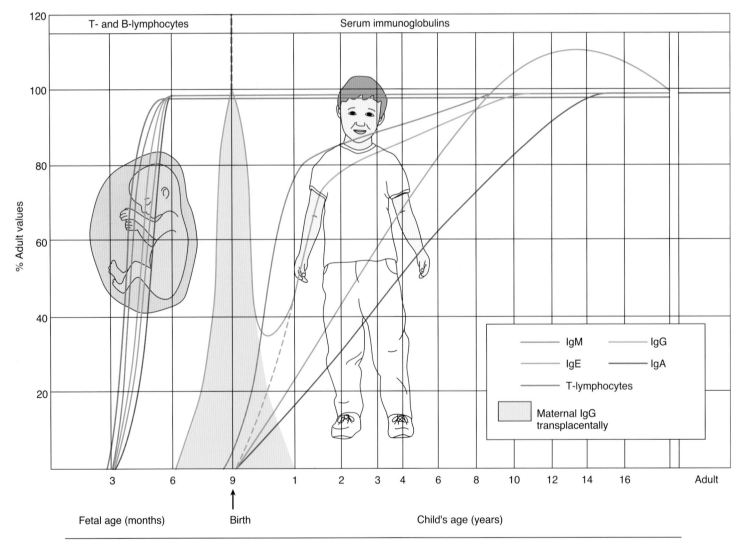

**Figure 20-3.** Both T-lymphocytes and B-lymphocytes appear in fetal tissues at as early as 8 to 12 weeks of development. B-lymphocytes capable of initiating immunoglobulin (Ig) G, IgA, and IgM synthesis are present by 12 weeks' gestation. Serum IgG, IgA, IgM, and IgE as percentages of the normal adult values in the fetus, child, adolescent, and adult are presented.

immunity as expressed by T-cell function is intact. Table 20-1 groups the humoral antibody deficiencies according to those with known gene defects and those clinically well-defined syndromes in which a genetic basis is not evident at this time.

## X-LINKED AGAMMAGLOBULINEMIA

This disease was the first primary immunodeficiency recognized and was described in 1952 by Colonel Bruton.[8] Thus, this condition is often called "Bruton's agammaglobulinemia." It is caused by a defect in a signal transducing protein known as Bruton's tyrosine kinase.[9] Bruton's tyrosine kinase transduces signals from the B-cell Ig receptor and is expressed in B-cells at all stages of development. In its absence, B-cell development is compromised early on at the pro–B-cell to pre–B-cell transition. Only males are affected, and females are the carriers of this congenital defect.[10] During the first few months of life, affected infants usually appear clinically well due to placentally acquired maternal antibodies, which provide passive immunity. As the maternal antibodies are catabolized with a half-life of 3 to 4 weeks, these infants develop recurrent or chronic infections at 6 to 12 months of age with virulent bacterial pathogens, such as *Streptococcus pneumoniae* and *Haemophilius influenzae*. Despite normal cell-mediated (T-cell) immunity, these children are prone to certain viral infections, especially enteroviruses and live vaccine-associated poliomyelitis. However, they are usually not susceptible to severe measles or fungal infections. Upper and lower respiratory tract infections, such as sinusitis, otitis media, and pneumonia, are most common. Sepsis, meningitis, and skin infections also occur. As a result of these infections, bronchiectasis can develop, with chronic cough, increased sputum production, and abnormal chest radiographs (Fig. 20-4A). These children have little adenoidal, tonsillar, and other lymphoid tissues (Fig. 20-5); what lymphoid tissues they do possess lack plasma cells able to produce Ig and lack the ability to form germinal follicles in response to antigen (see Fig. 20-4B). In any child who has recurrent infections with virulent bacterial pathogens, the diagnosis of hypogammaglobulinemia should be considered and confirmed by finding markedly decreased serum IgG, IgA, and IgM, as well as decreased circulating B-lymphocytes. Survival to adulthood is possible with early diagnosis and therapy with monthly γ-globulin replacement, accompanied by prompt antibiotic therapy directed against the infectious organisms.

## AUTOSOMAL-RECESSIVE AGAMMAGLOBULINEMIA

A few patients have been described who have agammaglobulinemia with autosomal-recessive inheritance. As shown in Table 20-1, several genetic mutations have been described that also can arrest B-cell development at an early stage.[11] Clinically, these patients are phenotypically similar to the X-linked agammaglobulinemia patients and also should be treated with monthly intravenous gammaglobulin replacement therapy and appropriate prompt antibiotics for infections.

**TABLE 20-1**

**Classification of Humoral Immunodeficiencies**

| Classification | Gene Defect |
|---|---|
| **Defined Genetic Basis** | |
| X-linked (Bruton's) agammaglobulinemia due to mutation of Bruton's tyrosine kinase (Btk) | *Btk* |
| Autosomal-recessive agammaglobulinemia due to | |
| Mutation of IgM constant region (Cμ) | *IGHM* |
| Mutation of signal transducing molecule Ig-α | *CD79A* |
| Mutation of surrogate light chain | *CD179B* |
| Mutation of B-cell linker protein | *BLNK* |
| Hyper-IgM syndrome | |
| X-linked due to mutation of tumor necrosis factor superfamily member 5 (CD154, CD40 ligand) | *TNFSF5* |
| Autosomal-recessive due to mutation of activation-induced cytidine deaminase | *AICDA* |
| **Unknown Genetic Basis** | |
| Common variable immunodeficiency | |
| IgA deficiency | |
| IgG subclass deficiency | |
| Specific antibody deficiency with normal immunoglobulins | |
| Transient hypogammaglobulinemia of infancy | |

Ig, immunoglobulin.

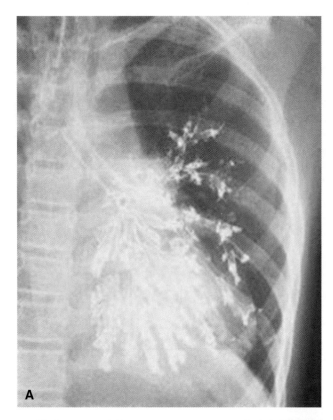

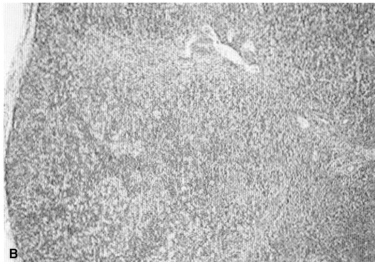

**Figure 20-4.** *A,* Bronchogram demonstrating bronchiectasis of the left lower lobe in an older child with hypogammaglobulinemia. Symptoms consisted of chronic cough and sputum production. The child was treated with antibiotics and γ-globulin replacement. *B,* Low-power photomicrograph of a lymph node biopsy from a 1-year-old child with hypogammaglobulinemia. No lymphoid follicles are visible, and no germinal centers are detected. Most of the node is paracortex, characterized by the presence of high-walled venules and a "starry sky" appearance. No immunoglobulin-producing plasma cells were detected in this section. (Hematoxylin and eosin stain, ×121.) (*A,* Reproduced from Skoner DP, Stillwagen PK, Friedman R, Fireman P: Pediatric Allergy and Immunology. In Zittelli BJ, Davis HW (eds.) Atlas of Pediatric Diagnosis. New York, Gower, 1987, p4.16; with permission. *B,* Courtesy of Dr. Ronald Jaffe, Children's Hospital, Pittsburgh, PA.

## IMMUNODEFICIENCY WITH HYPER-IMMUNOGLOBULIN M

This X-linked recessive disease of males, sometimes referred to as "hyper-IgM syndrome," is characterized by low IgG and low IgA but normal or elevated polyclonal IgM, with normal numbers of B-lymphocytes (see Table 20-1). The numbers of T-lymphocytes are also normal, but the interactions of T cells with antigen-presenting cells are impaired. Within the first 2 years of life, these patients have increased and recurrent pyrogenic respiratory tract infections and may also have neutropenia and manifest autoimmune disorders. They are prone to opportunistic infections from *Pneumocytosis* and fungal organisms. This immunodeficiency

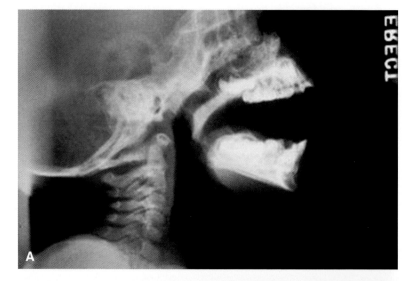

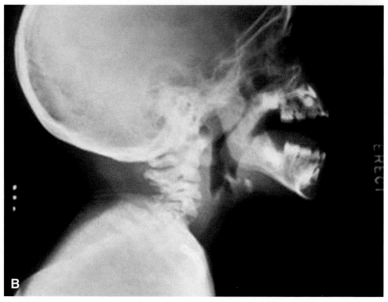

**Figure 20-5.** *A,* Lateral neck radiograph showing absent adenoid shadow in a child with congenital hypogammaglobulinemia. *B,* Lateral neck radiograph showing normal adenoid shadows in a child with no immunodeficiency. (Reproduced from Skoner DP, Stillwagen PK, Friedman R, Fireman P: Pediatric Allergy and Immunology. In Zittelli BJ, Davis HW (eds.) Atlas of Pediatric Diagnosis. New York, Gower, 1987, p4.16; with permission.)

is due to a mutation of the tumor necrosis factor super-family member 5 gene.[12] This molecule is also called CD154 or CD40 ligand. Because of this molecular defect of T cells that prevents Ig class switching from IgM to IgG, some immunologists would consider this disease to be a combined T- and B-cell immune deficiency. Therapy is the same as for X-linked agammaglobulinemia. An autosomal-recessive form of hyper-IgM syndrome has been described (see Table 20-1), but the pathophysiology is identical, and the same cellular interactions are affected.

## COMMON VARIABLE IMMUNODEFICIENCY

Patients with common variable immunodeficiency also present with recurrent infections (see Table 20-1). There is considerable variability in the clinical course of this syndrome, as well as in the serum IgG, IgA, and IgM levels (which, on occasion, may even appear normal).[13] This syndrome probably encompasses a group of potentially distinct conditions that have their onset most often in the 1st to 3rd decade of life. Widespread lymphoproliferation may be present with adrenopathy and splenomegaly. There is also an increased risk of gastrointestinal and lymphoid malignancy. Even though a familial pattern has been described in a few patients, no well-defined molecular defects have yet been established. Unlike X-linked agammaglobulinemia, B cells may be present in the blood and tissues of common variable immunodeficiency patients, even though tissue plasma cells are deficient. In addition to recurrent sinopulmonary infections, these patients frequently have gastrointestinal complaints and may manifest gastroenteropathy. They also have an increased number of auto-antibodies and may manifest symptoms of collagen-vascular disease. Documentation of functional antibody deficiency is helpful. Defective T-cell immunoregulation has been described in some patients, but clinical expression of T-cell deficiency is rarely observed. Replacement therapy with monthly intravenous gammaglobulin infusions is indicated and helpful in reducing infections and complications.

## IMMUNOGLOBULIN G SUBCLASS DEFICIENCY

Immunoglobulin G consists of four subclasses: $IgG_1$, $IgG_2$, $IgG_3$, and $IgG_4$. The $IgG_1$ subclass accounts for 67% of total IgG and shows antibody activity to most microbial protein antigens, such as tetanus and diphtheria. The $IgG_2$ subclass accounts for 23% of total IgG and contains antibodies to microbial polysaccharide antigens, such as *S. pneumoniae* and *H. influenzae* capsular antigens. $IgG_3$ antibody activities make up about 7% of the total IgG. $IgG_4$ antibodies (3% of total IgG) may mimic IgE antibody with its capacity to initiate histamine release from basophils and mast cells.

Some patients with recurrent infections and low-normal IgG levels have been found to have a deficiency of $IgG_1$ and/or $IgG_2$.[14] There is controversy with regard to this diagnosis because of variations in Ig subclass determination depending on differences in laboratory methodology as well as age and ethnicity of patients. These patients have recurrent infections of the respiratory tract but do not usually have a paucity of lymphoid tissue. Laboratory confirmation of these IgG subclass deficiencies also requires documentation of functional antibody deficiency prior to initiating a therapeutic program of prophylactic antibiotics and, if not successful, institution of replacement IgG therapy.

## SELECTIVE IMMUNOGLOBULIN A DEFICIENCY

Selective IgA deficiency is the most common humoral antibody deficiency, affecting about 1 of every 700 individuals.[4] Less than 50% of these affected individuals manifest recurrent infections, while the remainder, despite mucosal, secretory, and serum IgA deficiencies, are clinically well and asymptomatic. These patients typically have normal IgG and IgM levels. Most cases are sporadic, but siblings may manifest IgA or other immunodeficiencies. Recurrent infections of the sinuses (Fig. 20-6) and middle ear are frequent, but lower respiratory disease is unusual, unless another form of immunodeficiency, such as $IgG_2$ subclass deficiency, coexists with the IgA deficiency.[15] IgA-deficient patients have an increased incidence of allergy, chronic diarrhea, neoplasia, collagen vascular disorders, and autoimmune syndromes. Although IgA deficiency has been described in a few families, no genetic defect has been found. Gammaglobulin therapy is contraindicated because of risk of anaphylaxis due to presence or development of IgA antibodies.

## TRANSIENT HYPOGAMMAGLOBULINEMIA OF INFANCY

Transient hypogammaglobulinemia of infancy is a self-limiting antibody deficiency that begins at 3 to 6 months of age and usually resolves spontaneously by 24 to 48 months of age.[7] These infants may or may not have increased susceptibility to infection, and physical examination may reveal a paucity of tonsils and lymph

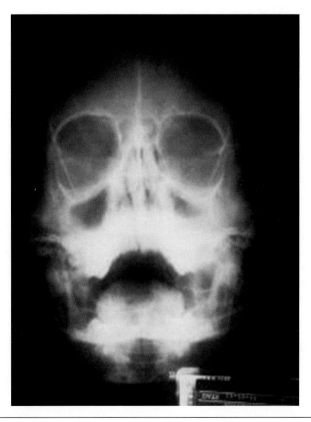

**Figure 20-6.** Maxillary sinusitis shown in this water's view x-ray of a child with immunoglobulin A deficiency. (Courtesy of Dr. Gilbert Friday, Children's Hospital, Pittsburgh, PA.)

nodes. This, however, is not always the case. Thrush is uncommon. These infants show the usual decline in placentally transferred Igs over the first months of life, but they fail to synthesize IgG until much later than normal. Serum IgM and IgA develop normally and help distinguish transient hypogammaglobulinemia from X-linked agammaglobulinemia. Circulating B cells are normal or near-normal in number and distribution, and a thymus is present on chest radiography. These patients have normal antibody responses to diphtheria and tetanus toxoids, usually well before the IgG levels become normal. Premature infants are especially prone to this disorder because of the lower levels of transplacental IgG at birth (see Fig. 20-3). While exogenous γ-globulin replacement therapy is occasionally used, it is temporary, as spontaneous recovery occurs. Levels of Igs become normal by 2 to 4 years of age. Following recovery, there is no recurrence or evidence of permanent immune system abnormality.

## SPECIFIC ANTIBODY DEFICIENCY WITH NORMAL IMMUNOGLOBULINS

There exists a rare group of patients with recurrent infections and poor antibody response, mostly to pneumococcal polysaccharide antigens, who have normal levels of serum IgG, IgA, IgM, and IgG subclasses. This syndrome has also been called functional antibody deficiency.[16] These patients typically have recurrent sinopulmonary infections and are clinically very similar to patients with IgG subclass deficiency. However, other immunologists categorize this condition as a variant of common variable immunodeficiency. No genetic defect has been identified.

# T-LYMPHOCYTE IMMUNODEFICIENCIES

T-lymphocytes are essential components of the immune response. Through cytolytic activity and Th1 cytokine (interferon) release, the T cells enhance innate resistance to intracellular pathogens. T cells also interact with B-lymphocytes and antigen presenting cells as well as generate soluble cytokines such as interleukin (IL)-4 and IL-10 to initiate and mount T-dependent antibody responses that contribute to the adaptive immune defense against extracellular pathogens. Defects in T-cell development can result in SCID, a life-threatening heterogeneous group of disorders with severe infections from early infancy. Unless reconstituted with stem cells or bone marrow transplantation, SCID patients typically die at an early age from repeated infections. In addition, there are several clinical syndromes in which there is impaired T-cell function but without severe compromise of T-cell development found in SCID.

## SEVERE COMBINED IMMUNODEFICIENCY DISEASE

Severe combined immunodeficiency disease consists of a heterogeneous group of immune deficiencies that present with distinct clinical and immunologic phenotype (Box 20-4). All forms of SCID are characterized by early onset of severe, recurrent, bacterial, viral, or fungal infections in infancy.[17] These infections include interstitial pneumonias, chronic diarrhea, and persistent

candidiasis (Fig. 20-7). Pneumonia due to *Pneumocystis carinii*, cytomegalovirus, or virulent bacteria is common, and the thymus is usually absent on chest radiography (Fig. 20-8). Hypoplasic tonsils and hypoplasic lymph nodes are common, as is absent or dysplasic thymus (Fig. 20-9). Skin manifestations are also common, with generalized erythroderma or eczemetoid eruption frequently occurring. These rashes may represent a manifestation of graft-versus-host disease caused by transplacental transfer of alloreactive maternal T-lymphocytes. Recurrent infections that are only partially responsive to antibiotic therapy often result in poor growth and failure to thrive. Laboratory results show peripheral blood lymphopenia with reduced numbers of circulatory CD3+ T-lymphocytes. Serum Igs (IgG, IgA, and IgM) are very low. In vitro lymphocyte proliferative response to phytohemoglutin is very low to absent. The phenotypic and laboratory findings in SCID are summarized in Box 20-4. As shown in Table 20-2, SCID is caused by different genetic mutations that manifest unique protein and/or enzyme deficiencies. Table 20-2 groups these variants of SCID based on the presence of T cells and B cells or defects in purine metabolism.

## SEVERE COMBINED IMMUNODEFICIENCY DISEASE WITH DECREASED T CELLS AND PRESENT B CELLS

X-linked severe combined immunodeficiency is the most common form of SCID, with an estimate incidence of 1:150,000 births. This X-linked disease is characterized by absence of both T-lymphocytes and natural killer lymphocytes with preserved B-lymphocytes. The disease is caused by a mutation in the gene that encodes for the IL-2 receptor common gamma chain (IL-2Rγc, γc) located on the X chromosome at Xq 12–13.1.[18] This defect affects not only the IL-2 receptor but also the IL-4, IL-7, IL-9, IL-15, and IL-21 receptors. This phenotype appears to be a complex association of

---

**BOX 20-4**
**Phenotypic Clinical and Laboratory Features in Severe Combined Immunodeficiency Disease**

**Clinical Features**
Presentation early in life (within the first 4–6 mo of age)
Severe respiratory infections (interstitial pneumonia)
Protracted diarrhea
Failure to thrive
Persistent candidiasis (oral thrush)
Skin rash, erythrodermia
Positive family history (X-linked, parental consanguinity)

**Laboratory Findings**
Lymphopenia (absolute lymphocyte count <2000/μL)
Reduced number (>1500/μL) of circulation CD3+ T cells
Very low to undetectable levels of serum immunoglobulins*
Very low to absent in vitro proliferative response to mitogens (such as phytohemagglutinin)

---

*Immunoglobulin G serum levels may initially be normal because of transplacental passage of maternal immunoglobulin G.

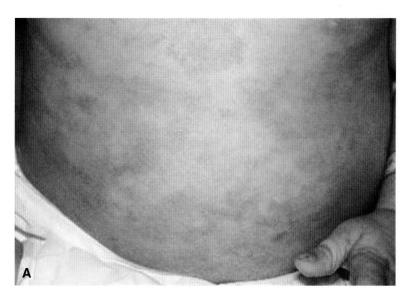

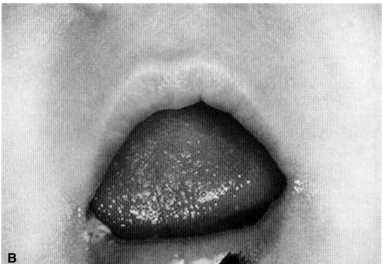

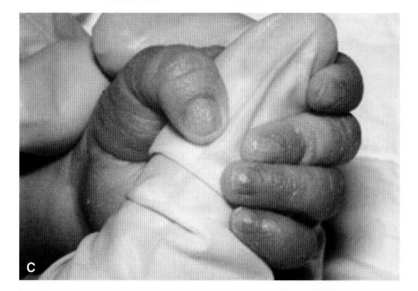

**Figure 20-7.** Disseminated *Candida albicans* fungal dermatitis on the trunk *(A)*, in the mouth *(B)*, and on the nails *(C)* of a child with severe combined immunodeficiency disease. Note the dystrophic appearance of the nails.

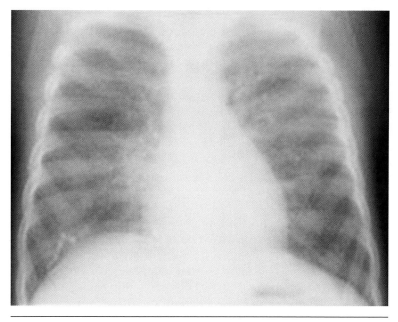

**Figure 20-8.** Chest radiograph of an infant with severe combined immunodeficiency disease. Note the absent thymic shadow and bilateral pulmonary infiltrates. Sutures indicate the site of lung biopsy, which documented the presence of *Pneumocystis carinii*.

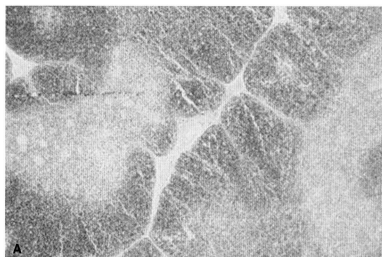

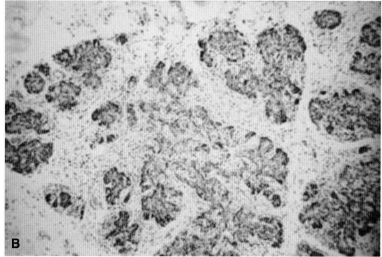

**Figure 20-9.** Histology of the normal thymus *(A)*, compared with that of the dysplastic thymus found in severe combined immunodeficiency disease *(B)*. Note the lack of normal lobulation and corticomedullary differentiation, the decreased numbers of lymphocytes, and the absence of Hassall's corpuscles in the thymus of severe combined immunodeficiency disease.

all of these cytokine receptor pathways. Some mutations in these pathways may impair but not completely abolish the cytokine signaling, which may result in atypical clinical presentation.

Severe combined immunodeficiency disease caused by *Jak-3* deficiency is clinically and immunologically undistinguishable from SCID-X, except that it follows an autosomal-recessive pattern of inheritance.[19] *Jak-3* is a cytoplasmic tyrosine kinase that is associated with the γc in all of the γc-containing cytokine receptors and mediates signaling through IL-2R, IL-4R, IL-7R, and several other ILs. The *Jak-3* gene is located in chromosome 19. Another autosomal-recessive form of SCID is caused by IL-7Ra deficiency.[20] Mutations that impair expression of IL-7R result in an early block in T-cell development with preserved development of B and natural killer cells. Two patients with SCID have been described in whom the disease was associated with a complete absence of the CD45 protein, a phosphatase that modulates signaling through the TCR/CD3 complex.[21,22] Deficiency of the intracellular tyrosine kinase, ZAP70, can also cause a variant of SCID.[23]

## SEVERE COMBINED IMMUNODEFICIENCY DISEASE WITH DECREASED T CELLS AND B CELLS

In humans, the second most common phenotype of SCID is characterized by a complete absence of T cells and B cells in peripheral blood. A subgroup of these patients have defects in the antigen recognition regions of the Ig and T-cell receptors, which are referred to as the variable/diverse/joining gene segments. This recognition process is initiated when the RAG1 and RAG2 proteins recognize signals of the variable/diverse/joining gene segments. A subset of SCID patients have mutations in either RAG1 or RAG2

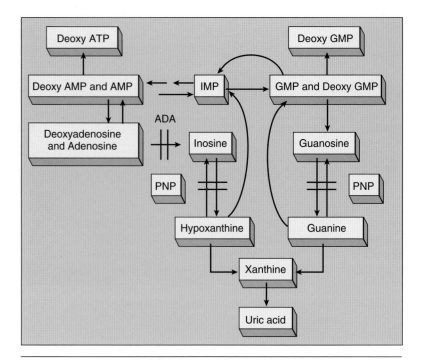

**Figure 20-10.** Steps in the purine catabolic pathway. One form of severe combined immunodeficiency is associated with a defect in adenosine deaminase (ADA), which catalyzes the conversions of adenosine into inosine and deoxyadenosine into deoxyinosine. In purine nucleoside phosphorylase (PNP) deficiency, the enzyme PNP that catalyzes the conversions of inosine into hypoxanthine and guanosine into guanine (and their deoxy derivatives) is absent or abnormal. AMP, adenosine monophosphate; ATP, adenosine triphosphate; GMP, guanosine triphosphate; GTP, guanosine triphosphate; IMP, inosine monophosphate.

**TABLE 20-2**

**Genetic and Immunologic Features of Selected Severe Combined Immunodeficiency Disease (SCID)**

| Disease | Gene Defect | Inheritance | Circulating Lymphocytes | | |
|---|---|---|---|---|---|
| | | | T | B | NK |
| T-cell decreased, B-cell present SCID | | | | | |
| X-linked SCID | *IL2RG* | XL | ↓↓ | N/↑ | ↓↓ |
| Jak-3 deficiency | *Jak-3* | AR | ↓↓ | N/↑ | ↓↓ |
| IL-7R deficiency | *IL7RA* | AR | ↓↓ | N/↑ | N |
| CD45 deficiency | *CD45* | AR | ↓↓ | ↑ | ↓ |
| ZAP-70 deficiency | *ZAP70* | AR | ↓ (↓↓ CD8) | N | N |
| CD25 deficiency | *IL2RA* | AR | ↓ | N | N |
| T-cell decreased, B-cell decreased SCID | | | | | |
| Reticular dysgenesis | ? | AR | ↓↓ | ↓↓ | ↓↓ |
| RAG deficiency, T⁻ B⁻ SCID | *RAG1, RAG2* | AR | ↓↓ | ↓↓ | N |
| Omenn syndrome | *RAG1, RAG2* | AR | ↓/N | ↓↓ | N/↑ |
| Radiation-sensitive T⁻ B⁻ SCID | *Artemis* | AR | ↓↓ | ↓↓ | N |
| Purine metabolism deficiency | | | | | |
| Adenosine deaminase deficiency | *ADA* | AR | ↓↓ | ↓ | ↓ |
| Nucleoside phosphorylase deficiency | *PNP* | AR | ↓↓ | ↓/N | ↓/N |

AR, autosomal recessive; N, normal; XL, X-linked; ↑, increased; ↓↓, decreased.

genes.[24] A second subgroup have a mutation in the Artemis gene, which participates in the later phase of variable/diverse/joining recombination.[25] In addition to the undue susceptibility to infection, typical for SCID, Omenn's syndrome patients present with an exudative erythrodermia, heptosplenomegaly, diarrhea, hypoproteinemia, and eosinophilia.[26] Omenn's syndrome has an autosomal-recessive inheritance and can express mutations in RAG1 and RAG2 genes.

Adenosine deaminase (ADA) deficiency, inherited as an autosomal-recessive trait, results in a variant of SCID.[27] ADA is an enzyme that converts adenosine into inosine and deoxyadenosine into deoxyinosine (Fig. 20-10). Deficiency of ADA results in the intracellular accumulation of deoxyinosine and its phosphorylated metabolites, which are toxic to lymphoid precursors. This leads to a deficiency of T and B cells with resultant consequences of SCID. Partial deficiency of ADA may result in a less severe clinical presentation of SCID with delayed or late onset of symptoms after infancy. The ADA gene maps to chromosome 20. A deficiency of the enzyme nucleoside phosphorylase (PNP) inherited as an autosomal-recessive trait can also cause a variant of SCID.[28] PNP deficiency results in the accumulation of phosphorylated deoxyguanine metabolites that inhibit DNA synthesis. PNP deficiency is especially deleterious to T-cell development, which manifests as a progressive T-cell lymphopenia; this is responsible for the clinical expression of this SCID genotype. The PNP gene maps to chromosome 20.

## OTHER T-CELL DEFICIENCIES

### DiGeorge Syndrome (Anomaly)

DiGeorge syndrome is characterized by deficient T-lymphocytes with normal or near-normal B-lymphocytes, serum IgG, IgA,

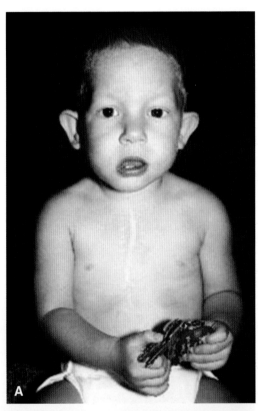

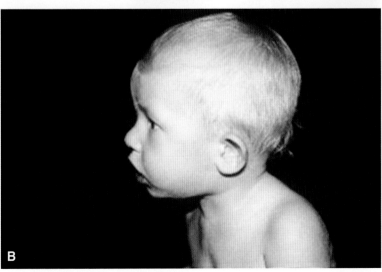

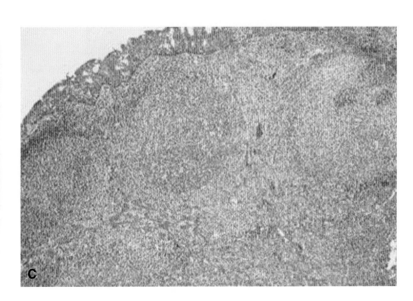

**Figure 20-11.** Frontal (*A*) and lateral (*B*) views of the facial features of a child with DiGeorge syndrome. Note the micrognathia, hyperteolorism, malformation of the ears, and midline thoracotomy scar following repair of a congenital heart defect. *C*, Photomicrograph of a resected adenoid from a child with an isolated T-cell defect associated with DiGeorge syndrome. The lymphoid follicles are well formed, having light and dark portions and a surrounding mantle of small cells. However, the paracortex between the follicles is virtually devoid of lymphoid T cells. Immunoglobulin-producing plasma cells are present. This lymphoid tissue is mirror image of that shown in Figure 20–4*B*. (Hematoxylin and eosin stain, ×121.) (*A* and *B*, Reproduced from Skoner DP, Stillwagen PK, Friedman R, Fireman P: Pediatric Allergy and Immunology. In Zittelli BJ, Davis HW (eds.) Atlas of Pediatric Diagnosis. New York, Gower, 1987, p.4.18; with permission. *C*, Courtesy of Dr. Ronald Jaffe, Children's Hospital, Pittsburgh, PA.)

and IgM. This pure T-cell deficiency results from the abnormal development of the third and fourth brachial pouches during embryogenesis and manifests thymic hypoplasia.[29] Because the parathyroid gland and the cardiovascular system also develop from the same brachial pouches, these patients frequently present with signs of hypocalcemic tetany, seizures, and congenital heart disease within the first few days of life. Associated abnormalities may include esophageal atresia, hypothyroidism, and unusual facies (Fig. 20-11). Because of these multiple anomalies, it has been proposed that this condition be designated DiGeorge anomaly; it may be a polytypic field defect of diverse etiology involving cephalic neural crest cells. This syndrome is also referred to as CATCH22 (Cardiac defect, Abnormal facies, Thymic hypoplasia, Cleft palate, Hypocalcemia, chromosome 22). Patients with this condition need to be tested for monosomy of chromosome 22q11 region by fluorescent in situ hybridization (FISH) assay.

The thymus provides the appropriate microenvironment for lymphoid tissue to mature into functioning T-lymphocytes. With a defective thymus, normal T-cell development does not occur and the T-cell immunodeficiency may manifest as overwhelming infection with fungi or viruses in a small subset of these patients. Often, the T-cell defect may be transient, resolving spontaneously. These infants have been successfully reconstituted with fetal thymus implants.[28]

## Wiskott-Aldrich Syndrome

Wiskott-Aldrich syndrome is an X-linked recessive disorder characterized by eczema and thrombocytopenia with cutaneous petechiae (Fig. 20-12). The recurrent infections usually begin in infancy. The most commonly reported immunologic defect is the inability to form antibodies to the T-cell–independent antigens, bacterial capsular polysaccharide antigens, but some patients also manifest a progressive decline in T-lymphocyte responses. The responsible defective gene, named *WASP*, encodes for a protein involved in the cytoskeletal reorganization in hematopoietic cells.[30] The only curative therapy is bone marrow transplantation.

## Ataxia Telangiectasia

Ataxia telangiectasia is an autosomal-recessive multisystem syndrome with telangiectasia, progressive ataxia, and variable immunodeficiency. Most patients develop ocular telangiectasia (Fig. 20-13) and cerebellar ataxia during the first 6 years of life. This progressive, variable immunodeficiency typically has depressed T-cell function. IgG, IgA, and IgG subclass deficiencies also have been reported. Sinusitis and pulmonary infections are quite frequent. These patients, as well as patients with other immunodeficiencies, have a high incidence of neoplasia. This disease is caused by mutation in the *ATM* gene, which encodes for a large protein that participates in the repair of DNA breakage and controls the cell cycle and cellular apoptosis.[31]

## Chronic Mucocutaneous Candidiasis

Chronic mucocutaneous candidiasis is characterized by superficial, persistent, and recurrent candidial infections of the mucous membranes, skin, and nails (Fig. 20-14). Endocrinopathy is often associated, and variants of this syndrome may include hypoparathyroidism and polyendocrinopathy. This illness may be sporadic or familial, and the age of onset of symptoms varies. Immunologic abnormalities include absence of delayed cutaneous hypersensitivity to *Candida* and lack of lymphokine production by *Candida*-stimulated T-lymphocytes. T-cell and B-cell enumeration, as well as serum Igs and functional antibodies, appear normal. Long-term antifungal therapy with ketoconazole, administered orally, has resulted in dramatic clinical improvement and decreased morbidity (Fig. 20-15).

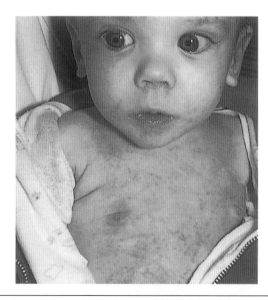

**Figure 20-12.** Child with Wiskott-Aldrich syndrome. The skin eruptions on the trunk and face are eczematoid and pruritic but not always similar to atopic dermatitis in flexural distribution. Many of these patients have thrombocytopenia, which results in petechiae of varying distribution and intensity.

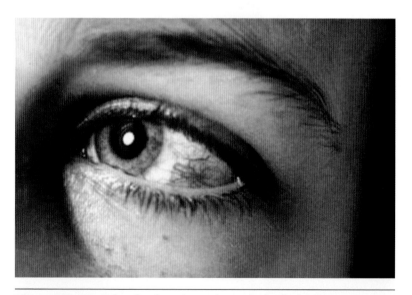

**Figure 20-13.** Scleral telangiectasia typical of ataxia-telangiectasia. Other findings characteristic of this disorder include cerebellar ataxia and variable T-cell and B-cell immunity. (Reproduced from Skoner DP, Stillwagen PK, Friedman R, Fireman P: Pediatric Allergy and Immunology. In Zittelli BJ, Davis HW (eds.) Atlas of Pediatric Diagnosis. New York, Gower, 1987, p4.19; with permission.)

# NEUTROPHIL DEFICIENCY DISEASES

Neutrophils mature in the bone marrow from a myeloid stem cell over 14 days, during which differentiation and proliferation takes place. Mature neutrophils contain granules in their cytoplasma and circulate in the vascular compartment for 6 to 8 hours. Adhesion to the vascular endothelium and diapedesis by neutrophils to sites of inflammation are facilitated by several leukocyte adhesion molecules, which are categorized as integrins and selectins. As part of the innate immune system, neutrophils have phagocytic and bactericidal activity. Deficient or defective neutrophil function will result in undue susceptibility to infection with recurrent severe bacterial or fungal infections, especially those caused by unusual organisms or in uncommon locations with abscess formation. Viral infections are not usually increased in these patients. Neutrophil deficiency diseases can be categorized into two groups: (1) quantitative disorders with neutropenia and (2) functional disorders with failure of specific metabolic activities (Box 20-5). Several of these neutrophil deficiency diseases are described in detail.

## NEUTROPHIL DEFICIENCY WITH NEUTROPENIA

### Severe Congenital Neutropenia (Kostmann's Syndrome)

Severe congenital neutropenia patients are a heterogeneous group of neutropenic infants whose infections begin by 1 month of age in 50% and by 6 months of age in 90%. Manifestations include omphalitis, skin and liver abscesses, as well as respiratory tract infections. Chronic neutropenia (fewer than 200 neutrophils per

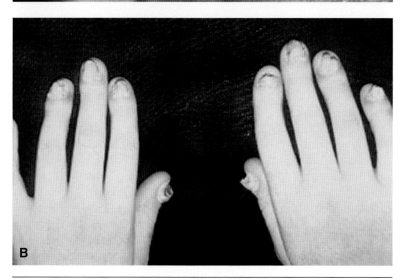

**Figure 20-14.** Diffuse mucocutaneous involvement with *Candida albicans* in a patient with chronic mucocutaneous candidiasis. Lesions involving the oral mucosal surfaces (*A*) and the nail beds (*B*) are almost always present and are recalcitrant to therapy with topical and antifungal agents.

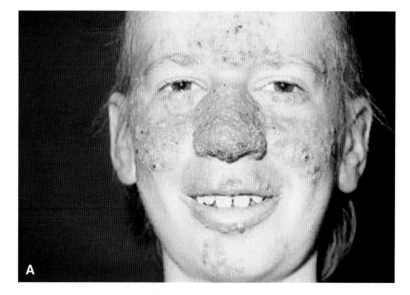

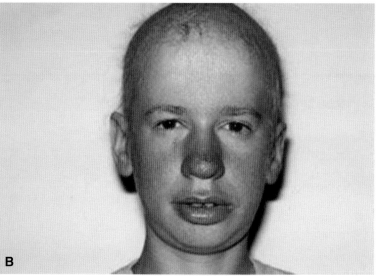

**Figure 20-15.** Patient with chronic mucocutaneous candidiasis before (*A*) and after (*B*) treatment with oral ketoconazole. (Reproduced from Skoner DP, Stillwagen PK, Friedman R, Fireman P: Pediatric Allergy and Immunology. In Zittelli BJ, Davis HW (eds.) Atlas of Pediatric Diagnosis. New York, Gower, 1987, p4.18; with permission.)

microliter) is due to bone marrow granulocyte maturation arrest at the promyelocyte or myelocyte stage with variable inheritance patterns. Some of these patients have mutations in the granulocyte colony–stimulating factor (G-CSF) receptor and also manifest an increased risk for the development of acute myeloid leukemia.[32] Another group of these patients has been found to have mutations in the gene encoding neutrophil elastase.[33] Treatment with recombinant G-CSF has improved the clinical outcome in some of these patients, with reductions in infections and some increase in life expectancy.

## Cyclic Neutropenia

Cyclic neutropenia is usually inherited as an autosomal-dominant trait with cyclic decreases in neutrophils as well as decreases in all hematopoietic lineages. Cycles of severe neutropenia (less than 200/µL) occur approximately every 3 to 4 weeks and last for 3 to 10 days. Oral ulcers, gingivitis, pharyngitis, tonsillitis, and skin abscesses are common beginning in early childhood. Gingivitis may cause loss of teeth. During periods of neutropenia, bone marrow will show maturation arrest at myelocyte stage. Mutation in genes for neutrophil elastase has been found in all patients studied thus far.[33] Therapy with G-CSF improves neutrophil counts and has improved clinical outcome of these patients.

## Warts, Hypogammaglobulinemia, Infections, and Myelokathexis (WHIM) Syndrome

This is a congenital autosomal syndrome with severe chronic neutropenia; however, during infections, neutrophil counts may increase. Unlike the other congenital neutropenic syndromes, the bone marrow shows myeloid hypercellularity at all stages of differentiation. Warts, hypogammaglobulinemia, infections, and myelokathexis (thus, WHIM syndrome) are frequently associated with this disorder.[34] G-CSF and granulocyte-macrophage colony-stimulating factor therapy has been shown to decrease infections, improve gammaglobulin levels, and mobilize mature neutrophils from the bone marrow.

---

**BOX 20-5**
## Neutrophil Deficiency Diseases

**Quantitative Disorders: Neutropenia**
Severe congenital neutropenia (Kostmann's syndrome)
Cyclic neutropenia
Warts, hypogammaglobulinemia, infections, and
    myelokathexis (WHIM) syndrome
Immune-mediated neutropenia

**Functional Disorders**
Chronic granulomatous disease
Reduced form of nicotinamide adenine dinucleotide
    phosphate oxidase defects
Leukocyte adhesion deficiency
Chédiak-Higashi syndrome
Hyper–immunoglobulin E (Job's) syndrome

---

## Immune-Mediated Neutropenia

Autoimmune neutropenia is a rare syndrome caused by destruction of neutrophils or their precursors by serum autoantibodies or mediated by sensitized T cells in the bone marrow. Autoimmune neutropenia can be primary or secondary to another immune-mediated disease such as systemic lupus erythematosus, viral infection (Epstein-Barr virus, cytomegalovirus, or HIV), leukemia, or Hodgkin's disease.[35] Neutrophil counts are below 1500/µL but higher than 500/µL. Patients present with skin infection, recurrent respiratory infection, and, occasionally, pneumonia. Despite low neutrophil counts, some patients may not manifest undue susceptibility to infection. Neutrophil counts can increase during infection, and bone marrow findings are normal or hypocellular. Antibodies have been found directed to several neutrophil antigens. Prognosis for primary autoimmune neutropenia is good because it is usually self-limited and resolves in several years. Treatment for severe infections now includes G-CSF as well as antibiotics. Secondary autoimmune neutropenia responds best to therapy directed at the underlying disease.

Autoimmune neonatal neutropenia is a form of immune-mediated neutropenia in which there is transplacental transfer of IgG maternal antibodies directed against an Ig receptor (FcγRIIIb) that causes destruction of the neonatal neutrophils. This syndrome appears in otherwise normal infants of apparently normal mothers. Omphalitis, cellulites, and pneumonia may occur, but many infants do not manifest infections. This neutropenia will improve with the catabolism of maternal antibodies but may take up to 6 months.

## DEFECTIVE NEUTROPHIL FUNCTION DISORDERS

### Chronic Granulomatous Disease

Chronic granulomatous disease is a genetically heterogeneous disease caused by defects in the reduced form of nicotinamide adenine dinucleotide phosphate oxidase, the enzyme responsible for phagocyte respiratory burst and generation of superoxide. The frequency of chronic granulomatous disease in the United States is estimated at 1:100,000. The most common genotype in two thirds of patients is X linked, and the remainder are autosomal recessive. Recurrent and chronic infections with granuloma formation occur in the skin, lung, lymph nodes, liver, gastrointestinal tract, and genitourinary tract. The most common infectious organisms are *Staphyloccocus aureus*, Burkholder's cepacia, *Serratia marcescens*, and *Nocardia* and *Aspergillus* spp. The diagnosis of chronic granulomatous disease is made by direct measurement of superoxide production, chemiluminescence, nitroblue tetrazolium reduction, or dihydrorhodamine oxidation. Precise gene defect should be sought in all cases for genetic counseling and prognosis, because the autosomal forms have a better prognosis than the X-linked disease.[36] Prophylactic trimethoprim/sulfamethoxazole reduces the frequency of major infections, especially the staphylococcal skin infections. Interferon gamma was shown in a multicenter placebo controlled study to reduce number and severity of infections in chronic granulomatous disease by 70%. Many clinicians also include prophylaxis with itraconazole along with the other two agents. Bone marrow transplantation has been successfully performed, but transplant-related complications limit this therapy to a few select patients with appropriate histocompatibility with donor bone marrow.

## Myeloperoxidase Deficiency

Myeloperoxidase deficiency is an autosomal-recessive trait and is the most common primary phagocyte disorder. In vitro studies have shown that myeloperoxidase deficiency–deficient neutrophils are markedly deficient compared with normal neutrophils in microbial killing; however, recurrent and serious infections due to myeloperoxidase deficiency are rare except in association with diabetes mellitus.

## Leukocyte Adhesion Deficiencies

Leukocyte adhesion to endothelium, to other leukocytes, and to microbes is critical for both the innate and adaptive immune responses. Different families of adhesion molecules facilitate these processes, which are essential for the expression of inflammation to fight infection.

Leukocyte adhesion deficiency (LAD) type I is an autosomal-recessive disease with a severe and moderate phenotype.[37] The severe phenotype manifests delayed umbilicus separation and omphalitis, severe gingivitis, and periodontitis with associated loss of dentition. Recurrent infections of skin, upper and lower airways, and rectal areas are commonly caused by *S. aureus* or gram-negative bacilli. Infections respond poorly to therapy, even through peripheral blood leucocytosis (715,000/μL), is evident. There is impaired healing of infections and traumatic or surgical wounds. In the severe phenotype, there is less than 1% of the normal expression of CD18 (β2 integrin) neutrophils. The moderate phenotype of LAD-1 has 1% to 30% of the normal expression of CD18 with fewer life-threatening infections. These patients live longer and have normal umbilical separation. However, they will manifest delayed wound healing, periodontal disease, and persistent leucocytosis. At present, bone marrow transplantation is the only definitive therapy when antibiotic therapy and antibiotic prophylaxis are inadequate.

Leukocyte adhesion deficiency type 2 is a very rare autosomal-recessive inherited disease that is characterized by delayed separation of the umbilical cord as well as poor pus formation; leucocytosis; and infections of the skin, lungs, and gums. There is also mental retardation and short stature. However, unlike with LAD-1, the frequency and severity of infections improve with age. These patients have a deficiency of the *GDP-fucose* transporter gene with a deficiency of the fucosylated proteins, which function as ligands for endothelial selectins that mediate the adhesion of neutrophils along the postcapillary venules.[38]

Leukocyte adhesion deficiency type 3 with deficient expression of E-selectin has been described in one female patient. This patient's clinical course is similar to that of LAD-1, except that the patient had mild neuropenia. LAD-4 with a deficiency of Rho GTP-ase enzyme activity has been reported in one male. The undue susceptibility to infection is similar to that in LAD-1, except that chemotaxis as well as superoxide production were impaired. This patient improved after bone marrow transplantation.

## Chédiak-Higashi Syndrome

Chédiak-Higashi syndrome is a rare, life-threatening autosomal-recessive disease characterized by oculocutaneous albinism, frequent pyogenic infections, and neutropenia. The disease is associated with a mutation in the lysosomal trafficking gene (*LYST*).[39] Giant azurophil granules formed from the fusion of primary granules are seen in the cytoplasm of neutrophils, eosinophils, and basophils. Neutrophil chemotaxis is diminished, phagocytosis is normal, but bacterial killing is delayed. Progressive neuropathy, seizures, and mental retardation have been reported. On occasion, this syndrome can progress to hemophagocytosis with fever, cytopenia, hepatosplenomegaly, and lymphadenopathy. Without bone marrow transplantation, this condition can worsen and lead to death.[39]

## Hyper-Immunoglobulin E and Recurrent Infection Syndrome

Hyper-IgE syndrome, or Job's syndrome, is a rare autosomal disorder in which patients have recurrent infection of the skin and respiratory tract, with eczema, high IgE levels, eosinophilia, and facial abnormalities with hypertelorism, protruding chin, and coarse facial features[40] (Fig. 20-16). Especially common are recurrent cutaneous staphylococcal skin infections as well as staphylococcal penumonia with lung abscesses and pneumatocele formation (Fig. 20-17). These patients have been described as having impaired in vitro leukocyte chemotaxis, but the mechanism or pathogenesis of this syndrome is unknown.

# COMPLEMENT DEFICIENCIES

Complement deficiencies are rare, but a failure to recognize a complement abnormality may have serious consequences for the patient. The complement system participates in both the innate

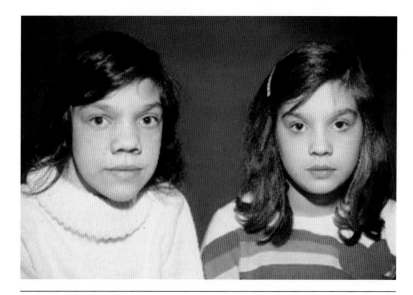

**Figure 20-16.** Coarse facial features of a girl with hyper–immunoglobulin E syndrome *(left)*. Her sister *(right)* has an immunoglobulin A deficiency. Although the syndromes are distinct, in this case they illustrate the frequency with which immune deficiencies are observed in family members of immunoglobulin A–deficient patients. (Reproduced from Skoner DP, Stillwagen PK, Friedman R, Fireman P: Pediatric Allergy and Immunology. In Zittelli BJ, Davis HW (eds.) Atlas of Pediatric Diagnosis. New York, Gower, 1987, p4.19; with permission.)

and adaptive immune systems in host defense against bacterial and certain viral infections, in scavenging cellular and molecular debris, as mediators of immune-based inflammation, and in amplifying specific immune responses. There are three separate pathways for activating the complement cascade. As shown in Figure 20-18, each pathway is triggered by a recognition phase. The classic pathway activation recognition is mediated by IgM and IgG antibodies of the adaptive immune response. These antibodies bind and activate the enzymes of the first component of complement (C1), which is a complex of three subunits, C1q, C1r, and C1s. Activated C1 then cleaves the fourth (C4) and second (C2) complement components. C4 and C2 associate into an enzyme that cleaves the most abundant complement component, C3, which then activates the complement cascade. The alternate activation pathway also summarized in Figure 20-18 shows the amplification of additional C3 cleavage by two proteins, factors B and D. The third and second activation pathways are part of the innate immune system. The binding of mannose lectin to mannose on microbial cell wall surfaces is the recognition phase for the third pathway. The enzymatic activities of two proteins, mannose-binding associate proteins (MASP1 and MASP2), amplifies this pathway. Cleavage fragments of C3 (C3a and C3b) mediate many aspects of inflammation. C3b can participate in cleaving the next protein in this cascade, C5. When this occurs, the remaining proteins, C6, C7, C8, and, finally, C9, are activated. The activation of these complement components promotes adherence and

recognition of particles by phagocytes, smooth muscle contraction, vascular permeability, mast cell and basophil degranulation, chemotaxis, and other proinflammatory effects.

As outlined in Table 20-3, genetic deficiencies of the complement system are characterized by four clinical symptom patterns: 1) undue susceptibility to infection; 2) rheumatologic manifestations; 3) hemolytic anemia; and 4) angioedema.[41] Patients with C3 deficiency suffer from repeated infections with encapsulated bacteria such as *S. pneumoniae* and *H. influenzae*.[42] This is an autosomal-recessive trait, and the heterozygous-deficient individuals are asymptomatic. Some C3-deficient patients also manifest immune complex–related disorders such as systemic lupus erythematosus. Deficiencies of complement proteins C5, C6, C7, C8, and C9 are each associated with increased susceptibility to neisserial infections, meningococcal meningitis, meningococcemia, and invasive gonococcal disease.[43] Deficiencies of the classic

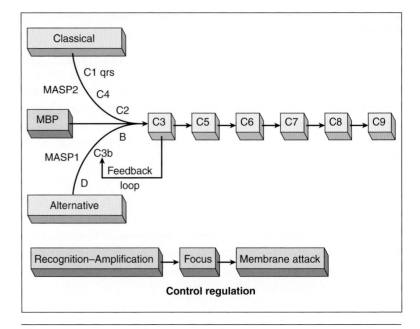

**Figure 20-18.** Complement cascade. C, component of complement; MBP, myelin basic protein.

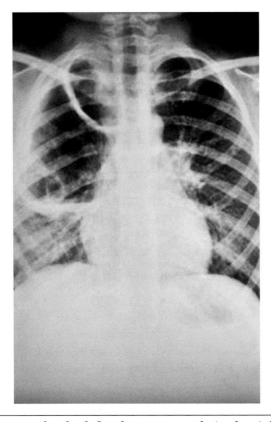

**Figure 20-17.** Clearly defined pneumatocele in the right lung of a patient with hyper–immunoglobulin E syndrome. This type of lesion is frequently associated with *Streptococcus aureus* pneumonia. (Reproduced from Skoner DP, Stillwagen PK, Friedman R, Fireman P: Pediatric Allergy and Immunology. In Zittelli BJ, Davis HW (eds.) Atlas of Pediatric Diagnosis. New York, Gower, 1987, p4.10; with permission.)

**TABLE 20-3**
**Genetic Deficiencies of the Complement System**

| Clinical Presentation | Genetic Deficiency |
|---|---|
| Recurrent infection | |
|   Encapsulated pyogenic bacteria | C3, factor I, CD11b/18 |
|   *Neisseria* sp. | C5, C6, C7, C8 properdin |
| Rheumatologic | Clq, Clr, Cls, C2, C4, factor H (nephritis) |
| Hemolytic anemia | CD59, PIG-A (acquired) |
| Angioedema | Cl inhibitor |

PIG-A, phosphatidylinositol glycan class A.

complement activation components C1, C2, and C4 are associated with lupus and other rheumatologic diseases.

# MUCOSAL AND SKIN BARRIER DISORDERS

Mucosa and skin are crucial barriers in preventing the entrance of microbes and antigens into the body. Host respiratory and gastrointestinal mucosal defense mechanisms are aided by secretory antibodies (predominantly IgA) in the pharynx, bronchi, and intestines. In addition, other factors such as salivary lysozyme, intestinal enzymes, and forceful coughing help in the removal of pathogens.

## *DYSFUNCTIONAL CILIA SYNDROME*

Initially called Kartagener syndrome, the dysfunctional cilia syndrome is characterized by defective mucociliary transport and the triad of chronic sinusitis, bronchiectasis, and situs inversus viscerum (Fig. 20-19), although situs inversus is not universal. Some patients are infertile, with poorly motile spermatozoa. The ciliary dysfunction impedes mucous clearance and produces the following: early onset of chronic rhinorrhea, chronic otitis media,

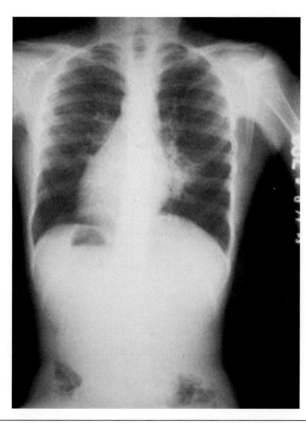

**Figure 20-19.** Dextrocardia and situs inversus of abdominal organs in a patient with Kartagener's syndrome and dysfunctional cilia syndrome. The abnormal ciliary motion is thought to result in malrotation during embryogenesis. (Reproduced from Skoner DP, Stillwagen PK, Friedman R, Fireman P: Pediatric Allergy and Immunology. In Zittelli BJ, Davis HW (eds.) Atlas of Pediatric Diagnosis. New York, Gower, 1987, p4.23; with permission.)

nasal polyps, chronic sinusitis with opaque sinuses on radiography, chronic productive cough, bronchiectasis, and digital clubbing. Electron microscopic analysis of cilia obtained from biopsy of the nasal or tracheobronchal mucosa (Fig. 20-20) or analysis of spermatozoa mobility and electron microscopy document the abnormality. Therapy with antibiotics is supportive.

# DIAGNOSIS

In all cases of immunodeficiency, laboratory tests are needed to confirm the diagnosis. If a B-cell or T-cell immunodeficiency is suspected, the initial laboratory tests (Fig. 20-20) include a complete blood count with differential and platelet count and measurement of IgG, IgM, and IgA serum levels. A complete blood count establishes anemia, thrombocytopenia, or neutropenia. A lymphopenia (less than 1500 cells/mL$^3$) suggests T-cell immunodeficiency. Serum Ig levels, as well as lymphocyte counts, must be interpreted carefully, with an eye toward age variations. In older children and adults, an IgG level of less than 300 mg/dL indicates a significant Ig deficiency.

Usually, if the screening tests are all normal, most B-cell immunodeficiency diseases can be excluded. However, if the history is unusually suspicious, further advanced testing must be done. In immunized subjects, antibody titers to tetanus, diphtheria, rubella, poliovirus, *H. influenza*, or *S. pneumoniae* antigens can be used to estimate IgG function. In nonimmunized patients, antibody titers should be obtained before and 4 weeks after tetanus or other immunizations. An inadequate response (less than a fourfold rise in titer) is suggestive of antibody deficiency, regardless of the Ig levels. Immunodeficient patients should never be immunized with live (attenuated) vaccines, because they may be unable to inactivate the attenuated organisms.

All humans, except young infants and individuals with blood type AB, have IgM isoagglutinins (anti-A and/or anti-B antibodies). These antibodies are selectively deficient in certain immunodeficiencies (e.g., Wiskott-Aldrich syndrome). IgG subclass determinations are indicated if IgG levels are normal or near normal but antibody function is deficient. These determinations should also be done in symptomatic, selective IgA deficiency, since IgG$_2$ subclass deficiency is present in some of these cases. If local infections are severe, secretory IgA levels (e.g., in tears or saliva) can be measured. If Ig levels are low, enumeration of B cells should be performed. Normally, 5% to 10% of peripheral blood lymphocytes are surface membrane Ig positive. Isolated absences of IgE are rare and not of much clinical significance. IgE levels are high in chemotactic disorders, partial T-cell immunodeficiencies, allergic disorders, and parasitism.

The presence of lymphopenia is suggestive of a T-cell immunodeficiency; however, lymphopenia may not always be present. An absent thymic shadow on a chest roentgenogram in the newborn period is suggestive of T-cell deficiency, particularly before the onset of infection or other stress that may shrink the thymus. Delayed hypersensitivity skin test with *Candida* is valuable in screening for T-cell deficiencies after 2 to 3 years of age.

In advanced evaluation of cellular immunodeficiencies, enumeration of T-lymphocytes is essential (Table 20-4). Most laboratories use various monoclonal antisera that react with T-cell surface receptors, thus allowing enumeration of T-cell subpopulations by automated fluorescent-activated cell sorting. CD8 monoclonal antibodies define suppressor/cytotoxic T-cells and

CD4 monoclonal antibodies define helper/inducer T-lymphocytes. The ratio between helper and suppressor T cells, which is normally about 2:1, may be characteristically reversed in AIDS, thus providing valuable diagnostic information. Monoclonal antibodies are also available to identify activated T cells, natural killer cells, and other T-cell receptors. Other useful "advanced" tests measure lymphocyte proliferation when cultured in the presence of mitogens (e.g., phytohemagglutinin, concanavalin A, irradiated allogeneic leukocytes) or antigens (e.g., tetanus, *Candida*) to which the patient has been previously exposed. T-cell immunodeficiencies manifest low proliferative responses. Procedures are also available to assess production of cytokines following mitogenic or antigenic. In some forms of T-cell immunodeficiency, enzymes of the purine pathway, ADA or PNP, are deficient and

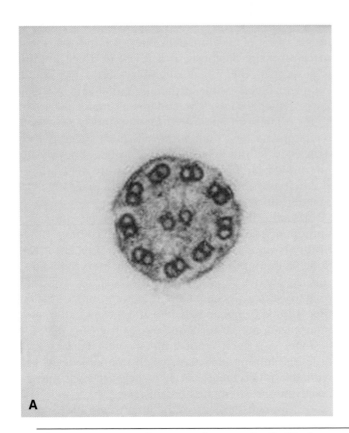
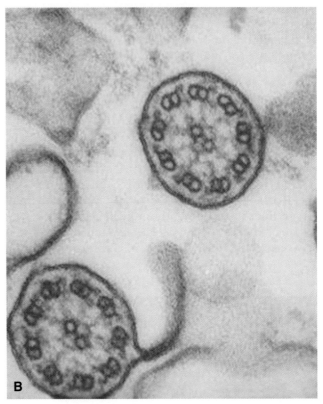

**Figure 20-20.** *A,* Electron micrograph of cilia from a patient with dysfunctional cilia syndrome. Note the absence of dynein arms from the outer doublets. *B,* Normal cilia with dynein arms. (Reproduced from Skoner DP, Stillwagen PK, Friedman R, Fireman P: Pediatric Allergy and Immunology. In Zittelli BJ, Davis HW (eds.) Atlas of Pediatric Diagnosis. New York, Gower, 1987, p4.23; with permission.)

**TABLE 20-4**
**Laboratory Tests for Diagnosis of B- and T-Cell Immunodeficiencies**

|  | Screening Tests | Advanced Tests |
|---|---|---|
| B-cell deficiency | IgG, IgM, IgA serum levels<br>Preexisting Ab (e.g., polio, rubella, tetanus, diphtheria, isoagglutinins) | B cell (CD19) enumeration<br>Lateral neck x-ray pharyngeal roentgenogram for adenoid size<br>Ab responses to vaccines, such as tetanus toxoids, killed polio, pneumococcal polysaccharide |
| T-cell deficiency | Lymphocye count and morphology<br>Thymic size by chest roentgenogram<br><br>Delayed skin tests (e.g., *Candida* spp, *trichophyton* spp, tetanus) toxoid | T-cell subsets: CD3, CD4, CD8, CD40, CD16<br>Proliferative responses to mitogens, antigens, allogenic cells<br>Cytokine assays (e.g., IL-2)<br><br>HIV serology |

Ab, antibodies; Ig, immunoglobulin.

can be assayed. A lymph node biopsy may be indicated in the presence of lymphadenopathy or to exclude malignancy. Finally, biopsy of the skin, liver, or thymus may be of value in certain patients.

Tests for phagocytic and complement deficiencies (Table 20-5) are indicated in patients with convincing histories of repeated infections who have normal B-cell and T-cell function. In addition to white blood cell and differential testing, initial screening should include determination of IgE levels and a nitro-blue tetrazolium dye test. The advanced tests include special staining of the granulocytes; bone marrow biopsy; and quantitative assays for myeloperoxidase, alkaline phosphatase, and esterase. Other specialized tests to define phagocytic defects include assays for granulocyte oxidant products, such as superoxide by chemoluminescence and granulocyte mobilization. Leukocyte adhesion deficiencies (e.g., CD18, CD15) are assayed by flow cytometry.

Screening for complement abnormalities is done by measuring total activity ($CH_{50}$). Low levels of this may be followed by the measurement of the individual components of complement. Assays of serum opsonic, chemotactic, or bactericidal activities also can be used to assess complement function.

# PREVENTION AND TREATMENT

## REPLACEMENT THERAPIES

The recognition of immunodeficiency as the basis for a patient's recurrent infections calls for prompt implementation of a treatment program that will not only reverse the clinical course of the current infection but also prevent the patient's undue susceptibility to future infection. As outlined in Table 20-6, this approach requires the availability of therapeutic procedures or agents that will correct, replace, or modulate the host's immune deficiency. The first such therapeutic agent was γ-globulin, pooled from human sera that showed antibody activity. In 1953, Colonel Bruton documented that intramuscular γ-globulin given monthly reduced the frequency and severity of the bacterial infections associated with functional antibody deficiency.[8] The development of γ-globulin for intravenous use represented another dimension of replacement therapy, as much larger amounts of IgG could be

administered. Patients with isolated serum IgA deficiency that is not accompanied by IgG subclass or functional antibody deficiency should not receive gammaglobulin therapy. It is contraindicated in the management of isolated IgA deficiency, as several instances of anaphylaxis following γ-globulin administration were attributed to IgE antibodies reacting with trace amounts of IgA in the IgG preparation.

## RECONSTITUTION THERAPIES

### Transplantation Therapies

The development of bone marrow transplantation has provided the opportunity to immunologically reconstitute certain patients with severe T-cell deficiencies. The use of such techniques has been very successful for the reconstitution of SCID patients when a histocompatibly similar sibling donor or donor bank cells are available. Because the SCID patient's T-cell and B-cell deficiencies markedly suppress their graft-rejection reaction, usually there is little need for immunosuppression prior to or after the bone marrow transplant. The use of a histocompatible-dissimilar bone marrow results in a fatal graft-versus-host reaction in the SCID recipient, unless mature T-lymphocytes are removed from the donor bone marrow cells by either lecithin-separation or monoclonal antibody techniques. The use of these T-cell–depleted bone marrow preparations has provided clinicians with the option of using one of the SCID patient's parents or haploid-identical siblings as a donor. Stem cells obtained from cord blood have also been utilized for reconstitution. The use of fetal thymic or liver implants for therapy of SCID is no longer recommended. However, fetal thymic implants have successfully reconstituted the immune systems of DiGeorge syndrome patients. The use of enzyme replacement with naturally occurring sources of ADA or PNP for these deficiencies had had limited clinical benefit but has provided the basis for future attempts using recombinant DNA engineering technology.

### Gene Therapy

The identification and cloning of specific genes involved in the pathogenesis of certain immunodeficiency diseases has enabled

---

**TABLE 20-5**
**Laboratory Tests for Phagocytic and Complement Deficiencies**

| | Screening Tests | Advanced Tests |
|---|---|---|
| Phagocytic deficiency | White blood cell and differential neutrophil morphology | Flow cytometry (CD18, CD15) |
| | Nitro-blue tetrazolium test or other tests of neutrophil oxidation activity | Myeloperoxidase |
| | Immunoglobulin E level | Cytokine assay (interferon gamma) |
| | | Bone marrow biopsy |
| Complement deficiency | Total ($CH_{50}$) activity | C2, C4, C5, C6, levels |
| | C3, C4 levels | Opsonization |

C, component of complement.

the initiation of a new era of potential gene reconstitution. The ADA gene has been cloned and inserted via a viral vector into the mature T cells, with limited success. The use of hematopoetic stem cells from cord blood has provided some preliminary promising results utilizing a retroviral vector containing γccDNA.[44]

## SUPPLEMENTAL TREATMENTS

Supplemental therapy with interferon has improved the clinical course of patients with chronic granulomatous disease. Additional cytokines, including the lymphocyte and granulocyte growth factors and ILs, have provided more potential therapeutic agents for immunodeficiency diseases.

The judicious use of appropriate antimicrobial agents continues to play an important role in the management of patients with recurring infections due to immunodeficiencies. Antimicrobials should be used in maximal dosages to reverse acute or recurrent infectious processes. In addition, prophylactic antibiotics, at times, deserve clinical trials to prevent infections.

**TABLE 20-6**

**Programs for the Treatment of Various Immunodeficiencies**

| Type of Therapy | Immunodeficiency |
|---|---|
| **Reconstitution** | |
| Bone marrow transplant | SCID |
| Thymus | DiGeorge syndrome |
| Gene therapy | SCID (experimental) |
| **Replacement** | |
| Intravenous γ-globulin | Hypogammaglobulinemia with deficient IgG |
| Enzymes (ADA, PNP) | Subclass or functional antibody ADA and PNP deficiencies |
| **Supplemental** | |
| ***Cytokines*** | |
| Interferon | Chronic granulomatous disease, neutropenia |
| ***Antimicrobial agents*** | |
| Antiviral | AIDS |
| Antifungal | Chronic mucocutaneous candidiasis |
| Antibacterial | Immune deficiency with severe bacterial infections |

ADA, adenosine deaminase; Ig, immunoglobulin; PNP, nucleoside phosphorylase; SCID, severe combined immunodeficiency disease.

# REFERENCES

1. Puck JM: Primary immunodeficiency diseases. JAMA 1997;278:1835–1840.
2. Louis DB, Tu Wen: Secondary immunodeficiencies. In Steihm ER, Ochs HD, Winkelstein JA (eds.). Immunologic Disorders in Infants and Children, 5th edition. Philadelphia, Saunders, 2004, pp 687–784.
3. International Union of Immunological Societies: Primary immunodeficiency diseases: Report of an IUIS scientific committee. Clin Exp Immunol 1999; 118(1):S1–S28.
4. Ropars C, Muller A, Paint N, et al: Large-scale detection of IgA-deficient blood donors. J Immunol Methods 1982;54(2):183–189.
5. Haynes BF, Martin ME, Kay HH, Kurtzberg J: Early events in human T cell ontogeny. Phenotypic characterization and immunohistologic localization of T cell precursors in early human fetal tissues. J Exp Med 1988; 168(3):1061–1080.
6. Royo C, Touraine JL, DeBonteiller O: Ontogeny of T lymphocyte differentiation in the human fetus acquisition of phenotype and functions. Thymus 1987;10(1–2):57–73.
7. Kilic SS, Tezcan I, Sanal O, et al: Transient hypogammaglobulinemia of infancy: Clinical and immunologic features of 40 new cases. Pediatr Int 2000; 42(6):647–650.
8. Bruton OC: Agammaglobulinemia. Pediatrics 1952;9:722–728.
9. Conley ME, Rohrer J, Minegishi Y: X-linked agammaglobulinemia. Clin Rev Allergy Immunol 2000;19(2):183–204.
10. Kanegane H, Futatani T, Wang Y, et al: Clinical and mutational characteristics of X-linked agammaglobulinemia and its carrier identified by flow cytometric assessment combined with genetic analysis. J Allergy Clin Immunol 2001; 108(6):1012–1020.
11. Yel L, Tezcan I, Hasturk H, et al: Oral findings, treatment and follow-up of a case with major aphthous stomatitis (Sutton's disease). J Clin Pediatr Dent 1994;19(1):49–53.
12. Ferrari S, Giliani S, Insalaco A, et al: Mutations of CD40 gene cause an autosomal recessive form of immunodeficiency with hyper IgM. Proc Natl Acad Sci U S A 2001;98(22):12614–12619.
13. Cunningham-Rundles C: Physiology of IgA and IgA deficiency. J Clin Immunol 2001;21(5):303–309.
14. Umetsu DT, Ambrosino DM, Quinti I, et al: Recurrent sinopulmonary infection and impaired antibody response to bacterial capsular polysaccharide antigen in children with selective IgG-subclass deficiency. N Engl J Med 1985;313(20): 1247–1251.
15. French MA, Denis KA, Dawkins R, Peter JB: Severity of infections in IgA deficiency: Correlation with decreased serum antibodies to pneumococcal polysaccharides and decreased serum IgG2 and/or IgG4. Clin Exp Immunol 1995;100(1):47–53.
16. Javier FC III, Moore CM, Sorensen RU: Distribution of primary immunodeficiency diseases diagnosed in a pediatric tertiary hospital. Ann Allergy Asthma Immunol 2000;84:25–30.
17. Fischer A: Severe combined immunodeficiencies (SCID). Clin Exp Immunol 2000;122:143–149.
18. Noguchi M, Yi H, Rosenblatt HM, et al: Interleukin-2 receptor gamma chain mutation results in X-linked severe combined immunodeficiency in humans. Cell 1993;73(1):147–157.
19. Macchi P, Villa A, Giliani S, et al: Mutations of Jak-3 gene in patients with autosomal severe combined immunodeficiency (SCID). Nature 1995; 377(6544):65–68.
20. Puel A, Ziegler SF, Buckley RH, Leonard WJ: Defective IL7R expression in T (−)B(+)NK(+) severe combined immunodeficiency. Nat Genet 1998;20(4): 394–397.
21. Kung C, Pingel JT, Heikinheimo M, et al: Mutations in the tyrosine phosphatase CD45 gene in a child with severe combined immunodeficiency disease. Nat Med 2000;6(3):343–345.
22. Tchilian EZ, Wallace DL, Wells RS, et al: A deletion in the gene encoding the CD45 antigen in a patient with SCID. J Immunol 2001;166(2):1308–1313.
23. Elder ME, Lin D, Clever J, et al: Human severe combined immunodeficiency due to a defect in ZAP-70, a T-cell tyrosine kinase. Science 1994;264(5165): 1596–1599.
24. Schwarz K, Gauss GH, Ludwig L, et al: RAG mutations in human B-cell–negative SCID. Science 1996;274(5284):97–99.
25. Moshous D, Callebaut I, de Chasseval R, et al: Artemis, a novel DNA double-strand break repair/V(D)J recombination protein, is mutated in human severe combined immune deficiency. Cell 2001;105(2):177–186.

26. de Saint-Basile G, Le Deist F, de Villartay JP, et al: Restricted heterogeneity of T lymphocytes in combined immunodeficiency with hypereosinophilia (Omenn's syndrome). J Clin Invest 1991;87(4):1352–1359.

27. Apasov SG, Blackburn MR, Kellems RE, et al: Adenosine deaminase deficiency increases thymic apoptosis and causes defective T cell receptor signaling. J Clin Invest 2001;108(1):131–141.

28. Markert ML, Finkel BD, McLaughlin TM, et al: Mutations in purine nucleoside phosphorylase deficiency. Hum Mutat 1997;9(2):118–121.

29. Greenberg F: DiGeorge syndrome: A historical review of clinical and cytogenetic features. J Med Genet 1993;30:803–806.

30. Thrasher AJ, Kinnon C: The Wiskott-Aldrich syndrome. Clin Exp Immunol 2000;120(1):2–9.

31. Stewart GS, Maser RS, Stankovic T, et al: The DNA double-strand break repair gene hMRE11 is mutated in individual with an ataxia-telangiectasia–like disorder. Cell 1999;99(6):577–587.

32. Dong F, Brynes RK, Tidow N, et al: Mutations in the gene for the granulocyte colony–stimulating-factor receptor in patients with acute myeloid leukemia preceded by severe congenital neutropenia. N Engl J Med 1995;333(8):487–493.

33. Dale DC, Person RE, Bolyard AA, et al: Mutations in the gene encoding neutrophils elastase in congenital and cyclic eutropenia. Blood 2000;96(7):2317–2322.

34. Gorlin RJ, Gelb B, Diaz GA, et al: WHIM syndrome, an autosomal dominant disorder: Clinical, hematological, and molecular studies. Am J Med Genet 2000;91(5):368–376.

35. Dale DC: Immune and idiopathic neutropenia. Curr Opin Hematol 1998;5(1):33–36.

36. Winkelstein JA, Marino MC, Johnston RB Jr, et al: Chronic granulomatous disease. Report on a national registry of 368 patients. Medicine 2000;79(3):155–169.

37. Fischer A, Lisowska-Grospierre B, Anderson DC, Springer TA: Leukocyte adhesion deficiency: Molecular basis and functional consequences. Immunodefic Rev 1988;1(1):39–54.

38. Phillips ML, Schwartz BR, Etzioni A, et al: Neutrophil adhesion in leukocyte adhesion deficiency syndrome type 2. J Clin Invest 1995;96(6):2898–2906.

39. Nagle DL, Karim MA, Woolf EA, et al: Identification and mutation analysis of the complete gene for Chediak-Higashi syndrome. Nat Genet 1996;14(3):307–311.

40. Grimbacher B, Holland SM, Gallin JL, et al: Hyper-IgE syndrome with recurrent infections—an autosomal dominant multisystem disorder. N Engl J Med 1999;340(9):692–702.

41. Sullivan KE, Winkelstein JA: Genetically determined deficiencies of complement. In Scriver CR, Beaudet AL, Sly WS, et al (eds): Metabolic Basis of Inherited Disease, 8th ed. New York, McGraw-Hill, 2001, pp 785–815.

42. Singer L, Colten HR, Wetsel RA: Complement C3 deficiency: Human, animal, and experimental models. Pathobiology 1994;62:14–28.

43. Ross SC, Densen P: Complement deficiency states and infections: Epidemiology, pathogenesis and consequences of neisserial and other infections in an immune deficiency. Medicine 1984;63:243–273.

44. Hacein-Bey-Abina S, Le Deist F, Carlier F, et al: Sustained correction of X-linked severe combined immunodeficiency by ex vivo gene therapy. N Engl J Med 2002;346(16):1185–1193.

*Christopher S. Baliga and William T. Shearer*

# *21* HIV and AIDS

In the latter half of the 20th century, it appeared that medicine had gained the upper hand in the war on microbial disease. With the aid of antibiotics and vaccines, infections like smallpox and tuberculosis has been largely eliminated from industrialized nations. A cluster of *Pneumocystis carinii* pneumonias in previously healthy homosexual men in Los Angeles and, subsequently, New York City in the summer of 1981 heralded the arrival of a new microbial onslaught. By 1982, it had a name, *acquired immunodeficiency syndrome*, or *AIDS*, and by 1983, the causative virus, human immunodeficiency virus, HIV, had been identified. More than 20 years later, the world is still struggling to reign in this modern epidemic.

## EPIDEMIOLOGY

### *GLOBAL PERSPECTIVE*

By the end of 2002, 42 million people were living with HIV/AIDS, of which 3 million were children (Fig. 21-1). Five million of those people were newly infected in 2002, and 3.1 million people died of AIDS that same year. Although certain regions of the globe have been affected more than others by the HIV/AIDS epidemic, none have been spared. Sub-Saharan Africa had 29.4 million people living with HIV/AIDS in 2002, giving it an 8.8% adult prevalence rate. North America, in comparison, had 980,000 infected individuals, giving it a 0.6% adult prevalence rate. By the start of 2003, there had been 28 million deaths due to AIDS since the epidemic began. Current estimates state that 14,000 individuals are newly infected each day. Adult prevalence rates exceed 20% in seven sub-Saharan African countries, with Botswana having the highest rate at 38.8%. South Africa, with 5 million infected citizens, has the largest HIV-positive population in the world. India ranks second with almost 4 million infected individuals.[1]

### *UNITED STATES PERSPECTIVE*

As of the end of 2001, there were 506,154 reported cases of HIV/AIDS in the United States, with an estimated prevalence of 900,000 HIV-infected individuals. The rates of AIDS per 100,000 population were highest in New York (39.3/100,000) and lowest in North Dakota (0.5/100,000) (Table 21-1). In a comparison of cities, Washington, DC, had the highest AIDS prevalence rate of 152.1 per 100,000 population, with New York (65.9/100,000) and Miami (53.8/100,000) rounding out the top three.

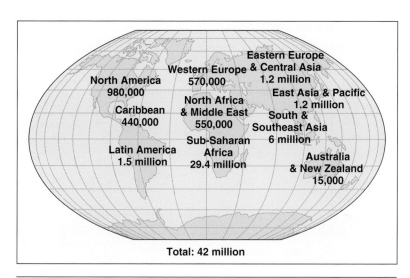

**Total: 42 million**

Figure 21-1. Global distribution of adults and children estimated to be living with HIV infections as of the end of 2002. (Modified from the United Nations Programme on HIV/AIDS.)

| **TABLE 21-1** |  |
| --- | --- |
| Top Five U.S. States/Commonwealths for AIDS Prevalence in 2001 | |
| **State/Commonwealth** | **AIDS Prevalence** |
| 1. New York | 39.3/100,000 |
| 2. Maryland | 34.6/100,000 |
| 3. Puerto Rico | 32.3/100,000 |
| 4. Florida | 31.3/100,000 |
| 5. Delaware | 31.1/100,000 |

It is estimated that 40,000 new cases of HIV infection occur every year in the United States. Male patients make up 60% of new infections, with the percentage of female patients becoming infected increasing each year. Forty-two percent of newly infected individuals are men who have sex with men (MSM), while heterosexual transmission and injection drug abuse account for 33% and 25%, respectively (Fig. 21-2). Racially, African Americans overwhelmingly bear the brunt of new infections, accounting for 54% of new cases even though they make up only 12% of the U.S. population. Whites and Hispanics account for 26% and 19% of new infections, respectively (Fig. 21-3).

The pattern of infection differs dramatically between the sexes. In women, 75% of new HIV cases come from heterosexual transmission, with injection drug abuse accounting for 25%. Of the newly infected women, 64% are African American, 18% are Hispanic, and 18% are white. In men, the pattern differs: Men who have sex with men make up 60% of new cases, and heterosexual transmission and injection drug abuse account for 15% and 25%, respectively. Fifty percent of new male patients are African American, 20% are Hispanic, and 30% are white.

Minorities, particularly African-American men who have sex with men, comprise the largest group of new HIV infections.

Initial successes at controlling the spread of HIV in the United States have faltered in recent years. Incidence rates of new AIDS cases in African Americans and Hispanics have plateaued and have even started to rise (Fig. 21-4). AIDS incidence rates among the MSM community and heterosexuals have also started to creep upward (Figs. 21-5 and 21-6), indicating the need to renew efforts at controlling the spread of HIV.[2]

## MODE OF TRANSMISSION

The three modes of acquiring HIV are sexual, perinatal, or parenteral (Table 21-2). An advanced clinical stage of the disease, a low CD4+ lymphocyte count, and a high HIV viral load are all positively correlated with the risk of HIV transmission.[3] For example, in a case of sexual transmission, the greater the viral load in the source person, the greater the risk of infecting the partner.

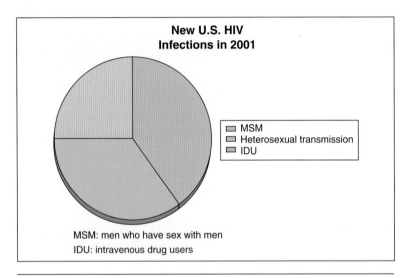

**Figure 21-2.** Route of infection of new HIV infections in the United States in 2001.

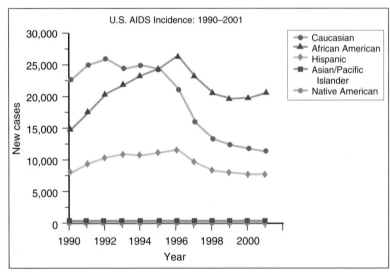

**Figure 21-4.** Incidence of AIDS in the United States broken down by race for 1990 to 2001.

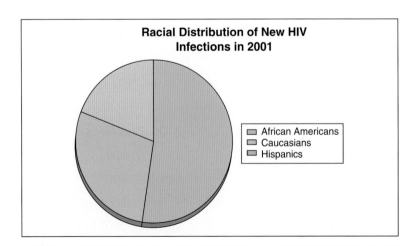

**Figure 21-3.** Racial distribution of new HIV infections in the United States in 2001.

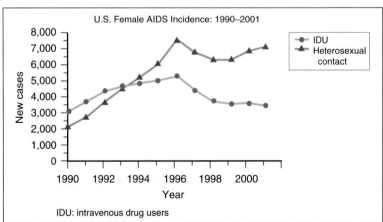

**Figure 21-5.** Incidence of AIDS in U.S. female patients broken down by route of infection for 1990 to 2001.

## Sexual Transmission

Sexual transmission, accounting for 75% of infections, is by far the most common route of infection worldwide.[1] In general, the recipient of penetrative intercourse has the greater risk of becoming infected.[4] Anal intercourse is more likely to spread the virus than vaginal intercourse, with oral intercourse being the least likely.[5] The presence of concomitant sexually transmitted disease, especially ulcerative types such as herpes simplex and syphilis, also increases the risk of HIV infection.[6] In the United States, homosexual transmission is still the most common mode of infection, although heterosexual transmission rates are increasing.[2]

## Perinatal Transmission

In the pediatric population, perinatal transmission represents the most common mode of HIV infection. There are three possible

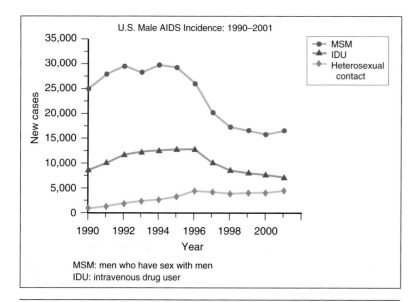

**Figure 21-6.** Incidence of AIDS in U.S. males broken down by route of infection for 1990 to 2001.

**TABLE 21-2**
**Global HIV Modes of Transmission**

| Mode of Transmission | Cases, % |
| --- | --- |
| **Sexual** | **70–80** |
| Vaginal intercourse | 60–70 |
| Anal intercourse | 5–10 |
| **Perinatal** | **5–10** |
| Intrapartum | 2.5–5.0 |
| Postpartum | 2.5–5.0 |
| **Parenteral** | **8–15** |
| IV drug abuse | 5–10 |
| Blood transfusions | 3–5 |

opportunities for perinatal infection to occur: in utero, intrapartum, and postpartum/during breastfeeding.

Babies born to HIV-infected mothers not on antiretroviral therapy have an approximately 25% chance of contracting HIV during gestation or during delivery.[7,8] The majority of these cases are thought to occur shortly before or during labor, although a number of studies have shown increased rates of spontaneous abortions and subfertility in HIV-infected populations.[9,10] This suggests that HIV can unfavorably alter the intrauterine environment and/or fatally infect fetuses during gestation. These in utero infections most likely represent transplacental passage of the virus early in gestation. Intrapartum transmission is defined clinically as negative HIV diagnostic tests within the first 48 hours of life with subsequent tests being positive.[11] These cases represent approximately half of perinatal HIV transmission and are due to fetal exposure to maternal blood and cervical and vaginal secretions during labor. Some studies indicate that the viral mode of entry may be due to fetal swallowing of HIV-infected fluids while traversing the birth canal or to fetal mucous membrane exposure.[12] The remainder of perinatal infections occurs through breast milk transmission. Breastfeeding by an HIV-positive mother adds another 15% to 29% increased risk of HIV infection for the baby.[13] Factors positively affecting breastfeeding transmission rates include maternal viral load, maternal acute retroviral syndrome, mastitis, cracked/ulcerated nipples, mixed bottle/breast feedings, the duration of breastfeeding, and prematurity of the infant.[14] HIV has been found in cell-free milk.[15] It is also known that breast milk contains macrophages and lymphocytes that potentially could be infected with HIV.

## Parenteral Transmission

Parenteral transmission, or direct inoculation of HIV into the host's body, represents the second most common mode of HIV transmission. Injection drug abuse, blood and blood product transfusion, improperly sterilized and reused needles, and needlestick injuries among health care workers are examples of parenteral transmission. In many areas of the world, injection drug abuse accounts for a large proportion, if not the majority, of newly infected cases. Eastern Europe and the Russian Federation's HIV epidemics, for example, are being spurred along by major outbreaks among their IV drug user populations. Official figures from Russia implicate injection drug use in 90% of their new HIV/AIDS cases. Prevalence studies in parts of South and South East Asia show that 50% of injection drug users are infected with HIV.[1] Thirty-six percent of cumulative U.S. AIDS cases can be attributed to injection drug use.[2] Improperly cleaned or reused injection needles/cannulas have resulted in epidemics of nosocomial HIV infections in Russia, China, and many developing countries. Contaminated blood products have resulted in numerous outbreaks around the world. The Romanian example is especially tragic: More than 8000 children became infected through mostly unnecessary HIV-contaminated blood transfusions.[16]

# CLINICAL PRESENTATION AND DIAGNOSIS

The natural history of HIV infection includes three stages: an acute retroviral syndrome, an asymptomatic phase, and a symptomatic phase that heralds the progression to AIDS.

## ACUTE RETROVIRAL SYNDROME

Following exposure to HIV, an incubation period of days to 6 weeks is followed by a period of high viral loads and the development of an immune response against HIV. This stage is characterized by a nonspecific viral illness lasting an average of 14 days. The majority of these patients seek medical attention for this illness; however, because its symptoms are somewhat generic, misdiagnosis by the care provider is common. Typical clinical features are listed in Box 21-1.[17] Any patient with a history of high-risk behavior or HIV exposure presenting with these symptoms should be screened for HIV. It is of note that the commonly used enzyme-linked immunosorbent assay tests for HIV diagnosis do not react until after this acute illness, usually 22 to 27 days following infection. In a case of suspected seroconversion illness, testing for HIV viral RNA or DNA levels is the diagnostic method of choice, although less-sensitive p24 antigen assays or more time-consuming viral cultures can be done.

## ASYMPTOMATIC PHASE AND PRE-AIDS SYNDROME

This is a period in which active HIV replication is occurring, with resultant loss of CD4+ T-cells, the helper T-lymphocytes that conduct the repertoire of immune responses.[18] The body is able to produce enormous numbers of CD4+ cells, which keep the infection in check for a variable length of time.[19] On average in untreated individuals, it takes 8 to 10 years to progress from the initial infection to AIDS.[20] The length of clinical latency is affected by age (with young children having a more rapid progression and adolescents having a longer asymptomatic period than adults) and the level of HIV viremia following the acute seroconversion illness, the viral set point. A higher set point positively correlates with a shorter period of clinical latency.[21] Initially, all infected individuals do not appreciate that they have HIV. Even though they feel fine, they are infectious and are capable of transmitting the disease to others.

Almost invariably in the absence of treatment, this period is characterized by declining CD4+ T-cell counts and relentlessly rising HIV levels in the blood. As the disease progresses, a so-called pre-AIDS develops. This is characterized by persistent generalized lymphadenopathy in 30% to 60% of patients, fatigue, fever, night sweats, diarrhea, and weight loss. Mucocutaneous manifestations become more common, including cutaneous fungal infections, aphthous ulcers, recurrent herpes simplex, molluscum contagiosum (Fig. 21-7), condyloma accuminata (Fig. 21-8), psoriasis, drug-induced skin eruptions, and sebhorrheic dermatitis. Recurrent bacterial infections become more common as antibody responses to antigens drop, despite a polyclonal increase in immunoglobulins. One bacterial disease in particular, tuberculosis, has become synonymous with HIV infection in many countries. Thrombocytopenia may also develop as platelets are destroyed in an autoimmune process. These pathologies illustrate the increasing dysregulation of the immune system.

As CD4+ T-cell levels progressively decrease, other more serious diseases emerge, such as bacillary angiomatosis, thrush, vulvovaginal candidiasis, cervical dysplasia, carcinoma in situ, fever or diarrhea lasting longer than 1 month, oral hairy leukoplakia (Fig. 21-9), recurrent and/or polydermatomal herpes zoster (Fig. 21-10), idiopathic thrombocytopenic purpura, listeriosis, pelvic inflammatory disease, peripheral neuropathy, and toxoplasmosis (Fig. 21-11).[22] In children, problems may include anemia, neutropenia, or thrombocytopenia lasting for more than

---

**BOX 21-1**
**Clinical Features of Acute HIV Infection**

**Symptoms**
Fever
Fatigue
Weight loss
Rash
Headache
Sore throat
Myalgia
Fleeting arthralgia
Nausea
Vomiting
Diarrhea

**Signs**
Tender lymphadenopathy
Pharyngitis
Features of aseptic meningitis
Oral or genital ulcers
Morbilliform or maculopapular nonpruritic rash of the face and trunk

**Laboratory Investigations**
Thrombocytopenia
Leucopenia
Elevated liver enzymes
Positive HIV RNA or DNA by polymerase chain reaction
p24 Antigen
Viral culture

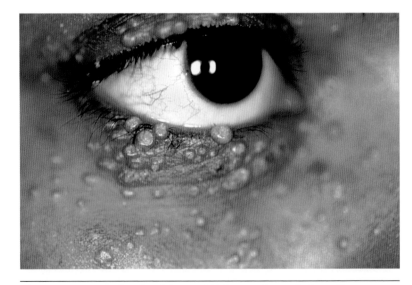

**Figure 21-7.** Multiple skin and lid margin nodules of molloscum contagiosum. (Courtesy of Richard Allen Lewis, MD, MS, Baylor College of Medicine, Houston, TX.)

1 month; bacterial meningitis, pneumonia, or sepsis; oropharyngeal candidiasis for longer than 2 months in children older than 6 months; cardiomyopathy; cytomegalovirus (CMV) infection with onset before 1 month of age; recurrent or chronic diarrhea; hepatitis; recurrent herpes simplex stomatitis; herpes simplex virus (HSV) bronchitis, pneumonitis, or esophagitis with onset before 1 month of age; polydermatomal, or two distinct episodes of, herpes zoster; leiomyosarcoma; lymphoid interstitial pneumonia or pulmonary lymphoid hyperplasia complex; nephropathy; nocardiosis; persistent fever lasting for more than 1 month; toxoplasmosis with onset before 1 month of age; and disseminated varicella.[23]

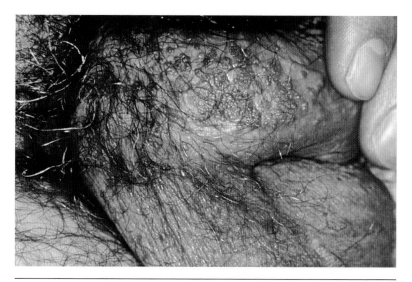

**Figure 21-8.** Multiple verrucous hyperkaratotic papules of condylomata acuminata along the dorsum of the penis. (Courtesy of the American Academy of Dermatology, Schaumburg, IL.)

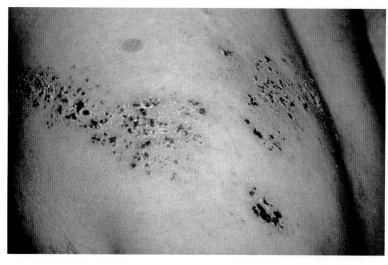

**Figure 21-10.** Numerous crusts in a polydermatomal distribution of herpes zoster with a psoriatic plaque. (Courtesy of the American Academy of Dermatology, Schaumburg, IL.)

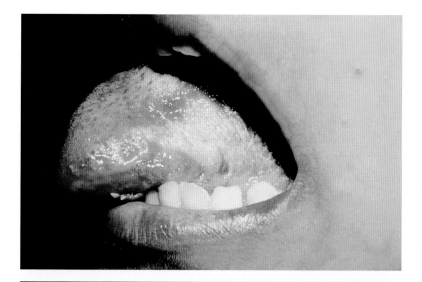

**Figure 21-9.** White adherent plaque of oral hairy leukoplakia located characteristically along the lateral border of the tongue. (Courtesy of Bruce Carter, DDS, Texas Children's Hospital, Houston, TX; Edina Moylett, MD, Baylor College of Medicine, Houston, TX; and the *Journal of Allergy and Clinical Immunology*.)

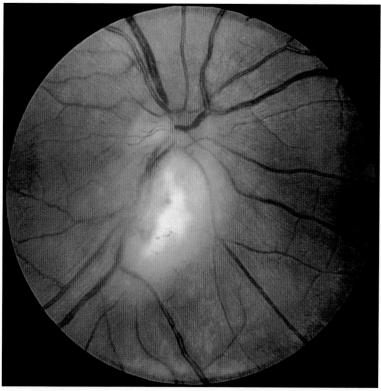

**Figure 21-11.** Acute central necrosis and surrounding neuroepithelial edema in toxoplasma retinitis. (Courtesy of Richard Allen Lewis, MD, MS, Baylor College of Medicine, Houston, TX.)

## BOX 21-2
## AIDS-Defining Illnesses

Candidiasis of the esophagus, bronchi, trachea, or lungs (Fig. 21-12)

Cervical cancer, invasive

Coccidioidomycosis, disseminated or extrapulmonary

Cryptococcosis, extrapulmonary (e.g., meningitis)

Cryptosporidiosis, chronic intestinal (longer than 1 mo duration)

Cytomegalovirus disease of any organ other than liver, spleen, or lymph nodes (Fig. 21-13)

Cytomegalovirus retinitis with loss of vision (Fig. 21-14)

Encephalopathy, HIV related

Herpes simplex: Chronic ulcer(s) (longer than 1 mo duration) or bronchitis, pneumonitis, or esophagitis

Histoplasmosis, disseminated or extrapulmonary

Isosporiasis, chronic intestinal (longer than 1 mo duration)

Kaposi's sarcoma (Fig. 21-15)

Burkitt's lymphoma

Non-Hodgkin's lymphoma (immunoblastic)

Primary lymphoma of the brain

*Mycobacterium avium* complex or *Mycobacterium kandasii*, disseminated or extrapulmonary (Fig. 21-16)

*Mycobacterium tuberculosis*, any site

*Mycobacterium* spp., other species, disseminated or extrapulmonary

*Pneumocystis carinii* pneumonia (Figs. 21-17 and 21-18)

Pneumonia recurrent

Progressive multifocal leukoencephalopathy

Salmonella septicemia, recurrent

Toxoplasmosis of the brain

Wasting syndrome due to HIV

## ACQUIRED IMMUNODEFICIENCY SYNDROME

Acquired immunodeficiency syndrome is an advanced stage of HIV infection that is characterized by CD4+ T-cell counts less than 200 cells per milliliter and certain defining illnesses, as listed in Box 21-2 and shown in Figures 21-12 through 21-18.[20,21] HIV infection can also directly damage several organ systems including the heart, brain, kidneys, and retinas (Fig. 21-19). Without therapy, most patients will develop AIDS 8 to 10 years after infection and will die 1.3 years after developing AIDS.[24,25]

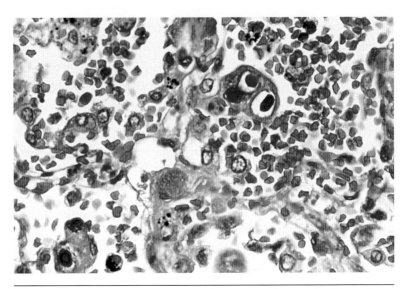

**Figure 21-13.** Characteristic "owl's eye" inclusion bodies of cytomegalovirus pneumonitis with hemorrhage into the alveolar spaces. (Courtesy of Edwina Popek, DO, Baylor College of Medicine, Houston, TX.)

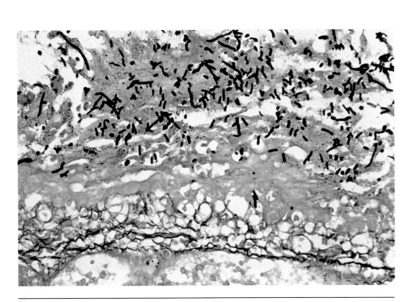

**Figure 21-12.** Numerous *Candida* hyphae infiltrating the esophageal epithelium. (Courtesy of Edwina Popek, DO, Baylor College of Medicine, Houston, TX.)

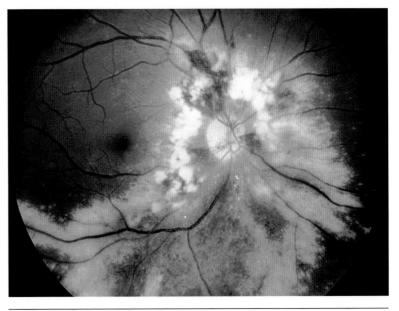

**Figure 21-14.** A classic pattern of cytomegalovirus retinitis, with acute necrotizing retinitis on the leading, expanding margins, some superficial hemorrhages, and central lucent zone of destroyed tissue. (Courtesy of Richard Allen Lewis, MD, MS, Baylor College of Medicine, Houston, TX.)

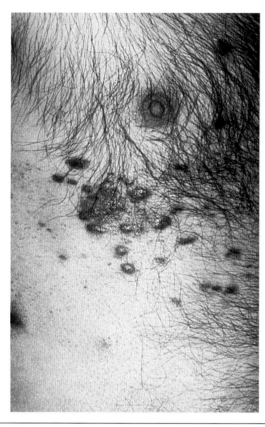

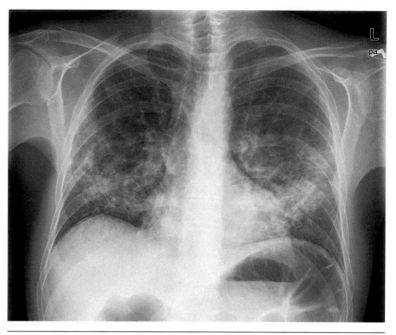

**Figure 21-17.** Chest x-ray demonstrating bilateral predominantly lower lobe diffuse infiltrates. Bronchoalveolar lavage confirmed the diagnosis of *Pneumocystis carinii* pneumonia. (Courtesy of Richard Hamill, MD, Baylor College of Medicine, Houston, TX.)

**Figure 21-15.** Multiple nodules of Kaposi's sarcoma in a follicular pattern along the chest wall. (Courtesy of the American Academy of Dermatology, Schaumburg, IL.)

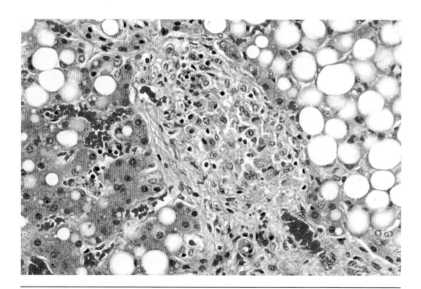

**Figure 21-16.** *Mycobacterium avium* complex infection of the liver demonstrating a granuloma and fatty changes and loss of normal architecture in the hepatic parenchyma. (Courtesy of Edwina Popek, DO, Baylor College of Medicine, Houston, TX.)

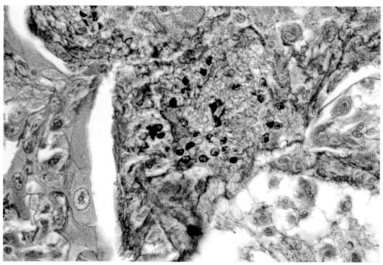

**Figure 21-18.** Numerous *Pneumocystis carinii* cysts visible in the alveolar spaces. (Courtesy of Edwina Popek, DO, Baylor College of Medicine, Houston, TX.)

# DIAGNOSIS

In a patient with a compatible history and clinical findings, the diagnosis of HIV should be confirmed. A variety of diagnostic tests are available (Box 21-3). In most cases, the initial test of choice is the simple, rapid, and inexpensive enzyme-linked immunosorbent assay. This test measures the presence of HIV envelope antibodies in the sera of patients. As it is a screening test, HIV enzyme-linked immunosorbent assays are designed to have a high sensitivity at the expense of specificity. That means that it is biased to detect false positives in lieu of false negatives. To confirm the diagnosis, a Western blot immunoassay for HIV envelope antibodies in the serum is ordered. Most patients seroconvert; that is, they develop measurable antibodies to HIV 6 to 8 weeks after infection, with 90% reacting by 3 months (Fig. 21-20). In cases of suspected acute infection or in infants born to HIV-infected mothers, other tests are used to support the diagnosis of HIV. HIV DNA polymerase chain reaction assays detecting cellular HIV DNA or HIV RNA polymerase chain reaction assays detecting plasma viral RNA are widely used tests. Polymerase chain reaction offers a highly sensitive and specific assay for the detection of HIV. Older assays that can still be employed, but that have less sensitivity or are harder to use, are viral p24 antigen assays and viral cultures.[26]

# PATHOPHYSIOLOGY

## ETIOLOGY

Human immunodeficiency virus is a member of the lentivirinae subfamily of retroviruses. It has a double-stranded RNA genome with a capsid and a lipid envelope (Fig. 21-21). HIV is thought to have arisen in Western Africa as the result of an HIV-like illness in chimpanzees caused by the simian immunodeficiency virus crossing species to humans.[27]

There are two main types of HIV, HIV-1 and HIV-2. HIV-1 is more common and is more pathogenic than its cousin. HIV-2 is found predominantly in West Africa and follows a more benign clinical course. HIV-1 is composed of three groups: M (major), O (outlier), and N (new or non-M, non-O). Group M is further subdivided into eight different clades, or subtypes. Clade B is the most common form of HIV-1 in the Americas, Western Europe, and Japan. Clade C, on the other hand, is the most common form worldwide, being widely prevalent in Africa and India. In South East Asia, clade E (also called AE) predominates.[28]

The HIV-1 genome consists of a 9.8-kbp double-stranded RNA, encoding structural proteins, accessory proteins, and regulatory proteins (Fig. 21-22). The structural proteins are encoded in the Gag, Pol, and Env genes. The Gag gene yields the protein p55, which aids in viral budding from infected cells. It is then cleaved into four components: matrix (p17), capsid (p24), nucleocapsid (p9), and p6. Pol encodes the viral reverse transcriptase, integrase, RNase H, and protease. Env leads to the production of gp160, which is further processed into gp120 and gp41. gp41 is the transmembrane domain of Env, and gp120 rests on the surface of the virion bound to gp41. The regulatory proteins, Tat and Rev, are

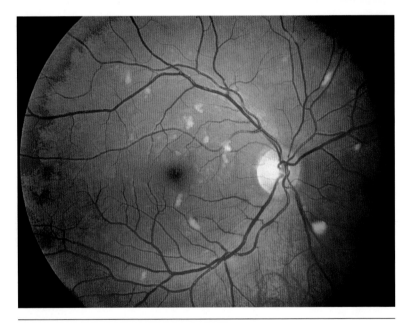

**Figure 21-19.** Numerous cotton-wool spots in primary HIV retinopathy. (Courtesy of Richard Allen Lewis, MD, MS, Baylor College of Medicine, Houston, TX.)

## BOX 21-3
### Diagnostic Tests for HIV Infection

ELISA
Western blot
DNA PCR
RNA PCR
p24 Antigen
Viral culture

ELISA, enzyme-linked immunosorbent assay; PCR, polymerase chain reaction.

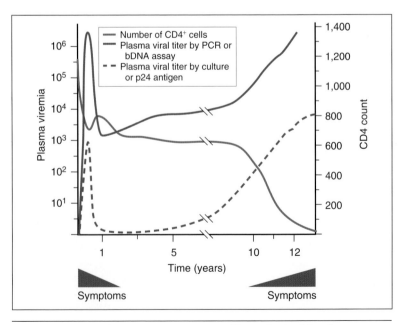

**Figure 21-20.** Changes in CD4+ T cells and viral load over time in an untreated case of HIV. PCR, polymerase chain reaction.

essential for HIV replication. Tat is a transcription activator, and Rev facilitates the transition from early- to late-phase HIV gene expression. The accessory proteins are not necessary for the survival of HIV, but they do increase the fitness of the virus. They include Nef, Vif, Vpr, and Vpu. Nef has many roles in increasing the virulence of the virus. These include downregulation of surface CD4 and major histocompatibility complex class I molecules, which interferes with signal transduction pathways and increases the infectivity of HIV virions by a factor of 10. Vpr aids HIV in infecting nondividing cells. Vif is believed to counteract an intracellular antiviral factor. Vpu downregulates CD4 expression and facilitates virion release from infected cells.[29,30]

## IMMUNOPATHOGENESIS

The majority of infections begin in mucosal Langerhans cells. The initial infection is predominantly by macrophage-tropic virus strains called M-tropic viruses or, more recently, R5 viruses. The name *R5* is derived from this strain's need to bind to chemokine receptor CCR5 on the macrophages.[31] HIV is phagocytosed by the Langerhans cells via an interaction with DC-SIGN (dendritic cell-specific intercellular adhesion molecule–grabbing nonintegrin) and viral gp120. This leads to internalization of the virus but not its fusion with the cell. As a result, HIV is endocytosed intact in phagosomes, and intact HIV virions are transported to the cell's

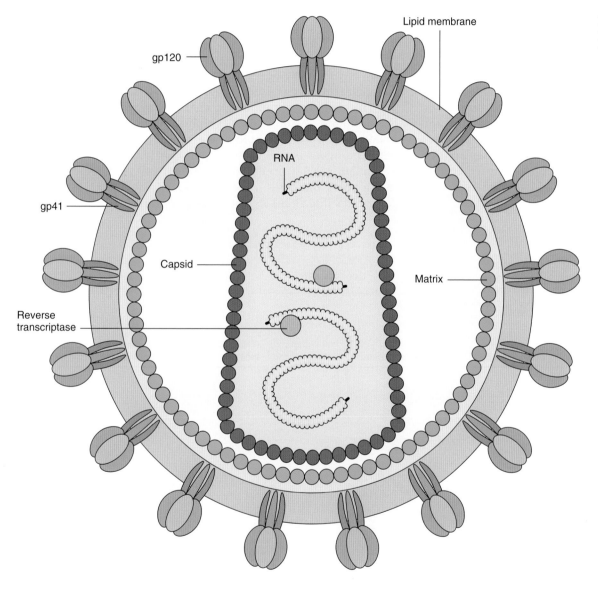

**Figure 21-21.** The structure of HIV.

**Figure 21-22.** Genomic sequence of HIV-1.

surface. It has been suggested that the acidic environment of the phagosome acts to prime or potentiate the infectivity of the virus.[32] Langerhans cells migrate to regional lymph nodes and in primate studies have been found in the pelvic draining internal iliac lymph nodes 3 days following infection.[33] Within 5 days, HIV can be cultured from the peripheral blood.[34] It is within the lymph nodes that the Langerhans cells present HIV virions to CD4+ T-cells.[28] HIV virion surface glycoprotein gp120 binds to the CD4+ receptor on T cells and then to the coreceptor CCR5. This induces a conformational change in HIV's envelope, allowing the fusion domain of gp41 to interact with the cell membrane. HIV gp41 is a coiled protein that when triggered "harpoons" the CD4+ cell like a spring. This allows the cell and the virus to interact in such a way that the viral contents enter into the cell's cytoplasm.[35] Once inside, the viral RNA is uncoated, and reverse transcriptase–mediated transcription into DNA takes place. The viral cDNA is then transported into the nucleus, where it integrates randomly with the host cell's DNA using the viral integrase enzyme. Following cell activation, viral DNA is transcribed into viral mRNA, which is then transported to the cytoplasm. Viral peptide chains are translated from the viral RNA and cleaved by viral proteinases. The virus is then assembled into a complete unit with proteins and RNA and released from the cell by budding or lysis (Fig. 21-23).[36]

Later in the course of infection, R5 viruses are replaced by X4 viruses. These T cell–tropic viruses bind to the coreceptor CXCR4 and are syncitium inducing. R5 viruses are non–syncitium inducing and more common in the early stages of infection.[37]

Whereas HIV can infect both activated and inactivated cells, it takes infection of activated CD4+ cells to yield productive HIV replication.[38] Studies suggest that the majority of virions present in the blood are produced from recently infected CD4+ cells in the lymph nodes and spleen.[39,40] As many as 10 billion virions a day can be produced in untreated patients, but most of these are uninfectious.[41,42] The plasma half-life of HIV is less than 6 hours, and the half-life of productively infected T cells is 1 to 2 days.[43]

One of the characteristics of HIV is its variability. At any given time, there may be thousands of genetically different strains of viruses in one person. This is due to the fact that reverse transcriptase has a high degree of infidelity and that HIV has a high degree of turnover. Reverse transcriptase fails to produce exact copies of the template genome, with nucleotide substitutions occurring as commonly as 1 in 1500 to 4000 bases.[27] Taken with the fact that as many as 10 billion virions a day are produced in untreated individuals, this means that every possible amino acid substitution can occur each day. These properties help HIV evade any effective host immune response, as well as allowing it to rapidly produce resistance to antiviral medications.

The defining immunologic characteristic of HIV infection is the profound loss of CD4+ T-lymphocytes in the body over time. Following an initial drop in CD4+ cell numbers that corresponds with the initial period of heavy viremia (viral loads higher than 10 million are not uncommon), CD4+ T-cell populations stabilize in numbers but with an extraordinary rise in cell turnover.[44] Active HIV infection kills not only infected HIV-specific T cells, but

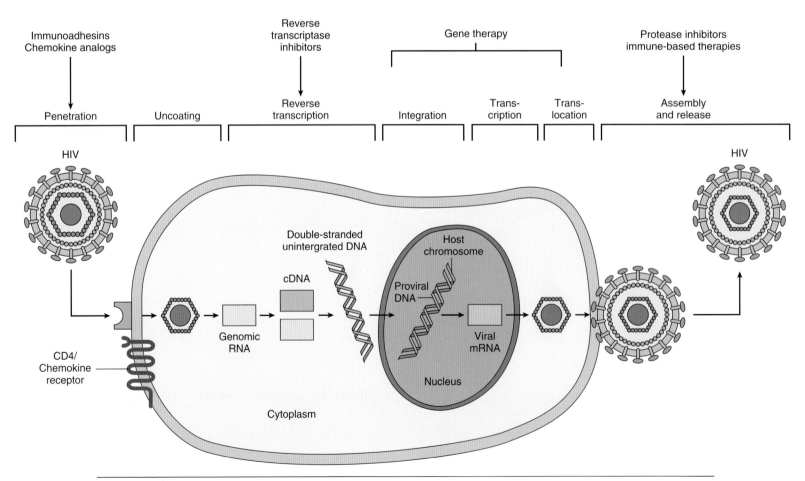

**Figure 21-23.** The life cycle of HIV, with the sites of actions of antiretroviral agents or anti-HIV therapies.

other CD4+ cells.[17] For a variable period of time, usually 7 to 10 years in untreated adults, the body is able to hold its own against the HIV onslaught, but the virus is relentless.

A poorly understood aspect of HIV infection is the concept of a viral set point. Following the initial stage of viremia, HIV viral loads stabilize at a level that they will maintain for several years.[45] A high HIV set point is a poor prognostic indicator, as patients with this condition tend to progress more rapidly to AIDS. Conversely, a low set point is a good prognostic indicator.[46] The correlates of what determines the set point are not known. It is believed that a high HIV set point indicates less initial control of the HIV infection by cytotoxic T-lymphocytes or neutralizing antibodies.[47]

In response to HIV infection, the body mounts a two-pronged attack, humoral and cell-mediated responses. Both ultimately fail. Neutralizing antibodies to a variety of HIV surface epitopes are produced.[48] However, the ability of HIV to mutate away from the body's selective immune pressure negates this response. Similarly, the body mounts an effective cytotoxic T-lymphocyte response to a variety of HIV epitopes. This positive pressure coupled with the virus' propensity to mutate pushes HIV toward the production of "escape mutants," which evade existing immune responses.[49] For a time (the asymptomatic period of HIV infection), T cells specific to the new mutants emerge. Eventually, the body's ability to regenerate the immune system is overwhelmed, possibly by clonal exhaustion or deletion through accelerated apoptosis, and what was once a gradual decline in CD4+ T-lymphocytes increases in rate.[50] As CD4 levels drop, the body tries to maintain the total number of T cells by increasing the numbers of CD8+ T cells.[17] But without the T-helper cell populations, the immune system ceases to mount an effective response to invading pathogens due to a lack of cell-mediated immunity. In particular, there is a failure of cytotoxic T-lymphocytes to fight infections due to the paucity of CD4+ T-lymphocyte–produced cytokines such as interleukin-2.[51] B cells also suffer derangement. There is a polyclonal activation of plasma cells, which in turn secrete antibodies. This nonspecific stimulation of B-lymphocytes and plasma cells is a result of gp120 acting as a superantigen and gp120's ability to induce tumor necrosis factor-α production.[52,53] There is also decreased ability to respond to recall antigens in vitro. In addition, the body loses its ability to mount an effective antibody response to new antigens.[54] Downregulation of the B-cell receptor by gp120 and loss of T-helper cells are possible explanations for these phenomena.[55] As a result, HIV-infected individuals become prone to infections. They suffer the same spectrum of disease as a person with a primary T-cell immunodeficiency, infection with organisms such as *P. carinii* and *Candida* spp. and the development of neoplasms such as

Kaposi's sarcoma and lymphoma. AIDS is a somewhat arbitrary definition of disease severity along HIV's spectrum of disease. But it is at CD4+ T-cell levels of less than 200 cells per milliliter that opportunistic infections begin their stranglehold on the patient.

CD4+ macrophages and microglia in the brain also become infected with HIV, usually by infected blood monocyte migration into the central nervous system. Neuronal injury is thought to occur as a result of macrophage, microglial, and astrocyte toxins, as HIV does not infect neurons.[56] Neuronal apoptosis has also been reported.[57] Eventually, neurologic sequelae, such as HIV-associated dementia and multifocal leukoencephalopathy, appear.

# TREATMENT

Despite the health care community's best efforts, HIV remains an incurable disease. The best therapy, therefore, is prevention. Barring that, the advent of highly active antiretroviral therapy (HAART) has revolutionized the care of HIV/AIDS in developed countries. Since its introduction in 1996, the incidence of AIDS has dropped 32%.[2] More experience managing opportunistic infections has also contributed to a decrease in AIDS mortality. With these two factors, there are more people living longer than ever before with HIV/AIDS. It is hoped that in compliant patients who tolerate HAART, HIV has been converted from a death sentence into a manageable chronic disease. Time will tell whether this is wishful thinking.

The cornerstone of HIV management is HAART, which is combination therapy for HIV. It consists of two nucleotide reverse transcriptase inhibitors (NRTIs) plus a protease inhibitor or two NRTIs plus a non-NRTI. These therapeutic cocktails lead to dramatic reductions in viral loads, rebounds in CD4+ T-cell counts, and, over time, a variable degree of immune reconstitution.

Ideally, the newly diagnosed HIV-infected patient should be introduced to the health care delivery system as quickly as possible for close follow-up. Time will be needed to counsel the patient on the risks and benefits of HAART and the need for full compliance. In addition, it will take some time to enroll indigent patients in local assistance programs so that the formidable financial hurdles associated with prescribing HAART can be overcome.

The question of when to begin HAART is not an easy one. Table 21-3 lists the current U.S. guidelines for initiating therapy.[58] Although few physicians would argue against the wisdom of starting therapy when the CD4+ counts are less than 200 cells per milliliter, the experts disagree when CD4+ counts are above 200. There is a 30% risk of developing AIDS in 3 years when viral

**TABLE 21-3**
**Indications for Initiating HAART: Adult Subjects**

| Clinical Status | CD4+ Cell Counts | Plasma HIV RNA | Recommendation |
|---|---|---|---|
| AIDS or symptomatic | <200 cells/mL | Any value | Treat |
| Asymptomatic | >200 cells/mL but < 350 cells/mL | Any value | Treat |
| | >350 cells/mL | >55,000 copies/mL | Treat or closely monitor |
| | >350 cells/mL | <55,000 copies/mL | Closely monitor |

HAART, highly active antiretroviral therapy.

RNA is above 55,000 copies per milliliter and CD4+ counts are more than 350 cells per milliliter. Alternatively, the 3-year risk of developing AIDS is less than 15% when CD4+ counts are above 350 cells per milliliter and plasma viral RNA is under 55,000. The national guidelines represent a starting point in the decision-making process, and each case should be considered individually. The actual decision to start HAART should be made only after considering a variety of factors. Unfortunately, practical concerns such as the patient's ability to afford therapy and his or her access to a pharmacy must be addressed. The practitioner should be satisfied that the patient will regularly take the antiretrovirals and thoroughly understands the therapeutic regime. The risks and benefits of either delaying therapy or starting therapy early should be discussed. These are outlined in Table 21-4.[56] Based on this information, patients should be allowed to make their own decisions whether to begin HAART. The regimens are not easy to follow, with many side effects, and the effects on the patient's quality of life are not trivial. If the patient is not fully convinced of the necessity of taking HAART regularly, there is a very real risk of HIV developing resistance to one or more antiretroviral drugs or class of drugs. Lack of adherence to medication regimens is perhaps the biggest factor in the development of drug resistance in the post-HAART era.

There are four classes of Food and Drug Administration–approved drugs for treating HIV: NRTIs, non-NRTIs, protease inhibitors, and fusion inhibitors. Table 21-5 lists the therapeutic agents licensed by the Food and Drug Administration.[59] Figure 21-23 shows their sites of action in the viral life cycle. NRTIs are also called nucleoside analogues. They act as competitive inhibitors of reverse transcriptase and can be incorporated into the transcribed cDNA. Once they are incorporated into the growing cDNA chain, further elongation is blocked. Non-NRTIs bind to reverse transcriptase and inhibit RNA- and DNA-dependent reverse transcriptase activities. They are specific for HIV-1, whereas all other antiretrovirals work for both HIV-1 and HIV-2. Protease inhibitors act to inhibit the HIV-protease, which cleaves the large polypeptide Gag-Pol into the functional proteins needed for HIV

to be infective.[60] The newest class of licensed antiretrovirals is fusion inhibitors, and monoclonal antibodies against HIV surface proteins are in clinical trials. These drugs and biologic agents act to prevent HIV penetration into susceptible cells.[61]

Human immunodeficiency virus's rapid ability to alter its genotype in such a way as to confer resistance to antiretrovirals has plagued clinicians since the first attempts to treat HIV. Monotherapy with NRTIs, non-NRTIs, protease inhibitors, and fusion inhibitors is associated with a rapid development of resistance.[62–65] As with other infections in which resistance is a problem, combination therapy is used to rapidly control viral replication.[66] While the chance of a mutation conferring resistance to one drug is high, the chance of multiple simultaneous mutations so that three drugs become ineffective is low. This strategy is successful in controlling HIV in most cases where the patient is compliant in taking medications regularly. This regimen is not easy to follow, as significant numbers of pills must be taken multiple times per day.[67] Failure of viral control, as evidenced by rising viral loads and dropping CD4+ cell counts, warrants a genotypic and a phenotypic evaluation of the virus to determine its drug sensitivities.[68] Using that information, a new combination of drugs can be devised to control the virus.

In well-controlled HIV cases where the CD4+ cell counts remain above 200 cells per milliliter, HAART is the mainstay of HIV treatment. The hallmark of AIDS and clinical progression is the appearance of opportunistic infections. These severely reduce the quality of life and in many cases are the cause of death in AIDS patients. To combat these infections, prophylactic guidelines, as shown in Table 21-6, have been developed.[69]

Following the introduction of HAART, many patients experience, to varying degrees, reconstitution of their battered immune systems.[70] In just a few days, viral loads drop precipitously and there is a rapid increase in peripheral lymphocyte counts. Most of this early increase is due to memory T- and B-lymphocytes, which are redistributing from the lymphoid compartment.[71] Over time, the thymus is able to repopulate the body with naïve T cells and B cells. Interestingly, this occurs in both adults and children.[72]

**TABLE 21-4**
**Risks and Benefits of Early Versus Delayed HAART**

|  | Benefits | Risks |
|---|---|---|
| Early therapy | Easier to control and maintain viral suppression | Reduces quality of life due to drug regimen |
|  | Delays or prevents immune system compromise | Increases risk of adverse events from the medication |
|  | Lowers the risk of resistance with complete viral suppression | Increases risk of earlier development of viral resistance if suppression is suboptimal |
|  | Decreases the risk of HIV transmission | Limits future antiretroviral options |
| Delayed therapy | Prevents decreased quality of life due to the therapeutic regimen | Increases risk of irreversible immune system damage |
|  | Prevents adverse events from the medication | Increases difficulty in achieving maximum viral suppression |
|  | Delays the development of drug resistance | May increase risk of HIV transmission |
|  | Preserves antiretroviral options for when risk is greatest |  |

**TABLE 21-5**
Antiretroviral Agents

## Food and Drug Administration–Approved Antiretroviral Drugs

|  | Generic Name | Abbreviation | Brand Name |
|---|---|---|---|
| **Nucleoside Reverse Transcriptase Inhibitors** | Zidovudine | AZT, ZDV | *Retrovir* |
|  | Didanosine | Ddl | *Videx* |
|  | Zalcitabine | DdC | *Hivid* |
|  | Stavudine | d4T | *Zerit* |
|  | Lamivudine | 3TC | *Epivir* |
|  | Abacavir | ABC | *Ziagen* |
|  | Tenofovir DF | TDF | *Viread* |
|  | Emtricitabine | FTC | *Emtriva* |
| **Fusion Inhibitor** | Enfuvirtide | T-20 | *Fuzeon* |
| **Non-Nucleoside Reverse Transcriptase Inhibitors** | Nevirapine | NVP | *Viramune* |
|  | Delavirdine | DLV | *Rescriptor* |
|  | Efavirenz | EFV | *Sustiva* |
| **Protease Inhibitors** | Saquinavir | SQV, hgc | *Invirase* |
|  |  | SQV, sgc | *Fortovase* |
|  | Ritonavir | RTV | *Norvir* |
|  | Indinavir | IDV | *Crixivan* |
|  | Nelfinavir | NFV | *Viracept* |
|  | Amprenavir | APV | *Agenerase* |
|  | Atazanavir |  | *Reyataz* |

**TABLE 21-6**
Opportunistic Infection Prophylaxis

| Risk Factor | Agent | Prophylactic Medication |
|---|---|---|
| CD4+ cell count <200 cells/mL | *Pneumocystis carinii* | Trimethoprim-sulfamethoxazole |
|  | Coccidioidomycosis | Fluconazole or itraconazole |
| CD4+ cell count <100 cells/mL | *Toxoplasma gondii* | Trimethoprim-sulfamethoxazole |
|  | Histoplasmosis | Itraconazole |
| CD4+ cell count <50 cells/mL | *Mycobacterium avium* complex | Macrolide (clarithromycin or azithromycin) |
|  | Cryptococcosis | Fluconazole or itraconazole |
|  | Cytomegalovirus | Ganciclovir |
| PPD >5 mm induration or recent tuberculosis contact | *Mycobacterium tuberculosis* | Rifampin + pyrizinamide or INH + pyridoxine |
| Contact with chickenpox or shingles in Varicella zoster–seronegative individuals | *Varicella zoster* | Varicella zoster immunoglobulins |
| HIV infected | *Streptococcus pneumoniae* | Pneumovax |
| Negative anti–hepatitis B core or anti–hepatitis B surface | Hepatitis B | Recombivax hepatitis B or Energex-B |
| Negative anti-hepatitis A serology | Hepatitis A | Havrix |

INH, isoniazid.

# PREVENTION

Prevention is the key to any AIDS control strategy, as HIV cannot be cured once infection has taken place. Sexual activity is the major mode of viral transmission worldwide, making an emphasis on safe sexual practices a necessity. Latex male condoms have been shown to be a cost-effective way to prevent the transmission of HIV. It has been estimated that condoms could reduce the risk of HIV transmission by 85%.[73] Directed interventions to high-risk populations have been shown to be more cost-effective than those aimed at the general public.[74] Ensuring sterile needle use by IV drug abusers and supplying condoms to the sexually promiscuous or to commercial sex workers are examples. Sources for nosocomial infection also must be eliminated. All blood products must be screened for HIV among other pathogens before they are administered to patients. Needles and surgical instruments must be sterile. It is estimated that 3.9% to 7% of new HIV cases worldwide are nosocomial, occurring due to the reuse of improperly sterilized needles, surgical instruments, and dialysis tubes or improperly screened blood products.[75]

## OCCUPATIONAL EXPOSURE

As of the end of 2001, there were 57 known cases of HIV infection resulting from occupational exposure in the United States.[76] Needlesticks, penetrating injuries, and body fluid exposure are real concerns for health care workers. Simple measures such as universal precautions, double gloving, not recapping needles, proper use of sharps containers, and wearing face shields in high-risk situations can reduce the likelihood of needlesticks or body fluid exposure. In the event of exposure, the risk of contracting HIV from a penetrating injury is 0.3%. Current recommendations for occupational postexposure prophylaxis are two NRTIs plus one protease inhibitor for 4 weeks following the exposure. Animal studies suggest that prophylactic therapy should begin within 1 to 2 hours of exposure and no later than 24 to 36 hours after exposure.[77]

## PERINATAL TRANSMISSION

In most countries, the main source of pediatric HIV infection is maternal transmission. The Pediatric AIDS Clinical Trial Group study 076 reported a striking 66% reduction in the transmission of HIV from mother to child, with a 27.5% transmission rate in the placebo arm of the study and a 7.9% transmission rate in the interventional arm.[78] This groundbreaking study forms the basis of current U.S. guidelines for the prevention of perinatal HIV transmission. The Public Health Service recommends a course of oral zidovudine starting at 14 to 36 weeks gestation, continuous intravenous zidovudine infusion during labor, and 6 weeks of oral zidovudine to the infant.[79] Simpler and less-expensive protocols have been designed for resource-poor settings. Examples include shorter courses of zidovudine, zidovudine/lamivudine combinations, and a two-dose regimen of nevirapine (one maternal dose at the onset of labor and one neonatal dose at 48 to 72 hours of life).[80–82] Although most of these alternative protocols are beneficial, they are all less efficacious than the Pediatric AIDS Clinical Trial Group 076 protocol.

Some controversy surrounds the optimal mode of infant delivery for an HIV-infected mother, mostly because the studies undertaken to answer the issue were conducted in the pre-HAART era and may not reflect today's realities. Evidence from older studies demonstrated that the rate of infection in an elective cesarean delivery before the onset of labor with intact membranes in a patient receiving zidovudine was 2%, compared with 7.3% for other delivery modalities, and if the mother did not receive zidovudine, the rate of infection was 3.4% to 10% versus 10.2% to 19%.[83,84] Current American College of Obstetricians and Gynecologists guidelines recommend considering an elective cesarean section only if the mother has an HIV viral load of more than 1000

---

**TABLE 21-7**
**Selected HIV Vaccine Strategies in Clinical Trials**

| Vaccine Name | Prime Component | Boost Component |
|---|---|---|
| ALVAC vCP1452 | Canarypox vector (clade B Env, Gag, Pro, RT, Nef) | Protein subunit (clade B Env) |
| NefTat + gp120W61 D | Protein (clade B Nef-Tat fusion protein, clade B Env subunit) | |
| PGA2/JS2 DNA | DNA plasmid (clade B Env, Gag, Pro, RT, Tat, Vpu, Rev) | MVA vector (clade B Env, Gag, Pro, RT, Tat, Vpu, Rev) |
| AVX-101 | VEE Vector (clade C Gag) | |
| HIVAX-GS | Heat-killed recombinant *Saccharomyces cerevisiae* (clade B Gag) | |
| VRC-HIVDNA-010 | Nonreplicating adenoviral vectors (clade B Gag-Pol-Nef; clades A, B, and C Env) | |
| TBC-M358; TBC-M335 | MVA vector (clade B Env, Gag, Tat, Rev, Pol, Nef) | Fowlpox vectors (clade B Env, Gag, Tat, Rev, Pol, Nef) |

MVA, modified vaccine ankara; VEE, Venezuelan equine encephalitis.

copies per milliliter, labor has recently started or not yet begun, and her membranes are intact or only recently ruptured. There is no evidence to support elective cesarean section for the purpose of HIV prophylaxis if the woman's viral load is less than 1000 copies per milliliter.[85]

An additional risk factor for HIV transmission is breastfeeding. Current World Health Organization recommendations advise against the breastfeeding of infants by an HIV-infected mother. In settings where no safe or affordable alternative to breast milk exists, the World Health Organization considers the health risks of not breastfeeding the infant greater than the risk of contracting HIV.[86]

## *VACCINES*

Current HAART therapy, while effective, is prohibitively expensive and logistically complex. It is an economic impossibility for developing countries to assume the enormous financial burden required. In some cases, treatment would involve more than 20% of a country's population. Considering that the majority of patients needing antiviral medications in underdeveloped countries are barely literate and unlikely to get close supervisory support, the need for an alternative solution is manifest. A successful vaccine holds the greatest hope for turning the tide of the epidemic, although years of effort and substantial resources have so far yielded only partial results in nonhuman models.

There are two possible endpoints for HIV vaccine developers: a prophylactic vaccine that protects the recipient from acquiring infection and a therapeutic vaccine that favorably alters the clinical course of HIV. The primary goal of a prophylactic vaccine, protection from infection, remains elusive. Only in Rhesus macaques has the goal been achieved with live-attenuated vaccines. Concerns over their ability to revert to pathogenic virus have prevented similar approaches with HIV from moving forward.[87] Therapeutic vaccines in nonhuman primate models, however, have succeeded in lowering the viral set point and prolonging the period of clinical latency.[88,89] Current strategies employed by vaccinologists against HIV include the use of whole-killed virus; live-attenuated virus; recombinant proteins like gp120 and gp160; peptide fragments like Nef and reverse transcriptase; DNA fragments or plasmids encoding Gag, Pol, or Env; replicons (i.e., viruses or bacteria genetically engineered to express various HIV components); and pseudovirions. Most current approaches focus on various combinations of these strategies. Table 21-7 lists examples of ongoing HIV vaccine trials.[90]

Human immunodeficiency virus has proven to be a formidable foe, especially with vaccine design. It has long been known that patients infected with HIV develop neutralizing antibodies as well as cytotoxic T-lymphocyte responses. HIV with its error-prone reverse transcriptase, ability to recombine with other HIV strains, and high rate of replication, is able to quickly evolve changes in its antigenic structure, thus enabling it to sidestep existing immune responses, possibly by creating glycan shields (glycoprotein coats of shifting character/location).[91] It is for these reasons that the body ultimately fails to control the virus. Vaccine designers are attempting to overcome these obstacles and to accomplish what the body could not, an effective immune response against HIV. One approach is to stimulate both a cellular and a humoral immune response against a few highly effective epitopes, such that following an exposure to the virus, the host's now primed immune system can block HIV from gaining a foothold in the body. This would not give HIV a chance to replicate and mutate away from immunologic control. Another approach is to induce neutralizing antibody and cytotoxic T-lymphocyte responses to HIV epitopes that do not change with virus replication. This should ensure that the vaccine-induced immunity will remain effective against the virus even as it mutates.[92]

# REFERENCES

1. Joint United Nations Program on HIV/AIDS: Report on the Global HIV/AIDS Epidemic. UNAIDS, Geneva, 2002.
2. Centers for Disease Control and Prevention: HIV/AIDS Surveillance Report. Vol. 13. Bethesda, MD, Centers for Disease Control and Prevention, 2001, pp 1–44.
3. Piot P, Plummer FA, Mhalu FS, et al: AIDS: An international perspective. Science 1988;239:573–579.
4. Winkelstein W, Lyman DM, Padian N, et al: Sexual practices and risk of infection by the human immunodeficiency virus. The San Francisco Men's Health Study. JAMA 1987;257:321–325.
5. European Study Group on Heterosexual Transmission of HIV: Comparison of female to male and male to female transmission of HIV in 563 stable couples. BMJ 1992;304:809–813.
6. Greenblatt RM, Lukehart SA, Plummer FA, et al: Genital ulceration as a risk factor for human immunodeficiency virus infection. AIDS 1988;2:47–50.
7. Sperling RS, Shapiro DE, Coombs RW, et al: Maternal viral load, zidovudine treatment, and the risk of transmission of human immunodeficiency virus type 1 from mother to infant: Pediatric AIDS Clinical Trials Group Protocol 076 Study Group. N Eng J Med 1996;335:1621–1629.
8. Pitt J, Brambilla D, Reichelderfer P, et al: Maternal immunologic and virologic risk factors for infant human immunodeficiency type 1 infection: Finding from the Women and Infants Transmission Study. J Infect Dis 1997;175:567–575.
9. Langston C, Lewis DE, Hammill HA, et al: Excess intrauterine fetal demise associated with maternal human immunodeficiency virus infection. J Infect Dis 1995;172:1451–1460.
10. Gray RH, Wawer MJ, Serwadda, et al: Population-bases study of fertility in women with HIV-1 infection in Uganda. Lancet 1998;351:98–103.
11. Bryson YJ, Luzuriaga K, Sullivan JL, et al: Proposed definitions for in utero versus intrapartum transmission of HIV-1. N Engl J Med 1992;327:1246–1247.
12. Nielsen K, Boyer P, Dillon M, et al: Presence of human immunodeficiency virus (HIV) type 1 and HIV-1–specific antibodies in cervicovaginal secretions of infected mothers and in the gastric aspirates of their infants. J Infect Dis 1996;173:1001–1004.
13. Kreiss J: Breastfeeding and vertical transmission of HIV-1. Acta Paediatr Suppl 1997;421:113–117.
14. Newell, M: Prevention of mother-to-child transmission of HIV: Challenges for the current decade. Bull World Health Organ 2001;79:1138–1144.
15. Thiry L, Sprecher-Goldberger S, Jonkheer T, et al: Isolation of AIDS virus from cell-free breast milk of three healthy virus carriers. Lancet 1985;2:891–892.
16. Patrascu IV, Dumitrescu O: The epidemic of human immunodeficiency virus infection in Romanian children. AIDS Res Hum Retroviruses 1993; 9:99–104.
17. Schacker T, Collier AC, Hughes J, et al: Clinical and epidemiological features of primary HIV infection. Ann Intern Med 1996;125:257–264.
18. Stein DS, Korvick JA, Vermund SH: CD4+ lymphocyte cell enumeration for prediction of clinical course of human immunodeficiency virus disease: A review. J Infect Dis 1992;165:352–363.
19. McCune JM, Hanley MB, Cesar D, et al: Factors influencing T-cell turnover in HIV-1–seropositive patients. J Clin Invest 2000;105:100–108.
20. Clark SJ, Shaw GM: The acute retroviral syndrome and the pathogenesis of HIV-1 infection. Semin Immunol 1993;5:149–155.
21. Mellors JW, Rinaldo CR Jr, Gupta P, et al: Prognosis in HIV-1 infection predicted by the quantity of virus in the plasma. Science 1996;272:1167–1170.
22. Centers for Disease Control and Prevention: 1993 revised classification system for HIV infection and expanded surveillance case definition for AIDS among adolescents and adults. MMWR 1992;41:RR–17.
23. Centers for Disease Control and Prevention: 1994 revised classification system for human immunodeficiency virus infection in children less than 13 years of age. MMWR 1994;43:RR–12.
24. Clark SJ, Shaw GM: The acute retroviral syndrome and the pathogenesis of HIV-1 infection. Semin Immunol 1993;5:149–155.

25. Bartlett JG, Gallant JE: Natural history and classification. In 2003 Medical Management of HIV Infection. Baltimore, Johns Hopkins University, Division of Infectious Disease and AIDS Service, 2003, pp 1–4.

26. Centers for Disease Control and Prevention: Revised guidelines for HIV counseling, testing and referral. MMWR 2001;50:RR–19.

27. Bailes E, Gao F, Bibollet-Ruche F, et al: Hybrid origin of SIV in chimpanzees. Science 2003;300:1713.

28. Hu DJ, Buvé A, Baggs J, et al: What role does HIV-1 subtype play in transmission and pathogenesis? An epidemiological perspective. AIDS 1999;13:873–881.

29. Chinen J, Shearer WT: Molecular virology and immunology of HIV infection. J Allergy Clin Immunol 2002;110:189–198.

30. Hope TJ, Trono D: Structure, Expression, and Regulation of the HIV Genome. HIV InSite Knowledge Base Chapter Website. Available at http://hivinsite.ucsf.edu/InSite.jsp?page=kb-02&doc=kb-02-01-02. Accessed July 31, 2003.

31. Kahn JO, Walker BD: Current concepts: Acute human immunodeficiency virus type 1 infection. N Engl J Med 1998;339:33–39.

32. Kwon, DS, Gregorio G, Bitton N, et al: DC-SIGN-mediated internalization of HIV is required for trans-enhancement of T cell infection. Immunity 2002;16:135–144.

33. Zhang Z, Schuler T, Zupancic M, et al: Sexual transmission and propagation of SIV and HIV in resting and activated CD4+ T cells. Science 1999;286:1353–1357.

34. Spira AI, Marx PA, Patterson BK, et al: Cellular targets of infection and route of viral dissemination after an intravaginal inoculation of simian immunodeficiency virus into rhesus macaques. J Exp Med 1996;183:215–225.

35. Wyatt R, Sodroski J: The HIV-1 envelope glycoproteins: Fusogens, antigens, and immunogens. Sceince 1998;280:1884–1888.

36. Greene WC, Peterlin BM: Charting HIV's remarkable voyage through the cell: Basic science as a passport to future therapy. Nat Med 2002;8:673–680.

37. Berger EA, Doms RW, Fenyo EM, et al: A new classification for HIV-1. Nature 1998;391:240.

38. Finzi D, Siliciano RF: Viral dynamics in HIV-1 infection. Cell 1998;93:665–671.

39. Embertson J, Zupancic J, Ribas JL, et al: Massive covert infection of T lymphocytes and macrophages by HIV during the incubation period of AIDS. Nature 1993;362:359.

40. Pantaleo G, Grazioso C, Demmarest JL, et al: HIV infection is active and progressive in lymphoid tissue during the clinically latent stage of disease. Nature 1993;362:355–358.

41. Geleziunas R, Greene WC: Molecular insights into HIV-1 infection and pathogenesis. In Sande MA, Volberding P (eds): The Medical Management of AIDS. Philadelphia, WB Saunders, 1999, pp 23–39.

42. Bourinbaiar AS: The ratio of defective HIV-1 particles to replication-competent infectious virions. Acta Virol 1994;38:59–61.

43. Perelson AS, Neumann AU, Markowitz M, et al: HIV-1 dynamics in vivo: Virion clearance rate, infected cell life-span, and viral generation time. Science 1996;271:1582–1586.

44. Wilson CC, Walker BD: Acquired immunodeficiency syndrome. In Rich RR (ed): Clinical Immunology: Principles and Practice, St Louis, Mosby, 2001, pp 38.1–38.28.

45. Henrad DR, Phillips JF, Muenz LR, et al: Natural history of HIV-1 cell-free viremia. JAMA 1995;274:554.

46. Lyles RH, Munoz A, Yamashita TE, et al: Natural history of human immunodeficiency virus type 1 viremia after seroconversion and proximal to AIDS in a large cohort of homosexual men. J Infect Dis 2000;181:872–880.

47. Connick E, Schlichtemeier RL, Purner MB, et al: Relationship between human immunodeficiency virus type 1 (HIV-1)–specific memory cytotoxic T lymphocytes and virus load after recent HIV-1 seroconversion. J Infect Dis 2001;184:1465–1469.

48. Burton DR, Montefiori DC: The antibody response in HIV-1 infection. AIDS 1997;11:S87–S98.

49. Goulder PJR, Rowland-Jones SL, McMichael AJ, Walker BD: Anti-HIV cellular immunity: Recent advances towards vaccine design. AIDS 1999;13:S121–S136.

50. McCune JM: The dynamics of CD4+ T-cell depletion in HIV disease. Nature 2001;410:974–979.

51. Rosenberg ES, Bilingsley JM, Caliendo AM, et al: Vigorous HIV-1–specific CD4+ T cell responses associated with control of viremia. Science 1997;278:1447–1450.

52. Goodglick L, Zevit N, Neshat MS, et al: Mapping the Ig superantigen site of HIV-1 gp120. J Immunol 1995;155:5151–5159.

53. Rieckman P, Poli G, Fox CH, et al: Recombinant gp120 specifically enhances tumor necrosis factor-α production and Ig secretion in B lymphocytes from HIV-infected individuals but not from seronegative donors. J Immunol 1991;147:2922–2927.

54. Shearer GM, Clerici M: Early T-helper cell defects in HIV infection. AIDS 1991;5:245–253.

55. Patke CL, Shearer WT: gp120 and TNF-α–induced modulation of human B cell function: Proliferation, cyclic AMP generation, Ig production, and B-cell receptor expression. J Allergy Clin Immunol 2000;105:975–982.

56. Kaul M, Garden GA, Lipton SA: Pathways to neuronal injury and apoptosis in HIV-associated dementia. Nature 2001;410:988–994.

57. Adle-Biassette H, Levy Y, Colombel M, et al: Neuronal apoptosis in HIV infection in adults. Neuropathol Appl Neurobiol 1995;21:218–227.

58. Panel on Clinical Practices for Treatment of HIV Infection convened by the Department of Health and Human Services (DHHS) and the Henry J. Kaiser Family Foundation: Considerations for initiating therapy for the patient with asymptomatic HIV-1 infection. In: Guidelines for the Use of Antiretroviral Agents in HIV-1–Infected Adults and Adolescents. Available at http://aidsinfo.nih.gov/guidelines/. Accessed August 8, 2003.

59. Food and Drug Administration: Drugs used in the treatment of HIV infection in HIV and AIDS Activities. Available at http://www.fda.gov/oashi/aids/hiv.html. Accessed August 8, 2003.

60. Weller IVD, Williams IG: ABC of AIDS: Antiretroviral drugs. BMJ 2001;322:1410–1412.

61. Kilby JM, Eron JJ: Novel therapies based on mechanisms of HIV-1 cell entry. N Engl J Med 2003;348:2228–2238.

62. Schuurman R, Nijhuis M, van Leeuwen R, et al: Rapid changes in human immunodeficiency virus type 1 RNA load and appearance of drug-resistant virus populations in persons treated with lamivudine (3TC). J Infect Dis 1995;171:1411–1419.

63. Saag MS, Emini EA, Laskin OL, et al: A short-term clinical evaluation of L-697,661, a non-nucleoside inhibitor of HIV-1 reverse transcriptase. New Engl J Med 1993;329:1065–1072.

64. Condra JH, Schleif WA, Blahy OM, et al: In vivo emergence of HIV-1 variants resistant to multiple protease inhibitors. Nature 1995;374:569–571.

65. Wei X, Decker JM, Liu H, et al: Emergence of resistant human immunodeficiency virus type 1 in patients receiving fusion inhibitor (T-20) monotherapy. Antimicrob Agents Chemother 2002;46:1896–1905.

66. Safrin S: Antiviral agents. In Katzang BG (ed): Basic and Clinical Pharmacology. St. Louis, Lange Medical Books/McGraw-Hill, 2001, pp 823–844.

67. Richman DD: HIV chemotherapy. Nature 2001;410:995–1001.

68. Panel on Clinical Practices for Treatment of HIV Infection convened by the Department of Health and Human Services (DHHS) and the Henry J. Kaiser Family Foundation: Using resistance assays in clinical practice. In Guidelines for the Use of Antiretroviral Agents in HIV-1–Infected Adults and Adolescents. Available at http://aidsinfo.nih.gov/guidelines/. Accessed August 8, 2003.

69. United States Public Health Service and the Infectious Disease Society of America: 2001 USPHS/IDSA Guidelines for the Prevention of Opportunistic Infections in Persons Infected with Human Immunodeficiency Virus. Available at http://aidsinfo.nih.gov/guidelines/. Accessed on August 9, 2003.

70. Gulick RM, Mellors JW, Havlir D, et al: 3-year suppression of HIV viremia with Indinavir, Zidovudine, and Lamivudine. Ann Intern Med 2000;133:35–39.

71. Lederman MM, Connick E, Landay A: Immunologic responses associated with 12 weeks of combination antiretroviral therapy consisting of zidovudine, lamivudine, and ritonavir: Results of AIDS clinical trial group protocol 315. J Infect Dis 1998;178:70–79.

72. Autran B, Carcelain G, Li TS, et al: Positive effects of combined antiretroviral therapy on CD4+ T cell homeostasis and function in advanced HIV disease. Science 1997;277:112–116.

73. Davis KR, Weller SC: The effectiveness of condoms in reducing heterosexual transmission of HIV. Fam Plann Perspect 1999;31:272–279.

74. Sweat M, Gregorich S, Sangiwa G, et al: Cost-effectiveness of voluntary HIV-1 counseling and testing in reducing sexual transmission of HIV-1 in Kenya and Tanzania. Lancet 2000;356:113–121.

75. Adler MW: ABC of AIDS: Development of the epidemic. BMJ 2001;322:1226–1229.

76. Preventing Occupational HIV Transmission to Healthcare Personnel. Centers for Disease Control and Prevention Website. Available at http://www.cdc.gov/hiv/pubs/facts/hcwprev.pdf. Accessed August 13, 2003.

77. Centers for Disease Control and Prevention: Updated U.S. Public Health Service Guidelines for the Management of Occupational Exposure to HBV, HCV, and HIV and Recommendations for Postexposure Prophylaxis. MMWR 2001;50:RR–11.

78. Connor EM, Sperling RS, Gelber R, et al: Reduction of maternal-infant transmission of human immunodeficiency virus type 1 with zidovudine treatment. N Engl J Med 1994;331(18):1173–1180.

79. Public Health Service Task Force: Recommendations for Use of Antiretroviral

Drugs in Pregnant HIV-1–Infected Women for Maternal Health and Interventions to Reduce Perinatal HIV-1 Transmission in the United States. Available at http://aidsinfo.nih.gov/guidelines/. Accessed August 12, 2003.

80. Shaffer N, Chuachoowong R, Mock PA, et al: Short-course zidovudine for perinatal HIV-1 transmission in Bangkok, Thailand: A randomised controlled trial. Bangkok Collaborative Perinatal HIV Transmission Study Group. Lancet 1999;353:773–780.

81. Guay LA, Musoke P, Fleming T, et al: Intrapartum and neonatal single-dose nevirapine compared with zidovudine for prevention of mother-to-child transmission of HIV-1 in Kampala, Uganda: HIVNET 012 randomised trial. Lancet 1999;354:795–802.

82. Petra study team: Efficacy of three short-course regimens of zidovudine and lamivudine in preventing early and late transmission of HIV-1 from mother to child in Tanzania, South Africa, and Uganda (Petra study): A randomized, double-blind, placebo-controlled trial. Lancet 2002;359:1178–1186.

83. The European Mode of Delivery Collaboration: Elective caesarean-section versus vaginal delivery in prevention of vertical HIV-1 transmission: A randomized clinical trial. Lancet 1999;353:1035–1039.

84. The International Perinatal HIV Group: The mode of delivery and the risk of vertical transmission of human immunodeficiency virus type 1—A meta-analysis of 15 prospective cohort studies. New Engl J Med 1999;340:977–987.

85. American College of Obstetricians and Gynecologists: Scheduled Cesarean Delivery and the Prevention of Vertical Transmission of HIV Infection. Int J Gynaecol Obstet 2001;73:279–281.

86. World Health Organization: Effect of Breastfeeding on Mortality among HIV-Infected Women: WHO Statement. Available at http://www.who.int/reproductivehealth/rtis/MTCT/WHO_Statement_on_breast_feeding_June_2001.html. Accessed August 13, 2003.

87. Johnson RP, Desrosiers RC: Protective immunity induced by live attenuated simian immunodeficiency virus. Curr Opin Immunol 1998;10:436–443.

88. Horton H, Vogel TU, Carter DK, et al: Immunization of rhesus macaques with a DNA prime/modified vaccinia virus Ankara boost regimen induces broad simian immunodeficiency virus (SIV)–specific T-cell responses and reduces initial viral replication but does not prevent disease progression following challenge with pathogenic SIVmac239. J Virol 2002;76:7187–7202.

89. Earl PL, Wyatt LS, Montefiori DC, et al: Comparison of vaccine strategies using recombinant env-gag-pol MVA with or without an oligomeric Env protein boost in the SHIV rhesus macaque model. Virology 2002;294:270–281.

90. HIV Vaccine Trials Network: Database of HIV vaccines in development. Available at http://chi.ucsf.edu/vaccines. Accessed August 13, 2003.

91. Malenbaum SE, Yang D, Cavacini L, et al: The N-terminal V3 loop glycan modulates the interaction of clade A and B human immunodeficiency virus type 1 envelopes with CD4 and chemokine receptors. J Virol 2000;74:1108–1116.

92. Letvin N: Strategies for an HIV vaccine. J Clin Invest 2002;110:15–20.

*Ira Finegold*

# 22 Immunotherapy: Vaccines for Allergic Diseases

## HISTORICAL PERSPECTIVE

The 19th century marked the beginning of the eruption of the vast knowledge of the immune system and how it both protects and harms us. When the 19th-century investigators discovered that the immune system could be harnessed to protect people from disease by vaccination, inoculation injections, and so on, it became a logical choice to try to do the same with regard to allergies.

Seasonal allergies were first described by Leonardo Botallo in Europe in 1565.[1] But it wasn't until 1819 that Bostock in London described a classic case of hay fever based on his own symptoms.[2] An American physician, Morrill Wyman, identified ragweed as a cause of "Autumnal Catarrh" by sniffing ragweed pollen in 1872.[3] One year later, Blackley published his observations that hay fever was caused by grass pollen.[4] By 1900, Curtis was using watery extracts of pollens to immunize patients with rhinitis and/or asthma.[5] Noon in 1910 began experiments with subcutaneous injections of pollen extracts using the first try at standardizing dose by establishing the Noon unit on a weight basis.[5] Cooke adopted and adapted Noon and Freeman's work and presented his results with injections of grass pollen extracts.[6]

The first 3 decades of the 20th century were noted for the discovery of various provocative agents that caused allergic illness. These included pollens, mold spores, insect stings, animal danders, and crude house dust. Eventually, it was found that the presence of dust mites was the major ingredient in the crude dust that caused allergic reactions to dust exposure. In the 1970s, dust mite extract preparations became available for diagnostic treatment and study. Dust mite extracts were among the earliest reagents (vaccines) for allergen immunotherapy to be standardized in the United States by the Food and Drug Administration (FDA). Currently, there are 19 allergens that are standardized by the Food and Drug Administration in use for treatment of allergies (Box 22-1). What standardization means to the physician and the patient is that potency can be ensured as long as the allergen vaccines are handled appropriately. This includes keeping these products refrigerated, observing the expiration date, and appropriately diluting them. Standardized allergen vaccines are also safer, as their potency is defined more accurately than the unstandardized material. Thus, with these newer, more specific and potent allergens, research investigations could be done to determine precisely what happens when patients are treated with specific allergen vaccine immunotherapy, often commonly referred to as "allergy shots."

In the past 5 years, there have been significant advances in the treatment of allergic diseases by immunotherapy. These involve the preparation and alteration of reagents, standardization, improved administration techniques, and understanding of the many processes involved in immunotherapy. Immunotherapy includes not only allergen vaccine therapy but also the recent introduction of a monoclonal anti-IgE antibody for the therapy of allergic asthma and other proposed therapies that could include anticytokine therapy or modified allergenic vaccines.

Recent studies using standardized materials and double-blinded placebo-controlled techniques have reaffirmed the efficacy of allergen vaccine immunotherapy for treatment of allergic rhinoconjunctivitis,[7] hymenoptera sting hypersensitivity,[8] and asthma.[9] In addition to efficacy reports, the role of specific allergen vaccine immunotherapy in preventing asthma is now well documented.[10,11]

## ALLERGEN VACCINE IMMUNOTHERAPY: MECHANISMS

A description of a typical allergic reaction will aid in understanding how allergies are modified by allergen vaccine immunotherapy. For example, ragweed pollen is inhaled and deposits on the nasal

---

**BOX 22-1**
**Currently Available Standardized Extracts Approved by the FDA**

Cat hair, cat pelt
Dust mites—*Dermatophagoides pteronyssinus, Dermatophagoides farinae*
Short ragweed
Bermuda grass, Kentucky bluegrass, perennial ryegrass, orchard grass, timothy grass, meadow fescue, red top, sweet vernal grass pollens
Hymenoptera venoms—yellowjacket, honeybee, wasp, yellow hornet, white-faced hornet

FDA, Food and Drug Administration.

mucosa; in turn, it is degraded as it is engulfed by cells lining the nasal passages or perhaps is passively absorbed into the nasal mucosa to reach the mast cells that have specific antiragweed immunoglobulin (Ig) E on their surface (Fig. 22-1). When a molecular fragment derived from ragweed pollen (or allergens for other allergies) link two specific anti-IgE antibodies on the mast cell, the release and generation of mediators of inflammation occur. These mediators, some preformed, others newly generated, include histamine, leukotrienes, prostaglandins, and others that provoke the various symptoms of allergic reactions: sneezing, itching, vasodilatation, watery nasal discharge, bronchospasm, angioedema, urticaria, and, in severe cases, anaphylactic shock and even death. Allergen vaccines or anti-IgE immunotherapy modify and may even abolish these reactions (Fig. 22-2).

Allergen vaccines are derived from the same allergens that cause the allergic reaction. They are injected subcutaneously, and their subsequent fate has been well studied but not yet completely understood. What *is* known is that the very substances capable of causing an allergic reaction when administered in gradually increasing doses result in a state of tolerance to the reacting substance (Fig. 22-3).[12] One of the earliest explanations of the mechanism for clinical improvement with allergen immunotherapy was the induction of blocking antibodies. Eventually, IgG$_4$ was identified as the blocking antibody. It was thought that blocking antibody competed for the determinants on the allergen and that the more blocking antibody present, from repeated injections, the better the clinical result. However, clinical response could not always be correlated with levels of blocking antibody. Studies also showed that as repeated injections were given, specific IgE increased as well and then subsequently decreased. There is also a blunting of the seasonal rise in specific IgE with treatment. At present, there are additional observations made concerning mechanisms of immunotherapy. Specifically, downregulation of T-helper (Th)2 lymphocytes and upregulation of Th1 cells are

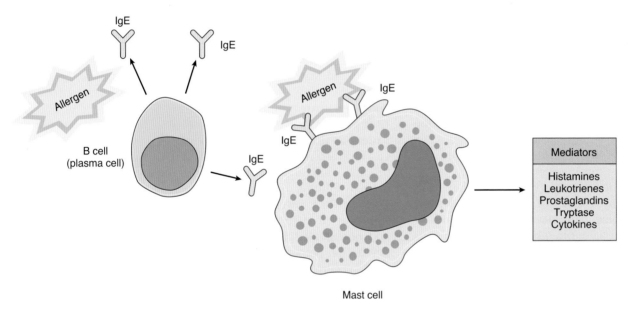

Figure 22-1. As a consequence of the immunoglobulin E–mediated allergic reaction, allergen bridges two immunoglobulin E molecules on the mast cell surface, which initiate mediator release.

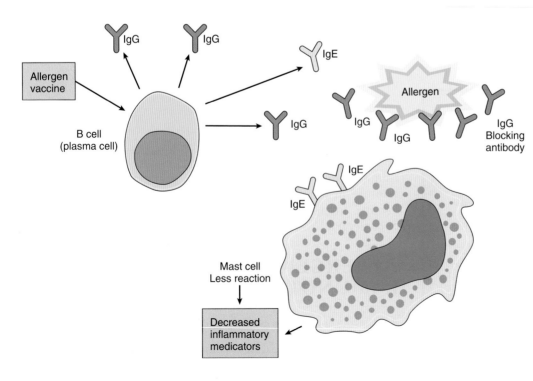

Figure 22-2. Among the many changes following allergen immunotherapy is the formation of blocking antibody or immunoglobulin IgG4. This IgG antibody reacts with the allergen, preventing mast cell reaction and therefore, release of mediator-caused illness. The plasma cell generates more IgG than IgE as immunotherapy progresses.

part of the process (Fig. 22-4). At present, some of the other observations associated with immunotherapy[13,14] are

- Reduction in the early and late responses to specific antigens in the skin, conjunctival, nasal, and bronchial tissues
- Reduction in nonspecific bronchial challenge with histamine
- Reduction in tissue inflammation, metachromatic cells, basophiles, and eosinophiles
- Initial increases and later decreases in specific IgE; seasonal rise is blunted
- Specific IgG increases—early, predominantly IgG$_1$; late, predominantly IgG$_4$
- Basophils: Nonspecific loss of immunologic responsiveness
- Changes in lymphocytes and peripheral blood mononuclear cells:
  - Decrease in lymphocyte proliferation

- Generation of allergen-specific CD8+ T cells
- Increase in cutaneous cells expressing human leukocyte antigen (HLA)-DR and CD25(IL-2 receptor)
- Decrease in stimulated release of macrophage inhibiting factor, histamine releasing factors, interleukin (IL)-4, IL-5, platelet-activating factor, and tumor necrosis factor
- Eosinophilic chemotactic activity
- Increase in stimulated mRNA levels, IL-2, IL-12, and interferon-γ
- Decrease in IL-5 expression and decrease in the seasonal rise of eosinophils, which correlates with improved symptoms and decreased medication requirements[15,16]
- Downregulation of IL-4 and IL-13–producing cells in peripheral blood[17]
- Decreases in median serum IL-1β and tumor necrosis factor-α levels during specific immunotherapy (SIT), together with increases in serum IL-2 and IL-6

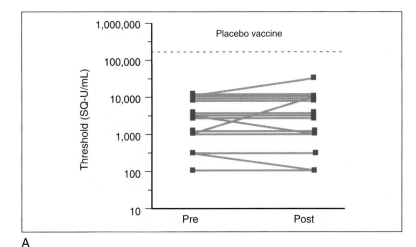

A

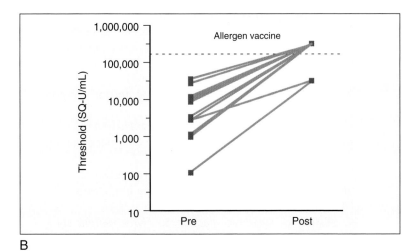

B

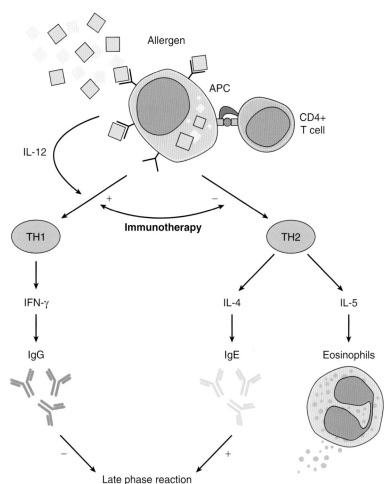

Figure 22-3. Conjunctival allergen provocation thresholds before and after allergen vaccine or placebo treatment. The *dotted line* represents threshold limit. Scores above this line represent no reaction at the maximum allergen concentration tested. Thus, the allergen vaccine therapy increased the level of allergen needed to provoke an allergic response and indicates evidence of desensitization. (Adapted from Varney VA, Edwards J, Tabbah K, et al: Clinical efficacy of specific immunotherapy to cat dander: A double-blind placebo-controlled trial. Clin Exp Allergy 1997;27:860–867; with permission.)

Figure 22-4. After the allergen is processed by the antigen-presenting cell, it in turn influences the CD4+ T cell to become either T-helper (Th)2 or Th1. As a consequence of the Th2 pathway, interleukin (IL)-4, as well as other cytokines, are produced. These stimulate IgE production, and IL-5 is produced, which stimulates eosinophils. On the other hand, immunotherapy pushes the system toward Th1 lymphocyte production, leading to cytokines that stimulate production of IgG. (Adapted from Durham SR, Till SJ: Immunologic changes associated with allergen immunotherapy. J Allergy Clin Immunol 1998;102:157–164; with permission.)

# INDICATIONS: ALLERGEN VACCINE

In the past few years, there have been numerous studies documenting the beneficial effect of immunotherapy on most but not all allergic diseases. The generally accepted allergic diseases that improve with immunotherapy are allergic rhinitis, allergic conjunctivitis, allergic asthma, and insect sting hypersensitivity. For such diseases as food allergy, urticaria, and atopic dermatitis, allergy immunotherapy is not indicated at present. It is quite evident that for immunotherapy to be effective, certain conditions need to be met. The first would be to diagnose the allergic disease. This is done after completion of the history, physical examination, skin testing, and/or in vitro allergen testing and other tests and procedures that are appropriate. These data are then summarized, and a treatment plan, which may involve allergen avoidance, medication, and, if appropriate, immunotherapy, is recommended. Box 22-2 lists the indications that are currently accepted for initiating immunotherapy for allergic rhinoconjunctivitis, allergic asthma, and stinging insect (hymenoptera) venom allergy.

The second condition is that the immunotherapy needs to be given in sufficient quantities so that an effective dose is reached. Table 22-1 gives examples of target doses for selected allergens.[11] These doses need to be repeated at weekly to monthly intervals for a suitable length of time. Current data suggest that a minimum of 3 years are probably needed.[18] At present, subcutaneous immunotherapy is the only Food and Drug Administration–approved route for administration of allergens in the United States.

The decision to begin immunotherapy rests on consideration of these factors as well as the need for the patient to be compliant and fulfill the course of treatment. The patient must know at the outset what this entails. Generally, treatment begins with 4 to 6 months of twice-weekly or weekly injections, administered in a physician's office, with progression of the injection intervals to every 4 weeks. At least 3 years of treatment should be completed. Generally, as the dose is increased, there may be localized tissue reactions, usually lasting less than 24 hours. Because these are biologic substances, the possibility of anaphylaxis from these injections is always present. Therefore, patients must wait at least 30 minutes in the physician's office after an injection. As increased activity may hasten absorption of the allergens, strenuous exercise is not recommended until several hours elapse after an injection. Systemic (anaphylactic) reactions are rare, but the patient must be advised of this possibility. There are also alternative methods of administering immunotherapy (rush immunotherapy) with abbreviated courses, allowing desensitization to be achieved in a number of hours or over several days. Rush immunotherapy might be used for patients who have allergies to stinging insects and need to be desensitized promptly because of occupational risk, that is, a farmer or bee keeper.

After an educational discussion and informed consent, immunotherapy is begun. The extract may be provided to the patient's primary practitioner for administration. The allergenic vaccine label should list its contents, the date it was prepared, the expiration date, and the patient's name and identification number or date of birth, so confusion does not occur with patients of the same name.

In the past 10 years research has determined the optimum allergen dose for many of the allergens; no longer is the dose advanced to the maximum tolerated. The current accepted optimum-dosing levels are listed in Table 22-1. Currently accepted procedure is to achieve optimal recommended doses if possible. However, extremely sensitive allergic patients may not be able to achieve these levels and experience uncomfortable local reactions or undesirable generalized allergic symptoms. Once optimal or maintenance levels are achieved, injections are spaced out to every 2 weeks and then, gradually, to every 4 to 6 weeks. In 1999, Durham and colleagues[18] showed that after 3 years of maintenance

---

**BOX 22-2**
## Clinical Indications for Immunotherapy

A. Indications for allergen immunotherapy in patients with allergic rhinoconjunctivitis:
   1. Symptoms of allergic rhinoconjunctivitis after natural exposure to aeroallergens and demonstrable evidence of clinically relevant specific IgE
        and (one or more of the following)
   2. Poor response to pharmacotherapy and/or allergen avoidance
   3. Unacceptable adverse effects of medications
   4. Wish to reduce or avoid long-term pharmacotherapy and the cost of medication
   5. Coexisting allergic rhinitis and asthma
   6. Pre-adolescent children, as immunotherapy may prevent the development of asthma in children (not accepted by all allergists)

B. Indications for allergen immunotherapy in patients with allergic asthma ($FEV_1$ of patients with asthma must be 70% of predicted values or greater):
   1. Symptoms of asthma after natural exposure to aeroallergens and demonstrable evidence of clinically relevant specific IgE
        and (one or more of the following)
   2. Poor response to pharmacotherapy and/or allergen avoidance
   3. Unacceptable adverse affects of medication
   4. Wish to reduce or avoid long-term pharmacotherapy and the cost of medications
   5. Coexisting allergic rhinitis and allergic asthma

C. Indication for allergen immunotherapy in patients with *Hymenoptera* stings:
   1. History of systemic reaction to *Hymenoptera* sting (respiratory and/or cardiovascular symptoms) with positive skin tests or serum-specific IgE
   2. Older than 16 years with systemic reactions limited to the skin (patients younger than 16 years of age who present with only cutaneous reactions may not require immunotherapy)
   3. Patients, including adults and children, with a history of systemic reaction to species including the imported fire ant and harvest ant

$FEV_1$, forced expiratory volume in 1 second; Ig, immunoglobulin.
From Li JT, Lockey RF, Portnoy JM, et al: Immunotherapy: A practice parameter. Ann Allergy Asthma Immunol 2003;90:S1–S4.

grass allergen therapy, injections may be discontinued in adult patients allergic to grass pollen, because 3 years is about how long the beneficial effects of treatment are achieved (Figs. 22-5 and 22-6). In general, immunotherapy should be maintained for a minimum of 3 years and possibly longer as the individual patient response requires. In clinical practice, longer durations of immunotherapy may be needed to achieve maximal benefit.

In addition to being effective for treating the illnesses mentioned here, allergy immunotherapy has been shown to prevent the development of asthma, especially in children with moderate to severe allergic rhinitis. This was the specific intent of the Preventive Allergy Treatment (PAT) study[19] of 205 children from six pediatric allergy clinics in Northern Europe ages 6 to 14 years (mean age, 10.7 years) with grass and/or birch pollen allergy. The

children were randomized either to receive SIT for 3 years or to be in a control group. The children who were diagnosed only with allergic rhinitis underwent methacholine challenge in the baseline evaluation. Twenty percent of these youngsters who had no diagnosis of asthma had abnormal methacholine challenge studies. The children who were treated with SIT had significantly fewer asthma symptoms after 3 years as evaluated by clinical diagnosis (odds ratio, 2.52; $P < 0.05$). Methacholine bronchial provocation test results improved in the active group ($P < 0.05$). The conclusion was that the patients who underwent specific immunotherapy had significantly less asthma than the untreated control groups (Fig. 22-7).

The hypothesis that asthma can be prevented by the use of SIT early in the course of allergic disease is not new. In 1968,

**TABLE 22-1**

**Effective Therapeutic Doses\* of Purified Allergens and Effective Concentration of Standardized and Unstandardized Extracts Based on Published Studies**

| Antigen | Potency | Effective Dose | Recommended Maintenance |
|---|---|---|---|
| Dust mite (Der pl) | 124 µg/10,000 BAU | 7–11.9 µg Der pl | 600 AU |
| Dust mite (Der fl) | 50 µg/10,000 BAU | 10 µg Der fl | 2000 AU |
| Cat | 57 µg/10,000 BAU | 11–17 Fel dl | 2000–3000 BAU |
| Grass pollen | 370 µg/100,000 BAU | 15 µg | 4000 BAU |
| Short ragweed pollen | 325 µg/1:10w/v | 6–24 µg Amb al | 1:30–1:250 w/v |
| Other pollen | | | 1:30–1:100 w/v |
| Molds | | | 1:30–1:100 w/v |

\*Assuming 0.5 mL per injection.
AU, allergy units; BAU, bioequivalent allergy units.

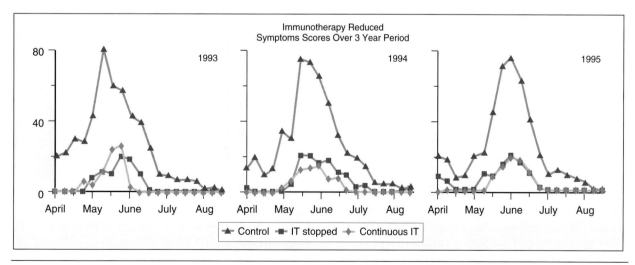

**Figure 22-5.** Immunotherapy (IT) was administered to grass- or tree-allergic patients for 3 or more years; symptoms were improved in those patients who continued to receive immunotherapy for years 4, 5, and 6 and in those who received placebo injections for the additional 3 years, compared with untreated patients for the years indicated. (Adapted from Durham S, Walker S, Varga E, et al: Long-term clinical efficacy of grass-pollen immunotherapy. N Engl J Med 1999;341:468–475; with permission.)

Johnstone and Dutton showed that after 4 years of immuno-therapy in the treated group, 70% of the 82 children were free of asthma, compared with 18% of 91 children in the placebo group.[20] However, the PAT study is the first study that utilized standardized extracts and methacholine challenges in a comparison population. Immunotherapy may decrease the tendency for allergic patients to develop additional allergies. This was demonstrated by Des Roches and associates in 1997[21] (Fig. 22-8) and by Pajno and others in 2001,[22] who showed that 52 of 69 children (75.4%) in the SIT group showed no new sensitization, compared with 18 of 54 children (33.3%) in the control group (P < 0.0002). A retrospective review suggested similar results.[23]

Another study investigated the development of new allergic sensitivities in patients who received only grass immunotherapy and were evaluated 6 years after discontinuing allergy vaccine therapy.[24] Whereas 61% of the initially pollen-monosensitized children had developed additional new sensitization to one or more perennial allergens, new allergies were documented in 100% in the control group (P < 0.05). Decreased symptom scores indicating significant clinical benefits from immunotherapy were documented 6 years after discontinuation of preseasonal grass pollen immunotherapy in children. Allergy vaccines are effective in relieving symptoms of allergic rhinoconjunctivitis and asthma, as well as decreasing medication requirement, improving pulmonary

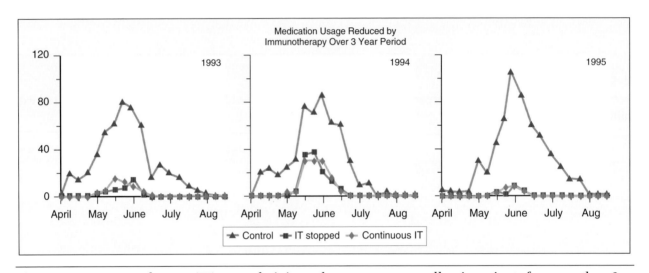

**Figure 22-6.** Immunotherapy (IT) was administered to grass- or tree-allergic patients for more than 3 years; medication usage was reduced in those patients who continued to receive immunotherapy for years 4, 5, and 6 and in those who received placebo injections for the additional 3 years, compared with untreated patients for the years indicated. (Adapted from Durham S, Walker S, Varga E, et al: Long-term clinical efficacy of grass-pollen immunotherapy. N Engl J Med 1999;341:468–475; with permission.)

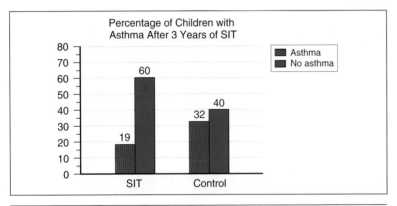

**Figure 22-7.** Children treated with specific immunotherapy (SIT) for 3 years developed less asthma, compared with a control group. The appearance of asthma occurred in 19 patients treated with immunotherapy compared with 32 patients in the untreated group, and there was no asthma in 60 treated patients compared with 40 in the control group. (Adapted from Moller C, Dreborg S, Ferdousi HA, et al: Pollen immunotherapy reduces the development of asthma in children with seasonal rhinoconjunctivitis (the PAT-study). J Allergy Clin Immunol 2002;109:251–256; with permission.)

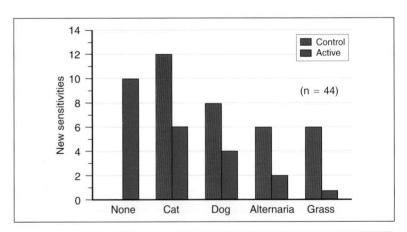

**Figure 22-8.** Fewer new allergic sensitivites developed to cat, dog, altenarea, and grass allergens in patients (active) treated with immunotherapy for 3 years compared to non-immunotherapy (control) treated subjects. (Adapted from Des Roches A, Paradis L, Menardo JL, et al: Immunotherapy with a standardized *Dermatophagoides pteronyssinus* extract. VI. Specific immunotherapy prevents the onset of new sensitizations in children. J Allergy Clin Immunol 1997;99:450–453; with permission.)

function in patients with asthma, and decreasing direct and indirect medical costs.[25] In addition, the development of new allergies is diminished and the likelihood of progression to asthma is decreased. Studies of longer duration have shown that there is less asthma in patients treated with allergen immunotherapy who discontinued the vaccines more than 10 years previously.[20,26] Thus, allergen immunotherapy has both long- and short-term beneficial effects.

# DISADVANTAGES: ALLERGEN VACCINE

Compliance is a significant problem. Patients may not comprehend and understand the necessity of continuing therapy for several years. At initiation of this treatment, it should be made clear that it is a prolonged treatment that will last at least 3 or more years. Although immunotherapy is considered safe, there is always the possibility of an anaphylactic reaction secondary to allergy injections. Box 22-3 is a list of actions to be taken to minimize this risk.

Patients also need to know that they must wait in the treating physician's office for 30 minutes in case a systemic allergic reaction (anaphylaxis) to the allergy vaccine develops. Lockey and coworkers[27] have shown that systemic allergic reactions generally occur within the first 30 minutes, but there are isolated instances of reactions occurring later. Treating physicians must have the appropriate materials necessary to treat anaphylaxis if they are to administer allergy shots to their patients. The overall incidence of systemic reactions is low.

Lin and associates[28] reported on a prospective 13-year study in a northeastern allergy practice involving 10,000 patients and 513,368 injections. They found that the probability of a systemic reaction from immunotherapy was 2.9% and that most of these reactions occurred with treatment using grass pollen. This study was conducted prior to grass extracts being standardized. Tinkelman and coworkers[29] found in a 1-year prospective study consisting of 151,837 patient visits for immunotherapy that there were 36 systemic reactions (1 in 1063 injections). Most reactions are easily controlled with the prompt use of epinephrine. There was an extremely low incidence of fatalities from systemic anaphylaxis: about 1 in 60 million injections.[30] Some fatalities occurred when epinephrine was either delayed or not given in appropriate quantities. Current dose recommendations for epinephrine are 0.3 to 0.5 mL of 1/1000 (1 mg/mL) injected in the lateral thigh intramuscularly and, in children, 0.01 mg/kg to a maximum of 0.5 mg. Beta-blockers interfere with the effects of epinephrine and should not be used in patients undergoing immunotherapy.

---

**BOX 22-3**
**Actions to Reduce the Risk of Anaphylaxis**

1. More dilute initial extracts should be used in selected patients who appear to have increased sensitivity on the basis of history and/or results of tests for specific immunoglobulin E antibodies.

2. Patients should be instructed to wait in the physician's office for at least 20–30 min after an immunotherapy injection. Patients who are at greater risk of reactions from allergen immunotherapy (e.g., those with increased allergen sensitivity, history of a previous systemic reaction) or patients who have a history of reactions that develop after 30 min may need to wait longer.

3. Patients with late reactions to immunotherapy injection should be carefully evaluated. The general medical condition of the patient should be assessed at the time of the injection (e.g., presence of an upper airway respiratory tract infection or asthma exacerbation).

4. Procedures to avoid clerical or nursing errors.

5. It should be recognized that dosage adjustments may be necessary with newly prepared extracts/vaccines if the patient has had a significant interruption in the immunotherapy schedule.

6. Adequate equipment and medication should be immediately available to manage anaphylaxis, if it should occur.

7. Before allergen immunotherapy is chosen as a treatment, the physician should educate the patient on the benefits and risks of immunotherapy and methods for minimizing risks. The patient should also be informed that despite appropriate precautions, reactions may occur without preceding warning signs or symptoms.

From Li JT, Lockey RF, Portnoy JM, et al: Immunotherapy: A practice parameter, Ann Allergy Asthma Immunol 2003;90:S1–S4.

---

# ALLERGY VACCINE IMMUNOTHERAPY FOR ALLERGIC ASTHMA

Despite two independent meta-analyses[9,31] demonstrating efficacy of allergy vaccines for patients with allergic asthma, there is still debate on this issue.[32,33] A conference held in New York in August 2000 addressed this issue. This consensus conference made the following conclusions[34]:

1. Specific allergen immunotherapy (allergy shots) has been shown, through documentation of well-controlled studies, to be effective for the treatment of allergic asthma.
2. There is emerging evidence that allergen immunotherapy can be an effective means of preventing the onset of asthma in children with allergic rhinitis.
3. Specific allergen immunotherapy should be considered as a mode of therapy in all patients with allergic asthma and disorders that predispose to asthma, such as hay fever, after appropriate diagnosis.
4. Environmental control, appropriate use of pharmacotherapy, and allergen immunotherapy are each treatment modalities to be considered carefully with respect to therapeutic intervention for the patient with allergic respiratory disease.
5. Future research in allergen standardization, appropriate dosage, treatment methods, improving safety, using new reagents, and quality of life issues and compliance was encouraged.

The current parameters[11] suggest that children younger than 5 years may have difficulty cooperating with an immunotherapy program and that the risks and benefits of immunotherapy should be carefully considered in this age group. A 2002 study by DiBernardino and colleagues[35] looked at 28 patients with dermatophagoides-induced asthma and rhinitis treated with subcutaneous immunotherapy compared with a control group. They confirmed the safety and the efficacy of SIT in children younger than 5 years.

Another form of allergen immunotherapy uses the sublingual route to deliver the desensitizing allergen and is being utilized in Europe. Low-dose immunotherapy had not been shown to be effective, but high-dose recently has shown improvement compared with placebo. Thus far, this method has not been shown to induce the long-term changes associated with subcutaneous immunotherapy and is not approved for use in the United States. A comprehensive review on allergen-specific sublingual immunotherapy for respiratory allergy was written by Passalacqua and Canonica.[36]

# ANTI-IGE IMMUNOTHERAPY FOR ASTHMA

Immunotherapy with omalizumab, anti-IgE recombinant humanized monoclonal antibody, has been approved for use in the United States only for the treatment of severe allergic asthma. This type of therapy offers a potential additional immunological method for the treatment of other IgE-mediated allergic disorders. Anti-IgE acts by *blocking IgE binding to mast cells* (Fig. 22-9) and also by the formation of IgE complexes that bind allergen, thus bypassing the mast cell. One of the pivotal clinical trials of omalizumab showed that the addition of omalizumab reduced asthma exacerbations by 9%. Inhaled corticosteroids were reduced in 75% of the omalizumab-treated group as compared to 50% in the placebo-treated group. General symptoms were improved in the treated group (61%) as compared to the placebo group (38%).[37] In addition, anti-IgE therapy has been reported to decrease symptoms of allergic rhinitis[38] and peanut food allergy but has not yet been approved for management of these allergic diseases at time of publication.[39] Immunotherapy has been combined with anti-IgE administration with synergistic results.[40]

# CONCLUSIONS

Specific allergen immunotherapy has been used for therapy for patients with allergic rhinoconjunctivitis and allergic asthma for nearly 100 years. Not only is efficacy for these diseases demonstrated, but also this treatment prevents the extension of these illnesses in the transition from allergic rhinitis to asthma and diminishes the appearance of new allergies. New data continuously emerge showing the beneficial changes affected by this treatment to the immune system.

The era of molecular and genetically engineered biology has introduced a new method of immunotherapy for allergic disease utilizing an anti-IgE recombinant humanized monoclonal antibody. Future molecular technology may employ the use of peptides of allergens or alter the allergens by linking DNA to them.[41] The purpose of these techniques is to produce a substance that is immunogenic without being allergenic. Thus, these may be safer products for future immunotherapy.

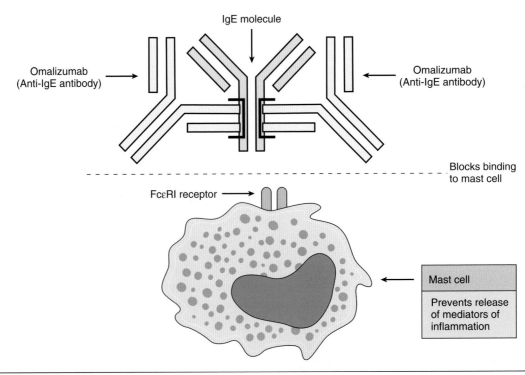

**Figure 22-9.** Omalizumab (anti-IgE antibody) combines with IgE molecules and blocks the IgE binding to the mast cell via the IgE ($F_{c\varepsilon} R_1$) receptor on the mast cell membranes. This blocks the release of mediators of allergy.

# REFERENCES

1. Simons FE: Ancestors of Allergy. New York, Global Medical Communications, 1994.

2. Bostock J: Case of periodical affection of the eyes and chest. Ann Allergy 1960;18:894–895.

3. Wyman M: Autumnal Catarrh. Cambridge, MA, Hurd & Houghton, 1872.

4. Blackley CH: Experimental researches on the causes and nature of Cattahrus Aestivus. London, Balliere, Tindall & Cox, 1873.

5. Cohen SG, Evans R: Allergen immunotherapy in historical perspective. In Lockey RF, Bukantz S (eds): Allergens and Allergen Immunotherapy. New York, Marcel Dekker, 1999, pp 1–37.

6. Cooke RA: The treatment of hay fever by active immunization. Laryngoscope 1915;25:108.

7. Ross RN, Nelson HS, Finegold I: Effectiveness of specific immunotherapy in the treatment of allergic rhinitis: A meta-analysis of prospective, randomized, double-blind, placebo-controlled studies. Clin Ther 2000;22:342–350.

8. Ross RN, Nelson HS, Finegold I: Effectiveness of specific immunotherapy in the treatment of hymenoptera venom hypersensitivity: A meta-analysis. Clin Ther 2000;22:351–358.

9. Ross RN, Nelson HS, Finegold I: Effectiveness of specific immunotherapy in the treatment of asthma: A meta-analysis of prospective, randomized, double-blind, placebo-controlled studies. Clin Ther 2000;22:329–341.

10. Moller C, Dreborg S, Ferdousi HA, et al: Pollen immunotherapy reduces the development of asthma in children with seasonal rhinoconjunctivitis (the PAT-Study). J Allergy Clin Immunol 2002;109:251–256.

11. Li JT, Lockey RF, Portnoy JM, et al: Immunotherapy: A practice parameter. Ann Allergy Asthma Immunol 2003;90:S1–S40.

12. Varney VA, Edwards J, Tabbah K, et al: Clinical efficacy of specific immunotherapy to cat dander: A double-blind placebo-controlled trial. Clin Exp Allergy 1997;27:860–867.

13. Nelson HS: Immunotherapy for inhalant allergens. In Adkinson NF, Yuninger JW, Busse WW, et al (eds): Middleton's Allergy Principles and Practice. Philadelphia, Mosby, 2003, pp 1455–1473.

14. Durham SR, Till SJ: Immunologic changes associated with allergen immunotherapy. J Allergy Clin Immunol 1998;102:157–164.

15. Wilson DR, Nouri-Aria KT, Walker SM, et al: Grass pollen immunotherapy: Symptomatic improvement correlates with reductions in eosinophils and IL-5 mRNA expression in the nasal mucosa during the pollen season. J Allergy Clin Immunol 2001;107(6):971–976.

16. Wilson DR, Irani AM, Walker SM, et al: Grass pollen immunotherapy inhibits seasonal increases in basophils and eosinophils in the nasal epithelium. Clin Exp Allergy 2001;31(11):1705–1713.

17. Gabrielsson S, Soderlund A, Paulie S, et al: Specific immunotherapy prevents increased levels of allergen-specific IL-4– and IL-13–producing cells during pollen season. Allergy 2001;56(4):293–300.

18. Durham S, Walker S, Varga E, Jacobson M, et al: Long-term clinical efficacy of grass-pollen immunotherapy. N Engl J Med 1999;341:468–475.

19. Moller C, Dreborg S, Ferdousi HA, et al: Pollen immunotherapy reduces the development of asthma in children with seasonal rhinoconjunctivitis (the PAT-study). J Allergy Clin Immunol 2002;109:251–256.

20. Johnstone DE, Dutton A: The value of hyposensitization therapy for bronchial asthma in children. Pediatrics 1968;42:793–802.

21. Des Roches A, Paradis L. Menardo JL, et al: Immunotherapy with a standardized *Dermatophagoides pteronyssinus* extract. VI. Specific immunotherapy prevents

22. the onset of new sensitizations in children. J Allergy Clin Immunol 1997;99:450–453.

23. Pajno GB, Barberio G, De Luca F, et al: Prevention of new sensitizations in asthmatic children monosensitized to house dust mite by specific immunotherapy. A six-year follow-up study. Clin Exp Allergy 2001;31(9):1392–1397.

24. Purello-D'Ambrosio F, Gangemi S, Merendino RA, et al: Prevention of new sensitizations in monosensitized subjects submitted to specific immunotherapy or not. A retrospective study. Clin Exp Allergy 2001;31(8):1295–1302.

25. Eng PA, Reinhold M, Gnehm HP: Long-term efficacy of preseasonal grass pollen immunotherapy in children. Allergy 2002;57:306–312.

26. Bernstein JA: Pharmacoeconmic considerations for allergen immunotherapy. In Lockey R, Bukantz S (eds): Allergens and Allergen Immunotherapy. New York, Marcel Dekker, 1999, pp 445–453.

27. Cools M, Van Bever HP, Weyler JJ: Long-term effects of specific immunotherapy administered during childhood, in asthmatic patients allergic to either house-dust mite or to both house-dust mite and grass pollen. Allergy 2000;55(1):69–73.

28. Lockey RF, Benedict LM, Turkeltaub PC, Bukantz SC: Fatalities from immunotherapy (IT) and skin testing (ST). J Allergy Clin Immunol 1987;79:660–677.

29. Lin MS, Tanner E, Lynn J, Friday GA: Non fatal systemic allergic reactions induced by skin testing and immunotherapy. Ann Allergy 1993;71:557–562.

30. Tinkelman DG, Cole W, Tunno J: Immunotherapy: A one year prospective study to evaluate risk factors of systemic reactions. J Allergy Clin Immunol 1995;95:8–14.

31. Immunotherapy Fact Sheet. www.allergy.mcg.edu.

32. Abramson M, Puy R, Weiner J: Immunotherapy in asthma: An updated systemic review. Allergy 1999;54:1022–1041.

33. Bousquet J: Pro: Immunotherapy is clinically indicated in the management of allergic asthma. Am J Respir Crit Care Med 2001;164(12):2139–2140.

34. Adkinson NF Jr: Con: Immunotherapy is not clinically indicated in the management of allergic asthma. Am J Respir Crit Care Med 2001;164(12):2140–2141.

35. Finegold I: Immunotherapy in Allergic Asthma Consensus Conference: An introduction to the presentations and conclusions. Ann Allergy Asthma Immunol 2001;87(suppl):1–2.

36. DiBernardino C, DiBernardino F, Colombo R, Angrisano A: A case control study of dermatophagoides immunotherapy in children below 5 years of age. Allergie Immunologie 2002;34(2):56–59.

37. Passalacqua G, Canonica GW: Allergen-specific sublingual immunotherapy for respiratory allergy. Biodrugs 2001;15(8):509–519.

38. Busse W, Corren J, Lanier R, et al: Omalizumab, anti-IgE recombinant humanized monoclonal antibody for the treatment of severe allergic asthma. J Allergy Clin Immunol 2001;108:184–190.

39. Casale TB, Condemi J, LaForce C, et al: Effect of omalizumab on symptoms of seasonal allergic rhinitis: A randomized controlled trial. JAMA 2001;286:2956–2967.

40. Leung DY, Sampson HA, Yuninger JW, et al: Effect of anti-IgE therapy in patients with peanut allergy. N Engl J Med 2003;348(11):986–993.

41. Kuehr J, Brauburger J, Zielen S, et al: Efficacy of combination treatment with anti-IgE plus specific immunotherapy in polysensitized children and adolescents with seasonal allergic rhinitis. J Allergy Clin Immunol 2002;109:274–280.

42. Tighe H, Takabayashi K, Schwartz D, et al: Conjugation of immunostimulatory DNA to the short ragweed allergen Amb a 1 enhances its immunogenicity and reduces its allergenicity. J Allergy Clin Immunol 2000;106:124–134.

*Klara M. Posfay-Barbe and David P. Greenberg*

# *23* Immunization

## HISTORY OF VACCINATION

The development of vaccines to protect humans against infectious diseases probably began around the 7th century in India and China, but the specifics of these attempts were not documented until the 17th century.[1] Variolation was successfully used to provide immunity against smallpox in England in 1721. It involved the introduction of infected material from smallpox pustules into the skin of healthy recipients, but the procedure's efficacy was unpredictable and at times caused smallpox, resulting in death. Edward Jenner used an animal virus, cowpox, to provide cross-protection, thus avoiding the severe complications of direct inoculation with the smallpox virus. Jenner published his work in 1798, marking the first attempt to systematically provide protection against an infectious disease by vaccination.

In the second half of the 19th century, Louis Pasteur's studies on chicken cholera and anthrax showed that animals could be protected against wild-type disease by vaccination with an attenuated organism that had been passaged in vitro. His success in creating these reproducible vaccines is considered by many to signal the beginning of modern scientific research in vaccinology. However, the concept of using potentially deadly, albeit attenuated, pathogens was met with strong opposition. Even after Pasteur's successful immunization against rabies in 1885, most scientists condemned vaccination. In the 1890s, killed vaccines were developed for use against human infections including typhoid, plague, and cholera. Simultaneously, important research in Europe and the United States contributed to an early understanding of passive and active immunity and humoral and cellular immunity.

At the beginning of the 20th century, new techniques to inactivate bacterial toxins led to the production of toxoid vaccines against diphtheria and tetanus. Also during this period, bacille Calmette-Guérin vaccine was first produced in an attempt to prevent tuberculosis. An important advance in the development of viral vaccines was made when investigators were able to grow human viruses in chick embryos. Viral vaccines against yellow fever and influenza were developed in the 1930s. Subsequently, in the late 1940s, human fibroblasts were successfully used to grow viruses in vitro. This technique opened the door for the development of many new viral vaccines.

**TABLE 23-1**
**Impact of Vaccination on Different Diseases in the United States**

| Disease | Baseline Annual Morbidity, yr | 2003 Morbidity* | Decrease, % |
|---|---|---|---|
| Smallpox | 48,164 (1900–1904) | 0 | 100 |
| Paralytic polio | 16,316 (1951–1954) | 0 | 100 |
| Tetanus | 1314 (<1947) | 20 | 98.5 |
| Diphtheria | 175,885 (1920–1922) | 1 | >99.9 |
| Pertussis | 147,271 (1922–1925) | 11,647 | 92.1 |
| *Haemophilus influenzae* type b <5 yr | 20,000 (<1985) | 32 | 99.8 |
| Measles | 503,282 (1958–1962) | 56 | >99.9 |
| Mumps | 152,209 (<1968) | 231 | 99.8 |
| Rubella | 47,745 (1966–1968) | 7 | >99.9 |
| Congenital rubella | 823 | 1 | 99.9 |

*Data from Centers for Disease Control and Prevention: Summary of Notifiable Diseases—United States, 2003. MMWR 2005;52(54):1–85.

In the past 50 years, more than 20 different vaccines have been developed.[2] Vaccination is recognized as the most cost-effective measure to prevent infectious diseases in all age groups.[3] The impact of vaccination on reducing the incidence of infectious diseases in the United States is shown in Table 23-1. In 1978, smallpox was successfully eradicated worldwide. The last case of endemic polio in the Western Hemisphere occurred in 1991, and the World Health Organization (WHO) is working toward global eradication by 2005.[4]

# IMMUNITY AGAINST INFECTIOUS AGENTS

There are two basic mechanisms of immunity against infectious organisms: passive and active immunity.[5,6] *Passive immunity* is provided by the administration of preformed antibody to a recipient. Examples include antibodies that an infant receives in utero during pregnancy and antibodies from animals or other humans that are administered to patients. Maternal immunoglobulin (Ig) G antibodies cross the placenta during the last 2 months of pregnancy. Full-term newborns have antibodies against a wide range of organisms and are protected against some infectious diseases for several months. Women previously immunized with tetanus toxoid transfer the antibody in utero, thereby passively protecting the newborn against neonatal tetanus. This transplacental passive immunization is temporary; the maternal IgG antibodies decrease gradually after several months because the catabolic half-life of IgG is approximately 23 days.

Sources of passive antibody used in clinical practice include homologous pooled human antibody (immune globulin), homologous human hyperimmune globulins, intravenous immune globulin (IVIG), and heterologous hyperimmune serum (antitoxin). Immune globulin consists of pooled plasma from thousands of donors (95% IgG) and is given by IM injection primarily for postexposure prophylaxis against measles and hepatitis A virus (HAV). Hyperimmune globulins are prepared from plasma donors who have high titers of antibodies against specific pathogens, as a result of either prior disease or vaccination. These preparations are administered IM and are used to prevent specific infections caused by tetanus, hepatitis B virus (HBV), rabies, varicella, cytomegalovirus, and respiratory syncytial virus. IVIG consists of pooled plasma from thousands of donors and is 95% IgG. Conditions for which IVIG is indicated include primary immunodeficiencies, Kawasaki disease, pediatric HIV infection, chronic B-cell lymphocytic leukemia, bone marrow transplantation, immune-mediated thrombocytopenia, and chronic inflammatory demyelinating polyneuropathy. Antitoxins derived from animals, usually horses, contain antibodies against a single pathogen. Equine antibodies have been used to prevent or treat rabies, tetanus, diphtheria, and botulism, but they are rarely used because of potential severe hypersensitivity reactions, and some of these products are no longer available in the United States.

*Active immunity* is acquired by stimulating the immune system to produce antigen-specific antibodies (humoral immunity) and/or lymphocyte responses (cellular immunity).[7] Active immunity is most commonly acquired by natural infection with the wild-type organism. However, similar immunity can be accomplished by the administration of all or part of a pathogen that has been purified or altered (e.g., cell surface polysaccharide or protein, or toxoid). In contrast to passive immunization, active immunization usually results in long-lasting protection that may persist for many years or for a lifetime. Similar to natural disease, vaccination induces immunologic memory. Upon reexposure to an antigen or organism, memory T and B cells are activated and result in enhanced protection by anamnestic humoral and/or cellular mechanisms. Responses to vaccines depend on host factors such as age, underlying medical conditions, and medications, as well as vaccine factors including the antigen content, delivery of the vaccine, number of doses given, and the presence of adjuvants.[8]

# CLASSIFICATION OF VACCINES

Vaccines can be divided in two groups: live attenuated and inactivated vaccines.[5,6,9]

## LIVE ATTENUATED VACCINES

Live attenuated vaccines are derived from wild-type viruses or bacteria that are weakened so as to cause little or no disease in the recipient yet induce protective immunity. Classically, attenuation was induced by serial passage in vitro, resulting in the introduction of point mutations that render the organism nonpathogenic. This empiric approach has led to successful vaccines for measles, mumps, rubella, varicella, and polio (oral polio vaccine). In an effort to produce live viral vaccines that are genetically more stable (e.g., less likely to revert to a virulent strain), site-directed mutagenesis has been utilized. By targeting specific genes, the mutations can be designed such that backmutation to the virulent form is nearly impossible. Molecular techniques are used to engineer viruses that produce peptides from other organisms. The immune system regards the recombinant protein as a live viral product, thereby inducing a broad immune response (e.g., vaccinia, canarypox, and adenovirus expressing HIV epitopes).

In some cases, animal viruses are similar antigenically to their human counterparts, but they cause little or no disease in the human host. Such strains are naturally attenuated in humans (e.g., cowpox [vaccinia], bovine rotavirus, and parainfluenza virus). Live reassortant vaccines have been derived from co-culture of two viruses, such as reassortant rotavirus composed primarily of genes from a rhesus strain and a gene encoding for surface glycoprotein that elicits serotype-specific neutralizing antibodies against human rotavirus. Although this rhesus reassortant rotavirus vaccine was highly effective against rotavirus disease, it was associated with intestinal intussusception and was withdrawn from the market.[10] Using another strategy, viral mutants can be propagated in the laboratory by selecting strains that grow at temperatures lower than 37°C (temperature-sensitive or cold-adapted strains). This technique was used to produce a recently licensed live attenuated influenza vaccine.

Live attenuated bacterial vaccines have been more difficult to produce. However, an example of a classically attenuated bacterium is the *Mycobacterium bovis* contained in bacille Calmette-Guérin vaccine. This organism was passaged 231 times in vitro over a 13-year period. Chemical mutagenesis has been used to produce attenuated bacteria (e.g., Ty21a of *Salmonella typhi* for the prevention of typhoid fever). As with viral vaccines, genetic engineering can produce attenuated bacterial strains, but the process is made more difficult because of the highly complex genome of bacteria. Techniques to delete specific virulence genes have been used to produce attenuated cholera and *Shigella* vaccines. More importantly, bacteria have been engineered to express foreign immunogens, such as polypeptides, of other organisms. Live attenuated vectors have been produced using *S. typhi*, *Shigella flexneri*, *Vibrio cholerae*, *Listeria monocytogenes*, bacille Calmette-Guérin, and others.

Compared with killed vaccines, the advantages of live attenuated vaccines are that they may elicit broader immune responses (including cell-mediated and mucosal immune responses), require fewer doses, and provide longer-lasting protection. Mucosal immunity has proved to be important in the control of polio worldwide, and it is likely to play a vital role in the protection against respiratory viruses, sexually transmitted diseases, and gastrointestinal infections. Live viral and bacterial vaccines must replicate in the recipient to induce an immune response. Replication of the vaccine strains of poliovirus in the gastrointestinal tract of children proved to be critically important in the control of the disease via herd immunity. That is, vaccinated children excrete the vaccine strains in their stool, thus exposing other children and adults to attenuated polioviruses despite their not having received the vaccine themselves. A disadvantage of live vaccines is that they may cause severe disease in immunocompromised individuals. Because vaccine recipients may shed the attenuated organisms, immunodeficient patients who are in close contact with the vaccinee can become infected, leading to severe consequences or even death (e.g., oral poliovirus vaccine or smallpox vaccine [vaccinia]). A common problem with live vaccines is that their replication can be inhibited by circulating humoral IgG, thus rendering the vaccine ineffective. For example, measles-mumps-rubella (MMR) and varicella vaccines cannot be given at an age younger than 12 months due to potential presence of maternally acquired IgG antibodies. An additional disadvantage is that live vaccine strains potentially may revert back to a pathogenic form. Such reversion of the oral polio vaccine strains led to vaccine-associated paralytic poliomyelitis. One in every 2 to 3 million oral polio vaccine recipients or contacts in the United States developed vaccine-associated paralytic poliomyelitis, and it is because of this complication that the oral live attenuated vaccine has been replaced by inactivated poliovirus vaccine in this nation. A list of currently used live attenuated vaccines is found in Box 23-1.

## INACTIVATED VACCINES

Inactivated vaccines contain killed whole viruses or bacteria or inactivated antigens derived from the organism. Killed vaccines have a number of important advantages over live vaccines, including the relative ease in manufacturing and reproducibility. They are generally very safe and cause few adverse reactions. In contrast to live vaccines, immunologic responses to inactivated vaccines generally are not inhibited by passively acquired antibodies. In addition, killed vaccines pose no risk of infection to immunocompromised individuals. Disadvantages include the necessity to administer multiple doses over a prolonged period to achieve long-lasting immunity. Inactivated vaccines often elicit humoral immune responses without cell-mediated responses. In addition, it is necessary to add an adjuvant to some of the killed vaccines to achieve antibody concentrations high enough to provide significant protection.

The first inactivated vaccines were derived from killing whole organisms with heat or chemicals. Killed whole bacterial vaccines

undergo little if any purification; thus, the final product contains a wide array of cellular constituents that contribute significantly to systemic and injection-site adverse effects (e.g., killed whole-cell pertussis vaccine). In contrast, killed whole viral vaccines are generally well tolerated, in part because the viral particles are easily purified. A list of whole-cell inactivated vaccines is found in Box 23-2.

Subunit vaccines can be either protein or polysaccharide based (Table 23-2). Protein-based vaccines are very useful, particularly when specific epitopes are known to induce protective antibodies. The first vaccines for HBV contained hepatitis B surface antigen (HBsAg) purified from the plasma of chronically infected patients. Subunit protein-based vaccines for pertussis have replaced the earlier versions of whole-cell vaccines because they are significantly less reactogenic and are equally protective. Other protein-based vaccines are composed of inactivated bacterial toxins

---

**BOX 23-1**
**Live Attenuated Vaccines**

**Viral**
Measles
Mumps
Rubella
Vaccinia (smallpox)
Varicella
Yellow fever
Oral polio*
Rotavirus†
Influenza‡

**Bacterial**
BCG
Oral typhoid

*No longer available in the United States.
†No longer distributed because of its association with intussusception.
‡Vaccine administered by nasal spray.
BCG, bacille Calmette-Guérin.

---

**BOX 23-2**
**Inactivated Vaccines: Whole-Cell Vaccines**

**Viral**
Influenza
Polio
Rabies
Hepatitis A

**Bacterial**
Pertussis*
Typhoid*
Cholera*
Plague*

*No longer available in the United States.

(toxoids). For example, tetanus and diphtheria vaccines are made up of purified toxins that are detoxified with chemicals such as formalin or glutaraldehyde. The antitoxins induced by these vaccines do not prevent infection but rather neutralize the pathologic effects of the excreted toxins. An alternative to chemical inactivation of toxins is genetic inactivation (introduction of mutations in the genome), which has the advantage of producing more stable toxoids that are less likely to revert to a pathologic form. Using molecular techniques, genetic sequences can be expressed in a host cell (e.g., *Escherichia coli*) and the recombinant polypeptide used for immunization (e.g., recombinant HBV vaccine). The S gene of HBV encoding HBsAg was cloned and introduced into baker's yeast (*Saccharomyces cerevisiae*). Recombinant technology is being used to produce a wide array of polypeptides including HIV and herpes simplex virus glycoproteins.

Bacterial polysaccharide-based vaccines are composed of either pure cell-wall polysaccharides or a conjugate in which the polysaccharide is linked to a carrier protein. Plain polysaccharide vaccines licensed in the United States include 23-valent pneumococcal and quadrivalent meningococcal vaccines. They are composed of long chains of capsular polysaccharides that are located on the surface of the bacteria. Antibodies to the capsule mediate opsonization of the bacteria, providing protective efficacy against the invasive pathogen. Polysaccharides are T cell–independent antigens; they stimulate B cells without the assistance of T-helper cells, and they are poorly immunogenic in children younger than 2 years because of young childrens' relatively immature immune system. At any age, plain polysaccharide vaccines do not elicit immunologic memory, no booster response is induced with repeated doses, the immune response is short lived and has no effect on nasopharyngeal carriage of the organism, and the antibodies have less functional activity than those induced by proteins. To enhance their immunogenicity, polysaccharides have been covalently linked (conjugated) to protein carriers. Polysaccharide-protein conjugate vaccines have been licensed in the United States for *H. influenzae* type b, *Streptococcus pneumoniae* (7-valent), and *Neisseria meningitidis* (serogroups A, C, Y, and W-135). Conjugation converts the immune response to T cell–dependent, increasing the immunogenicity in infants and young children. These vaccines induce T- and B-cell memory (providing longer-lasting protection than plain polysaccharides), generate high-affinity and high-avidity antibodies, induce booster responses to repeated doses, and decrease nasopharyngeal carriage of the organism.

In recent years, DNA vaccines have been developed for a variety of pathogens. Mammalian cells can be transformed with a plasmid containing DNA encoding for an antigen of interest. The mammalian cells transcribe and secrete the antigen, thereby inducing an immunologic response. In animal studies and clinical trials, uncoated DNA has been administered IM, resulting in humoral and cellular immune responses. Advantages of this technique include the ease of producing these vaccines and the ability to induce synthesis of multiple copies of a single antigen or direct the synthesis of multiple antigens simultaneously. In addition, DNA vaccines induce cytotoxic T-lymphocyte responses more efficiently than other types of vaccines.[11]

# ADJUVANTS AND DELIVERY SYSTEMS

Adjuvants are substances that enhance the humoral and/or cellular responses to antigens contained in a coadministered vaccine. Aluminum salts are the only adjuvants licensed for human use in the United States. Aluminum supports T-helper cell (Th) type 2 antibody responses but not cytotoxic lymphocyte responses. This adjuvant is included in diphtheria-tetanus–acellular pertussis (DTaP) and HBV vaccines, but it is not useful for many other vaccines, especially those intended for mucosal delivery. Many other adjuvants are under development or have been tested in clinical trials. For example, monophosphoryl lipid A induces a Th1 response, which may be very important in stimulating interferon-γ and cellular immunity. Some vaccines delivered to mucosal sites (e.g., oral, intranasal, or vaginal), cholera toxin and heat labile toxin of *E. coli*, have been shown to be potent adjuvants.

In recent years, new and expanded methods of vaccine delivery have been explored.[12] Mucosal immunity is important to protect against respiratory and intestinal viruses and some sexually transmitted infections. For example, FluMist (MedImmune Vaccines, Inc., Gaithersburg, MD) is a recently licensed live attenuated influenza vaccine administered by intranasal spray. The vaccine induces both humoral (mucosal and systemic) and cell-mediated immune responses. Another approach to vaccine delivery is to stimulate dendritic cells in the dermis by transcutaneous administration. Antigens such as tetanus toxoid have been evaluated by applying them to the skin along with certain adjuvants (e.g., labile

**TABLE 23-2**
Inactivated Vaccines: Fractional Protein- and Polysaccharide-Based Vaccines

| Protein Based | | Polysaccharide Based | |
|---|---|---|---|
| **Subunit** | **Toxoid** | **Pure polysaccharide** | **Conjugate polysaccharide** |
| Hepatitis B | Diphtheria | Pneumococcal (23-valent) | Pneumococcal (7-valent) |
| Influenza | Tetanus | Meningococcal (4-valent) | Meningococcal (4-valent) |
| Acellular pertussis | | *Haemophilus influenzae* type b* | *Haemophilus influenzae* type b |
| | | Typhoid Vi | |

*No longer available in the United States.

toxin) using a patch. In addition, vaccine antigens (e.g., HBsAg) have been expressed in plants. Animal studies have shown good immunologic responses, and clinical trials are in progress to assess whether edible vaccines could be a practical approach for humans.

## UNIVERSAL CHILDHOOD IMMUNIZATION

A harmonized schedule for routine immunization of children is published each year by several physicians' organizations (Fig. 23-1). Updated recommendations for routine and catch-up immunizations of children, adolescents, and adults can be found at www.cdc.gov/nip/home-hcp.htm.

The most recent harmonized schedule can be found on the American Academy of Pediatrics website at www.aap.org. (See Box 23-5 for other useful websites.) Information from the WHO for the Expanded Program on Immunization can be found on the WHO website at www.who.int/vaccines/.

## UNIVERSAL ADULT IMMUNIZATION

The Centers for Disease Control and Prevention (CDC) publishes recommendations for adult immunization that are summarized in Figure 23-2A for healthy adults and in Figure 23-2B for adults with medical conditions. The most recent schedules can be accessed at the National Immunization Program website at www.cdc.gov/nip.

## CLINICAL DESCRIPTION OF DISEASES PREVENTED BY ROUTINE VACCINATION

The following is a brief description of the infectious diseases for which vaccines are routinely administered to children, and sometimes adults, in the United States.[13,14]

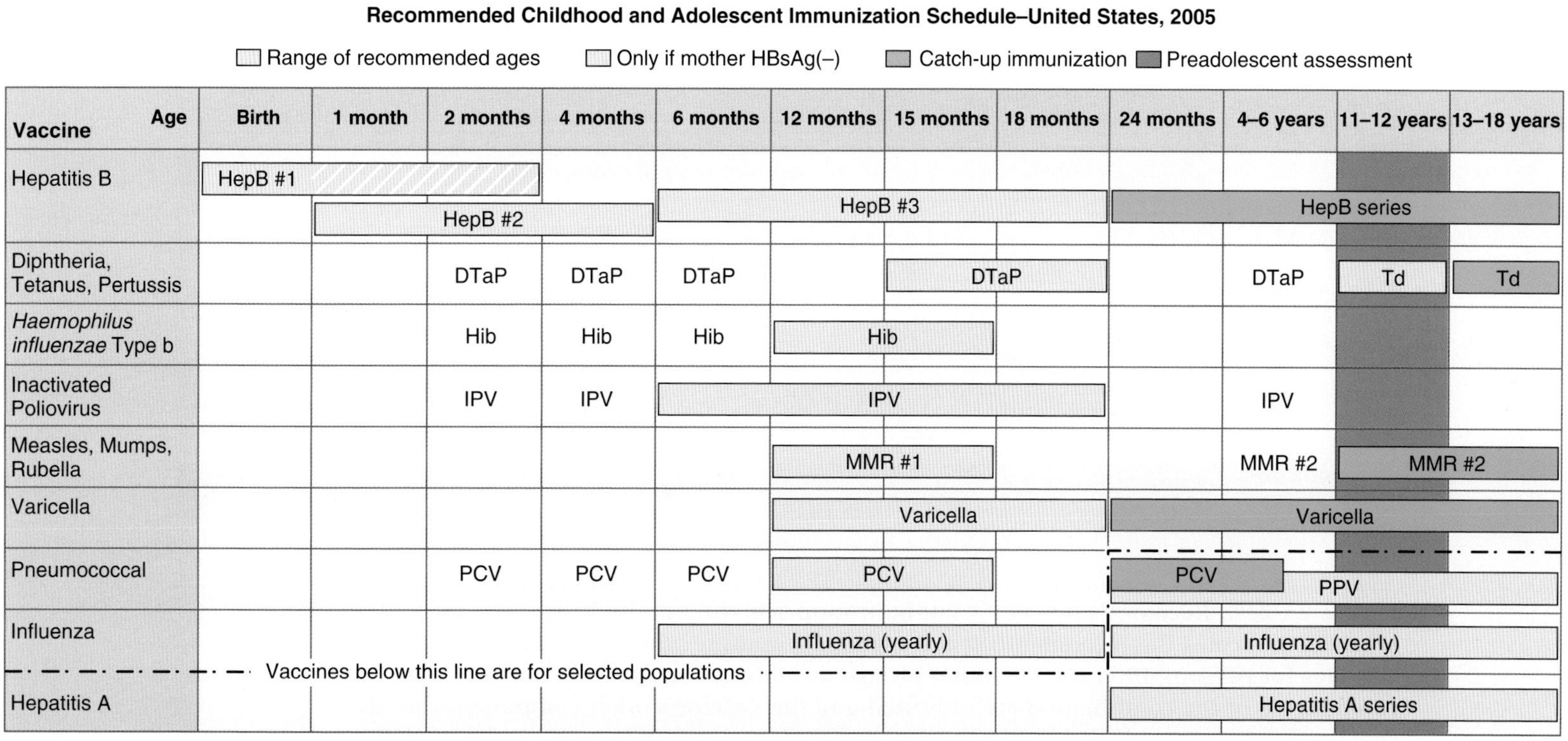

### Recommended Childhood and Adolescent Immunization Schedule–United States, 2005

☐ Range of recommended ages ☐ Only if mother HBsAg(–) ☐ Catch-up immunization ■ Preadolescent assessment

| Vaccine \ Age | Birth | 1 month | 2 months | 4 months | 6 months | 12 months | 15 months | 18 months | 24 months | 4–6 years | 11–12 years | 13–18 years |
|---|---|---|---|---|---|---|---|---|---|---|---|---|
| Hepatitis B | HepB #1 | | HepB #2 | | | HepB #3 | | | | HepB series | | |
| Diphtheria, Tetanus, Pertussis | | | DTaP | DTaP | DTaP | | DTaP | | | DTaP | Td | Td |
| *Haemophilus influenzae* Type b | | | Hib | Hib | Hib | Hib | | | | | | |
| Inactivated Poliovirus | | | IPV | IPV | | IPV | | | | IPV | | |
| Measles, Mumps, Rubella | | | | | | MMR #1 | | | | MMR #2 | MMR #2 | |
| Varicella | | | | | | Varicella | | | | Varicella | | |
| Pneumococcal | | | PCV | PCV | PCV | PCV | | | PCV | | PPV | |
| Influenza | | | | | | Influenza (yearly) | | | | Influenza (yearly) | | |
| Hepatitis A | | | | | | | | | | Hepatitis A series | | |

Vaccines below this line are for selected populations

For additional information about the vaccines listed here and their contraindications, visit the National Immunization Program website at www.cdc.gov/nip or call the National Immunization hotline at 800-232-2522 (English) or 800-232-0233 (Spanish). Clinically significant adverse events that follow immunization should be reported to the Vaccine Adverse Event Reporting System (VAERS). Guidance about how to obtain and complete VAERS form are available at vaers.hhs.gov or by telephone, 800-822-7967.

**Figure 23-1.** Recommended adolescent and adult immunization schedule in the United States, 2005. The schedule indicates the recommended ages for routine administration of currently licensed childhood vaccines, as of December 1, 2004, for children through 18 years of age. Any dose not given at the recommended age should be given at any subsequent visit when indicated and feasible. The *cross-hatched shaded bar* represents age groups that warrant special effort in administering those vaccines not previously given. Additional vaccines may be licensed and recommended during the year. Licensed combination vaccines may be used whenever any components of the combination are indicated and the vaccine's other components are not contraindicated. Providers should consult the manufacturer's package inserts for detailed recommendations. (From the Centers for Disease Control and Prevention, Atlanta, GA.)

## DIPHTHERIA

Diphtheria is caused by *Corynebacterium diphtheriae*, an aerobic gram-positive bacillus. Humans are the only reservoir; carriers are usually asymptomatic. Transmission is person to person via respiratory secretions. In the 1920s, up to 200,000 cases and 15,000 deaths occurred annually in the United States. In the past 20 years, an average of only two to three cases has been reported each year. Forty-three percent of cases occur in persons older than 40 years. Universal vaccination has rendered the disease rare in industrialized countries; however, major epidemics have occurred in countries of the former Soviet Union, with more than 157,000 cases and over 5000 deaths reported since 1990.

Nasal diphtheria causes mucopurulent nasal discharge and mild systemic disease. Pharyngeal diphtheria produces a white membrane on the tonsils and soft palate, and anterior neck lymphadenopathy and edema give the appearance of a "bull neck." Effects of toxin absorption include severe prostration,

**Recommended Adult Immunization Schedule–United States, 2004–2005**

| | For all persons in this group | | For persons lacking documentation of vaccination or evidence of disease | | For persons at risk (i.e., with medical/exposure indications) |

| Age group (yrs)<br>Vaccine | 19–49 | 50–64 | ≥ 65 |
|---|---|---|---|
| Tetanus, Diphtheria (Td)* | 1 dose booster every 10 years | | |
| Influenza | 1 dose annually | | 1 dose annually |
| Pneumococcal (polysaccharide) | 1 dose | 1 dose | |
| Hepatitis B* | 3 doses (0, 1–2, 4–6 months) | | |
| Hepatitis A* | 2 doses (0, 6–12 months) | | |
| Measles, Mumps, Rubella (MMR)* | 1 or 2 doses | | |
| Varicella* | 2 doses (0, 4–8 weeks) | | |
| Meningococcal (polysaccharide) | 1 dose | | |

**A**

**Figure 23-2.** *A,* Recommended adult immunization schedule in the United States, 2004–2005. This schedule indicates the recommended age groups for routine administration of currently licensed vaccines for persons 19 years and older. Licensed combination vaccines may be used whenever any components of the combination are indicated and the vaccine's other components are not contraindicated. Providers should consult the manufacturers' package inserts for detailed recommendations. Report all clinically significant postvaccination reactions to the Vaccine Adverse Event Reporting System. Reporting forms and instructions for filing a report are available by calling 800-822-7967 or at vaers.hhs.gov. For additional information about the vaccines listed here and their contraindications, visit the National Immunization Program website at www.cdc.gov/nip or call the National Immunization hotline at 800-232-2522 (English) or 800-232-0233 (Spanish). The *asterisk* indicates that the disease is covered by the Vaccine Injury Compensation Program. For information on how to file a claim, call 800-338-2382 or 202-219-9657, visit www.hrsa.gov/osp/vicp, or write to the United States Court of Federal Claims, 717 Madison Place, NW, Washington, DC 20005.

**Recommended Adult Immunization Schedule by Vaccine and Medical and Other Indications–United States, October, 2004–September, 2005**

☐ For all persons in this group  ☐ For persons lacking documentation of vaccination or evidence of disease  ☐ For persons at risk (i.e, with medical/exposure indications)  ☐ Contraindicated

| Indication / Vaccine | Pregnancy | Diabetes, heart disease, chronic pulmonary disease, chronic liver disease (including chronic alcoholism) | Congenital immunodeficiency, cochlear implants, leukemia, lymphoma, generalized malignancy, therapy with alkylating agents, antimetabolites, CSF** leaks, radiation or large amounts of corticosteroids | Renal failure/end stage renal disease, recipients of hemodialysis or clotting factor concentrates | Asplenia (including elective splenectomy and terminal complement component deficiencies) | HIV*** infection | Health-care workers |
|---|---|---|---|---|---|---|---|
| Tetanus-Diphtheria (Td)* | | | | | | | |
| Influenza | | A, B | | | C | | |
| Pneumococcal (polysaccharide) | | B | D | | D, E, F | D, G | |
| Hepatitis B* | | | | H | | | |
| Hepatitis A* | | I | | | | | L |
| Measles, Mumps, Rubella (MMR)* | | | | | | J | |
| Varicella* | | | K | | | | |

*Covered by the Vaccine Injury Compensation Program. **Cerebrospinal fluid. ***Human immunodeficiency virus. See Special Notes for Medical and Other Indications below. Also see Footnotes for Recommended Adult Immunization Schedule.

Special Notes for Medical and Other Indications

A. Although chronic liver disease and alcoholism are not indications for influenza vaccination, administer 1 dose annualy if the patient is aged ≥ 50 years, has other indications for influenza vaccine, or requests vaccination.

B. Asthma is an indication for influenza vaccination but not for pneumococcal vaccination.

C. No data exist specifically on the risk for severe or complicated influenza infections among persons with asplenia. However, influenza is a risk factor for secondary bacterial infections that can cause severe disease among persons with asplenia.

D. For persons aged < 65 years, revaccinate once after ≥ 5 years have elapsed since initial vaccination.

E. Administer meningococcal vaccine and consider *Haemophilus influenzae* type b vaccine.

F. For persons undergoing elective splenectomy, vaccinate ≥ 2 weeks before surgery.

G. Vaccinate as soon after diagnosis as possible.

H. For hemodialysis patients, use special formulation of vaccine (40 µg/mL) or two 20 µg/mL doses administered at one body site. Vaccinate early in the course of renal disease. Assess antibody titers to hepatitis B surface antigen (anti-HB) levels anually. Administer additonal doses if anti-HB levels decline to < 10 mIU/mL.

I. For all persons with chronic liver disease.

J. Withhold MMR or other measles-containing vaccines from HIV-infected persons with evidence of severe immunosuppression (see *MMWR* 1998;47 [No. RR-8]:21–2 and *MMWR* 2002;51 [No.RR-2]:22–4).

K. Persons with impaired humoral immunity but intact cellular immunity may be vaccinated (see *MMWR* 1999;48[No. RR-6]).

L. No data to support a recommendation.

**B**

**Figure 23-2.** *B,* Recommended immunization for adults with medical conditions in the United States, 2004–2005. For additional information about the vaccines listed here and their contraindications, visit the National Immunization Program website at www.cdc.gov/nip or call the National Immunization hotline at 800-232-2522 (English) or 800-232-0233 (Spanish).

pallor, tachycardia, myocarditis, neuritis, altered mental status, coma, and death. Cutaneous diphtheria manifests with a scaling rash or ulcers with clearly demarcated borders and a membrane.

Diphtheria toxoid contained in the vaccine is produced by treating the toxin with formaldehyde. The toxoid is adsorbed onto aluminum salts and combined with tetanus toxoid (pediatric DT or adult Td) or tetanus toxoid and pertussis antigens (pediatric DTP and DTaP). The adult Td vaccine (for persons older than 7 years) contains approximately one quarter to one third of the quantity of diphtheria toxoid as the pediatric formulations (for children younger than 7 years). Diphtheria vaccine has an estimated efficacy of 97%. The schedule of vaccinations in children includes a four-dose primary series at 2, 4, 6, and 15 to 18 months of age, a booster dose at 4 to 6 years of age, and additional booster doses every 10 years in adults (see Figs. 23-1 and 23–2A and B).

## TETANUS

Tetanus is caused by *Clostridium tetani,* a gram-positive, anaerobic spore-forming bacillus that is present in soil. Transmission occurs by contamination of wounds with dirt, feces, soil, or saliva. Also, necrotic or gangrenous wounds, frostbite, crush and avulsion

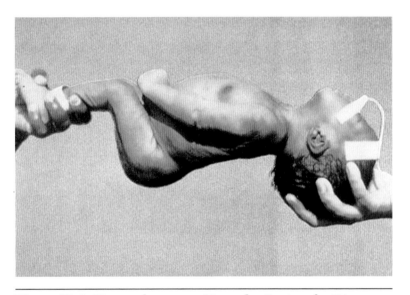

**Figure 23-3.** Neonatal tetanus. (From the Centers for Disease Control and Prevention, Atlanta GA.)

injuries, and burns are prone to *C. tetani* infection. The number of cases occurring in the United States was 500 to 600 annually in the 1940s and 25 to 50 annually since 1992. Neonatal tetanus is common in some developing countries; more than 270,000 cases occur worldwide annually. Tetanus occurs most commonly in young injecting drug users and in otherwise healthy persons older than 40 years. Risk factors other than injecting drug use include never having been vaccinated or not having had a booster dose in the past 10 years and a recent history of puncture wound (especially stepping on a nail), lacerations, abrasions, body piercing, tattooing, animal bites, and splinter injury.

Localized tetanus presents with muscle spasms confined to the area of the injury, and generalized tetanus manifests with trismus (lockjaw), stiffness of the neck, difficulty swallowing, and rigid abdominal muscles. Complications include laryngospasm, tetanic seizures, fractures of the spine or long bones, hypertension, cardiac arrhythmias, aspiration pneumonia, and death. Neonatal tetanus occurs when the mother has not received immunization and the umbilical stump becomes contaminated (Fig. 23-3).

Tetanus toxoid vaccine is manufactured by treatment of the toxin with formaldehyde. The toxoid is available adsorbed to aluminum salts (precipitated) or as a fluid toxoid preparation. The vaccine is manufactured as a stand-alone product, combined with diphtheria toxoid (pediatric DT or adult Td), or combined with diphtheria toxoid and pertussis antigens (pediatric DTP and DTaP). The quantity of tetanus toxoid is similar in all preparations. Vaccine efficacy is thought to be nearly 100%. The schedule of immunizations is the same as for diphtheria toxoid, as discussed previously (see Figs. 23-1 and 23-2). In addition to routine immunizations, tetanus toxoid vaccine is indicated following wound injuries (Table 23-3).

## PERTUSSIS

Pertussis (whooping cough) is a highly contagious disease caused by *Bordetella pertussis,* an aerobic gram-negative rod. Humans are the only known reservoir, and transmission occurs by direct contact with airborne droplets of infected persons. Adolescents and adults are often the source of infection for unvaccinated or undervaccinated infants. As many as 80% of susceptible household contacts develop the disease. Before availability of vaccine, as many as 200,000 cases were reported annually in the United States. The number of reported cases decreased to only 1000 to

**TABLE 23-3**
Wound Management Guidelines

| History of absorbed tetanus toxoid | Clean, Minor Wound | | All Other Wounds* | |
|---|---|---|---|---|
| | Td[1] | TIG | Td[1] | TIG |
| Unknown or <3 doses | Yes | No | Yes | Yes |
| ≥3 doses | No[2] | No | No[3] | No |

[1]If younger than 7 yr, diphtheria-tetanus–acellular pertussis is preferred to tetanus toxoid alone. Use DT (pediatric-strength diphtheria and tetanus toxoids) if pertussis vaccine is contraindicated.
[2]Yes, if 10 yr since last dose of tetanus toxoid.
[3]Yes, if >5 yr since last dose of tetanus toxoid
Td, adult-strength tetanus and diphtheria toxoids; TIG, tetanus immunoglobulin.
*Contaminated with soil, feces, saliva, dirt; puncture wounds; avulsions; or wounds resulting from missiles, crushing, burns, or frostbite.
From the Centers for Disease Control and Prevention, Atlanta GA.

2000 cases annually in the 1970s, but the incidence has increased steadily since 1980. In 2004, the provisional number of cases reported to the CDC was 18,957. The number of reported cases has increased most significantly among adolescents and adults and may be due to increased recognition and diagnosis in these age groups. Worldwide, at least 20 million cases of pertussis occur annually, with a majority in developing countries, resulting in an estimated 200,000 to 300,000 fatalities each year.

The three clinical phases of classic pertussis are described here. In the catarrhal phase, the clinical symptoms are not unlike a routine upper respiratory tract infection. The paroxysmal phase is heralded by sudden bursts of severe coughing fits (paroxysmal coughing) followed by a high-pitched inspiratory whoop. Cyanosis and post-tussive vomiting may occur. The patient appears normal between episodes of coughing. After a 2- to 6-week period, the coughing gradually improves during convalescence. Young infants may not have cough but instead present with apnea. Adolescents and adults may have milder forms of the disease, but some will cough for weeks to months. Complications occur most commonly in young infants and include primary or secondary pneumonia, seizures, encephalopathy, and malnutrition. Nearly all deaths due to pertussis are among infants younger than 6 months.

Whole-cell pertussis vaccines (combined with diphtheria and tetanus toxoids) were used from the 1940s until they were replaced in the United States with acellular pertussis vaccines (DTaP) in 1991 (booster doses) and 1996 (primary series). Three DTaP vaccines are currently licensed and available in the United States—DAPTACEL (Sanofi Pasteur Inc.), Tripedia (Sanofi Pasteur Inc.), and Infanrix (GlaxoSmithKline). Each vaccine contains a different number of pertussis antigens and varying quantities of each antigen. All three of the currently available vaccines have demonstrated efficacy rates against severe pertussis between 84% and 93%. The schedule of immunizations is the same as for diphtheria and tetanus toxoids, as discussed previously (see Fig. 23-1). In addition, two combination vaccines contain DTaP components. Tripedia is available in a combination vaccine with ActHIB (Hib vaccine, Sanofi Pasteur Inc), marketed as TriHIBit but can be given only for the fourth booster dose to toddlers. Infanrix is available in a combination vaccine with HBV vaccine and inactivated polio vaccine (IPV) (Pediarix; GlaxoSmithKline) licensed for the primary series. Historically, pertussis vaccines were not available in the United States for individuals older than 7 years. However, in 2005, two acellular pertussis vaccines combined with Td (Tdap) were licensed in the United States. Boostrix (GlaxoSmithKline) is indicated for adolescents aged 10–18 years and Adacel (Sanofi Pasteur Inc.) is indicated for adolescents and adults aged 11–64 years.

## POLIOMYELITIS

Poliovirus belongs to the *Enterovirus* subgroup of the *Picornaviridae* family. There are three serotypes of poliovirus (types 1, 2, and 3). Poliomyelitis is neurotropic and infects cells of the central nervous system. The virus is spread predominantly by the fecal-oral route. It is highly contagious, with infection rates of nearly 100% among susceptible household contacts. In the United States before vaccine availability, yearly summer epidemics of polio occurred, with as many as 20,000 cases of paralytic polio reported annually. The disease incidence fell sharply with the introduction of IPV vaccine in 1955 and with the oral poliovirus (OPV) vaccine in 1961.

The last case of endemic wild-type poliomyelitis in the United States occurred in 1979. Wild poliovirus transmission has ceased in almost all industrialized countries and much of the developing world as a result of aggressive vaccination programs. In 2004, most of the 1227 cases reported worldwide occurred in Nigeria, India, Sudan, and Pakistan. Unfortunately, an outbreak in northern Nigeria has resulted in importation of wild poliovirus to 13 previously polio-free countries, 5 of which have reestablished transmission. This outbreak has placed additional strain on the efforts to achieve global eradication of poliomyelitis.

Up to 95% of persons who acquire polio infection are asymptomatic, although they can transmit the infection to others. Approximately 4% to 8% of cases involve a minor illness (abortive poliomyelitis) without central nervous system disease. About 1% to 2% of infections result in nonparalytic aseptic meningitis, and less than 1% of infections result in flaccid paralysis. The paralysis is asymmetrical and is without loss of sensation or cognition. Many individuals experience a complete recovery, some regain partial function, and others suffer permanent sequelae. Figure 23-4 shows deformation of a limb following poliomyelitis.

Only one stand-alone IPV is available in the United States—IPOL (Sanofi Pasteur Inc). IPV contains all three poliovirus serotypes inactivated with formaldehyde: type 1 (Mahoney, 40 D-antigen units), type 2 (MEF1, 8 D-antigen units), and type 3 (Saukott, 32 D-antigen units). The vaccine is nearly 100% immunogenic and effective after three doses. The schedule consists of three primary doses at 2, 4, and 6 to 18 months of age and a booster dose at 4 to 6 years of age (see Fig. 23-1).[15] IPV is also available in combination with DTaP and HBV (Pediarix), given in the primary series at 2, 4, and 6 months of age. Occasionally, adults need one or more doses of IPV because of travel to an endemic area or other exposure to the virus (see www.cdc.gov/ travel/diseases/polio.htm).

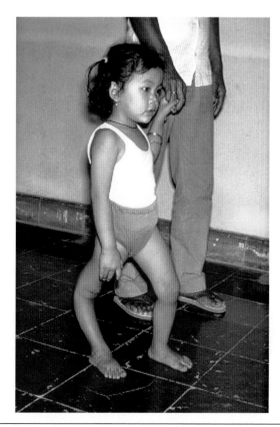

**Figure 23-4.** Deformed leg after polio infection in a little girl. (From World Health Organization.)

## HAEMOPHILUS INFLUENZAE TYPE B

*Haemophilus influenzae* is a gram-negative, aerobic coccobacillus. Nonencapsulated strains cause primarily noninvasive infections such as otitis media, sinusitis, and bronchitis. Encapsulated strains are coated with a polysaccharide, polyribosylribitol phosphate (PRP). Six serotypes of this organism exist, designated a through f, but type b (Hib) is the most common type of *H. influenzae* that causes invasive disease in children. Transmission occurs by respiratory droplet spread; humans are the only reservoir. Prior to the late 1980s, approximately 20,000 cases of invasive Hib disease occurred annually in the United States in children younger than 5 years. The incidence of disease fell dramatically after the introduction of Hib conjugate vaccines (Fig. 23-5). Currently, less than 100 cases of invasive Hib disease in children younger than 5 years are reported annually in the United States.[16] The most common manifestations of invasive Hib disease are meningitis, sepsis, pneumonia, facial cellulitis, epiglottitis, osteomyelitis, and septic arthritis. Neurologic sequelae occur in 15% to 30% of patients, and death in 2% to 5%.

Three Hib vaccines are currently licensed and available in the United States. Each vaccine contains PRP conjugated to a protein carrier. ActHIB (Sanofi Pasteur Inc.) contains PRP polysaccharide conjugated to tetanus toxoid (PRP-T); HibTITER (Wyeth Lederle Vaccines) contains PRP oligosaccharide conjugated to $CRM_{197}$, a mutant form of diphtheria toxoid (HbOC); and PedvaxHIB (Merck & Co., Inc.) contains PRP polysaccharide conjugated to the outer membrane protein complex of serogroup B *N. meningitidis* (PRP-OMP). In addition, PRP-OMP is available in a combination vaccine with HBsAg (Comvax, Merck & Co., Inc.). The schedule of immunizations includes a primary series of two (PedvaxHIB or Comvax) or three (ActHIB or HibTITER) doses within the first 6 months of life and a booster dose at 12 to 15 months of age (see Fig. 23-1).

## PNEUMOCOCCAL DISEASE

*Streptococcus pneumoniae* is a lancet-shaped, encapsulated, facultative anaerobic organism. More than 90 serotypes have been identified based on the structure of their capsular polysaccharide and binding of type-specific antisera. Asymptomatic nasopharyngeal colonization with pneumococci is common (up to 70%), especially in children who attend daycare. Infection is acquired by direct person-to-person contact via respiratory droplets. Known risk factors for invasive pneumococcal disease are provided in Box 23-3. Until recently, *S. pneumoniae* caused an estimated 570,000 cases of pneumonia, 55,000 cases of bacteremia, 6000 cases of meningitis, and 5 million cases of otitis media annually. The highest rates of invasive pneumococcal disease occur in children younger than 2 years. The number of episodes of invasive disease in children has decreased significantly since licensure of pneumococcal conjugate vaccine in 2000.

*Streptococcus pneumoniae* causes a variety of clinical illnesses, including pneumonia, meningitis, and bacteremia. In adults, mortality rates are 5% to 7% with pneumonia, 20% with bacteremia, and 30% with meningitis, but the rates are much higher in the elderly, persons with asplenia, and others with significant underlying medical conditions. Noninvasive diseases commonly caused by pneumococci in children include otitis media, sinusitis, and bronchitis.

Two types of pneumococcal vaccines are available in the United States: 23-valent plain polysaccharide and 7-valent polysaccharide-protein conjugate vaccines. The plain polysaccharide vaccine is available from Merck & Co, Inc. (Pneumovax 23). It contains purified capsular polysaccharide of 23 serotypes, accounting for approximately 90% of the strains causing invasive disease in adults in the United States. The vaccine consists of 25 μg polysaccharide of each serotype (total = 575 μg). It is not immunogenic in children younger than 2 years due to the T cell–independent nature of the capsular polysaccharide. The

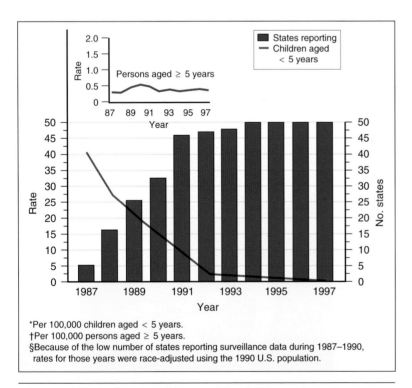

*Per 100,000 children aged < 5 years.
†Per 100,000 persons aged ≥ 5 years.
§Because of the low number of states reporting surveillance data during 1987–1990, rates for those years were race-adjusted using the 1990 U.S. population.

**Figure 23-5.** Incidence of *Haemophilus influenzae* invasive disease among children 5 years or younger and number of states reporting *H. influenzae* surveillance data in the United States from 1987 to 1997. (From Centers for Disease Control and Prevention, Atlanta GA.)

**BOX 23-3**
**Risk Factors for Invasive Pneumococcal Disease in Children**

Age <24 mo
Attendance at a daycare center during the preceding 3 mo
Certain ethnic groups (African American, Native Alaskan, Native American)
Sickle cell disease and other hemoglobinopathies
Asplenia or splenic dysfunction
HIV infection
Congenital or acquired antibody or complement deficiencies
Cerebrospinal fluid leak

overall efficacy of the 23-valent vaccine against invasive pneumococcal disease is 60% to 70%. The vaccine should be administered to all adults older than 65 years and all persons older than 2 years with high-risk medical conditions (Box 23-4). Revaccination is not recommended for most individuals; however, a single revaccination is recommended for persons at highest risk for serious pneumococcal disease and for those likely to experience a rapid decline of their antibody titers (see Figs. 23-1 and 23-2).

The 7-valent conjugate vaccine is available from Wyeth Lederle Vaccines (Prevnar). It contains the capsular polysaccharides of seven serotypes that account for approximately 80% of the strains causing invasive disease in U.S. children younger than 5 years.[17] Each polysaccharide is covalently bound to a mutant diphtheria toxoid ($CRM_{197}$). In contrast to the plain polysaccharide vaccine, this conjugate vaccine is highly immunogenic in infants and young children. In a large clinical trial in northern California, the efficacy of the vaccine was approximately 95% against invasive disease, 18% against pneumonia with positive radiologic findings, and 6% to 7% against otitis media (all causes).[18,19] The conjugate vaccine is recommended for use in all children younger than 24 months and in children 24 to 59 months of age who have high-risk conditions.[20] The infant series is given at 2, 4, 6, and 12 to 15 months of age. For some high-risk children (e.g., those who are HIV positive or asplenic or have sickle cell disease), a mixed regimen is recommended: two doses of 7-valent conjugate vaccine separated by 8 weeks, followed 8 weeks later with one dose of 23-valent polysaccharide and a second dose of 23-valent vaccine 3 to 5 years later.[21]

## HEPATITIS B

Hepatitis B virus (HBV) is a partially double-stranded DNA virus of the *Hepadnaviridae* family. Humans are the only known natural host, and transmission occurs by contact with infected body fluids. HBV is transmitted through sexual contact, percutaneous inoculation by contaminated needles or syringes (e.g., illegal injection drug use, needle-stick injuries, tattooing, piercing, and acupuncture), and direct contact of contaminated blood or serum onto skin with fresh breaks or on to mucosal surfaces. Perinatal transmission may occur from an infected mother to her baby. The estimated number of cases of acute HBV infection in the United States peaked in the mid-1980s at about 300,000 cases annually but has since declined to about 80,000 cases per year. There are approximately 1 to 1.25 million chronic carriers of HBV in the United States, with 5000 to 8000 new carriers added each year. The most common risk factors of HBV infection in the United States are heterosexual (41%) or homosexual contact (9%), injection drug use (15%), household contact (2%), and exposed health care workers (1%); about 30% of patients have no known risk of exposure.

Hepatitis B virus infection can be asymptomatic, especially in infants and children but also in about one half of adults. Clinical hepatitis manifests with malaise, anorexia, abdominal discomfort, nausea, vomiting, headache, myalgia, arthralgia or arthritis, rash, and dark urine followed by the development of jaundice in some cases. Fulminant hepatitis occurs in 1% to 2% of cases. The risk of chronic HBV infection is related to age at acquisition; 5% to 10% of adults, 30% to 50% of children 1 to 5 years of age, and 90% of perinatally infected newborns develop chronic HBV infection. Such individuals carry a 15% to 25% lifetime risk of developing liver failure and death secondary to chronic active hepatitis, cirrhosis, or hepatocellular carcinoma.

---

**BOX 23-4**
**Pneumococcal Polysaccharide Vaccine Recommendations**

Adults ≥65 yr
Persons ≥2 yr with
    Chronic illness
        Cardiovascular disease (congestive heart failure, cardiomyopathy)
        Pulmonary disease (chronic obstructive pulmonary disease, emphysema)
        Diabetes mellitus
        Alcoholism
        Liver disease (cirrhosis)
        Cerebrospinal fluid leak
    Anatomic or functional asplenia (sickle cell disease, splenectomy)
    Native Alaskan, Native American
    Immunocompromised
        HIV infection
        Leukemia, lymphoma, Hodgkin's disease, multiple myeloma, generalized malignancy
        Chronic renal failure, nephrotic syndrome
        Other conditions associated with immunosuppression or immunosuppressive therapy

---

**TABLE 23-4**
**Postexposure Prophylaxis for Hepatitis B Virus Infection in Susceptible Persons (e.g., Previously Not Immunized)**

| Type of Exposure | Immunization | HBIG |
|---|---|---|
| Perinatal | Yes | Yes |
| Sexual, partner with acute infection | Yes | Yes |
| Sexual, partner with chronic infection | Yes | No |
| Household contact HBsAg-positive person | Yes | No |
| Household contact is acute case and exposure to blood | Yes | Yes |
| Infant, acute case in primary caretaker | Yes | Yes |
| Percutaneous or mucosal exposure to blood | Yes | +/− |

HBIG, hepatitis B immune globulin; HBsAg, hepatitis B surface antigen.

Two HBV vaccines are licensed and available in the United States: Engerix-B (GlaxoSmithKline) and Recombivax HB (Merck & Co., Inc.). Both vaccines are produced using recombinant DNA technology in which the gene encoding for HBsAg has been inserted via a plasmid into *S. cerevisiae*; there is no infectious virus contained in the vaccines. The quantity of HBsAg differs in the two vaccines. In addition, Engerix-B is included in a combination DTaP–Hep B–IPV vaccine, Pediarix, and in a combination hepatitis A–Hep B vaccine (adult use only), Twinrix (GlaxoSmithKline). Recombivax HB is included in a combination Hib–Hep B vaccine, Comvax (Merck & Co., Inc.). HBV vaccines induce protective immunity in more than 90% of infants, children, and young adults; however, the proportion decreases to about 75% in adults older than 40 years. Efficacy of the vaccine is estimated at 80% to 100% in children and adults and approximately 95% in perinatally exposed infants when the vaccine is given at birth along with hepatitis B immune globulin (HBIG) given within the first 12 hours after birth. The routine schedule for infants is dependent on the HBsAg status of the mother (see Fig. 23-1). Adolescents not previously immunized should be given a HBV vaccine series at age 11 to 12 years. Adults should be immunized if they are at high risk of exposure to the virus (see Fig. 23-2). In addition, HBV vaccine is recommended as prophylaxis in certain postexposure situations (Table 23-4; CDC website: www.cdc.gov/mmwr/preview/mmwrhtml/rr5011a1.htm).

## MEASLES

Measles is a highly contagious infection caused by a paramyxovirus, a single-stranded RNA virus. Humans are the only source of infection; transmission occurs person-to-person via large respiratory droplets and by airborne transmission of aerosolized droplet nuclei. Secondary attack rates of more than 90% occur among exposed susceptible individuals. In the prevaccine era, nearly all children acquired measles (3 to 4 million cases per year), resulting in 500 deaths annually in the United States. The measles vaccine was introduced in 1963; the number of annual cases decreased to about 1500 in 1982. However, in 1989 to 1991, as a result of low rates of vaccination, an outbreak of more than 55,000 cases occurred, resulting in more than 11,000 hospitalizations and 123 deaths. Improved immunization rates led to a decline of cases to only 56 reported in 2003. However, in developing countries, measles is responsible for nearly 1 million deaths annually.

The disease typically presents with a prodrome of fever, followed by cough, coryza, conjunctivitis, and a transient enanthem of Koplik's spots (bluish-white spots) on mucous membranes. The skin rash of measles is a maculopapular eruption that starts on the face and neck and proceeds down the body and out to the hands and feet over a 5- to 6-day period. Common complications include diarrhea, otitis media, and pneumonia. Rarely, seizures, encephalitis, and death may occur acutely, and subacute sclerosing panencephalitis may be seen as a late complication.

Measles vaccine is available in a combination MMR vaccine (M-M-R-II) and as a stand-alone product in limited supply (Merck & Co., Inc.). The vaccine consists of live attenuated Edmonston-Enders strain. The vaccine induces protective immunity in 95% of children vaccinated at 12 months of age and in 98% of those vaccinated at 15 months of age. Two doses after the first birthday confer protection in more than 99% of recipients and probably provide lifelong immunity. The schedule of MMR vaccine involves two doses separated by at least 4 weeks; the first dose on or after the first birthday.[22] The second dose is commonly given at age 4 to 6 years, before entry into kindergarten (see Fig. 23-1). Adults born in 1957 or later who are at increased risk of exposure should make sure that they have had two doses of MMR vaccine or that there is acceptable evidence of immunity (see Fig. 23-2).

## MUMPS

Mumps is caused by a paramyxovirus, a single-stranded RNA virus. Humans are the only source of infection; transmission occurs person-to-person via large respiratory droplets and by airborne transmission of aerosolized droplet nuclei. In the 1960s, approximately 200,000 cases were reported annually in the United States. Mumps vaccine was licensed in 1967, and the number of annual cases in the United States has now decreased to the lowest ever recorded (231 cases in 2003).

Following a prodrome of nonspecific symptoms (fever, malaise, headache, myalgia, and anorexia), approximately 30% to 40% of patients develop unilateral or bilateral parotitis and swelling of one or more salivary glands. As many as 20% of mumps infections are asymptomatic, and 40% to 50% manifest only with nonspecific symptoms. As many as 60% of patients with mumps develop asymptomatic aseptic meningitis, and another 15% of patients develop aseptic meningitis with typical symptoms. Encephalitis is a rare complication. Orchitis occurs in as many as 50% of postpubertal male patients. Approximately one half of patients with orchitis develop testicular atrophy, but sterility is rare. Oophoritis occurs in 5% of postpubertal female patients. Other complications include myocarditis, pancreatitis, deafness, arthralgia/arthritis, and nephritis.

Mumps vaccine is available in the combination MMR vaccine or as a stand-alone vaccine (in limited supply from Merck and Co., Inc.). The vaccine consists of live attenuated Jeryl Lynn strain. It is immunogenic in 97% of recipients, and the estimated efficacy is approximately 95%. Immunity is probably lifelong. The schedule of MMR vaccine was described previously and is shown in Figures 23-1 and 23-2.[22]

## RUBELLA

Rubella is caused by a togavirus, an enveloped RNA virus. Humans are the only source of infection; transmission occurs person-to-person via large respiratory droplets and direct contact. In 1964 and 1965, approximately 12.5 million cases of rubella and 20,000 cases of congenital rubella syndrome (CRS) occurred in the United States. Rubella vaccine was licensed in 1969, and by 1983 the number of annual cases decreased to fewer than 1000. Since 1980, the number of CRS cases has averaged five or six cases per year. The majority of infants with CRS are born to mothers from countries where rubella vaccination is not routine.

Children with rubella usually have a mild illness with rash as the first manifestation. Adolescents and adults may experience a prodrome with low-grade fever, malaise, lymphadenopathy, and upper respiratory symptoms preceding the rash. The rash starts on the face and progresses down the body. It lasts about 3 days and is less intense compared with measles. Lymphadenopathy often involves the postauricular, posterior cervical, and suboccipital nodes. Complications are more common in adults; as many as 70% of adult women experience arthralgia or arthritis. Other complications include orchitis, neuritis, encephalitis, thrombocytopenia, and vascular damage resulting in gastrointestinal, cerebral, or intrarenal hemorrhage.

In the fetus, rubella has devastating effects when the infection occurs during the first trimester. In CRS, rubella can cause defects in any organ system but the most common are ophthalmologic (e.g., cataracts), cardiac (e.g., patent ductus arteriosus), auditory (e.g., deafness), and neurologic (e.g., mental retardation). Additional manifestations of CRS include hepatitis, splenomegaly, thrombocytopenia, and purpura.

Rubella vaccine is available in the combination MMR vaccine or as a stand-alone vaccine (in limited supply from Merck and Co., Inc.). The vaccine consists of live attenuated RA 27/3 strain. The vaccine is immunogenic in 95% of recipients, and the estimated efficacy is greater than 90%. Immunity is probably lifelong. The schedule of MMR vaccine was described previously and is shown in Figures 23-1 and 23-2.[22]

## VARICELLA

Varicella zoster virus (VZV) is a highly contagious DNA virus of the herpes group. The virus can persist in a latent form in sensory nerve ganglia and reemerge to cause herpes zoster years after the primary infection. The only reservoir of VZV is humans. Transmission is person-to-person from infected airborne droplets, direct contact, or inhalation of aerosols from vesicular fluid of skin lesions. The attack rate among susceptible household contacts of an individual with chickenpox is approximately 90%. In the prevaccine era, nearly all children in the United States developed chickenpox (approximately 4 million cases annually). The peak incidence occurs in children 1 to 9 years of age. In 2000, the incidence of chickenpox decreased 71% to 84% (depending on the age group) compared with that in 1995, when varicella vaccine was licensed.[23] It is estimated that approximately 300,000 cases of zoster occur annually. The risk increases with advancing age.

Primary VZV (chickenpox) may present with a brief prodrome, and then a pruritic rash begins on the scalp and trunk and spreads outward onto the extremities. Macules progress to papules and vesicles that open and form scabs. Typically 200 to 500 lesions develop over a 4-day period, including on any mucous membrane. Complications of chickenpox include secondary bacterial infections, pneumonia, central nervous system disease, and Reye syndrome. Before vaccine was available, chickenpox resulted in approximately 11,000 hospitalizations and 100 deaths annually. In immunocompromised individuals, varicella can cause severe illness, with case fatality rates as high as 7% to 10%. Neonatal infection due to maternal onset near the time of delivery is associated with a 30% mortality rate. Congenital infection may cause multiple abnormalities, including limb atrophy, scarring of the skin on the extremity, encephalitis, chorioretinitis, and microcephaly.

Herpes zoster (commonly called "shingles") is due to reactivation of latent VZV infection. Shingles appears unilaterally in a dermatomal distribution. A prodrome of pain and paresthesia may precede the onset of the vesicular eruption. Complications include ocular involvement and postherpetic neuralgia (pain) in the area of the rash, which may persist for up to 1 year after the rash resolves.

Varicella vaccine contains a live attenuated VZV (Oka strain) (VARIVAX, Merck & Co., Inc.). It is immunogenic in 97% of children 12 months to 12 years of age given a single dose and in 99% of adolescents and adults given two doses. The efficacy is estimated to be approximately 80% against all severities of disease and 95% against severe disease. The duration of immunity is unknown, although some experts believe it is lifelong. Nevertheless, approximately 1% to 3% of vaccinated individuals develop breakthrough VZV each year. Breakthrough disease is usually mild with no fever and often less than 50 lesions that may not become vesicular. Varicella vaccine should be given to all healthy children at 12 to 18 months of age (see Fig. 23-1). Only one dose is needed for any child younger than 13 years of age, but two doses given 4 to 8 weeks apart are required for adolescents and adults 13 years of age and older.[24]

## INFLUENZA

Influenza is a single-stranded RNA virus belonging to the orthomyxovirus family. Type A strains are subtyped by their hemagglutinin (H) and neuraminidase (N) antigens; they infect humans, pigs, and birds. Type B influenza tends to cause milder disease than type A, and it only infects humans. Antigenic shift occurs because of recombination of human and animal strains leading to major changes to the H and/or N surface antigens of type A influenza, and may result in worldwide pandemics. Antigenic drift occurs because of point mutations and may involve type A or B strains. Such minor changes cause annual epidemics in the United States and elsewhere. As a result of the rapid changes in surface antigens, the influenza strains included in the vaccine are evaluated each year so that they will be effective against the strains expected to circulate the following winter season. Transmission occurs by the airborne route or by direct contact with respiratory droplets.

The clinical disease can vary from asymptomatic infection to fatal disease. Patients usually experience rapid onset of fever, chills, sore throat, and dry cough, often accompanied by headache, coryza, myalgia, and prostration. Complications include pneumonia and Reye syndrome (rare). Influenza leads to approximately 200,000 hospitalizations and 36,000 deaths in the United States annually.

Inactivated influenza vaccine consists of "split virus," called this because the whole virus is treated with solvents and detergents that disrupt its structure. Influenza vaccine includes two type A strains (H1N1 and H3H2) and one type B strain. Efficacy rates against influenza infection have been as low as 30% in immunologically naïve young children and in the elderly and as high as 90% in healthy young adults. Vaccination is most protective against severe illness, hospitalization, and death. Because protection from the vaccine generally lasts for only one season, revaccination is required yearly. Only one dose is needed each year, except for children 6 months to 9 years of age, who need two doses given 1 month apart if they have never received a previous dose (see Figs. 23-1 and 23-2).[25] Persons who should be vaccinated yearly include those 50 years of age or older and those of any age with chronic underlying medical conditions (see Figs. 23-1 and 23-2). The Advisory Committee on Immunization Practices recommends the use of influenza vaccine in all children 6 to 23 months of age (and their household contacts) because of increased risk of hospitalization secondary to influenza illness in this young age group.

In addition to the parenteral inactivated vaccines, a live attenuated influenza vaccine (FluMist, MedImmune) administered by intranasal spray was licensed in 2003 for healthy persons 5 to 49 years of age. The vaccine contains a whole virus that has been attenuated by adaptation to cold temperatures. It replicates in the cooler upper airway, inducing broad systemic and mucosal immune responses but does not replicate in the warmer lower airway. The cold-adapted master strain is cultured with prevailing wild-type strains to produce reassortants that contain the H and N antigens of the wild-type strains. The efficacy of the vaccine has been approximately 85% to 95% in the clinical trials conducted so far. The Food and Drug Administration has requested further information regarding safety and immunogenicity before considering licensure for children younger than 5 years and adults older than 49 years.[26,27]

## HEPATITIS A

Hepatitis A virus (HAV) is a nonenveloped RNA picornavirus. Humans are the only natural host, and transmission occurs by the fecal-oral route. Acquisition of HAV occurs either by close contact with an infected person or by consumption of contaminated food or drinking water. Risk factors include household or sexual contact with an infected person, illegal injection drug use, daycare attendance or employment, recent foreign travel, and association with a recent outbreak. However, approximately one half of infected persons have no identifiable exposure to the virus. An estimated 180,000 cases of HAV occur annually in the United States. Until recently, the highest incidence rates occurred in the western areas of the United States; 11 western states (22% of the U.S. population) accounted for 50% of all cases. Widespread use of HAV vaccines has dramatically reduced the incidence of this infection in western states.

An acute infection with HAV virus manifests with an abrupt onset of fever, malaise, anorexia, nausea, and abdominal discomfort, followed by the development of jaundice and dark urine a few days later. Symptoms occur in as many as 90% of adult patients (70% with jaundice) but in a minority of young children. Complications include fulminant hepatitis, resulting in about 100 deaths annually in the United States. The case fatality rate increases with age and reaches 4% for those older than 60 years. Hospitalization rates vary between 11% and 22%, and adults miss an average of 27 days from work due to the disease.

Two inactivated HAV vaccines are available in the United States: Havrix (GlaxoSmithKline) and VAQTA (Merck & Co., Inc.) vaccines consist of whole virus that is lysed, purified, and treated with formalin to ensure complete inactivation, and it is adsorbed to an aluminum adjuvant. These products induce protective antibody responses in more than 95% of persons after one dose and nearly 100% after two doses. Efficacy was estimated at 94% for Havrix in a study in Thailand and at an estimated 100% for VAQTA in a study in New York. Protection is likely maintained for at least 20 years after the two-dose series. The two doses of vaccine should be given 6 to 12 months apart (see Figs. 23-1 and 23-2). The Advisory Committee on Immunization Practices and American Academy of Pediatrics recommend vaccination for all children 2 years of age and older in states, counties, or communities where the average annual incidence of HAV during 1987 to 1997 was more than 20 cases per 100,000 population per year, and vaccination should be considered for areas where the average annual incidence during 1987 to 1997 was between 10 and 20

cases per 100,000 persons per year.[28,29] In addition, other persons at increased risk of acquiring HAV (see previous and Fig. 23-2) or those at higher risk of complications (e.g., anyone with chronic liver disease) should be vaccinated. No HAV vaccine is available for children younger than 2 years; maternal antibody interferes with the immune response to vaccine. A combination HAV and HBV vaccine, Twinrix, is available for individuals 18 years of age and older.

## MENINGOCOCCAL DISEASE

*Neisseria meningitidis* is an encapsulated gram-negative diplococcus. At least 13 serogroups have been identified by agglutination with antisera. In the United States, most meningococcal disease is caused by serogroups B, C, and Y, with a few cases due to group W135. Transmission occurs by direct person-to-person contact by spread of respiratory droplets. Asymptomatic carriage of *N. meningitidis* occurs in as many as 15% to 25% of adults and at lower rates in infants and children. Approximately 2600 cases of meningococcal disease occur annually in the United States, with about half being meningitis. The highest attack rates occur in infants younger than 1 year, and a second peak occurs in adolescents and young adults. Risk factors associated with this illness include overcrowding, low socioeconomic status, African-American race, smoking, a preceding respiratory infection (especially influenza), C3 and C5–9 complement deficiencies, asplenia, hypogammaglobulinemia, and HIV infection. In addition, attack rates are higher in college students, particularly freshmen living in dormitories. In sub-Saharan Africa, large epidemics caused by serogroup A occur in a zone stretching across the continent from Senegal to Ethiopia (the "meningitis belt").

Meningococcal meningitis has a sudden onset of intense headache, fever, nausea, vomiting, photophobia, stiff neck, and neurologic signs. The disease is fatal in 5% to 10% of cases, even with prompt antimicrobial therapy. Among individuals who survive, as many as 20% have permanent neurologic sequelae. Meningococcemia develops suddenly with fever, lethargy, and a nonspecific rash that progresses rapidly to petechiae and purpura, circulatory collapse, and death. Mortality rates of 40% have been observed in some studies. Additional complications include necrosis of large areas of skin, digits or extremities, and involvement of other organ systems with pneumonia, myocarditis, pericarditis, arthritis, endophthalmitis, and neurologic sequelae.

Until recently, the only licensed meningococcal vaccine in the United States was Menomune (Sanofi Pasteur Inc.), containing polysaccharides of serogroups A, C, Y, and W-135 (50 µg of polysaccharide of each serogroup). This is a plain polysaccharide and T cell–independent vaccine; therefore, it is not highly immunogenic in persons younger than 2 years. Menomune is 80% to 100% efficacious against the development of invasive disease due to the serogroups contained in the vaccine. In January 2005, a quadrivalent meningococcal-diphtheria toxoid conjugate vaccine was licensed in the United States (Menactra, Sanofi Pasteur Inc.) for use in persons 11–55 years of age. This vaccine contains the same four serogroups as Menomune, but each polysaccharide is conjugated to diphtheria toxoid. Protein conjugation induces T-cell help, immunologic memory, long-term protection and booster responses with revaccination. Menactra may reduce nasopharyngeal carriage of the organism leading to herd immunity. The American Academy of Pediatrics and the Centers for Disease Control and Prevention recommend that one dose of Menactra vaccine be given to all adolescents.[30] Convenient times to administer the dose are at 11–12 years of age (pre-adolescent visit) or at entry into high school. In addition, all persons who are at high risk of disease should be given Menactra (ages 11–55 years) or Menomune (ages 2–10 and >55 years). Persons at high risk include those in the military, college freshman living in dormitories, and individuals who travel to endemic regions (e.g., sub-Saharan Africa), have deficiencies of C3 or C5–9, have functional or anatomic asplenia, or are exposed to *N. meningitidis* as part of their employment.

# HYPERSENSITIVITY REACTIONS TO VACCINES

Adverse reactions to vaccines can be divided in three categories: local, systemic, and allergic. The most common adverse reactions (as many as 50% of vaccine doses) are injection site reactions, which are also the least severe. They manifest as mild to moderate pain, swelling, and redness at the site of injection. These reactions are most common with inactivated vaccines, particularly if they contain an adjuvant (e.g., DTaP). They occur within a few hours

---

**TABLE 23-5**
**Potential Causes of Hypersensitivity Reactions to Vaccines***

| Potential Hypersensitivity to | Vaccine |
| --- | --- |
| Neomycin | MMR, varicella, IPV, rabies |
| Polymyxin B | IPV |
| Streptomycin | IPV |
| Gentamicin | Influenza |
| Amphotericin B | Rabies |
| Tetracycline | Rabies |
| Gelatin | MMR, varicella, DTaP, yellow fever, rabies, typhoid |
| Egg protein | Influenza, yellow fever, measles, mumps, rabies |
| Yeast protein | Hepatitis B |
| Alum | Hepatitis A, hepatitis B, pneumococcal conjugate, DTaP, DT, tetanus |
| 2-Phenoxyethanol | Hepatitis A IPV DTaP |
| Thimerosal | Pneumococcal polysaccharide, influenza, meningococcal polysaccharide, rabies, Japanese encephalitis virus |

*This is nonexhaustive list; there are many components not listed here. Check the package insert for each vaccine to see all of the contents.
DT, pediatric-strength diphtheria and tetanus toxoids; DTaP, diphtheria-tetanus–acellular pertussis; IPV, inactivated polio vaccine; MMR, measles, mumps, and rubella.

of injection and are usually mild and self-limited. Rarely, these reactions can be severe: Some severe cases are believed to be due to high titers of preexisting antibody, especially after repeated doses of vaccine, and appear most commonly with tetanus- and diphtheria-containing vaccines. About 1% to 4% of children given booster doses of DTaP vaccine develop diffuse swelling of the thigh or upper arm. This is a self-limited reaction of unknown etiology.

Systemic reactions to vaccines can include fever, malaise, muscle pain, headache, loss of appetite, and others. Fever and rash following vaccination with live attenuated vaccines may represent symptoms produced from replication of the vaccine virus. These symptoms usually appear 1 to 2 weeks after vaccination.

Many national public health organizations and vaccine manufacturers have hotlines to report adverse events possibly related to vaccines. In the United States, the CDC monitors these through the Vaccine Adverse Events Reporting System, which can be reached by dialing 800-822-7967 or visiting vaers.hhs.gov.

Allergic reactions are very rare (less than 1 per 500,000 doses) but can be life threatening. They may be caused by the vaccine antigen itself or some other component of the vaccine (e.g., cell culture antigens, stabilizer, or preservatives). Potential causes of hypersensitivity reactions are summarized in Table 23-5.[31]

Individuals with egg allergy, even those with severe hypersensitivity reaction to eggs, are at low risk of anaphylaxis to measles- and mumps-containing vaccines. Such individuals can be immunized with MMR vaccine without prior skin testing; skin testing with dilute MMR vaccine is not predictive of allergic reactions. On the other hand, persons with severe anaphylactic reactions to eggs should not be immunized with influenza vaccine because of the risk of inducing a severe reaction, the need for yearly immunization, and the availability of chemoprophylaxis to prevent influenza infection.

Thimerosal is a mercury-containing preservative and is used in some vaccines to prevent bacterial and fungal contamination. However, it has been removed from almost all vaccines recommended for children and adolescents. Some individuals have had hypersensitivity reactions to this preservative. Antibiotics, including those in IPV, MMR, and varicella vaccines, can possibly induce allergic reactions. No currently recommended vaccine contains penicillin. Gelatin is a stabilizer in some vaccines, and people with history of food allergy to gelatin should be skin tested before administration of such vaccines. Persons with significant hypersensitivity to yeast may experience an allergic reaction to HBV vaccine, although this has not been well documented.

# IMMUNOCOMPROMISED PATIENTS

The number of immunocompromised patients has dramatically increased in recent decades. This is a heterogeneous population of patients for whom experience with specific vaccines may be limited.[32] In general, severely immunocompromised patients can be given killed, inactivated, and subunit vaccines but not live vaccines. Unfortunately, their immune responses to inactivated vaccines may be inadequate to provide long-term protection.[33]

## PRIMARY IMMUNODEFICIENCIES

Patients with B- and T-lymphocyte deficiencies should not be given live vaccines, although measles and varicella vaccines can be considered for patients with isolated B-cell disorders. Patients incapable of mounting antibody responses to vaccines should be given routine doses of IVIG, and they may require specific immune globulin preparations for postexposure prophylaxis. Some patients with an isolated IgA defect may be given live vaccines (except oral poliovirus) with caution. There are no restrictions to the use of live vaccines for persons with complement deficiencies, but patients with phagocytic disorders should not be immunized with live bacterial vaccines.

## SECONDARY IMMUNODEFICIENCIES

Most patients with secondary immunodeficiencies should not be given live vaccines. However, patients with HIV infection should be given MMR vaccine if their CD4 cell count is above 15% of total lymphocytes, and varicella vaccine should be considered if their CD4 cell count is above 25%. Varicella vaccine can be considered for patients with acute lymphocytic leukemia in remission.[34] Live viral vaccines should be withheld for at least 3 months after immunosuppressive chemotherapy is discontinued. Some patients will benefit from vaccination against *H. influenzae, S. pneumoniae,* and *N. meningitidis,* particularly those with asplenia, splenic dysfunction, or complement deficiencies. Household contacts of patients with immunodeficiencies should not be given oral poliovirus vaccine but should be given MMR and inactivated influenza vaccines. Varicella vaccine is recommended for susceptible household contacts, because transmission of the vaccine virus

from a healthy recipient is rare, and the consequences of wild-type varicella in an immunocompromised host may be severe. However, if the vaccinee develops a varicella-like rash postvaccination, the recipient should avoid direct contact with the immunocompromised host until the rash has resolved.

Individuals taking corticosteroids may be immunosuppressed. In general, persons taking more than 2 mg/kg/day of prednisone or equivalent or more than 20 mg/day for those weighing more than 10 kg should be considered immunosuppressed and not be given live viral vaccines. If the corticosteroids have been administered for less than 14 days, live viral vaccines can be considered once the corticosteroids have been discontinued, but if the steroids have been given for more than 14 days, then the live viral vaccines should be delayed for at least 1 month after discontinuation. Patients with Hodgkin's disease should be given Hib, meningococcal, and pneumococcal vaccines. The vaccines should be given at least 2 weeks before initiating therapy for Hodgkin's disease, but if that is not possible, then the vaccines can be given as early as 3 months after discontinuation of chemotherapy.

The ability of bone marrow transplant (BMT) recipients to respond to vaccinations depends on the donor's immunologic experience, source of the transplant (e.g., autologous, allogeneic, stem cell), time since the transplant, immunosuppressive therapy, and presence of graft-versus-host disease. BMT patients respond well to immediate post-transplant administration of diphtheria and tetanus toxoids if the donor was given the same vaccines pretransplant. Similar responses should be expected to other inactivated vaccines. BMT patients respond adequately to DTaP,

---

**TABLE 23-6**
**Vaccines in HIV-Positive Patients***

|  | Suggested | Comments |
|---|---|---|
| DTaP | Yes | |
| OPV | No | Do not give to household contacts |
| IPV | Yes | |
| MMR | Yes | Except in severely immunosuppressed patients |
| *Haemophilus influenzae* type b | Yes | |
| Pneumococcal | Yes | |
| Influenza (inactivated) | Yes | Yearly + household contacts |
| VZV | Consider | If CD4 ≥ 25% of total lymphocytes |
| Hepatitis A | Yes | |
| Hepatitis B | Yes | |
| BCG | No | If exposed to TB, use tuberculosis preventive therapy |
| Typhoid (live) | No | Use Typhoid Vi vaccine if needed |
| Yellow fever | No | Vaccine may cause encephalitis |
| Vaccinia | No | Vaccine may cause fatal disease |

*Suboptimal response to recommended vaccines may be induced in HIV-infected patients.
BCG, bacille Calmette-Guérin; DTaP, diphtheria-tetanus–acellular pertussis; IPV, inactivated polio vaccine; MMR, measles, mumps, rubella; OPV, oral poliovirus; TB, tuberculosis; VZV, varicella zoster virus.

Td, IPV, HBV, and Hib vaccines when administered 12, 14, and 24 months after transplant. The optimal schedule for pneumococcal vaccine is unknown. Autologous BMT recipients maintain good levels of Hib antibody when they are immunized before bone marrow harvest. MMR vaccine may be given 2 years after BMT if the patient is immunocompetent. Similarly, varicella vaccine should be considered 2 years after transplant under protocol. Beginning 6 months after BMT, these patients should receive yearly influenza vaccination. Less information is known about immunization of patients who have undergone solid organ transplantation. Whenever possible, transplant candidates should be fully immunized for age before the transplant is performed. MMR and varicella vaccines should be given at least 1 month before transplantation, and titers should be evaluated 1 or more years after transplantation. There is very limited data concerning live viral vaccines after transplantation, so they should only be given in research protocols. Household and other close contacts of transplant recipients should be fully immunized and receive yearly influenza vaccine.

The immune status of HIV-infected patients often deteriorates over time; thus, vaccines that may be appropriate early in the course of disease may not be appropriate later on. Advancing immunologic deterioration may lead to a higher risk of complications from vaccination (e.g., replication of live attenuated viruses) or decreased immune responses to vaccine components. Table 23-6 lists the vaccines that should be given to children and adults with HIV. Two doses of MMR vaccine should be given 1 month apart unless the patient has severe immunodeficiency.

HIV patients with a CD4 cell count of more than 25% of total lymphocytes should be considered to receive varicella vaccine if they are susceptible. Yearly inactivated influenza vaccine should also be given. Household and close contacts should be immunized as described previously.

Patients with congenital, surgical, or functional asplenia are at higher risk for fatal sepsis due to encapsulated organisms including Hib, *S. pneumoniae*, and *N. meningitidis*. All asplenic patients should be given Hib and pneumococcal vaccines, and meningococcal vaccine should be provided to patients 2 years and older.

# VACCINES FOR TRAVELERS

Travelers should not assume that they are free of the risk of developing the disease(s) against which they have been vaccinated. All other preventative measures should be followed carefully. Many local health departments and travel clinics offer expert and updated health advice for travelers. The CDC maintains a telephone hotline (888-232-3299) and website (www.cdc.gov/travel) that serve as excellent resources for health care providers and the general public who need up-to-date travel and health information for all regions of the world. In addition, the WHO has a comprehensive website found at www.who.int/ith. A list of vaccines commonly administered to travelers is provided in Table 23-7. A review of the indications and proper use of travel vaccines is beyond the scope of this chapter, so the reader is encouraged to consult the websites given here and in Box 23-5, review specific

**TABLE 23-7**
**Vaccines for Travelers**

| Category | Vaccine |
|---|---|
| Routine vaccination | Diphtheria-tetanus–pertussis (DTaP), DT, or Td |
| | Hepatitis B |
| | *Haemophilus influenzae* type b |
| | Measles (MMR) |
| | Poliomyelitis (IPV) |
| Selective use for travelers | Influenza |
| | Hepatitis A |
| | Japanese encephalitis |
| | Meningococcal |
| | Pneumococcal |
| | Rabies |
| | Tick-born encephalitis |
| | Tuberculosis (BCG) |
| | Typhoid fever |
| | Yellow fever (for individual protection) |
| Mandatory vaccination | Yellow fever (for protection of vulnerable countries) |
| | Meningococcal (for Mecca) |

BCG, bacille Calmette-Guérin; IPV, inactivated poliomyelitis vaccine; MMR, measles, mumps, rubella; Td, adult-strength tetanus-diphtheria vaccine.
Adapted from the WHO recommendations: www.who.int/ith/

**BOX 23-5**
**Useful Websites**

www.cdc.gov/nip: CDC's National Immunization Program website (general information, updates, handouts)
www.aap.org: American Academy of Pediatrics (yearly updated schedule for children and information)
www.cispimmunize.org: American Academy of Pediatrics (immunization initiatives)
www.who.int/vaccines: WHO general vaccine website
www.vaccinealliance.org: Global Alliance for Vaccines & Immunization (WHO; worldwide projects, general information)
www.cdc.gov/travel/index.htm: CDC (recommendations for travelers)
www.who.int/ith/: WHO (recommendations for travelers)
vaers.hhs.gov: Vaccine Adverse Event Reporting System (CDC and FDA; postmarketing safety surveillance program; downloadable report forms)
www.niaid.nih.gov: National Institutes of Health Infectious Diseases website (information on vaccine-preventable illnesses)
www.vaccinesafety.edu: Institute for Vaccine Safety, John Hopkins (safety issues)
www.immunize.org: Immunization Action Coalition (nonprofit organization that gives information on vaccines for all ages)

resources such as the American Academy of Pediatrics *Red Book,* or seek assistance from local or state health departments.

Travelers should be immunized with vaccines that are provided routinely to children and adults, recommended for travel to high-risk areas, and mandatory for entrance into specific countries. In planning for travel, the individual should allow ample time (at least 4 to 6 weeks) to attain adequate protection from vaccination, depending on the type and number of doses of vaccine and whether he or she has previously been vaccinated.

Some childhood vaccines (i.e., tetanus and diphtheria toxoids) require periodic booster doses throughout life to maintain an effective level of immunity. Pretravel planning should include booster doses of previously administered vaccines or a full course of primary immunizations for persons who have never been vaccinated. To assess which vaccines should be given before a trip, the health care provider should take into account the patient's age, health status, vaccination history, special risk factors, reactions to previous vaccine doses, and allergies.

Mandatory vaccination, as authorized by International Health Regulations, currently includes yellow fever and meningococcal vaccines. Travelers should be vaccinated if they plan to visit a country endemic for yellow fever and they *must* be vaccinated if they visit a country that requires yellow fever vaccination as a condition of entry. Vaccination against meningococcal disease is required by Saudi Arabia for pilgrims visiting Mecca and by some countries for returning pilgrims. Travelers should be provided with a written record of all vaccines administered, including the international vaccination certificate, required in the case of yellow fever vaccination.

# REFERENCES

1. Plotkin S, Plotkin SA: A short history of vaccination. In Plotkin SA, Orenstein WA (eds): Vaccines. Philadelphia, W.B. Saunders, 1999, pp 1–12.
2. Peltola H: Vaccines and worldwide utilization. Int J Clin Pract Suppl 2000;115:30–31.
3. Salisbury DM, Beverley PC, Miller E: Vaccine programmes and policies. Br Med Bull 2002;62:1201–1211.
4. Peltola H: What would happen if we stopped vaccination? Lancet 2000;356(suppl):s22.
5. Active immunization. In Pickering LK (ed): 2003 Red Book: Report of the Committee on Infectious Diseases. Elk Grove Village, IL, American Academy of Pediatrics, 2003, pp 7–66.
6. Principles of vaccination. In Atkinson W, Wolfe C (eds): Epidemiology and Prevention of Vaccine-Preventable Diseases. The Pink Book, 8th ed. Atlanta, GA, Centers for Disease Control and Prevention, 2005, pp 1–7.
7. Beverley PC: Immunology of vaccination. Br Med Bull 2002;62:15–28.
8. Levine MM, Campbell JD, Kotloff KL: Overview of vaccines and immunisation. Br Med Bull 2002;62:1–13.
9. Ellis RW: New technologies for making vaccines. In Plotkin SA, Orenstein WA (eds): Vaccines. Philadelphia, W.B. Saunders, 1999, pp 881–901.
10. Centers for Disease Control and Prevention: Withdrawal of rotavirus vaccine recommendation. JAMA 1999;282:2113–2114.
11. Moingeon P, Leclerc C: Challenges and issues in new vaccine development. Trends Immunol 2002;23:173–175.
12. Moingeon P, De Taisne C, Almond J: Delivery technologies for human vaccines. Br Med Bull 2002;62:29–44.
13. Summaries of infectious diseases. In Pickering LK (ed): 2003 Red Book: Report of the Committee on Infectious Diseases. Elk Grove Village, IL, American Academy of Pediatrics, 2003, pp 189–692.
14. In Atkinson W, Wolfe C (eds): Epidemiology and Prevention of Vaccine-Preventable Diseases. The Pink Book, 8th ed. Atlanta, GA, Centers for Disease Control and Prevention, 2005, pp 55–295.
15. Centers for Disease Control and Prevention: Poliomyelitis prevention in the United States: Introduction of a sequential vaccination schedule of inactivated poliovirus vaccine followed by oral poliovirus vaccine. Recommendations of the Advisory Committee on Immunization Practices (ACIP). MMWR 1997;46(RR-3):1–25.
16. Peltola H: Worldwide *Haemophilus influenzae* type b disease at the beginning of the 21st century: Global analysis of the disease burden 25 years after the use of the polysaccharide vaccine and a decade after the advent of conjugates. Clin Microbiol Rev 2000;13:302–317.
17. Pelton SI, Klein JO: The future of pneumococcal conjugate vaccines for prevention of pneumococcal diseases in infants and children. Pediatrics 2002;110:805–814.
18. Black S, Shinefield H, Fireman B, et al: Efficacy, safety and immunogenicity of heptavalent pneumococcal conjugate vaccine in children. Northern California Kaiser Permanente Vaccine Study Center Group. Pediatr Infect Dis J 2000; 19:187–195.
19. Black SB, Shinefield HR, Ling S, et al: Effectiveness of heptavalent pneumococcal conjugate vaccine in children younger than five years of age for prevention of pneumonia. Pediatr Infect Dis J 2002;21:810–815.
20. Preventing pneumococcal disease among infants and young children. Recommendations of the Advisory Committee on Immunization Practices (ACIP). MMWR 2000;49(RR-9):1–35.
21. Schutze GE, Mason EO Jr, Barson WJ, et al: Invasive pneumococcal infections in children with asplenia. Pediatr Infect Dis J 2002;21:278–282.
22. Centers for Disease Control and Prevention: Measles, mumps, and rubella—vaccine use and strategies for elimination of measles, rubella, and congenital rubella syndrome and control of mumps: Recommendations of the Advisory Committee on Immunization Practices (ACIP). MMWR 1998;47(RR-8):1–57.
23. Seward JF, Watson BM, Peterson CL, et al: Varicella disease after introduction of varicella vaccine in the United States, 1995–2000. JAMA 2002;287:606–611.
24. Centers for Disease Control and Prevention: Prevention of varicella. Updated recommendations of the Advisory Committee on Immunization Practices (ACIP). MMWR 1999;48(RR-6):1–5.
25. Centers for Disease Control and Prevention: Prevention and control of influenza. Recommendations of the Advisory Committee on Immunization Practices (ACIP). MMWR 2004;53(RR-6):1–39.
26. Nichol KL, Mendelman PM, Mallon KP, et al: Effectiveness of live, attenuated intranasal influenza virus vaccine in healthy, working adults: A randomized controlled trial. JAMA 1999;282:137–144.
27. Belshe RB, Mendelman PM, Treanor J, et al: The efficacy of live attenuated, cold-adapted, trivalent, intranasal influenzavirus vaccine in children. N Engl J Med 1998;338:1405–1412.
28. Centers for Disease Control and Prevention: Prevention of hepatitis A through active or passive immunization: Recommendations of the Advisory Committee on Immunization Practices (ACIP). MMWR 1999;48(RR-12):1–37.
29. Prevention of hepatitis A infections: Guidelines for use of hepatitis A vaccine and immune globulin. American Academy of Pediatrics Committee on Infectious Diseases. Pediatrics 1996;98:1207–1215.
30. Centers for Disease Control and Prevention: Prevention and Control of Meningococcal Disease. Recommendations of the Advisory Committee on Immunization Practices (ACIP). 2005;54(RR-7):1–21.
31. Hypersensitivity reactions to vaccine constituents. In Pickering LK (ed): 2003 Red Book: Report of the Committee on Infectious Diseases. Elk Grove Village, IL, American Academy of Pediatrics, 2003, pp 46–49.
32. Hibberd PL, Rubin RH: Approach to immunization in the immunosuppressed host. Infect Dis Clin North Am 1990;4:123–142.
33. Centers for Disease Control and Prevention: Recommendations of the Advisory Committee on Immunization Practices (ACIP): Use of vaccines and immune globulins for persons with altered immunocompetence. MMWR 1993;42(RR-4):1–18.
34. Varicella-zoster infections: Immunocompromised Patients. In Pickering LK (ed): 2003 Red Book: Report of the Committee on Infectious Diseases. Elk Grove Village, IL, American Academy of Pediatrics, 2003, pp 684–685.

# Index

Note: Page numbers followed by b refer to boxed material; those followed by f refer to tables; those followed by t refer to tables.

## A

*Acer saccharum,* 47, 48f, 48t
Acetonide, for allergic rhinitis, 164t
Acneiform irritant contact dermatitis, 227
Acquired immunity, 1, 1b
Acquired immunodeficiency syndrome. *See*
    HIV/AIDS.
ActHIB, 388
Active immunity, 380
Adaptive immunity, 1, 1b
Adenosine deaminase deficiency, 338f, 339
Adhesive bandages, contact dermatitis due to,
    233
Adjuvants, for vaccines, 382–383
Adrenergic agents, for urticaria and
    angioedema, 291
Adult immunization, universal, 383, 384f, 385f
Adverse food reactions. *See* Food *entries.*
Aero-allergens
    animal, 52t, 52–53
    asthma and, 88, 90f
    detection of, 35–36, 36t
    environmental dusts as, 53
    fungi as, 49t, 49–51, 50f
    indoor, 51b, 51f, 51–52, 52b, 52f
    nomenclature for, 36–37
    pollens as, 37, 37b, 37f–42f
        of grasses, 44, 45t, 45f–47f, 47
        of trees, 47, 48f, 48t, 49f
        of weeds, 37–38, 38t, 43f, 43–44, 44f
Agammaglobulinemia
    autosomal-recessive, 333
    X-linked, 333, 334f
*Agrostis gigantean,* 45t, 46f
AIDS. *See* HIV/AIDS.
Albuterol, for anaphylaxis, 72b
Albuterol, for asthma, 108
Alder trees, 47
Allergen(s), 1, 35–53. *See also specific allergens.*
    classification of, 35, 35b
    inhalant. *See* Aero-allergens.
Allergen vaccines. *See* Vaccine(s), allergen.
Allergic bronchopulmonary aspergillosis, 137b,
    137f, 137–145
    defenses against *Aspergillus* and, 137–138
    diagnostic criteria for, 138b, 138–139, 139b
    differential diagnosis of, 144, 144t, 145b
    laboratory testing for, 139–140, 140f
    lung biopsy in, 143, 144f

Allergic bronchopulmonary aspergillosis—*cont'd*
    pathogenesis of, 138, 138f
    prognosis of, 145
    pulmonary function tests in, 140
    radiographic findings in, 140–141,
        141f–143f, 143
    signs and symptoms of, 139
    skin testing for, 139, 139f
    sputum in, 143, 143f
    treatment of, 144–145, 145b
Allergic conjunctivitis, 44, 199t, 199–200, 200t
Allergic contact dermatitis, 225, 227, 228f,
    228t, 229b, 229f, 230t, 231f–233f,
    232–233
Allergic eosinophilic gastroenteropathy, 217b,
    217f, 217–218, 218f
Allergic reactions, immunogenetics of, 31–32,
    32f
Allergic rhinitis, 147–166
    clinical presentation of, 151, 153t,
        153f–156f, 154
    diagnosis of, 156–158, 156f–158f, 157b
    differential diagnosis of, 158b, 158–159, 159f
        nonallergic rhinitis and, 159, 160t
        obstructions and, 158–159, 159f
    epidemiology of, 147–148, 148f
    etiology of, 148–149
    immunopathology of, 149–151, 150f
    pathophysiology of, 151, 152f
    seasonal, 151, 154
    treatment of, 160–165, 161b
        environmental control for, 160–161
        pharmacologic, 161t, 161–165, 162t
Allergic "shiners," 154, 156f
    in atopic dermatitis, 251f
Allergy, definition of, 1, 2f
Alterative complement pathway, 30, 31f
*Alternaria,* 49, 49t, 50f
Alveolar hemorrhage, in systemic lupus
    erythematosus, 306
*Amaranthus retroflexus,* 43, 44f
*Ambrosia artemisiifolia,* 37–38, 43f
*Ambrosia trifida,* 37, 43f
Aminophylline, for anaphylaxis, 72b
Aminophylline, for asthma, 108
Ampicillin, drug eruption caused by, 275
Anaphylactic, definition of, 65
Anaphylactic reaction(s), 5
Anaphylactoid, definition of, 65

Anaphylaxis
    clinical presentation of, 66–69, 67b
        cardiovascular and neurovascular, 67, 68t,
            69
        cutaneous and respiratory, 66–67, 67f
    definition of, 65
    diagnosis of, 71
        laboratory evaluation in, 71
        physical evaluation in, 71, 71b
    disorders confused with, 71
    drug-induced, 273–274
        treatment of, 278
    epidemiology of, 65
    etiology of, 65–66
        IgE-mediated reactions in, 65
        non-IgE-mediated reactions in, 65
        nonimmune mechanisms in, 66, 67b
    idiopathic, 66
    immunologically mediated, 73–76
        *Hymenoptera,* 73, 73t, 74t, 74f–76f, 75
        penicillin, 75–76, 77t, 78t
    with immunotherapy, reducing risk of, 375,
        375b
    non—immune-mediated, 77
        exercise-induced, 77
        radiocontrast media, 77, 77b
    pathogenesis of, 69–70
        immunoglobulin E mediation in, 68f, 69,
            69b, 69f
        mediator release in, 69–70, 70f
    pathology of, 70f, 70–71, 71f
    prevention of, 73, 73b
    treatment of, 72b, 72f, 72–73
Andersen sampler, 36b
Angioedema, 286–291
    in acquired complement 1 esterase inhibitor
        deficiency, 288
    in angioedema-eosinophilia syndrome,
        288
    differential diagnosis of, 283, 288, 289b
    epidemiology of, 279
    etiology of, 280–281
    in food hypersensitivity, 216, 216f
    hereditary, 286–288, 288f
    histologic changes in, 281–282
    pathogenesis of, 282–283
    patient evaluation in, 288–290, 289f,
        290f
    treatment of, 290–291

Angiotensin-converting enzyme inhibitors, allergy to, 276
Animal allergens, 52t, 52–53
Antazoline phosphate/naphazoline hydrochloride (Vasocon-A), for allergic conjunctivitis, 199, 200t
*Anthoxanthum odoratum*, 45t
Antibiotics. *See also* Antimicrobials; *specific antibiotics.*
    anaphylactic reactions to, 65
    for sinusitis, 175, 175t
Antibodies. *See* Immunoglobulin(s).
Anticholinergics, intranasal, for rhinitis, 161t
Antidepressants, tricyclic, for urticaria and angioedema, 291
Antigens
    binding of, 29, 29f
    causing hypersensitivity pneumonitis, 126, 126t
Antihistamines. *See also specific drugs.*
    intranasal, for rhinitis, 161t
    oral
        for allergic rhinitis, 162–163, 163t
        for atopic dermatitis, 256
        for rhinitis, 161t
        for urticaria and angioedema, 291
    topical, for atopic dermatitis, 256
Anti-IgE antibody, for asthma, 109
Anti-inflammatory agents, topical. *See also* Nonsteroidal anti-inflammatory drugs.
    for contact dermatitis, 239b, 240, 240f
Antimicrobial agents. *See also* Antibiotics; *specific drugs.*
    oral
        for atopic dermatitis, 256
        for immunodeficiency diseases, 348
    topical, for atopic dermatitis, 256
Antineutrophil cytoplasmic antibodies, in vasculitis, 321, 322f
Antipruritics, topical, for contact dermatitis, 239
Antiretroviral therapy, highly active, for HIV/AIDS, 361–362, 361t–363t
Antisynthetase syndrome, 315, 315f
Arachidonic acid metabolites, in anaphylaxis, 70
Arterial blood gases, in asthma, 98, 98t
Arthritis. *See* Rheumatoid arthritis.
Ash trees, 47, 48f, 48t
Aspergillosis, bronchopulmonary. *See* Allergic bronchopulmonary aspergillosis.
*Aspergillus,* chronic granulomatous disease and, 342
*Aspergillus flavus,* 50f
Aspirin
    allergy to, 276
    anaphylactic reactions to, 66
    avoidance of, for urticaria and angioedema, 291
Aspirin challenge testing, 63
Asteatotic eczema, 227, 227f
Asthma, 81f, 81–113, 82f
    allergic
        allergy vaccine immunotherapy for, 375–376
        anti-IgE immunotherapy for, 376, 376f

Asthma—*cont'd*
    clinical presentation and differential diagnosis of, 89–90, 91t, 92f, 92–99, 93t, 94f–98f, 98t
    death related to, identification of patients at risk for, 110b, 113
    epidemiology of, 81, 82f–85f, 83–85, 84t
    exacerbations of
        pathophysiology of, 89
        severity estimation of, 93t
    exercise-induced, challenge testing for, 60, 62f
    extrinsic, 84
    genetic basis for, 88, 89f
    intrinsic, 84, 84f
    leukotriene receptor antagonists for, 104, 107, 109t
    occupational. *See* Occupational asthma.
    pathophysiology of, 85–89
        of acute exacerbations, 89
        general, 85, 85t, 86f–90f, 87–89
    severity of
        control of factors contributing to, 100–101
        tailoring therapy to, 102, 103f–105f, 104
    sinusitis and, 176–177, 177b, 177t
    treatment of, 99b, 99–113
        adherence and, 109–110
        anticholinergic agents for, 109
        anti-IgE antibody for, 109
        assessment and monitoring in, 99f, 99–100, 100f
        beta-2 agonists for, 108, 109t
        chromones for, 107–108
        controlling factors contributing to asthma severity and, 100–101
        for exacerbations, 110, 111f, 112f
        general approach for, 101b, 101–105, 103b, 103f–105f
        goals of, 101, 102t
        immunotherapy for, 109
        inhaled corticosteroids for, 105–107, 106f, 109t
        methylxanthines for, 108
        oral corticosteroids for, 108–109, 110f
        patient education for, 101
        during pregnancy, 110, 113
    as whole-airway disease component, 113
Ataxia telangiectasia, 340, 340f
"Athlete's foot," 250f
Atopic conjunctivitis, 199t, 201–202, 202f
Atopic dermatitis, 243–257
    complications of, 253, 253f, 254f
    diagnosis of, 245–251, 246b
        atopy and, 245–247, 247b, 247f
        eczema and, 248–249, 248f–251f, 251
        pruritus and, 247t, 247–248, 248b
    differential diagnosis of, 253–254, 254b
    epidemiology of, 243, 243t, 244b, 244f
    epidermal antimicrobial peptide deficiency in, 245
    food-induced, 216–217
    impetiginized, 253f
    management of, 254–256
        antihistamines in, 256
        antimicrobials in, 256
        emollients in, 254–255

Atopic dermatitis—*cont'd*
    phototherapy for, 256
    systemic options for, 256
    topical corticosteroids in, 255, 255b
    topical immunomodulators in, 256, 256f
    pathogenesis of, 243–244, 244b
        environmental factors in, 244, 245b
        genetics in, 243–244
        pharmacological and vascular abnormalities in, 245, 246b
        pruritus in, 244–245, 246t
    psychological aspects and impact on quality of life of, 256–257
    spectrum of, 251, 251b, 251f, 252f
    thermal sweating abnormalities in, 245
    xerosis in, 245
Atopic keratoconjunctivitis, 201–202, 202f
Atopic triad, 243
Atopy
    in atopic dermatitis, 245–247, 247b, 247f
    definition of, 1
Audiometry, in otitis media, 190, 190f
Autocrine actions, of cytokines, 17, 17f
Autoimmune urticaria, 280
Autoimmunity, definition of, 1
Autosomal-recessive agammaglobulinemia, 333
Azelastine hydrochloride (Optivar), for allergic conjunctivitis, 200t

**B**
Bacille Calmette-Guérin, 380, 381
Bahia grass, 45t
Baker's cyst, in rheumatoid arthritis, 296
Balsam of Peru, contact dermatitis due to, 230t
Basophils, 6f, 14, 16, 16f
    activation of, 20–21, 21f, 22f
B-cells. *See* B-lymphocytes.
Beclomethasone
    for allergic rhinitis, 164t
    for asthma, 103t
Beclomethasone dipropionate (Beconase AQ; Vancenase AQ), for allergic rhinitis, 164t
Benzocaine, contact dermatitis due to, 230t
Benzylpenicillopolylysine challenge, 76, 77t
Bermuda grass, 45t, 47, 47f
Beta-2 agonists, for asthma, 108, 109t
*Betula populifolia,* 47, 48f, 48t
Birch trees, 47, 48f, 48t
"Black mold," 50
Black oak trees, 48t, 49f
Black rubber mix, contact dermatitis due to, 230t
Black willow trees, 48t
*Blomia tropicalis,* 51, 51f
Blood transfusions, anaphylactic reactions to, 65
Bluegrass, 45t, 46f
B-lymphocytes, 6f, 8, 11f, 12f
    deficiency of, 332–336, 333t
        laboratory tests for, 345, 346t
    hyperactivated, in systemic lupus erythematosus, 302b
Bone marrow transplantation
    for immunodeficiency diseases, 347
    vaccines and, 394–395

*Bordetella pertussis*, vaccine for, 379t, 382t, 386–387
Bronchial challenge testing, 61–62, 62f
in occupational asthma, 121–122, 122f
Bronchiolitis, asthma differentiated from, 84, 84t
Bronchoconstriction, exercise-induced, 105
Bronchoprovocation tests, in hypersensitivity pneumonitis, 129, 129f
Budesonide (Rhinocort AQ)
for allergic rhinitis, 164, 164t
for asthma, 103t
Burkard trap, 36b
Burkholder's cepacia, chronic granulomatous disease and, 342
Burning bush, 43, 44f
*p-tert*-Butylphenol, contact dermatitis due to, 230t

**C**

Calcinosis, in dermatomyositis, 314f
Calcium, for idiopathic inflammatory myopathies, 316
*Candida* hypersensitivity, 64
Candidiasis
in HIV/AIDS, 356f
mucocutaneous, chronic, 340, 341f
in severe combined immunodeficiency disease, 336, 337f
Carba mix, contact dermatitis due to, 230t
Cardiac manifestations
in idiopathic inflammatory myopathies, 314
in rheumatoid arthritis, 299
in systemic sclerosis, 311
Cardiopulmonary arrest, during anaphylaxis, 72–73
Cardiopulmonary manifestations, in systemic lupus erythematosus, 306
Cardiovascular manifestations, in anaphylaxis, 67, 68t, 69
*Carya alba*, 48t
Cat allergens, 52
immunotherapy dose for, 373t
Cataracts, in atopic keratoconjunctivitis, 201, 202f
Catarrhal marginal infiltrates, 204, 204f
CD4 cells, 6f, 7, 8f–10f
CD8 cells, 6f, 7, 8f
Cefuroxime, oral, for atopic dermatitis, 256
Celecoxib (Celebrex), allergy to, 276
Celiac disease, 218, 219f, 220
Cetirizine (Zyrtec), for allergic rhinitis, 163t, 165
Challenge testing, 60–63, 62t
benzylpenicillopolylysine, 76, 77t
bronchial, 61–62, 62f
in hypersensitivity pneumonitis, 129, 129f
in occupational asthma, 121–122, 122f
exercise, 60, 62f
food, double-blind, placebo-controlled, 220, 221
injections for, 63, 63t
nasal, 62
for allergic rhinitis, 157
oral, 62–63, 63f
Chédiak-Higashi syndrome, 343

Cheilitis, atopic, 250f
Chemokines, 19–20, 20f
*Chemopodium album*, 43, 44f
"Chicken" skin, in atopic dermatitis, 251f
Chickenpox, vaccine for, 391
Childhood immunization, universal, 383, 383f
Chlorpheniramine (Chlor-Trimeton), for allergic rhinitis, 163t
Cholera vaccine, 380, 381
Cholesteatoma, congenital, 187, 188f
Choroiditis, 208–209, 210f
Chromium, hexavalent, dermatitis due to, 230, 232f
Churg-Strauss syndrome, 320b, 325, 325f
Cimetidine
for radiocontrast media anaphylaxis prevention, 77b
for urticaria and angioedema, 291
Cinnamic aldehyde, contact dermatitis due to, 230t
*Cladosporium*, 49, 49t, 50f
Classical complement pathway, 30, 31f
*Clostridium tetani*, vaccine for, 379t, 382t, 386, 386f, 386t
Cockroaches, 52, 52b
Colchicine, for urticaria and angioedema, 291
Cold-induced urticaria, 289, 289f
Colophony, contact dermatitis due to, 230t
Common variable immunodeficiency, 335
Complement deficiencies, 343–345, 344f, 344t
Complement system, 29–31, 30f, 31f
activation of, 31
biologic effects of C3a and C5a anaphylatoxins and, 31
enzyme cascades of, 30, 31f
proteins of, 30–31, 31f
Comvax, 388, 390
Condyloma acuminata, in HIV/AIDS, 354, 355f
Conjunctiva, normal anatomy of, 195, 197, 197f
Conjunctivitis, 198–202. *See also* Dermatoconjunctivitis; Keratoconjunctivitis.
allergic, 44, 199t, 199–200, 200t
atopic, 199t, 201–202, 202f
giant papillary, 202, 203f
vernal, 199t, 200–201, 201f
Connective tissue diseases. *See also* Idiopathic inflammatory myopathies; Rheumatoid arthritis; Sjögren's syndrome; Systemic lupus erythematosus; Systemic sclerosis; Vasculitis.
relationship among, 293, 293f
Contact dermatitis, 225b, 225–241
allergic, 225, 227, 228f, 228t, 229b, 229f, 230t, 231f–233f, 232–233
diagnosis of, 234–239
history in, 234
patch testing for, 235, 235b, 235f–238f, 236t, 237–238, 238t
physical examination in, 234b, 234f, 234–235, 235f, 235t
differential diagnosis of eczema and, 238–239, 239b
irritant, 225–227, 226b, 226f, 227f

Contact dermatitis—*cont'd*
patient education about, 240
treatment of, 239b, 239–240
avoidance in, 239
systemic anti-inflammatory agents in, 240
topical anti-inflammatory agents in, 239b, 240, 240b
topical antipruritics in, 239
Contact dermatoconjunctivitis, 202, 203f
Cornea, normal anatomy of, 197–198
Corticosteroids. *See also specific drugs.*
growth suppression related to, 106–107
inhaled, for asthma, 105–107, 106f, 109t
intranasal, for allergic rhinitis, 163–164, 164t
systemic
for allergic rhinitis, 165
for asthma, 108–109, 110f
for urticaria and angioedema, 291
topical
for atopic dermatitis, 255, 255b
for contact dermatitis, 239b, 240
vaccines and, 394
*Corynebacterium diphtheriae*, vaccine for, 379t, 382t, 384, 386
Cotton-wool spots, in HIV retinopathy, 358f
Cromolyn sodium (Crolom)
for allergic conjunctivitis, 200t
for asthma, 107–108
for rhinitis, 161t, 165
Cromolyn sodium (Opticrom), for allergic conjunctivitis, 200t
Cross-reaction, in rhus dermatitis, 227, 229f
Cryoglobulinemic vasculitis, essential, 320b
Cutaneous leukocytoclastic vasculitis, 320b
Cutaneous manifestations
in anaphylaxis, 66–67, 67f
in idiopathic inflammatory myopathies, 313, 313f, 314f
in systemic sclerosis, 309, 309f
Cyclophosphamide, for systemic lupus erythematosus, 307
Cyclosporine
for atopic dermatitis, 256
for contact dermatitis, 240
for urticaria and angioedema, 291
*Cynadon dactylin*, 45t, 47, 47f
Cyproheptadine, for urticaria and angioedema, 291
Cytokines, 17, 17b, 17f–20f, 19–20
reactions to, 276
Cytolytic reaction, 5
Cytomegalovirus pneumonitis, in HIV/AIDS, 356f
Cytomegalovirus retinitis, in HIV/AIDS, 356f
Cytotoxic reaction, 5
Cytotoxic T-cells, 6f, 7, 8f
Cytotoxic testing, 63–64

**D**

*Dactylis glomerata*, 45t, 46f
Dalens-Fuchs nodules, 209, 210f
Dancer, 52
Dapsone, for urticaria and angioedema, 291
DAPTACEL, 387
Death, asthma-related, identification of patients at risk for, 110b, 113

Decongestants
    for allergic rhinitis, 164–165
    for rhinitis, 161t
Delayed hypersensitivity reaction, 3–4, 4f, 5–6
Delivery systems, for vaccines, 382–383
Dendritic cells, 6f, 13, 14f, 15f
Dennie's lines, in allergic rhinitis, 154, 155f
Dermatitis
    atopic. *See* Atopic dermatitis.
    contact. *See* Contact dermatitis.
    eyelid, 250f
Dermatitis herpetiformis, 286, 287f
Dermatoconjunctivitis, contact, 202, 203f
Dermatographism, 289, 289f
Dermatomyositis. *See* Idiopathic inflammatory
    myopathies.
*Dermatophagoides*, 51, 51f, 52f
Dermographism, 58
Desensitization
    for anaphylaxis prevention, 73
    for drug allergy, 277, 277b, 277t
Desloratadine (Clarinex), for allergic rhinitis,
    163t
Diagnostic tests, 55–64. *See also* Pulmonary
    function tests; *specific tests.*
    enzyme immunoassay as, 59
        allergen-specific immunoglobulin E
            antibody determination using, 59, 61f
        serum-specific immunoglobulin E
            antibody levels versus using, skin tests
            versus, 59, 61t
        total serum immunoglobulin E
            determination using, 59, 60f
    patch testing as, 235, 235b, 235f–238f, 236t,
        237–238, 238t
    provocative challenge tests as. *See* Challenge
        testing.
    skin tests as, 55f, 55t, 55–59, 56f
        epicutaneous, 55, 57t
        false-negative results with, 57–58, 58t
        false-positive results with, 58t, 58–59, 59t
        intercutaneous, 57, 57f
    unproven techniques and theories for, 63t,
        63–64
Diet(s), elimination, 220
Diet diaries, 220
Dietary protein enterocolitis, 218, 218b
Dietary protein proctitis, 218
DiGeorge syndrome, 339f, 339–340
Diphenhydramine hydrochloride (Benadryl)
    for allergic rhinitis, 163t
    for anaphylaxis, 72b
    for drug allergy, 278
    for radiocontrast media anaphylaxis
        prevention, 77b
Diphtheria, vaccine for, 379t, 382t, 384, 386
DNA vaccines, 382
Dog allergens, 52
Dopamine hydrochloride, for anaphylaxis, 72b
Double-blind, placebo-controlled food
    challenge, 220, 221
Doxepin (Zonalon)
    for atopic dermatitis, 256
    contact dermatitis due to, 233, 233f
    for urticaria and angioedema, 291
*Drechslera*, 49, 49t, 50f

Drug(s). *See also specific drugs and drug types.*
    skin tests and, 58, 58b
    topical, contact dermatitis due to, 232–233,
        233f
Drug allergy, 271t, 271–278, 272b, 272t, 273f
    clinical presentation of, 273–275, 274b,
        275b, 275f, 276f
    diagnosis of, 276b, 276–278, 277b, 277t
    epidemiology of, 272–273, 274b
    immunogenicity of drugs and, 273
    new agents and, 275–276
    reporting of, 278
    treatment and prevention of, 278, 278b
Dry eye, in Sjögren's syndrome, 317, 317f, 319
Dry mouth, in Sjögren's syndrome, 317–318,
    318f, 319
Dry skin, in atopic dermatitis, 245
DTaP vaccines, 387
Durham sampler, 36b
Dust(s), environmental, 53
Dust mite allergen, immunotherapy dose for,
    373t
Dye(s)
    anaphylactic reactions to, 66
    for hair, contact dermatitis due to, 230, 232f
Dysfunctional cilia syndrome, 345, 345f
Dysphagia, in Sjögren's syndrome, 318

**E**

Eardrum, perforation of, 188f, 190
Eastern cottonwood, 48t
Eczema
    antecubital, 249f
    asteatotic, 227, 227f
    in atopic dermatitis, 248–249, 248f–251f, 251
    differential diagnosis of, 238–239, 239b
    facial, 249f
    of nipple, 250f
    popliteal, 249f
Edema. *See also* Angioedema.
    laryngeal, in anaphylaxis, 70, 70f
Eggs, allergy to, vaccines and, 393
Elimination diets, 220
Elm trees, 47, 48t
Emedastine difumerate (Emadine), for allergic
    conjunctivitis, 200t
Emollients, for atopic dermatitis, 254–255
Emphysema, pulmonary, in anaphylaxis, 70,
    70f
Endocrine actions, of cytokines, 17, 17f
Engerix-B, 390
English plantain, 43, 43f
Enterocolitis, dietary protein, 218, 218b, 219f
Environmental control, for allergic rhinitis,
    160–161
Environmental dusts, 53
Enzyme(s), as aeroallergens, 53
Enzyme immunoassay, 59
    allergen-specific immunoglobulin E antibody
        determination using, 59, 61f
    sandwich, 59, 61f
    serum-specific immunoglobulin E antibody
        levels versus using, skin tests versus, 59,
        61t
    total serum immunoglobulin E
        determination using, 59, 60f

Eosinophil(s), 6f, 13–14, 15f
Eosinophilia, in atopic dermatitis, 247
Ephedrine, for radiocontrast media
    anaphylaxis prevention, 77b
*Epicoccum*, 50
Epicutaneous skin tests, 55, 57t
Epinephrine, for anaphylaxis, 72b, 72–73
Epi-Pen, for food hypersensitivity, 223
Epi-Pen Jr., for food hypersensitivity, 223
Episcleritis, 205–207
    clinical presentation of, 205, 206f, 207f
    pathogenesis of, 207
    treatment of, 207
Epoxy resin, contact dermatitis due to, 230t
Erythema annulare centrifugum, 286, 287f
Erythema multiforme, 275, 286, 287f
Essential cryoglobulinemic vasculitis, 320b
Ethylenediamine, contact dermatitis due to,
    230t
*Euroglyphus maynei*, 51, 51f
Eustachian tube
    dysfunction of, otitis media and, 182
    obstruction of, otitis media and, 182, 182f
Excoriation, in atopic dermatitis, 250f, 251f
Exercise
    anaphylaxis due to, 77
    asthma induced by, challenge testing for, 60,
        62f
    bronchoconstriction induced by, 105
Extrinsic allergic alveolitis. *See* Hypersensitivity
    pneumonitis.
Eye(s), normal anatomy of, 195, 195f, 196f,
    197–198
Eyelid dermatitis, 250f

**F**

Fab fragments, 26
Facial allergic contact dermatitis, 230
False-negative results, with skin tests, 57–58, 58t
False-positive results, with skin tests, 58t,
    58–59, 59t
*Festica pratensis*, 45t
Fetal development, immunoglobulins and,
    27–28
Fexofenadine (Allegra), for allergic rhinitis,
    163t, 165
Fire ants. *See Hymenoptera* allergy.
Fixed drug eruption, 275
Floppy thumb sign, in idiopathic inflammatory
    myopathy, 315, 315f
FluMist, 382, 392
Flunisolide
    for allergic rhinitis, 164, 164t
    for asthma, 103t
Fluticasone, for asthma, 103t
Fluticasone propionate (Flonase), for allergic
    rhinitis, 164, 164t
Food(s)
    as aeroallergens, 53
    anaphylactic reactions to, 65
Food hypersensitivity, 213b, 213–224
    diagnosis of, 220b, 220–223, 221t, 222b,
        222t, 223t
    immunoglobulin E-mediated
        clinical manifestations of, 215–216, 216b
        pathophysiology of, 214f, 214–215, 215f

Food hypersensitivity—*cont'd*
   mixed immunoglobulin E-mediated and
      non—immunoglobulin E-mediated,
      clinical manifestations of, 5b, 5f, 5–6, 6f
   non—immunoglobulin E-mediated
      clinical manifestations of of, 218, 218b,
      219f, 220
   pathophysiology of, 214–215
   prevalence of, 213
   prevention of, 222b
   prognosis of, 224
   treatment of, 223
Food intolerance, definition of, 213
Formaldehyde, contact dermatitis due to,
   230t
Formoterol, for asthma, 108
Fragrance allergy, contact dermatitis due to,
   230
*Fraxinus Pennsylvania,* 47, 48f, 48t
Fungi, 49t, 49–51, 50f
   immunotherapy dose for, 373t

**G**

Gastroenteropathy, eosinophilic, allergic, 217b,
   217f, 217–218, 218f
Gastrointestinal food hypersensitivity
   reactions, 215–216, 216b
Gastrointestinal manifestations, in idiopathic
   inflammatory myopathies, 314
Gell and Coombs classification schema, 4f, 4–5
Gene therapy, for immunodeficiency diseases,
   347–348
Giant papillae, 200, 201f
Giant papillary conjunctivitis, 202, 203f
Giant ragweed, 37, 43f
Giant-cell arteritis, 321b, 322–323, 323f
Glucagon, for anaphylaxis, 72
Gottron's changes, in dermatomyositis, 314f
Granulocytes, 13–16. *See also* Basophils;
   Eosinophils; Neutrophils.
Granulomatous disease, chronic, 342–343
Grass pollen allergen, immunotherapy dose
   for, 373t
Ground-glass opacities, in hypersensitivity
   pneumonitis, 128, 128f
*Haemophilus influenzae*
   in otitis media, 182, 183f
   sinusitis due to, 170, 170t

**H**

*Haemophilus influenzae* type b, vaccine for,
   379t, 382, 388, 388f
Hair dye, contact dermatitis due to, 230, 232f
Hairy leukoplakia, in HIV/AIDS, 354, 355f
Hand dermatitis, 230, 231f
Havrix, 392
Hay fever, 44, 199t, 199–200, 200t
Hazel trees, 47
Heavy chains, 26f, 26–27, 27t
*Helminthosporium,* 49, 49t, 50f
Helper T-cells, 6f, 7, 8f–10f
Hematologic manifestations, in systemic lupus
   erythematosus, 304
Hematopoietic family cytokines, 17, 18f, 19
Hematopoietic stem cells, 6f
   pluripotent, 331f, 331–332, 332f

Henoch-Schönlein purpura, 320b, 327
Hepatitis A, vaccine for, 392
Hepatitis B, vaccine for, 382t, 389t, 389–390
Herpes simplex infection
   in atopic dermatitis, 253f
   lesions of, 286, 287f
Herpes zoster infection
   in HIV/AIDS, 354, 355f
   lesions of, 286, 287f
   vaccine for, 391
Hertoe's sign, 250f
*Hevea brasiliensis,* 259–260, 260f. *See also* Latex
   allergy.
Hib vaccines, 379t, 382, 388, 388f
HibTITER, 388
Hickory trees, 48t
Highly active antiretroviral therapy, for HIV/
   AIDS, 361–362, 361t–363t
Histamine, anaphylaxis and, 66, 69, 70f
HIV/AIDS, 351–367
   clinical presentation of, 353–356
      in acute retroviral syndrome, 354, 354b
      in AIDS, 356, 356b, 356f–358f
      in asymptomatic phase and pre-AIDS
      syndrome, 354f, 354–355, 355f
   diagnosis of, 358, 358b, 358f
   epidemiology of, 351f, 351–353
      global perspective on, 351, 351f
      mode of transmission and, 352–353, 353t
      United States perspective on, 351t,
      351–352, 352f, 353f
   etiology of, 358–359, 359f
   immunopathogenesis of, 359–361, 360f
   prevention of, 364–365
      occupational exposure and, 364
      perinatal transmission and, 364–365
      vaccines for, 364t, 365
   treatment of, 361–362, 361t–363t
   vaccines in, 394t, 395
Hives. *See* Urticaria.
Hodgkin's disease, vaccines in, 394
Homocytotopic reaction, 5
Honeybees. *See Hymenoptera* allergy.
*Hormodendrum,* 49, 49t, 50f
Hornets. *See Hymenoptera* allergy.
Host immune system, 1b, 2–3, 3b
House dust mites, 51b, 51f, 51–52, 52f
Human immunodeficiency virus. *See*
   HIV/AIDS.
Hydrocortisone, for anaphylaxis, 72b
Hydroxyzine (Atarax), for allergic rhinitis,
   163t
*Hymenoptera* allergy, 63, 65
   anaphylaxis due to, 73, 73t, 74t, 74f–76f
Hyper-immunoglobulin E syndrome, 343,
   343f, 344f
Hyper-immunoglobulin M, immunodeficiency
   with, 334–335
Hypersensitivity, definition of, 1, 2f
Hypersensitivity pneumonitis, 125t, 125–135
   bronchoprovocation tests in, 129, 129f
   clinical presentation of, 126, 127t
   diagnosis of, 131–132, 132b
   differential diagnosis of, 132–133, 133b
   epidemiology of, 125–126, 126b, 126t
   pathogenesis of, 130–131, 131b, 131f, 132f

Hypersensitivity pneumonitis—*cont'd*
   pathology of, 130f, 130–131
   prevention of, 133, 133b, 134f
   prognosis of, 134
   pulmonary function studies in, 128
   radiographic findings in, 126–128, 127f–129f
   treatment of, 133–134, 134b
Hypersensitivity vasculitis, 326, 327f
Hypogammaglobulinemia, of infancy,
   transient, 335–336

**I**

Idiopathic inflammatory myopathies, 312–316
   classification of, 312
   clinical features of, 313–315
      antisynthetase syndrome as, 315, 315f
      cardiac, 314
      cutaneous, 313, 313f, 314f
      gastrointestinal, 314
      inclusion body myositis as, 314
      in joints, 314
      muscular, 313, 313f
      pulmonary, 314
      vascular, 314, 314f
   diagnosis of, 312, 312b
   epidemiology of, 312
   management of, 316, 316f
   natural history of, 315, 316f
   pathogenesis of, 315, 315b
Idiopathic thrombocytopenic purpura, in
   HIV/AIDS, 354
Idiopathic urticarial vasculitis, 283, 285, 285f
Imidazolidinyl urea, contact dermatitis due to,
   230t
Immediate gastrointestinal hypersensitivity,
   215–216, 216b
Immediate hypersensitivity reactions, 2f, 3
Immediate reaction, 5
Immune deficiency syndrome, otitis media
   versus, 190, 190f
Immune response, T-cell-mediated, 5–6
Immune system, 1b, 2–3, 3b
   development of, 331f, 331–332, 332f
Immune-complex injury, 5
Immune-mediated neutropenia, 342
Immunity
   active, 380
   adaptive (acquired; specific), 1, 1b
   innate (natural), 1, 1b
   passive, 380
Immunization. *See* Vaccine(s).
Immunocompromised patients. *See also*
   HIV/AIDS; Immunodeficiency diseases.
   vaccines for, 393–395
      with primary immunodeficiencies,
      393–394
      with secondary immunodeficiencies, 394t,
      394–395
Immunodeficiency diseases, 329b, 329–349,
   330b. *SEe also* HIV/AIDS.
   B-lymphocyte deficiencies and, 332–336,
   333t
   complement deficiencies and, 343–345,
   344f, 344t
   diagnosis of, 345–347, 346f, 346t, 347t
   epidemiology of, 330, 330f

Immunodeficiency diseases—*cont'd*
  immune system development and, 331f,
    331–332, 332f
  mucosal and skin barrier disorders and, 345
  neutrophil deficiencies and, 341–343, 342b
  T-lymphocyte deficiencies and, 336–340
  treatment of
    reconstitution therapies for, 347–348
    replacement therapies for, 347, 348t
    supplemental, 348
Immunogenetics, of allergic reactions, 31–32,
  32f
Immunoglobulin(s), 25f, 25–29
  antigen binding and, 29, 29f
  concentrations of, 27, 27f, 28f
  deficiencies of, 332–336, 333t
  fetal development and, 27–28
  heavy and light chains of, 26f, 26–27, 27t
  for idiopathic inflammatory myopathies, 316
  isotypes of, 26, 26f
    biologic activity of, 28t, 28–29
  mast cell interactions of, 29
  normal, specific antibody deficiency with,
    336
Immunoglobulin A, selective deficiency of,
  335, 335f
Immunoglobulin E
  allergen-specific
    in atopic dermatitis, 246–247, 247f
    EIA determination of, 59, 61f
  in anaphylaxis, 68f, 69, 69b, 69f
  concentration of, 27, 28f
  serum-specific levels of, EIA versus skin tests
    for determining, 59, 61t
  total serum level of, EIA determination of,
    59, 60f
Immunoglobulin G
  concentration of, 27, 27f, 28f
  subclass deficiency of, 335
Immunologic abnormalities, in idiopathic
  inflammatory myopathies, 315, 315b
Immunomodulators, topical, for atopic
  dermatitis, 256
Immunopathologic mechanisms, Gell and
  Coombs classification schema for, 4f,
  4–5
Immunoregulatory abnormalities, in systemic
  lupus erythematosus, 302b
Immunotherapy. *See also* Vaccine(s).
  for allergic bronchopulmonary aspergillosis,
    145
  for asthma, 109
  for food hypersensitivity, 223
  oral, 165t, 165–166, 166b
  for rhinitis, 161t
Inactivated vaccines, 381b, 381–382, 382t
Inclusion body myositis, 314
Indoor allergens, 51b, 51f, 51–52, 52b, 52f
Infancy, transient hypogammaglobulinemia of,
  335–336
Inflammation
  airway, in asthma, 85, 87–88, 87f–89f
  immune pathways of, 18f, 19
Influenza, vaccine for, 382t, 391–392
Inhalant allergens. *See* Aero-allergens.
Injections, for challenge testing, 63, 63t

Innate immunity, 1, 1b
Intercutaneous skin tests, 57, 57f
Interferon
  for immunodeficiency diseases, 348
  reactions to, 276
Intestinal manifestations, in systemic sclerosis,
  310, 310f
Iodine, contact dermatitis due to, 233
Ipratropium bromide, for asthma, 109
IPV vaccine, 387
Iridocyclitis, 208, 208f
Iritis, 208
Irritant contact dermatitis, 225–227, 226b,
  226f, 227f
Isoproterenol, for anaphylaxis, 72
Itraconazole, for allergic bronchopulmonary
  aspergillosis, 145

**J**
Jaccoud's arthropathy, 304
Job's syndrome, 343, 343f, 344f
Johnson grass, 45t, 47, 47f
Joints
  in idiopathic inflammatory myopathies, 314
  in systemic sclerosis, 309–310
*Juglans nigra,* 48t
*Juniperus oshei,* 47, 48t, 49f
Juvenile plantar dermatosis, 250f

**K**
Kapok, 53
Kaposi herpetiform eruption, in atopic
  dermatitis, 253f
Kaposi's sarcoma, in HIV/AIDS, 357f
Kawasaki disease, 320b
Kentucky bluegrass, 45t, 46f
Keratitic precipitates, 209, 211f
Keratoconjunctivitis
  atopic, 201–202, 202f
  phlyctenular, 202, 203f, 204
Keratosis pilaris, in atopic dermatitis, 251f
Ketorolac tromethamine (Acular), for allergic
  conjunctivitis, 200t
Ketotifen fumarate (Zaditor), for allergic
  conjunctivitis, 200t
Koeppe nodules, 209, 211f
Kostmann's syndrome, 341–342
Kramer-Collins trap, 36b
Lacrimal glands, normal anatomy of, 197, 198f
Lamb's quarter, 43, 44f
Lanolin, contact dermatitis due to, 232, 232f
Laryngeal edema, in anaphylaxis, 70, 70f
Late-phase responses, 3–4, 4f, 88
Latex allergy, 259f, 259–270
  biology of latex and, 259–261, 259t–261t, 260f
    common enzymes and structural proteins
      of latex and, 261
      plant defense related function and, 261
      polyisoprene elongation and latex
        coagulation and, 260
  clinical issues in, 264, 265f–268f, 266–268
  diagnostic testing in, 268–269
  management of, 269b, 269–270
  manufacture of latex products and,
    261–262, 262f–264f, 262t, 264, 264t
Lectin complement pathway, 30, 31f

Lens, normal anatomy of, 198
Leukocyte adhesion deficiencies, 343
Leukocytoclastic vasculitis, cutaneous, 320b
Leukotriene receptor antagonists
  for allergic rhinitis, 165
  for asthma, 104, 107, 109t
Leukotrienes, in anaphylaxis, 70
Levalbuterol, for anaphylaxis, 72b
Levocarbastine (Livostin), for allergic
  conjunctivitis, 199, 200t
Light chains, 26f, 26–27, 27t
*Lilium perenne,* 45t, 46f
*Listeria monocytogenes* vaccine, 380, 381
Live attenuated vaccines, 380–381, 381b
Local anesthetic challenge, 63, 63t
Lodoxamide tromethamine (Alomide), for
  allergic conjunctivitis, 200t
Loratadine (Claritin), for allergic rhinitis, 163t,
  165
Loteprednol etabonate (Alrex), for allergic
  conjunctivitis, 200t
Lung biopsy, in allergic bronchopulmonary
  aspergillosis, 143, 144f
Lupus. *See* Systemic lupus erythematosus.
Lymphocyte(s), 7f, 7–9. *See also* B-lymphocytes;
  T-lymphocytes.
  large, 6f, 8–9
Lymphocyte infiltration, in Sjögren's
  syndrome, 318
Lymphocyte predominant urticaria, 281, 282f
Lymphoid precursors, 6f

**M**
Macrophages, 6f, 9, 12f, 13, 13f
Mammalian animal allergens, 52t, 52–53
Mannose binding complement pathway, 30, 31f
Maple trees, 47, 48f, 48t
Masks, disposable, 133, 134f
Mast cell(s), 6f, 16f, 16–17, 17t
  activation of, 20–21, 21f, 22f
  immunoglobulin interactions with, 29
Mast cell stabilizers, for allergic rhinitis, 165
Mastocytosis, 285, 286f
Mattress mites, 51b, 51f, 51–52, 52f
Meadow fescue, 45t
Measles, vaccine for, 379t, 390
"Mechanic's hands," in idiopathic
  inflammatory myopathy, 315, 315f
Megakaryocytes, 6f
Menactra, 392–393
Meningococcal disease, vaccine for, 382,
  392–393
Menomune, 392
Mercapto mix, contact dermatitis due to, 230t
Mercaptobenzothiole, contact dermatitis due
  to, 230t
Methacholine challenge testing, 61, 62f
Methylprednisolone
  for anaphylaxis, 72b
  oral, for atopic dermatitis, 256
Methylxanthines, for asthma, 108
Microscopic polyangiitis, 320b, 324–325, 325f
Middle ear, structure and function of,
  179–180, 180f, 181f
Mites, 51b, 51f, 51–52, 52f
MMR vaccine, 390

Molds, 49t, 49–51, 50f
    immunotherapy dose for, 373t
Molluscum contagiosum, in HIV/AIDS, 354, 354f
Mometasone furoate (Nasonex), for allergic rhinitis, 164, 164t
Monoclonal antibodies, reactions to, 276
Monocytes, 6f
Mooren's ulcer, 204, 205f
*Moraxella catarrhalis*
    in otitis media, 183, 183f
    sinusitis due to, 170, 170t
Mountain cedar trees, 47, 48t, 49f
Mucocutaneous candidiasis, chronic, 340, 341f
Mucosal barrier disorders, 345
Multiple-chemical sensitivity, 64
Multitest applicator, 57, 57f
Mumps, vaccine for, 379t, 390
Mupirocin (Bactroban), topical, for atopic dermatitis, 256
Musculoskeletal manifestations
    in idiopathic inflammatory myopathies, 313, 313f
    in systemic lupus erythematosus, 304
    in systemic sclerosis, 310
*Mycobacterium avium* complex infection, in HIV/AIDS, 357f
*Mycobacterium bovis,* 380
Myeloid precursors, 6f
Myeloperoxidase deficiency, 343
Myopathies, inflammatory, idiopathic. *See* Idiopathic inflammatory myopathies.
Myositis, inclusion body, 314

N
Naphazoline (Naphcon-A), for allergic conjunctivitis, 200t
Naphazoline hydrochloride/pheniramine maleate (Opcon-A), for allergic conjunctivitis, 200t
Naphazoline/pheniramine (OcuHist), for allergic conjunctivitis, 200t
Nasal challenge testing, 62
    for allergic rhinitis, 157
Nasal obstruction(s)
    differential diagnosis of, 158–159, 159f
    in otitis media, 184
Natural immunity, 1, 1b
Natural killer cells, 6f, 8–9
Nedocromil (Alocril), for allergic conjunctivitis, 200t
Nedocromil sodium, for asthma, 107
*Neisseria meningitidis,* vaccine for, 382, 392–393
Neomycin, contact dermatitis due to, 230t, 233
Neurologic symptoms, in anaphylaxis, 69
Neuropsychiatric manifestations, in systemic lupus erythematosus, 306, 306f
Neutropenia
    congenital, severe, 341–342
    cyclic, 342
    immune-mediated, 342
Neutrophils, 6f, 13, 15f
    deficiency of, 341–343, 342b
        with defective neutrophil function, 342–343
        with neutropenia, 341–342

Nickel, contact dermatitis due to, 229–230, 230t, 231f
Nifedipine, for urticaria and angioedema, 291
Nipples, eczema of, 250f
Nitric oxide, in anaphylaxis, 70
*Nocardia,* chronic granulomatous disease and, 342
Nonerythematous irritant contact dermatitis, 227
Nonsteroidal anti-inflammatory drugs
    allergy to, 276
    avoidance of, for urticaria and angioedema, 291
    for Sjögren's syndrome, 319

O
Oak trees, 47, 48t
Oakleaf poison ivy, 228t. *See also* Rhus dermatitis.
Occupational asthma, 115b, 115–123, 116f
    allergic, 117, 118b, 118f
    diagnosis of, 119–122
        bronchial provocation studies in, 121–122, 122f
        imaging studies in, 121
        laboratory studies in, 120–121
        medical history and examination in, 119, 119b, 120f
        physical examination in, 120
        pulmonary function studies in, 121, 122f
        site visit for, 119, 120f, 121f
    differential diagnosis of, 122–123, 123b
    epidemiology of, 115–116
    nonallergic, 117–118, 119b
    pathogenesis of, 117, 117f
    predisposing factors for, 116b, 116–117
    prevention and management of, 123
    prognosis of, 123, 123b
Ocular manifestations. *See also specific conditions.*
    in Sjögren's syndrome, 317, 317f
*Olea europaea,* 48t
Olive trees, 48t
Olopatadine hydrochloride (Patanol), for allergic conjunctivitis, 200t
Omalizumab, for allergic asthma, 376, 376f
Ophthalmia, sympathetic, 209, 210f
Oral allergy syndrome, 215, 216b
Oral challenge testing, 62–63, 63f
Oral manifestations, in Sjögren's syndrome, 317–318, 318f
Oral poliovirus vaccine, 387
Orchard grass, 45t, 46f
Organic dusts, 53
Otitis media, 179f, 179–193
    diagnosis of, 184–190
        allergy and, 190
        audiometry in, 190, 190f
        history in, 184f, 184–186
        immune deficiency syndrome and, 190
        pneumatic otoscopy in, 185f–188f, 186–187, 190
        tympanometry in, 189f, 190
    epidemiology of, 180–181, 181b
    middle ear structure and function and, 179–180, 180f, 181f
    for otitis media with perfusion, 192f, 193

Otitis media—*cont'd*
    pathogenesis of, 181–184
        allergy in, 183f, 183–184
        eustachian tube dysfunction in, 182
        eustachian tube obstruction in, 182, 182f
        infection in, 182–183, 183f
    treatment of, 191–193
        for acute otitis media, 191, 191f
Otoscopy, pneumatic, in otitis media, 185f–188f, 186–187, 190

P
Palms, hyperlinearity of, 252f
Paracrine actions, of cytokines, 17, 17f
Paraphenylenediamine, contact dermatitis due to, 230, 230t, 232f
*Paspalum notatum,* 45t
Passive immunity, 380
Patch testing, for contact dermatitis, 235, 235b, 235f–238f, 236t, 237–238, 238t
Pathogen-associated molecular patterns, 3
Patient education
    about contact dermatitis, 240
    about food hypersensitivity, 223
    for asthma management, 100
Peak expiratory flow rate, in asthma monitoring, 99f, 99–100, 100f
Pediarix, 387, 390
PedvaxHIB, 388
Pemirolast potassium (Alamast), for allergic conjunctivitis, 200t
Penicillin
    allergy to, diagnosis of, 277t
    anaphylaxis due to, 75–76, 77t, 78t
*Penicillium,* 50, 50f
Pericarditis, in systemic lupus erythematosus, 306
Pertussis, vaccine for, 379t, 382t, 386–387
Phagocytes, in systemic lupus erythematosus, 302b
Phenylpropanolamine, for allergic rhinitis, 164
*Phleum pretense,* 45t, 45t
Phlyctenular keratoconjunctivitis, 202, 203f, 204
Phototherapy, for atopic dermatitis, 256
Pigweed, 43, 44f
Pimecrolimus (Elidel) cream
    for atopic dermatitis, 256
    for contact dermatitis, 240
Pityriasis alba, 252f
Plasma cells, 6f
Plasmapheresis, for urticaria and angioedema, 291
*Platanus accidentelis,* 48t
Platelets, 6f
Pluripotent hematopoietic stem cells, 331f, 331–332, 332f
Pneumatic otoscopy, in otitis media, 185f–188f, 186–187, 190
Pneumococcal disease, vaccine for, 388b, 388–389, 389b
*Pneumocystis carinii* infection, in HIV/AIDS, 357f
Pneumonitis
    cytomegalovirus, in HIV/AIDS, 356f
    hypersensitivity. *See* Hypersensitivity pneumonitis.
    lupus, 306

Pneumovax 23, 388
*Poa pretensis,* 45t, 46f
Poison ivy, 228t. *See also* Rhus dermatitis.
Poison sumac, 228t. *See also* Rhus dermatitis.
Poliomyelitis, vaccine for, 379t, 380, 381, 387, 387f
Pollen(s), 37, 37b, 37f–42f
    of grasses, 44, 45t, 45f–47f, 47
    immunotherapy dose for, 373t
    of trees, 47, 48f, 48t, 49f
    of weeds, 37–38, 38t, 43f, 43–44, 44f
Polyangiitis, microscopic, 320b, 324–325, 325f
Polyarteritis nodosa, 320b, 324, 324f
Polyisoprene, 260
Polymyositis. *See* Idiopathic inflammatory myopathies.
Popliteal cysts, in rheumatoid arthritis, 296
*Populus alba,* 48t
*Populus deltoids,* 48t
Potassium dichromate, contact dermatitis due to, 230t
Prednisone
    for allergic bronchopulmonary aspergillosis, 144, 145b
    for asthma, 108–109, 110f
    for atopic dermatitis, 256
    for contact dermatitis, 240
    for drug allergy, 278
    for idiopathic inflammatory myopathies, 316
    for radiocontrast media anaphylaxis prevention, 77b
    for systemic lupus erythematosus, 307
    vaccines and, 394
Pregnancy
    asthma management during, 110, 113
    urticaria in, 283, 285f
Prevnar, 389
Proctitis, dietary protein, 218
Propranolol, anaphylaxis management and, 72
Prostaglandins, in anaphylaxis, 70
Protein(s), anaphylactic reactions to, 65
Protein intolerance, 218, 218b, 219f
PRP-OMP, 388
Pruritic urticarial papules and plaques of pregnancy, 283, 285f
Pruritus, in atopic dermatitis, 244–245, 246t, 247t, 247–248, 248b
Pseudoallergy, 273
Pseudoephedrine, for allergic rhinitis, 164–165
Pulmonary emphysema, in anaphylaxis, 70, 70f
Pulmonary fibrosis, in hypersensitivity pneumonitis, 128, 129f
Pulmonary function tests
    for allergic bronchopulmonary aspergillosis, 140
    in asthma, 97, 98f
    in hypersensitivity pneumonitis, 128
    in occupational asthma, 121, 122f
Pulmonary hypersensitivity syndrome. *See* Hypersensitivity pneumonitis.
Pulmonary manifestations
    in idiopathic inflammatory myopathies, 314
    in rheumatoid arthritis, 299
    in systemic sclerosis, 310f, 310–311

"Pulseless disease," 321b, 323, 323f
Purpura, idiopathic thrombocytopenic, in HIV/AIDS, 354
Pustular irritant contact dermatitis, 227

**Q**

Quaternium, contact dermatitis due to, 230t
*Quercus alba,* 48t, 49f
*Quercus velutina,* 48t, 49f

**R**

Radioallergosorbent tests, for food hypersensitivity, 221
Radiocontrast media
    allergy to, treatment of, 278
    anaphylaxis due to, 77, 77b
RADS, 118, 119b
Ragweeds, 37–38, 43, 43f
    immunotherapy dose for, 373t
Ranitidine
    for anaphylaxis treatment, 72b
    for radiocontrast media anaphylaxis prevention, 77b
    for urticaria and angioedema, 291
Raynaud's phenomenon, in systemic sclerosis, 309, 309f
Recombivax HB, 390
Red maple trees, 51f
Redtop grass, 45t, 46f
Refecoxib (Vioxx), allergy to, 276
Regulatory T-lymphocytes, 7, 10f
Renal manifestations
    in systemic lupus erythematosus, 304, 305f
    in systemic sclerosis, 311
Respiratory food hypersensitivity reactions, 216, 216f
Respiratory symptoms, in anaphylaxis, 66–67
Respiratory syncytial virus, asthma differentiated from, 84, 84t, 85f
Retinal arteritis, occlusive, 208
Retinitis, 208–209, 210f
    cytomegalovirus, in HIV/AIDS, 356f
Rheumatoid arthritis, 293–300
    clinical manifestations of, 295–299
        articular, 296, 297f, 298, 298f
        extra-articular, 298t, 298–299, 299f
    diagnosis of, 300, 300t
    epidemiology of, 293
    pathogenesis of, 293, 294f, 295, 295f, 296t
    treatment of, 300, 301f
Rheumatoid factors, diseases associated with, 293, 295, 296t
Rheumatoid nodules, in rheumatoid arthritis, 298, 299f
Rheumatologic diseases. *See also* Idiopathic inflammatory myopathies; Rheumatoid arthritis; Sjögren's syndrome; Systemic lupus erythematosus; Systemic sclerosis; Vasculitis.
    relationship among, 293, 293f
Rhinomanometry, in allergic rhinitis, 157f, 157–158, 158f
Rhus dermatitis, 227, 228f, 228t, 229, 229f
Rodent allergens, 52–53
Rosin, contact dermatitis due to, 233, 234f
Rotorod sampler, 36b

Rubber compounds. *See also* Latex allergy.
    contact dermatitis due to, 233, 234f
Rubber elongation factor, 260
Rubella, vaccine for, 379t, 390–391
Ryegrass, perennial, 45t, 46f

**S**

Sagebrush, 43, 44f
Salivary glands, in Sjögren's syndrome, 318, 318f
*Salix migra,* 48t
Salmeterol, for asthma, 108
*Salmonella typhi* vaccine, 380, 381
Salt grasses, 47, 47f
Schirmer test, in Sjögren's syndrome, 317, 317f
Schnitzler's syndrome, 286
Scleral diseases, 204–207, 205b, 206f
Scleritis, 205–207
    clinical presentation of, 205, 206f, 207f
    pathogenesis of, 207
    treatment of, 207
Scleroderma. *See also* Systemic sclerosis.
    classification of, 308b
"Scleroderma facies," 309, 309f
Scleromalacia perforans, 205, 207f
*Serratia marcescens,* chronic granulomatous disease and, 342
Serum sickness-like reactions, to drugs, 274
Severe combined immunodeficiency disease, 336, 336b, 337f, 338t
    with decreased T cells and B cells, 338f, 338–339
    with decreased T cells and present B cells, 336, 338
*Shigella* vaccine, 381
"Shingles," vaccine for, 391
Sialometry, in Sjögren's syndrome, 318
Sick building syndrome, 53
Sinus aspiration, 174f, 174–175, 175b
Sinusitis, 167–177
    asthma and, 176–177, 177b, 177t
    defense mechanisms against, 168, 168b, 170, 170t
    diagnosis of, 171–175
        ancillary laboratory tests for, 175, 175b
        computed tomography in, 172, 174, 174b, 174f
        nasal secretions and, 171, 172f
        radiographs in, 172, 173f
        sinus aspiration in, 174f, 174–175, 175b
    history and physical examination in, 170–171, 171b, 171f, 172b
    microbiology of, 170, 170t
    paranasal sinus structure and function and, 167f, 167–168, 168b, 168t, 169f
    treatment of
        medical, 175, 175b
        surgical, 175–176, 176f
Sjögren's syndrome, 317–319
    classification and diagnosis of, 317, 317b
    clinical features of, 317–319
        exocrine, 318
        extraglandular, 318–319
        ocular, 317, 317f
        oral, 317–318, 318f

Sjögren's syndrome—*cont'd*
  epidemiology of, 317
  laboratory abnormalities in, 319
  management of, 319
  natural history of, 319
  pathogenesis of, 319, 319f
Skeletal muscle, in systemic sclerosis, 310
Skin, dry, in atopic dermatitis, 245
Skin barrier disorders, 345
Skin food hypersensitivity reactions, 216–217, 217b
Skin manifestations
  drug-induced, 274, 275b, 275f, 276f
    treatment of, 278
  in systemic lupus erythematosus, 303–304, 304f, 305f
Skin testing, 55f, 55t, 55–59, 56f
  for *Aspergillus*, 139, 139f
  with benzylpenicillopolylysine, 76, 77t
  epicutaneous, 55, 57t
  false-negative results with, 57–58, 58t
  false-positive results with, 58t, 58–59, 59t
  intercutaneous, 57, 57f
  intradermal, for food hypersensitivity, 221
  prick, for food hypersensitivity, 220–221
Smallpox
  in atopic dermatitis, 253f
  vaccine for, 379t
Solar-induced urticaria, 289, 289f
Solu-Medrol, for systemic lupus erythematosus, 307
*Sorgham halepense*, 45t, 47, 47f
Specific immunity, 1, 1b
Sputum, in allergic bronchopulmonary aspergillosis, 143, 143f
*Stachybotrys*, 50
*Staphylococcus aureus*
  in atopic dermatitis, 245
  chronic granulomatous disease and, 342
Stem cells, hematopoietic, pluripotent, 331f, 331–332, 332f
Steroids. *See also* Corticosteroids; *specific steroids.*
  nasal, for rhinitis, 161t
*Streptococcus pneumoniae*
  in otitis media, 182, 183f
  penicillin-resistant, otitis media due to, 191
  sinusitis due to, 170, 170t
  vaccine for, 382, 388b, 388–389, 389b
Subjective irritant contact dermatitis, 227
Subpleural nodules, in hypersensitivity pneumonitis, 128, 129f
Sugar maple trees, 47, 48f, 48t
Sweet vernal grass, 45t
Sycamore trees, 48t
Sympathetic ophthalmia, 209, 210f
Systemic lupus erythematosus, 300–307
  clinical manifestations of, 303–306
    cardiopulmonary, 306
    hematologic, 304
    mucocutaneous, 303–304, 304f, 305f
    musculoskeletal, 304
    neuropsychiatric, 306, 306f
    renal, 304, 305f
  diagnosis of, 307, 307f, 308b
  discoid, 304
  epidemiology of, 300–301

Systemic lupus erythematosus—*cont'd*
  management of, 307
  pathogenesis of, 301, 302b, 302f, 303, 303f
  urticaria in, 285–286, 286b, 286f, 287f
Systemic sclerosis, 307–312
  clinical features of, 309–311
    cardiac, 311
    cutaneous, 309, 309f
    intestinal, 310, 310f
    in joints and tendons, 309–310
    pulmonary, 310f, 310–311
    renal, 311
    in skeletal muscle, 310
    vascular, 309, 309f
  diagnosis of, 311, 312f
  epidemiology of, 308
  management of, 311–312, 312t
  natural history of, 311, 311f
  pathogenesis of, 308f, 308–309

**T**

Tacrolimus (Protopic), topical
  for atopic dermatitis, 256
  for contact dermatitis, 240
Takayasu's arteritis, 321b, 323, 323f
Tartrazine, anaphylactic reactions to, 66
T-cell(s). *See* T-lymphocytes.
T-cell-mediated immune response, 5–6
Temporal arteritis, 321b, 322–323, 323f
Tendons, in systemic sclerosis, 309–310
Tetanus, vaccine for, 379t, 382t, 386, 386f, 386t
Th1 and Th2 subsets, 7, 9f
Theophylline, for asthma, 108
Thermoregulation, abnormalities of, in atopic dermatitis, 245
Thimerosal, in vaccines, 393
Thistle, 43, 44f
Thiuram mix, contact dermatitis due to, 230t
3M disposable masks, 133, 134f
Thymus, 6f
  in severe combined immunodeficiency disease, 336, 337f
Thyroxine, for urticaria and angioedema, 291
Timothy grass, 45f, 45t
Tissue damage, 5
T-lymphocytes, 6f, 7, 8f–10f
  activation of, 21–22, 23f
  deficiencies of, 336–340
  deficiency of, laboratory tests for, 345, 346t
  differentiation of, 22, 23f, 24, 24f
  hyperactivated, in systemic lupus erythematosus, 302b
  regulatory (Tr-), 7, 10f
  T-cell-mediated immune response and, 5–6
TNF cytokines, 19, 19f
Tourniquets, in anaphylaxis, 72
Toxoplasmosis, in HIV/AIDS, 354, 355f
Toynbee phenomenon, 184
Transient hypogammaglobulinemia of infancy, 335–336
Traumatic irritant contact dermatitis, 227
Travelers, vaccines for, 395b, 395t, 395–396
Triamcinolone, for allergic rhinitis, 164t
Triamcinolone acetonide, for asthma, 103t
Tricyclic antidepressants, for urticaria and angioedema, 291

"Trigger finger," in rheumatoid arthritis, 296
TriHIBit, 387
Tripedia, 387
Tr-lymphocytes, 7, 10f
Tryptases, in anaphylaxis, 69
Twinrix, 390
Tympanic membrane, perforation of, 188f, 190
Tympanometry, in otitis media, 189f, 190
Tympanostomy tubes, for otitis media, 188f, 190
Type I cytokines, 17, 18f, 19
Type I reactions, 5
Type II cytokines, 19
Type II reactions, 5
Type III reactions, 5
Type IV reactions, 5–6

**U**

Ulcerative keratitis, peripheral, 204, 204f
*Ulmus americaria*, 47, 48t
Universal adult immunization, 383, 384f, 385f
Universal childhood immunization, 383, 383f
Urticaria, 279–286
  animal allergens and, 52
  autoimmune, 280
  clinical presentation of, 279–280, 279f–281f
  cold-induced, 289, 289f
  differential diagnosis of, 283, 285–288, 286b, 286f, 287f
  epidemiology of, 279
  etiology of, 280b, 280–281, 281b
  in food hypersensitivity, 216
  giant. *See* Angioedema.
  histologic changes in, 281, 282f
  in idiopathic urticarial vasculitis, 283, 285, 285f
  in latex allergy, 265f, 266
  lymphocyte predominant, 281, 282f
  pathogenesis of, 282–283, 283b, 284f
  in pregnancy, 283, 285f
  pressure, 289, 289f
  in serum sickness, 285
  solar-induced, 289, 289f
  in systemic lupus erythematosus, 285
  treatment of, 290–291
Urticaria pigmentosa, 285
Uveitis, 208b, 208f–210f, 208–212, 209t
  clinical manifestations of, 209, 211f, 212, 212f
  treatment of, 212

**V**

Vaccine(s), 379–396
  adjuvants and delivery systems for, 382–383
  allergen, 369–377
    for allergic asthma, 375–376
    disadvantages of, 375, 375b
    historical perspective on, 369, 369b
    indications for, 372b, 372–375, 373f, 373t, 374f
    mechanism of action of, 369–371, 370f, 371f
  for diphtheria, 384, 386
  DNA, 382
  for *Haemophilus influenzae* type B, 379t, 382, 388, 388f

Vaccine(s)—*cont'd*
   for hepatitis A, 392
   for hepatitis B, 382t, 389t, 389–390
   historical perspective on, 379t, 379–380
   for HIV/AIDS, 364t, 365
   hypersensitivity reactions to, 393, 393t
   immunity against infectious agents and, 380
   in immunocompromised patients, 393–395
     with primary immunodeficiencies,
       393–394
     with secondary immunodeficiencies, 394t,
       394–395
   inactivated, 381b, 381–382, 382t
   for influenza, 391–392
   live attenuated, 380–381, 381b
   for measles, 379t, 390
   for meningococcal disease, 382, 392–393
   for mumps, 379t, 390
   for pertussis, 379t, 382t, 386–387
   for pneumococcal disease, 388b, 388–389,
     389b
   for poliomyelitis, 379t, 380, 381, 387, 387f
   for rubella, 379t, 390–391
   for tetanus, 379t, 382t, 386, 386f, 386t
   for travelers, 395b, 395t, 395–396
   universal adult immunization and, 383,
     384f, 385f
   universal childhood immunization and, 383,
     383f
   for varicella, 391
Vaccinia, in atopic dermatitis, 253f
VAQTA, 392

Varicella, vaccine for, 391
VARIVAX, 391
Vascular manifestations. *See also specific*
     *conditions.*
   in idiopathic inflammatory myopathies, 314,
     314f
Vasculitis, 319, 320f, 320t, 321–327
   cryoglobulinemic, essential, 320b
   epidemiology of, 321
   hypersensitivity, 326, 327f
   large-vessel, 320b, 322–323, 323f
   leukocytoclastic, cutaneous, 320b
   management of, 327
   medium-vessel, 320b, 324, 324f
   pathogenesis of, 321, 321f, 322f
   retinal, 209, 212f
   in rheumatoid arthritis, 298–299
   in Sjögren's syndrome, 318–319
   small-vessel, 320b, 324–327, 325f–327f
   urticarial, idiopathic, 283, 285, 285f
Vasoconstriction, in atopic dermatitis, 245,
    246b
Venom immunotherapy, for *Hymenoptera*
    allergy, 75
Vernal conjunctivitis, 199t, 200–201, 201f
*Vibrio cholerae* vaccine, 380, 381
Viral infections. *See also specific infections.*
   respiratory
    asthma differentiated from, 84, 84t, 85f
    pathophysiology of asthma and, 88–89
    Sjögren's syndrome and, 319
Vogt-Koyanagi-Harada syndrome, 209, 210f

**W**
Walnut trees, 48t
Warts, in atopic dermatitis, 254f
Warts, hypogammaglobulinemia, infections,
    and myelokathexis syndrome, 342
Wasps. *See Hymenoptera* allergy.
Wegener's granulomatosis, 320b, 325–326,
    326f
Western poison ivy, 228t. *See also* Rhus
    dermatitis.
Wheal-and-flare reaction, 2f
Wheezing, 83. *See also* Asthma.
   diagnostic tests for, 91t
   differential diagnosis of, 91t
   of infancy, transient, benign, 83, 83f
White birch trees, 47, 48t, 49f
White poplar, 48t
Wiskott-Aldrich syndrome, 340, 340f
Wool wax alcohol, contact dermatitis due to,
    230t

**X**
Xerophthalmia, in Sjögren's syndrome, 317,
    317f, 319
Xerosis, in atopic dermatitis, 245
Xerostomia, in Sjögren's syndrome, 317–318,
    318f, 319
X-linked agammaglobulinemia, 333, 334f

**Y**
Yellow jackets. *See Hymenoptera* allergy.

## TERM

This Agreement will remain in effect until terminated pursuant to the terms of this Agreement. You may terminate this Agreement at any time by removing from Your system and destroying the CD-ROM Product. Unauthorized copying of the CD-ROM Product, including without limitation, the Proprietary Material and documentation, or otherwise failing to comply with the terms and conditions of this Agreement shall result in automatic termination of this license and will make available to Elsevier legal remedies. Upon termination of this Agreement, the license granted herein will terminate and You must immediately destroy the CD-ROM Product and accompanying documentation. All provisions relating to proprietary rights shall survive termination of this Agreement.

## LIMITED WARRANTY AND LIMITATION OF LIABILITY

NEITHER ELSEVIER NOR ITS LICENSORS REPRESENT OR WARRANT THAT THE INFORMATION CONTAINED IN THE PROPRIETARY MATERIAL IS COMPLETE OR FREE FROM ERROR, AND NEITHER ASSUMES, AND BOTH EXPRESSLY DISCLAIM, ANY LIABILITY TO ANY PERSON FOR ANY LOSS OR DAMAGE CAUSED BY ERRORS OR OMISSIONS IN THE PROPRIETARY MATERIAL, WHETHER SUCH ERRORS OR OMISSIONS RESULT FROM NEGLIGENCE, ACCIDENT, OR ANY OTHER CAUSE. IN ADDITION, NEITHER ELSEVIER NOR ITS LICENSORS MAKE ANY REPRESENTATIONS OR WARRANTIES, EITHER EXPRESS OR IMPLIED, REGARDING THE PERFORMANCE OF YOUR NETWORK OR COMPUTER SYSTEM WHEN USED IN CONJUNCTION WITH THE CD-ROM PRODUCT.

If this CD-ROM Product is defective, Elsevier will replace it at no charge if the defective CD-ROM Product is returned to Elsevier within sixty (60) days (or the greatest period allowable by applicable law) from the date of shipment.

Elsevier warrants that the software embodied in this CD-ROM Product will perform in substantial compliance with the documentation supplied in this CD-ROM Product. If You report a significant defect in performance in writing to Elsevier, and Elsevier is not able to correct same within sixty (60) days after its receipt of Your notification, You may return this CD-ROM Product, including all copies and documentation, to Elsevier and Elsevier will refund Your money.

**YOU UNDERSTAND THAT, EXCEPT FOR THE 60-DAY LIMITED WARRANTY RECITED ABOVE, ELSEVIER, ITS AFFILIATES, LICENSORS, SUPPLIERS AND AGENTS, MAKE NO WARRANTIES, EXPRESSED OR IMPLIED, WITH RESPECT TO THE CD-ROM PRODUCT, INCLUDING, WITHOUT LIMITATION THE PROPRIETARY MATERIAL, AND SPECIFICALLY DISCLAIM ANY WARRANTY OF MERCHANTABILITY OR FITNESS FOR A PARTICULAR PURPOSE.**

If the information provided on this CD-ROM contains medical or health sciences information, it is intended for professional use within the medical field. Information about medical treatment or drug dosages is intended strictly for professional use, and because of rapid advances in the medical sciences, independent verification of diagnosis and drug dosages should be made.

IN NO EVENT WILL ELSEVIER, ITS AFFILIATES, LICENSORS, SUPPLIERS OR AGENTS, BE LIABLE TO YOU FOR ANY DAMAGES, INCLUDING, WITHOUT LIMITATION, ANY LOST PROFITS, LOST SAVINGS OR OTHER INCIDENTAL OR CONSEQUENTIAL DAMAGES, ARISING OUT OF YOUR USE OR INABILITY TO USE THE CD-ROM PRODUCT REGARDLESS OF WHETHER SUCH DAMAGES ARE FORESEEABLE OR WHETHER SUCH DAMAGES ARE DEEMED TO RESULT FROM THE FAILURE OR INADEQUACY OF ANY EXCLUSIVE OR OTHER REMEDY.

## U.S. GOVERNMENT RESTRICTED RIGHTS

The CD-ROM Product and documentation are provided with restricted rights. Use, duplication or disclosure by the U.S. Government is subject to restrictions as set forth in subparagraphs (a) through (d) of the Commercial Computer Restricted Rights clause at FAR 52.22719 or in subparagraph (c)(1)(ii) of the Rights in Technical Data and Computer Software clause at DFARS 252.2277013, or at 252.2117015, as applicable. Contractor/Manufacturer is Elsevier Science Inc., 360 Park Avenue South, New York, NY 10010-5107 USA.

## GOVERNING LAW

This Agreement shall be governed by the laws of the State of New York, USA. In any dispute arising out of this Agreement, you and Elsevier Science each consent to the exclusive personal jurisdiction and venue in the state and federal courts within New York County, New York, USA.